Pathophysiology of Heart Disease

An Introduction to Cardiovascular Medicine

EDITION 7

Pathophysiology of Heart Disease

An Introduction to Cardiovascular Medicine

EDITOR

Leonard S. Lilly, MD
Professor of Medicine
Harvard Medical School
Chief, Brigham and Women's/Faulkner Cardiology
Brigham and Women's Hospital
Boston, Massachusetts

Philadelphia • Baltimore • New York • London
Buenos Aires • Hong Kong • Sydney • Tokyo

Senior Acquisitions Editor: Crystal Taylor
Senior Development Editor: Amy Millholen
Senior Editorial Coordinator: Emily Buccieri
Editorial Assistant: Parisa Saranj
Marketing Manager: Phyllis Hitner
Senior Production Project Manager: Alicia Jackson
Design Coordinator: Holly McLaughlin
Manufacturing Coordinator: Margie Orzech
Prepress Vendor: SPi Global

Seventh Edition

Cataloging-in-Publication Data available on request from the Publisher

ISBN: 978-1-9751-2059-7

Dedicated to

**CAROLYN, JONATHAN, REBECCA, DOUGLAS, DEBORAH,
AND NORMA LILLY**

List of Contributors

David D. Berg, MD, MPH
Instructor in Medicine
Harvard Medical School
Cardiovascular Division
Brigham and Women's Hospital
Boston, Massachusetts

Ankeet S. Bhatt, MD, MBA
Fellow in Cardiovascular Medicine
Brigham and Women's Hospital
Harvard Medical School
Boston, Massachusetts

Ron Blankstein, MD
Associate Professor of Medicine
    and Radiology
Harvard Medical School
Associate Director, Cardiovascular Imaging
    Program
Co-Director, Cardiovascular Imaging Training
    Program
Director, Cardiac Computed Tomography
Brigham and Women's Hospital
Boston, Massachusetts

David W. Brown, MD
Associate Professor of Pediatrics
Harvard Medical School
Director, Fellowship Training Program
Department of Cardiology
Boston Children's Hospital
Boston, Massachusetts

Jenifer M. Brown, MD
Fellow in Cardiovascular Medicine
Brigham and Women's Hospital
Harvard Medical School
Boston, Massachusetts

Mark A. Creager, MD
Anna Gundlach Huber Professor of Medicine
Geisel School of Medicine at Dartmouth
Director, Heart and Vascular Center
Dartmouth-Hitchcock Medical Center
Lebanon, New Hampshire

Jonathan W. Cunningham, MD
Fellow in Cardiovascular Medicine
Brigham and Women's Hospital
Harvard Medical School
Boston, Massachusetts

Sanjay Divakaran, MD
Instructor in Medicine
Harvard Medical School
Cardiovascular Division
Brigham and Women's Hospital
Boston, Massachusetts

Ershela Durresi, MD, PhD
Resident in Internal Medicine/Clinical
    Investigator Track
New York University School of Medicine
New York, New York

Lauren A. Eberly, MD, MPH
Fellow in Cardiovascular Medicine
Perelman School of Medicine at the University of
    Pennsylvania
Hospital of the University of Pennsylvania
Philadelphia, Pennsylvania

Elazer R. Edelman, MD, PhD, FACC
Poitras Professor of Medical Engineering and
    Science, Massachusetts Institute of Technology
Director, MIT Institute of Medical Engineering
    and Science
Professor of Medicine, Harvard Medical School
Cardiovascular Division, Brigham and Women's
    Hospital
Boston, Massachusetts

Stanislav Henkin, MD, MPH
Assistant Professor of Medicine
Geisel School of Medicine at Dartmouth
Heart and Vascular Center
Dartmouth-Hitchcock Medical Center
Lebanon, New Hampshire

Bruce A. Koplan, MD, MPH
Assistant Professor of Medicine
Harvard Medical School
Director, Electrophysiology Laboratories
Cardiovascular Division
Brigham and Women's Hospital
Boston, Massachusetts

Vivek T. Kulkarni, MD, MHS, EdM
Fellow in Cardiovascular Medicine
Perelman School of Medicine at the University of
    Pennsylvania
Hospital of the University of Pennsylvania
Philadelphia, Pennsylvania

Neal K. Lakdawala, MD
Assistant Professor of Medicine
Harvard Medical School
Cardiovascular Genetics and Center for Advanced
    Heart Disease
Cardiovascular Division
Brigham and Women's Hospital
Boston, Massachusetts

Eldrin F. Lewis, MD, MPH
Professor of Medicine
Stanford University School of Medicine
Chief, Cardiovascular Medicine
Stanford Health
Stanford, California

Peter Libby, MD
Mallinckrodt Professor of Medicine
Harvard Medical School
Senior Physician
Cardiovascular Division
Brigham and Women's Hospital
Boston, Massachusetts

Leonard S. Lilly, MD
Professor of Medicine
Harvard Medical School
Chief, Brigham and Women's/Faulkner
    Cardiology
Brigham and Women's Hospital
Boston, Massachusetts

Mathew S. Lopes, MD
Fellow in Cardiovascular and Critical Care
    Medicine
Brigham and Women's Hospital
Harvard Medical School
Boston, Massachusetts

Diana M. Lopez, MD
Fellow in Cardiovascular Medicine
Brigham and Women's Hospital
Harvard Medical School
Boston, Massachusetts

Victor Nauffal, MD
Fellow in Cardiovascular Medicine
Brigham and Women's Hospital
Harvard Medical School
Boston, Massachusetts

Patrick T. O'Gara, MD
Professor of Medicine
Harvard Medical School
Watkins Family Distinguished Chair in Cardiology
Cardiovascular Division
Brigham and Women's Hospital
Boston, Massachusetts

Siddharth M. Patel, MD
Fellow in Cardiovascular Medicine
Brigham and Women's Hospital
Harvard Medical School
Boston, Massachusetts

Daniel C. Pipilas, MD
Fellow in Cardiovascular Medicine
Massachusetts General Hospital
Harvard Medical School
Boston, Massachusetts

Marc S. Sabatine, MD, MPH
Professor of Medicine
Harvard Medical School
Lewis Dexter, MD, Distinguished Chair in
    Cardiovascular Medicine and Chair, TIMI
    Study Group
Brigham and Women's Hospital
Boston, Massachusetts

Gordon H. Williams, MD
Professor of Medicine
Harvard Medical School
Senior Physician
Endocrinology, Diabetes, and Metabolism
Brigham and Women's Hospital
Boston, Massachusetts

Foreword

When designing any product or service, the needs of the prospective user must receive primary consideration. Regrettably, this is rarely the case with medical textbooks. Most of these are written for a wide audience so as to attract as many readers (and buyers) as possible. Most medical textbooks are tomes written either for the specialist or advanced trainee or they are technical "how to" manuals. This lack of textbooks designed *specifically* for medical students often forces faculty at medical schools around the world to spend countless hours preparing and duplicating voluminous lecture notes and providing students with custom-designed "camels" (a camel is a cow created by a committee!).

Pathophysiology of Heart Disease: An Introduction to Cardiovascular Medicine represents a refreshing and innovative departure in the preparation of a medical text. Medical students need to understand the pathophysiology of cardiovascular disorders, how the pathophysiology leads to key clinical and laboratory findings and to the rationale for management. The editor is Dr. Leonard Lilly, a Professor of Medicine at Harvard Medical School, who is a brilliant teacher and a respected cardiologist at the Brigham and Women's and Faulkner Hospitals. He has brought together a group of talented residents and cardiology fellows from the Brigham and Women's Hospital and Harvard Medical School, and senior faculty who have collaborated closely. Under Dr. Lilly's leadership, they have produced this superb introductory text *specifically* designed to meet the needs of medical students during their initial encounters with patients with heart disease. Dr. Lilly, who was a coauthor of many of the chapters, made certain that there were no repetitions or major gaps, as so often occurs with multi-authored texts. While *Pathophysiology of Heart Disease: An Introduction to Cardiovascular Medicine* is not meant to be encyclopedic or all inclusive, it is remarkably thorough.

The first six editions of this fine book were received enthusiastically, and *Pathophysiology of Heart Disease: An Introduction to Cardiovascular Medicine* is now a required or recommended text at many medical schools not only in the United States and Canada but in other countries as well. It has been translated into several languages, has received two awards of excellence from the American Medical Writers Association, and has inspired several other student-faculty collaborative book projects at Harvard and at other medical schools. This seventh edition is completely updated, as is essential for a field as dynamic as cardiology. The figures have been upgraded, are in full color, and they display complex concepts in uncomplicated ways. This edition will prove to be even more valuable than its predecessors.

Dr. Lilly and his colleagues—faculty, cardiology fellows, and medical residents—have made a significant and unique contribution in preparing this important book. Future generations of medical educators and students, and ultimately the patients that they serve, will be indebted to them for this important contribution.

Eugene Braunwald, MD
Distinguished Hersey Professor of Medicine
Harvard Medical School
Chair Emeritus, Department of Medicine
Brigham and Women's Hospital
Boston, Massachusetts

Preface

This textbook is a comprehensive introduction to diseases of the cardiovascular system. Although excellent cardiology reference books are available, their encyclopedic content can overwhelm the beginning student. Therefore, this text was created to serve as a simplified bridge between courses in basic physiology and the care of patients in clinical settings. It is intended to help medical students and physicians-in-training form a solid foundation of knowledge of diseases of the heart and circulation and is designed to be read in its entirety during standard courses in cardiovascular pathophysiology. Emphasis has been placed on the basic mechanisms by which cardiac illnesses develop, in order to facilitate later in-depth study of clinical diagnosis and therapy.

The motivation for writing this book was the need for such a text voiced by our medical students, as well as their desire to participate in its creation and direction. Consequently, the book's development is unusual in that it arose from a close collaboration between Harvard medical students and cardiology faculty, who shared in the writing and editing of the original manuscript. The goal of this pairing was to focus the subject matter on the needs of the student, while providing the expertise of our faculty members. Similar collaboration between medical students and faculty continued through the first six editions of the text. In this updated and rewritten seventh edition of *Pathophysiology of Heart Disease: An Introduction to Cardiovascular Medicine*, another collaborative effort has been undertaken, this time between a select group of postgraduate trainees (cardiology fellows and internal medical residents) and our cardiovascular faculty. This new pairing was designed to extend the coverage of clinically relevant material and to create a series of pertinent questions and answers in each chapter to reinforce the reader's learning.

The introductory chapters of the book consider basic cardiac anatomy and physiology and describe tools needed for understanding clinical aspects of subsequent material. The remainder of the text addresses the major groups of cardiovascular diseases. The chapters are designed and edited to be read in sequence but are sufficiently cross-referenced so that they can also be used out of order. The final chapter describes the major classes of cardiovascular drugs and explains the physiologic rationale for their uses.

It has been a great privilege for me to collaborate with the 118 talented and creative medical students and physicians-in-training who have contributed to the seven editions of this book. Their intelligence, enthusiasm, energy, and dedication have made the production of each manuscript enjoyable and intellectually stimulating. I am also indebted to my faculty colleague coauthors for their time, their expertise, and their continued commitment to this project.

I sincerely appreciate the thoughtful comments received from faculty and students around the globe pertaining to previous editions of this book. These communications have been very helpful in directing the current revision. I also acknowledge with gratitude several individuals who provided images, comments, reviews, or other support to this edition: Suhny Abbara, Lauren Bayer, J. Phillip Bowen, Marcelo DiCarli, Sharmila Dorbala, Marie Gerhard-Herman, Andetta Hunsaker, Raymond Kwong, Gillian Lieberman, Robert Padera, Helmut Rennke, Frank Rybicki, Christian Sampson, Frederick Schoen, Pinak Shah, Michael Steigner, Scott Streckenbach, and Yee-Ping Sun.

It has been a pleasure to work with the editorial and production staffs of our publisher, Lippincott

Williams & Wilkins/Wolters Kluwer. Most notably, I thank Emily Buccieri, Amy Millholen, Crystal Taylor, Holly McLaughlin, Alicia Jackson and Gayathri Govindarajan (of SPi Global) for their skill and professionalism in bringing this edition to completion.

Finally, a project of this magnitude could not be undertaken without the support and patience of my family, and for that, I am very grateful.

On behalf of the contributors, I hope that this book enhances your understanding of cardio-vascular diseases and provides a solid founda-tion for further learning and clinical care of your patients.

LEONARD S. LILLY, MD
Boston, Massachusetts

Table of Contents

1 Normal Cardiac Structure and Function

Ershela Durresi | Elazer R. Edelman | Leonard S. Lilly

Knowledge of normal structure and function of the heart is crucial to understand diseases that afflict the cardiovascular system. The purpose of this chapter is to describe the heart's basic anatomy, its electrical system, and the cellular and molecular mechanisms of contraction that allow the heart to serve its critical functions.

CARDIAC ANATOMY AND HISTOLOGY

Although the study of cardiac anatomy dates back to ancient times, interest in this field has gained renewed momentum. The application of sophisticated cardiac imaging techniques such as coronary angiography, echocardiography, computed tomography, and magnetic resonance imaging requires an intimate knowledge of the spatial relationships of cardiac structures. Such information also proves helpful in understanding the pathophysiology of heart disease. This section emphasizes the aspects of cardiac anatomy that are important to the clinician.

PERICARDIUM

The heart and roots of the great vessels are enclosed by a fibroserous sac called the pericardium (Fig. 1-1). This structure consists of two layers: a strong outer fibrous layer and an inner serosal layer. The inner serosal layer adheres to the external wall of the heart and is called the *visceral pericardium*. The visceral pericardium reflects back on itself and lines the outer fibrous layer, forming the *parietal pericardium*. The space between the visceral and parietal layers contains a thin film of pericardial fluid that allows the heart to beat in a minimal-friction environment.

The pericardium is attached to the sternum and the mediastinal portions of the right and left pleurae. Its many connections to the surrounding structures keep the pericardial sac firmly anchored within the thorax and thereby help to maintain the heart in its normal position.

Emanating from the pericardium in a superior direction are the aorta, the pulmonary artery, and the superior vena cava (see Fig. 1-1). The inferior vena cava projects through the pericardium inferiorly.

1

SURFACE ANATOMY OF THE HEART

The heart is shaped roughly like a cone and consists of four muscular chambers. The right and left ventricles are the main pumping chambers. The less muscular right and left atria deliver blood to their respective ventricles.

Several terms are used to describe the heart's surfaces and borders (Fig. 1-2). The **apex** is formed by the tip of the left ventricle, which points inferiorly, anteriorly, and to the left. The base or **posterior** surface of the heart is formed by the atria, mainly the left, and lies between the lung hila. The **anterior** surface of the heart is shaped by the right atrium and ventricle. Because the left atrium and ventricle lie more posteriorly, they form only a small strip of this anterior surface. The **inferior** surface of the heart lies along the diaphragm and is formed by both ventricles, primarily the left.

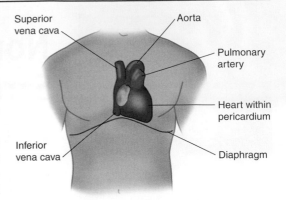

Figure 1-1. The position of the heart in the chest. The superior vena cava, aorta, and pulmonary artery exit superiorly, whereas the inferior vena cava projects inferiorly.

Observing the chest from an anteroposterior view (as on a chest radiograph; see Chapter 3, Fig. 3-1), four recognized borders of the heart are apparent. The right border is established by the right atrium and is almost in line with the superior and inferior venae cavae. The inferior border is nearly horizontal and is formed mainly by the right ventricle, with a slight contribution from the left ventricle near the apex. The left ventricle and a portion of the left atrium make up the left border of the heart, whereas the superior border is shaped by both atria. From this description of the surface of the heart emerges two basic "rules" of normal cardiac anatomy: (1) right-sided structures lie mostly anterior to their left-sided counterparts and (2) atrial chambers are located mostly to the right of their corresponding ventricles.

INTERNAL STRUCTURE OF THE HEART

Four major valves in the normal heart direct blood flow in a forward direction and prevent backward leakage. The atrioventricular (AV) valves (tricuspid and mitral) separate the atria and ventricles, whereas the semilunar valves (pulmonic and aortic) separate the ventricles from the great arteries (Fig. 1-3). All four heart valves are attached to the fibrous **cardiac skeleton**, which is composed of dense connective tissue. The cardiac skeleton also serves as a site of attachment for the ventricular and atrial muscles.

The surface of the heart valves and the interior surface of the chambers are lined by a single layer of endothelial cells, termed the **endocardium**. The subendocardial tissue contains fibroblasts, elastic and collagenous fibers, veins, nerves, and branches of the conducting system and is continuous with the connective tissue of the heart muscle layer, the myocardium. The **myocardium** is the thickest layer of the heart and consists of bundles of cardiac muscle cells, the histology of which is described later in the chapter. External to the myocardium is a layer of connective tissue and adipose tissue through which pass the larger blood vessels and nerves that supply the heart muscle. The **epicardium** is the outermost layer of the heart and is identical to, and just another term for, the visceral pericardium previously described.

Right Atrium and Ventricle

Opening into the **right atrium** are the superior and inferior venae cavae and the coronary sinus (Fig. 1-4). The venae cavae return deoxygenated blood from the systemic veins into

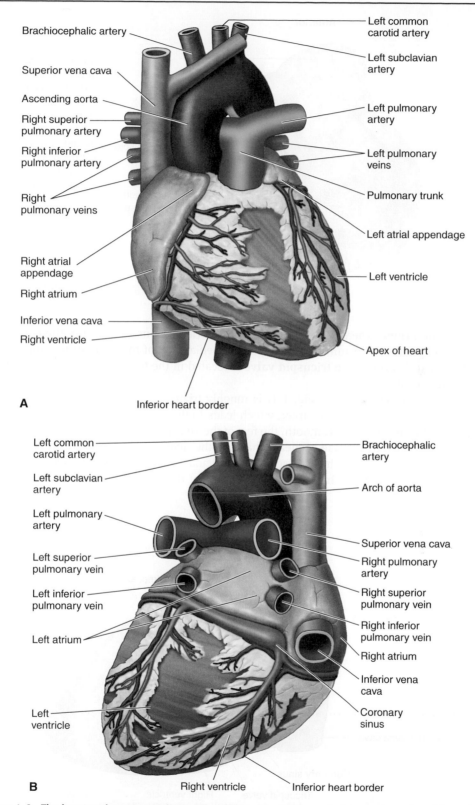

Figure 1-2. The heart and great vessels. A. The anterior view. **B.** The posterior aspect, as viewed from the back. (From Moore KL, Dalley AF, Agur AMR. *Clinically Oriented Anatomy*. 7th ed. Philadelphia, PA: Lippincott Williams & Wilkins; 2014:137-138.)

Anterior

Aortic valve

Mitral valve

Annulus fibrosus

Pulmonic valve

Tricuspid valve

Annulus fibrosus

Posterior

Figure 1-3. The four heart valves viewed from above with atria removed. The figure depicts the period of ventricular filling (diastole) during which the tricuspid and mitral valves are open and the semilunar valves (pulmonic and aortic) are closed. Each annulus fibrosus surrounding the mitral and tricuspid valves is thicker than those surrounding the pulmonic and aortic valves; all four contribute to the heart's fibrous skeleton, which is composed of dense connective tissue.

the right atrium, whereas the coronary sinus carries venous return from the coronary arteries. The interatrial septum forms the posteromedial wall of the right atrium and separates it from the left atrium. The **tricuspid valve** is located in the floor of the atrium and opens into the right ventricle.

The **right ventricle** (see Fig. 1-4) is roughly triangular in shape, and its superior aspect forms a cone-shaped outflow tract, which leads to the pulmonary artery. Although the inner wall of the outflow tract is smooth, the rest of the ventricle is covered by a number of irregular bridges (termed **trabeculae carneae**) that give the right ventricular wall a spongelike appearance. A large trabecula that crosses the ventricular cavity is called the **moderator band**. It carries a component of the right bundle branch of the conducting system to the ventricular muscle.

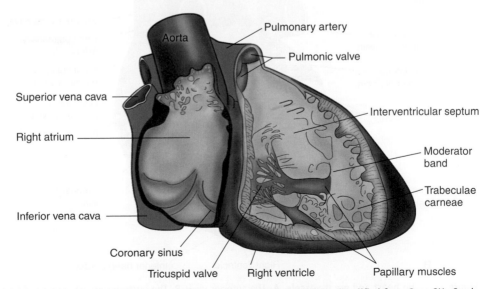

Aorta

Pulmonary artery

Pulmonic valve

Superior vena cava

Right atrium

Interventricular septum

Moderator band

Trabeculae carneae

Inferior vena cava

Coronary sinus

Tricuspid valve

Right ventricle

Papillary muscles

Figure 1-4. Interior structures of the right atrium and right ventricle. (Modified from Goss CM. *Gray's Anatomy*. 29th ed. Philadelphia, PA: Lea & Febiger; 1973:547.)

The right ventricle contains three **papillary muscles**, which project into the chamber and via their thin, stringlike **chordae tendineae** attach to the edges of the tricuspid valve leaflets. The leaflets, in turn, are attached to the fibrous ring that supports the valve between the right atrium and ventricle. Contraction of the papillary muscles prior to other regions of the ventricle tightens the chordae tendineae, helping to align and restrain the leaflets of the tricuspid valve as they are forced closed. This action prevents blood from regurgitating into the right atrium during ventricular contraction.

At the apex of the right ventricular outflow tract is the **pulmonic valve**, which leads to the pulmonary artery. This valve consists of three cusps attached to a fibrous ring. During relaxation of the ventricle, elastic recoil of the pulmonary arteries forces blood back toward the heart, distending the valve cusps toward one another. This action closes the pulmonic valve and prevents regurgitation of blood back into the right ventricle.

Left Atrium and Ventricle

Entering the posterior half of the **left atrium** are the four pulmonary veins (Fig. 1-5). The wall of the left atrium is about 2 mm thick, being slightly greater than that of the right atrium. The mitral valve opens into the left ventricle through the inferior wall of the left atrium.

The cavity of the **left ventricle** is approximately cone shaped and longer than that of the right ventricle. In a healthy adult heart, the wall thickness is 9-11 mm, roughly three times that of the right ventricle. The aortic vestibule is a smooth-walled part of the left ventricular cavity located just inferior to the aortic valve. Inferior to this region, most of the ventricle is covered by trabeculae carneae, which are finer and more numerous than those in the right ventricle.

The left ventricular chamber (see Fig. 1-5B) contains two large papillary muscles. These are larger than their counterparts in the right ventricle, and their chordae tendineae are thicker but less numerous. The chordae tendineae of each papillary muscle distribute to both leaflets of the **mitral valve**. Similar to the case in the right ventricle, tensing of the chordae tendineae during left ventricular contraction helps restrain and align the mitral leaflets, enabling them to close properly and preventing the backward leakage of blood.

The **aortic valve** separates the left ventricle from the aorta. Surrounding the aortic valve opening is a fibrous ring to which is attached the three cusps of the valve. Just above the right and left aortic valve cusps in the aortic wall are the origins of the right and left coronary arteries (see Fig. 1-5B).

Interventricular Septum

The interventricular septum is the thick wall between the left and right ventricles. It is composed of a muscular and a membranous part (see Fig. 1-5B). The margins of this septum can be traced on the surface of the heart by following the anterior and posterior interventricular grooves. Owing to the greater hydrostatic pressure within the left ventricle, the large muscular portion of the septum bulges toward the right ventricle. The small, oval-shaped membranous part of the septum is thin and located just inferior to the cusps of the aortic valve.

To summarize the functional anatomic points presented in this section, the following is a review of the path of blood flow: deoxygenated blood is delivered to the heart through the inferior and superior venae cavae, which enter into the right atrium. Flow continues through the tricuspid valve orifice into the right ventricle. Contraction of the right ventricle propels the blood across the pulmonic valve to the pulmonary artery and lungs, where carbon dioxide is released and oxygen is absorbed. The oxygen-rich blood returns to the heart through the pulmonary veins to the left atrium and then passes across the mitral valve into the left ventricle. Contraction of the left ventricle pumps the oxygenated blood across the aortic valve into the aorta, from which it is distributed to all other tissues of the body.

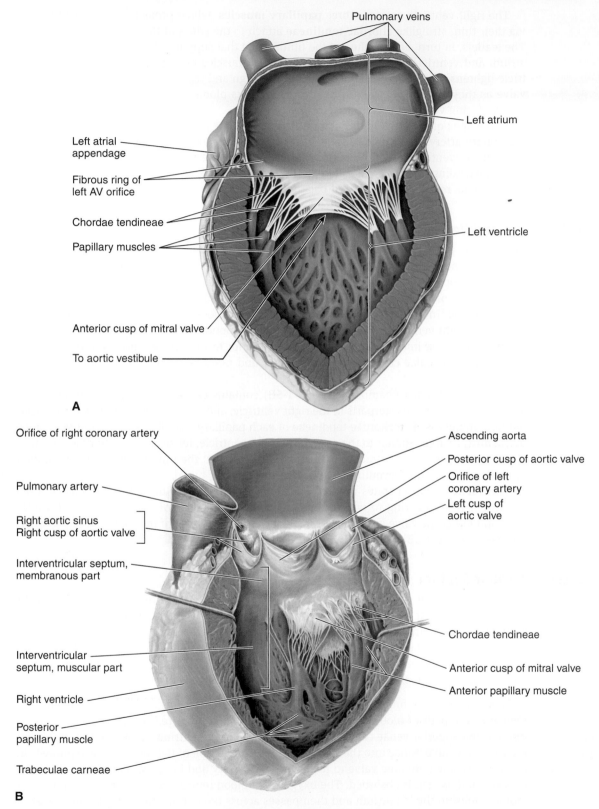

Figure 1-5. Interior structures of the left atrium and left ventricle. A. The left atrium and left ventricular (LV) inflow region. **B.** Interior structures of the LV cavity. (Modified from Moore KL, Dalley AF, Agur AMR. *Clinically Oriented Anatomy*. 7th ed. Philadelphia, PA: Lippincott Williams & Wilkins; 2014:142–143.)

IMPULSE-CONDUCTING SYSTEM

The impulse-conducting system (Fig. 1-6) consists of specialized cells that initiate the heart-beat and electrically coordinate contractions of the heart chambers. The **sinoatrial (SA) node** is a small mass of specialized cardiac muscle fibers in the wall of the right atrium. It is located to the right of the superior vena cava entrance and normally initiates the electrical impulse for contraction. The **atrioventricular (AV) node** lies beneath the endocardium in the infero-posterior part of the interatrial septum.

Distal to the AV node is the **bundle of His**, which perforates the interventricular septum posteriorly. Within the septum, the bundle of His bifurcates into a compact, cablelike structure on the right side, known as the **right bundle branch**, and a broad sheet of fibers that continues over the left side of the septum, the **left bundle branch**.

The right bundle branch is thick and deeply buried in the muscle of the interventricular septum and continues toward the apex. Near the junction of the interventricular septum and the anterior wall of the right ventricle, the right bundle branch becomes subendocardial and bifurcates. One branch travels across the right ventricular cavity in the moderator band, whereas the other continues toward the tip of the ventricle. These branches eventually arborize into a finely divided anastomosing plexus that travels throughout the right ventricle.

Functionally, the left bundle branch is divided into an anterior and a posterior fascicle and a small branch to the septum. The anterior fascicle runs anteriorly toward the apex, forming a subendocardial plexus in the area of the anterior papillary muscle. The posterior fascicle travels to the area of the posterior papillary muscle; it then divides into a subendocardial plexus and spreads to the rest of the left ventricle.

The subendocardial plexuses of both ventricles send distributing **Purkinje fibers** to the ventricular muscle. Impulses within the His-Purkinje system are transmitted first to the papillary muscles and then throughout the walls of the ventricles, allowing papillary muscle contraction to precede that of the ventricles. This coordination prevents regurgitation of blood flow through the AV valves, as discussed earlier.

Figure 1-6. Main components of the cardiac conduction system. This system includes the sinoatrial node, atrioventricular node, bundle of His, right and left bundle branches, and the Purkinje fibers. The moderator band carries a large portion of the right bundle (IV, interventricular).

Cardiac Innervation

The heart is innervated by both parasympathetic and sympathetic afferent and efferent nerves. Preganglionic *sympathetic* neurons, with cell bodies located within the upper five to six thoracic levels of the spinal cord, synapse with second-order neurons in the cervical sympathetic ganglia. Traveling within the cardiac nerves, these fibers terminate in the heart and great vessels. Preganglionic *parasympathetic* fibers originate in the dorsal motor nucleus of the medulla and pass as branches of the vagus nerve to the heart and great vessels. Here, the fibers synapse with second-order neurons located in ganglia within these structures. A rich supply of vagal afferents from the inferior and posterior aspects of the ventricles mediates important cardiac reflexes, whereas the abundant vagal efferent fibers to the SA and AV nodes are active in modulating electrical impulse initiation and conduction.

Cardiac Vessels

The cardiac vessels consist of the coronary arteries and veins and the lymphatics. The largest components of these structures lie within the loose connective tissue in the epicardial fat.

Coronary Arteries

The heart muscle is supplied with oxygen and nutrients by the right and left coronary arteries, which arise from the root of the aorta just above the aortic valve cusps (Fig. 1-7; see also Fig. 1-5B). After their origin, these vessels pass anteriorly, one on each side of the pulmonary artery (see Fig. 1-7).

The large **left main coronary artery** passes between the left atrium and the pulmonary trunk to reach the AV groove. There it divides into the **left anterior descending (LAD) coronary artery** and the circumflex artery. The LAD travels within the anterior interventricular groove toward the cardiac apex. During its descent on the anterior surface, the LAD gives off *septal branches* that supply the anterior two-thirds of the interventricular septum and the apical portion of the anterior papillary muscle. The LAD also gives off *diagonal branches* that supply the anterior surface of the left ventricle. The **circumflex artery** continues within the left AV groove and passes around the left border of the heart to reach the posterior surface. It gives off large *obtuse marginal branches* that supply the lateral and posterior wall of the left ventricle.

The **right coronary artery (RCA)** travels in the right AV groove, passing posteriorly between the right atrium and ventricle. It supplies blood to the right ventricle via *acute marginal branches*. In most people, the distal RCA gives rise to a large branch, the **posterior descending artery** (see Fig. 1-7C). This vessel travels from the inferoposterior aspect of the heart to the apex and supplies blood to the inferior and posterior walls of the ventricles and the posterior one-third of the interventricular septum. Just before giving off the posterior descending branch, the RCA usually gives off the **AV nodal artery**.

The posterior descending and AV nodal arteries arise from the RCA in 85% of the population, and in such people, the coronary circulation is termed *right dominant*. In ~8%, the posterior descending artery arises from the circumflex artery instead, resulting in a *left dominant* circulation. In the remaining population, the heart's posterior blood supply is contributed to from branches of both the RCA and the circumflex, forming a *codominant* circulation.

The blood supply to the SA node is also most often (70% of the time) derived from the RCA. However, in 25% of normal hearts, the **SA nodal artery** arises from the circumflex artery, and in 5% of cases, both the RCA and the circumflex artery contribute to this vessel.

From their epicardial locations, the coronary arteries send perforating branches into the ventricular muscle, which form a richly branching and anastomosing vasculature in the walls of all the cardiac chambers. From this plexus arise a massive number of capillaries that form an elaborate network surrounding each cardiac muscle fiber. The muscle fibers located just

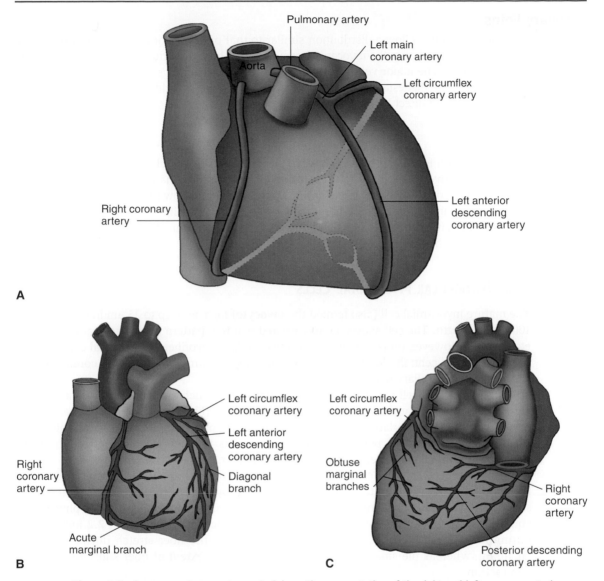

Figure 1-7. Coronary artery anatomy. A. Schematic representation of the right and left coronary arteries demonstrates their orientation to one another. The left main artery bifurcates into the circumflex artery, which perfuses the lateral and posterior regions of the left ventricle (LV), and the anterior descending artery, which perfuses the LV anterior wall, the anterior portion of the intraventricular septum, and a portion of the anterior right ventricular (RV) wall. The right coronary artery (RCA) perfuses the right ventricle and variable portions of the posterior left ventricle through its terminal branches. **B.** Anterior view of the heart demonstrating the coronary arteries and their major branches. **C.** Posterior view of the heart demonstrating the terminal portions of the right and circumflex coronary arteries and their branches. The posterior descending artery most often arises from the RCA.

beneath the endocardium, particularly those of the papillary muscles and the thick left ventricle, are supplied either by the terminal branches of the coronary arteries or directly from the ventricular cavity through tiny vascular channels, known as **thebesian veins**.

Collateral connections, usually <200 µm in diameter, exist at the subarteriolar level between the coronary arteries. In the normal heart, few of these collateral vessels are visible. However, they may become larger and functional when atherosclerotic disease obstructs a coronary artery, thereby providing blood flow to distal portions of the vessel from a nonobstructed neighbor.

Coronary Veins

The coronary veins follow a distribution similar to that of the major coronary arteries. These vessels return blood from the myocardial capillaries to the right atrium predominantly via the coronary sinus. The major veins lie in the epicardial fat, usually superficial to their arterial counterparts. The thebesian veins, described earlier, provide an additional potential route for a small amount of direct blood return to the cardiac chambers.

Lymphatic Vessels

The heart lymph is drained by an extensive plexus of valved vessels located in the subendocardial connective tissue of all four chambers. This lymph drains into an epicardial plexus from which are derived several larger lymphatic vessels that follow the distribution of the coronary arteries and veins. Each of these larger vessels then combines in the AV groove to form a single lymphatic conduit, which exits the heart to reach the mediastinal lymphatic plexus and ultimately the thoracic duct.

HISTOLOGY OF VENTRICULAR MYOCARDIAL CELLS

The mature myocardial cell (also termed the **myocyte**) measures up to 25 μm in diameter and 100 μm in length. The cell shows a cross-striated banding pattern similar to that of the skeletal muscle. However, unlike the multinucleated skeletal myofibers, myocardial cells contain only one or two centrally located nuclei. Surrounding each myocardial cell is connective tissue with a rich capillary network.

Each myocardial cell contains numerous **myofibrils**, which are long chains of individual **sarcomeres**, the fundamental contractile units of the cell (Fig. 1-8). Each sarcomere is made up of two groups of overlapping filaments of contractile proteins. Biochemical and biophysical interactions occurring between these myofilaments produce muscle contraction. Their structure and function are described later in the chapter.

Within each myocardial cell, the neighboring sarcomeres are all in register, producing the characteristic cross-striated banding pattern seen by light microscopy. The relative densities of the cross bands identify the location of the contractile proteins. Under physiologic conditions, the overall sarcomere length (Z-to-Z distance) varies between 2.2 and 1.5 μm during the cardiac cycle. The larger dimension reflects the fiber stretch during ventricular filling, whereas the smaller dimension represents the extent of fiber shortening during contraction.

The myocardial cell membrane is named the **sarcolemma**. A specialized region of the membrane is the **intercalated disk**, a distinct characteristic of cardiac muscle tissue. Intercalated disks are seen on light microscopic study as darkly staining transverse lines that cross chains of cardiac cells at irregular intervals. They represent the gap junction complexes at the interface of adjacent cardiac fibers and establish structural and electrical continuity between the myocardial cells.

Another functional feature of the cell membrane is the **transverse tubular system** (or **T tubules**). This complex system is characterized by deep, fingerlike invaginations of the sarcolemma (Fig. 1-9; see also Fig. 1-8). Similar to the intercalated disks, transverse tubular membranes establish pathways for rapid transmission of the excitatory electrical impulses that initiate contraction. The T-tubule system increases the surface area of the sarcolemma in contact with the extracellular environment, allowing the transmembrane ion transport accompanying excitation and relaxation to occur quickly and synchronously.

The **sarcoplasmic reticulum (SR**, the myocyte analog of the endoplasmic reticulum) is an extensive intracellular tubular membrane network that complements the T-tubule system

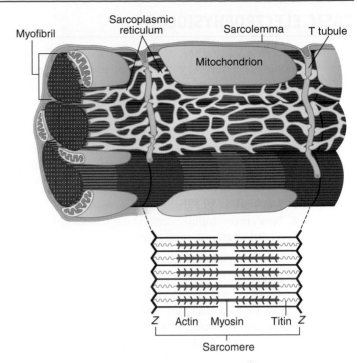

Figure 1-8. Myocardial cell. Top. Schematic representation of the ultrastructure of the myocardial cell. The cell consists of multiple parallel myofibrils surrounded by mitochondria. The T tubules are invaginations of the cell membrane (the sarcolemma) that increase the surface area for ion transport and transmission of electrical impulses. The intracellular sarcoplasmic reticulum houses most of the intracellular calcium and abuts the T tubules. (Modified from Katz AM. *Physiology of the Heart*. 2nd ed. New York, NY: Raven Press; 1992:21). **Bottom.** Expanded view of a sarcomere, the basic unit of contraction. Each myofibril consists of serially connected sarcomeres that extend from one *Z* line to the next. The sarcomere is composed of alternating thin (actin) and thick (myosin) myofilaments. Titin is a protein that tethers myosin to the *Z* line and provides elasticity.

both structurally and functionally. The SR abuts the T tubules at right angles in lateral sacs, called the terminal cisternae (see Fig. 1-9). These sacs house most of intracellular calcium stores; the release of these stores is important in linking membrane excitation with activation of the contractile apparatus. Lateral sacs also abut the intercalated disks and the sarcolemma, providing each with a complete system for excitation-contraction coupling.

To serve the tremendous metabolic demand placed on the heart and the need for a constant supply of high-energy phosphates, the myocardial cell has an abundant concentration of mitochondria. These organelles are located between the individual myofibrils and constitute ∼35% of cell volume (see Fig. 1-8).

Figure 1-9. Schematic view of the tubular systems of the myocardial cell. The T tubules, invaginations of the sarcolemma, abut the sarcoplasmic reticulum at right angles at the terminal cisternae sacs. This relationship is important in linking membrane excitation with intracellular release of calcium from the sarcoplasmic reticulum.

BASIC ELECTROPHYSIOLOGY

Rhythmic contraction of the heart relies on the organized propagation of electrical impulses along its conduction pathway. The marker of electrical stimulation, the **action potential**, is created by a sequence of ion fluxes through specific channels in the sarcolemma. To provide a basis for understanding how electrical impulses lead to cardiac contraction, the process of cellular depolarization and repolarization is reviewed here. This material serves as an important foundation for topics addressed later in the book, including electrocardiography (see Chapter 4), cardiac arrhythmias (see Chapters 11 and 12), and the actions of antiarrhythmic drugs (see Chapter 17).

Cardiac cells capable of electrical excitation are of three electrophysiologic types, the properties of which have been studied by intracellular microelectrode and patch-clamp recordings:

1. Pacemaker cells (eg, SA node, AV node)
2. Specialized rapidly conducting tissues (eg, Purkinje fibers)
3. Ventricular and atrial muscle cells

The sarcolemma of each of these cardiac cell types is a phospholipid bilayer that, by itself, is largely impermeable to ions. There are specialized proteins interspersed throughout the membrane that serve as ion channels, passive cotransporters, and active transporters (Fig. 1-10). These help to maintain ionic concentration gradients and charge differentials between the inside and the outside of the cardiac cells. Note that normally the Na^+ and Ca^{++} concentrations are much higher outside the cell, and the K^+ concentration is much higher inside.

Figure 1-10. Ion channels, cotransporters, and active transporters of the myocyte. A. Sodium entry through the fast sodium channel is responsible for the rapid upstroke (phase 0) of the action potential (AP) in nonpacemaker cells. **B.** Calcium enters the cell through calcium channel during phase 2 of the Purkinje fiber and muscle cell AP and is the main channel responsible for depolarization of pacemaker cells. **C.** Potassium exits through a number of different potassium channels to repolarize the cell, and open potassium channels contribute to the resting potential (phase 4) of nonpacemaker cells. **D.** Sodium-calcium exchanger helps maintain the low intracellular calcium concentration. **E.** Sodium-potassium ATPase maintains concentration gradients for these ions. **F, G.** Active calcium transporters aid removal of calcium to the external environment and into the sarcoplasmic reticulum, respectively.

ION MOVEMENT AND CHANNELS

The movement of specific ions across the cell membrane serves as the basis of the action potential. Passive ion movement depends on two major factors: (1) the energetic favorability and (2) the permeability of the membrane for the ion.

Energetics

The two major forces that drive the direction of passive ion flux are the *concentration gradient* and the *transmembrane potential* (voltage). Molecules diffuse from areas of high concentration to areas of lower concentration, and the gradient between these values is a determinant of the rate of ion flow. For example, the extracellular Na^+ concentration is normally 145 mM, while the concentration inside the myocyte is 15 mM. As a result, a strong diffusive force tends to drive Na^+ into the cell, down its concentration gradient.

The transmembrane potential of cells exerts an electrical force on ions (ie, like charges repel one another, and opposite charges attract). The transmembrane potential of a myocyte at rest is about −90 mV (the inside of the cell is negative relative to the outside). Extracellular Na^+, a positively charged ion, is therefore attracted to the relatively negatively charged interior of the cell. Thus, there is a strong tendency for Na^+ to enter the cell and remain there, because of the steep concentration gradient and the electrical attraction.

Permeability

If there is such a strong force driving Na^+ into the cell, what keeps this ion from actually moving inside? The membrane of the cell at its resting potential is *not permeable* to sodium. The phospholipid bilayer of the cell membrane is composed of a hydrophobic core that does not allow simple passage of charged, hydrophilic particles. Instead, permeability of the membrane is dependent on the opening of specific **ion channels**, specialized proteins that span the cell membrane and contain hydrophilic pores through which certain charged atoms can pass under specific circumstances. Typically, one cell's sarcolemma contains a million or more such channels. Each type of channel is normally *selective* for a specific ion, which is a manifestation of the size and structure of its pore. For example, in cardiac cells, some channels permit the passage of sodium ions, some are specific for potassium, and others allow only calcium to transit through.

Ions can pass through their specific channels only at certain times. That is, ion channels are *gated*—at any given moment, a channel is either open or closed. The more time a channel is in its open state, the larger the number of ions that can pass through it and therefore, the greater the transmembrane current. The voltage across the membrane determines what fraction of channels is open at a given time. Therefore, the gating of channels is said to be **voltage sensitive**. As the membrane voltage changes during depolarization and repolarization of the cell, specific channels open and close, with corresponding alterations in the ion fluxes across the sarcolemma.

An example of voltage-sensitive gating is apparent in the cardiac channel known as the **fast sodium channel**. The transmembrane protein that forms this channel assumes various conformations depending on the cell's membrane potential (Fig. 1-11). At a voltage of −90 mV (the typical resting voltage of a ventricular muscle cell), the channels are predominantly in a closed, *resting state*, such that Na^+ ions cannot pass through (Fig. 1-11A). In this resting state, the channels are available for conversion to the open configuration.

A rapid wave of depolarization renders the membrane potential less negative, and this activates the resting channels to change conformation to the *open state* (see Fig. 1-11B). Na^+ ions readily permeate through the open channels, constituting an inward Na^+ current that further depolarizes the cell. However, the activated channels remain open for only a brief time, a few thousandths of a second, and then spontaneously close to an *inactive state* (see Fig. 1-11C). Channels in the inactivated conformation cannot be directly converted back to the open state.

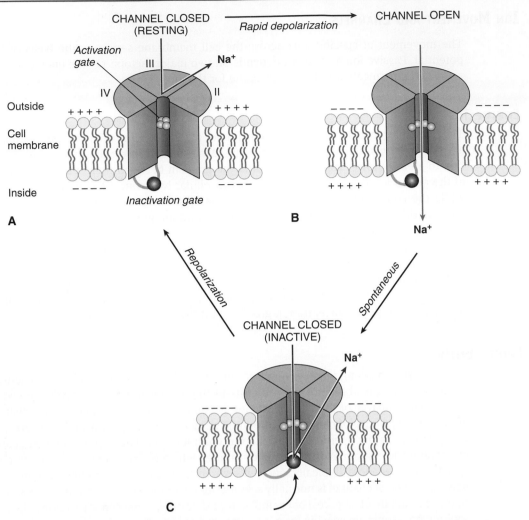

Figure 1-11. Gating of fast sodium channels. A. Four covalently linked transmembrane domains (*I, II, III,* and *IV*) form the sodium channel, which is guarded by activation and inactivation gates, schematically represented here. (Here, domain *I* is cut away to show the transmembrane pore.) In the resting membrane, most channels are in a closed state. Even though the inactivation gate is open, Na⁺ ions cannot easily pass through because the activation gate is closed. **B.** A rapid depolarization changes the cell membrane voltage and forces the activation gate to open, presumably mediated by translocation of the charged portions of a segment in each domain. With the channel in this conformation (in which both the activation and inactivation gates are open), Na⁺ ions permeate into the cell. **C.** As the inactivation gate spontaneously closes, the sodium current ceases. The inactivation gating function is thought to be achieved by a peptide loop that connects domains III and IV, which translocates into the intracellular opening of the channel pore (*black arrow*). The channel cannot reopen directly from this closed, inactive state. Cellular repolarization returns the channel to the resting condition **(A).** During repolarization, as more negative membrane voltages are achieved, the activation gate closes and the inactivation gate reopens.

The inactivated state persists until the membrane voltage has been repolarized nearly back to its original resting level. Until then, the inactivated channel conformation maintains a closed pore that prevents any flow of sodium ions. Thus, during normal cellular depolarization, the voltage-dependent fast sodium channels conduct for a short period and then inactivate, unable to conduct current again until the cell membrane has nearly fully repolarized, and the channels recover from the inactivated to the closed resting state.

Another important attribute of cardiac fast sodium channels should be noted. If the transmembrane voltage of a cardiac cell is *slowly* depolarized and maintained chronically at levels less negative than the usual resting potential, inactivation of channels occurs *without* initial opening and current flow. Furthermore, as long as this partial depolarization exists, the closed, inactive channels cannot recover to the resting state. Thus, the fast sodium channels in such a cell are persistently unable to conduct Na$^+$ ions. This is the typical case in cardiac pacemaker cells (eg, the SA and AV nodes) in which the membrane voltage is generally less negative than −70 mV throughout the cardiac cycle. As a result, the fast sodium channels in pacemaker cells are persistently inactivated and do not play a role in the generation of the action potential in these cells.

Calcium and potassium channels in cardiac cells also act in voltage-dependent fashions, but they behave differently than the sodium channels, as described later.

Resting Potential

In nonpacemaker cardiac cells at rest, prior to excitation, the electrical charge differential between the inside and outside of a cell corresponds to the **resting potential**. The magnitude of the resting potential of a cell depends on two main properties: (1) the concentration gradients for all the different ions between the inside and outside of the cell and (2) the relative permeabilities of ion channels that are open at rest.

As in other tissues such as nerve cells and skeletal muscle, the potassium concentration is much greater inside cardiac cells compared with outside. This is attributed mainly to the cell membrane transporter Na$^+$K$^+$-ATPase (see Fig. 1-10). This protein "pump" actively extrudes 3 Na$^+$ ions out of the cell in exchange for the inward movement of 2 K$^+$ ions in an ATP-dependent process. This acts to maintain intracellular Na$^+$ at low levels and intracellular K$^+$ at high levels.

Cardiac myocytes contain a set of potassium channels (termed *inward rectifier* potassium channels) that are open in the resting state, at a time when other ionic channels (eg, sodium and calcium) are closed. Therefore, the resting cell membrane is much more permeable to potassium than to other ions. As a result, K$^+$ flows in an outward direction down its concentration gradient, removing positive charges from the cell. As potassium ions exit the cell, negatively charged anions that are impermeant to passage are left behind, causing the interior of the cell to become electrically negative with respect to the outside.

As the interior of the cell becomes more *negatively* charged by the outward flux of potassium, the *positively* charged K$^+$ ions are attracted back by the electrical potential toward the cellular interior, slowing their net exit from the cell. Thus, the K$^+$ concentration gradient and the electrostatic force oppose each other (Fig. 1-12). At equilibrium, these forces are balanced, and there is zero net movement of K$^+$ across the membrane. The electrical potential

Figure 1-12. The resting potential of a cardiac muscle cell is determined by the balance between the concentration gradient and electrostatic forces for potassium, because only potassium channels are open at rest. The concentration gradient favors outward movement of K$^+$, whereas the electrical force attracts the positively charged K$^+$ ions inward. The resting potential is approximated by the Nernst equation for potassium, as shown here.

Equilibrium (Nernst) potential = $-26.7 \ln ([K^+]_{in}/[K^+]_{out}) = -91$mV

at which that occurs is known as the *potassium equilibrium potential* and in ventricular myocytes is −91 mV, as calculated by the Nernst equation, shown in Figure 1-12. Since at rest the membrane is almost exclusively permeable to potassium ions alone, this value closely approximates the cell's resting potential.

The permeability of the cardiac myocyte cellular membrane for sodium is minimal in the resting state because the channels that conduct that ion are essentially closed. However, there is a slight leak of sodium ions into the cell at rest. This small inward current of positively charged ions explains why the actual resting potential is slightly less negative (−90 mV) than would be predicted if the cell membrane were truly only permeable to potassium. The sodium ions that slowly leak into the myocyte at rest (and the much larger amount that enters during the action potential) are continuously removed from the cell and returned to the extracellular environment by Na^+K^+-ATPase, as previously described.

ACTION POTENTIAL

When the cell membrane's voltage is altered, its permeability to specific ions changes because of the voltage-gating characteristics of the ion channels. Each type of channel has a characteristic pattern of activation and inactivation that determines the progression of the electrical signal. The ionic currents that pass through the channels discussed in this chapter are listed in Table 1-1. This description begins by following the development of the action potential in a typical cardiac muscle cell (Fig. 1-13). The unique characteristics of action potentials in cardiac pacemaker cells are described thereafter.

Cardiac Muscle Cell

Until stimulated, the resting potential of a cardiac muscle cell remains stable, at approximately −90 mV. This resting state before depolarization is known as **phase 4** of the action potential. Following phase 4, four additional phases characterize depolarization and repolarization of the cell (see Fig. 1-13).

Phase 0

At the resting membrane voltage, sodium and calcium channels are closed. Any process that makes the membrane potential less negative than the resting value causes some sodium channels to open. As these channels open, sodium ions rapidly enter the cell, flowing down their concentration gradient toward the negatively charged cellular interior. The entry of Na^+ ions into the cell causes the transmembrane potential to become progressively less negative, which in turn causes more sodium channels to open and promotes

TABLE 1-1	**Transmembrane Cardiac Ionic Currents Described in This Chapter**	

Current	Description	
I_f	Pacemaker current; responsible for phase 4 depolarization in pacemaker cells	
I_{Na}	Na^{++} current; responsible for phase 0 rapid depolarization in nonpacemaker cells	
$I_{Ca.L}$	Slow, long-lasting Ca^{++} current; responsible for phase 0 depolarization in pacemaker cells and major contributor to inward current during phase 2 of nonpacemaker cells	
I_{K1}	Maintains resting potential; current of the inward rectifying potassium channel	
I_{to}	Transient outward potassium current; responsible for phase 1 of action potential	
I_{Ks}, I_{Kr}	Delayed rectifier potassium currents of slow (I_{Ks}) and rapid (I_{Kr}) types; repolarizing currents that are active during phases 2 and 3 of action potential	

further sodium entry into the cell. When the membrane voltage approaches the **threshold potential** (approximately −70 mV in cardiac muscle cells), enough of these fast Na$^+$ channels have opened to generate a self-sustaining inward Na$^+$ current (termed I_{Na}). The entry of positively charged Na$^+$ ions at and beyond threshold exceeds the exit of K$^+$ ions through the open inward rectifier channels, such that the cell continues to depolarize, transiently to a net positive potential.

The prominent influx of sodium ions is responsible for the rapid upstroke, or phase 0, of the action potential. However, the Na$^+$ channels remain open for only a few thousandths of a second and are then quickly inactivated, preventing further influx (see Fig. 1-13). Thus, while activation of these fast Na$^+$ channels causes the rapid early depolarization of the cell, the rapid inactivation makes their major contribution to the action potential short lived.

Phase 1

Following rapid phase 0 depolarization into the positive voltage range, a brief current of repolarization during phase 1 returns the membrane potential to ~0 mV. The responsible current (termed I_{to}) is carried by the outward flow of K$^+$ ions through a type of transiently activated potassium channel.

Phase 2

This relatively long "**plateau**" phase of the action potential is mediated by the balance of outward K$^+$ currents (known as I_{Ks} and I_{Kr}) carried through voltage-gated *delayed rectifier* K$^+$ channels, in competition with an inward Ca^{++} current, which flows through specific L-type calcium channels. The latter channels begin to open during phase 0, when the membrane voltage reaches approximately −40 mV, allowing Ca^{++} ions to flow down their concentration gradient into the cell (this current is termed $I_{ca.L}$). Ca^{++} entry proceeds in a more gradual fashion than the initial influx of sodium, because with calcium channels, activation is slower and the channels remain open much longer compared with sodium channels (see Fig. 1-13). During this phase, the near equality of current from inward Ca^{++}

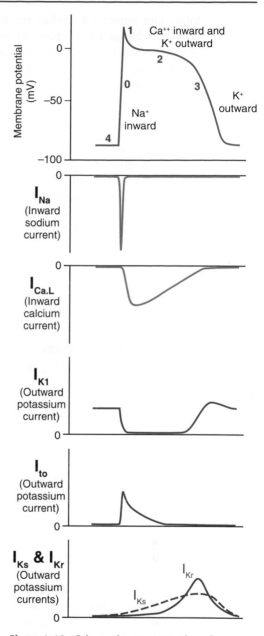

Figure 1-13. Schematic representation of a myocyte action potential (AP) and major ionic currents. The resting potential is represented by phase 4 of the AP. During depolarization, Na$^+$ influx (I_{Na}) results in the rapid upstroke of phase 0; a transient outward potassium current (I_{to}) is responsible for partial repolarization during phase 1; slow Ca^{++} influx ($I_{ca.L}$) balanced by K$^+$ efflux (I_{Ks} and I_{Kr}) results in the plateau of phase 2; and final rapid repolarization results largely from further K$^+$ efflux during phase 3. The resting potential of phase 4 is maintained primarily by the current I_{K1} through inward rectifier potassium channels.

influx and outward K⁺ efflux results in nearly zero net current, and the membrane voltage does not change for a prolonged period, which accounts for the flat plateau portion of the action potential curve. Calcium ions that enter the cell during this phase play a critical role in triggering additional internal calcium release from the SR, which is important in initiating myocyte contraction, as discussed later in this chapter. As the Ca⁺⁺ channels gradually inactivate and the charge efflux of K⁺ begins to exceed the charge influx of calcium, phase 3 begins.

Phase 3

This is the final phase of repolarization that returns the transmembrane voltage back to the resting potential of approximately −90 mV. A continued outward potassium current exceeds the low inward current of other cations and is thus responsible for this period of rapid repolarization. Phase 3 completes the action potential cycle, with a return to resting phase 4, preparing the cell for the next stimulus for depolarization.

To preserve normal transmembrane ionic concentration gradients, sodium and calcium ions that enter the cell during depolarization must be returned to the extracellular environment, and potassium ions must return to the cell interior. As shown in Figure 1-10, Ca⁺⁺ ions are removed by the sarcolemmal Na⁺-Ca⁺⁺ exchanger and to a lesser extent by the ATP-energized calcium pump (sarcolemmal Ca⁺⁺-ATPase). The corrective exchange of Na⁺ and K⁺ across the cell membrane is mediated by Na⁺K⁺-ATPase, as described earlier.

Specialized Conduction System

The process described in the previous sections applies to the action potential of cardiac muscle cells. The cells of the specialized conduction system (eg, Purkinje fibers) behave similarly, although the resting potential is slightly more negative and the upstroke of phase 0 is even more rapid, due to a greater presence of Na⁺ channels in these tissues.

Pacemaker Cells

The upstroke of the action potential of cardiac muscle cells does not normally occur spontaneously. Rather, when a wave of depolarization reaches the myocyte through the electrical junctions with neighboring cells, its membrane potential becomes less negative and an action potential is triggered.

Conversely, certain heart cells do not require external provocation to initiate their action potential. Rather, they are capable of self-initiated depolarization in a rhythmic fashion and are known as **pacemaker cells**. They are endowed with the property of **automaticity**, by which the cells undergo spontaneous depolarization during phase 4. When the threshold voltage is reached in such cells, an action potential upstroke is triggered (Fig. 1-14).

Cells that display pacemaker behavior include the SA node (the "natural pacemaker" of the heart) and the AV node. Although atrial and ventricular muscle cells do not normally display automaticity, they may do so under disease conditions.

Figure 1-14. Action potential of a pacemaker cell. Phase 4 is characterized by gradual, spontaneous depolarization owing to the pacemaker current (I_f). When the threshold potential is reached, at about −40 mV, the upstroke of the action potential follows. The upstroke of phase 0 is less rapid than in nonpacemaker cells because the current represents Ca⁺⁺ influx through the relatively slow calcium channels ($I_{ca.L}$). Repolarization occurs with inactivation of the calcium channels and K⁺ efflux from the cell through potassium channels (I_{Ks} and I_{Kr}).

The action potential of a pacemaker cell is different from that of a ventricular muscle cell in three ways:

1. The maximum negative voltage of pacemaker cells is approximately −60 mV, substantially less negative than the resting potential of ventricular muscle cells (−90 mV). The persistently less negative membrane voltage of pacemaker cells causes the fast sodium channels within these cells to remain inactivated.
2. Unlike that of cardiac muscle cells, phase 4 of the pacemaker cell action potential is not flat but has an upward slope, representing spontaneous gradual depolarization. This spontaneous depolarization is the result of an ionic flux known as the **pacemaker current** (denoted by I_f, also known as the "funny current;" see Table 1-1). The pacemaker current is carried predominantly by Na^+ ions, but the ion channel through which the pacemaker current passes is different from the fast sodium channel responsible for phase 0 of the action potential. Importantly, this pacemaker channel opens in the very negative voltage ranges reached during repolarization of the cell. The influx of positively charged Na^+ ions through the pacemaker channel causes the membrane potential to become progressively less negative during phase 4, ultimately depolarizing the cell to its threshold voltage (see Fig. 1-14).
3. The phase 0 upstroke of the pacemaker cell action potential is less rapid and reaches a lower amplitude than that of a cardiac muscle cell. These characteristics result from the fast sodium channels of the pacemaker cells being inactivated and the upstroke of the action potential relying solely on Ca^{++} influx through the relatively slow calcium channels.

Repolarization of pacemaker cells occurs in a fashion similar to that of ventricular muscle cells and relies on inactivation of the calcium channels and increased activation of potassium channels with enhanced K^+ efflux from the cell.

Refractory Periods

Compared with electrical impulses in nerves and skeletal muscle, the cardiac action potential is much longer in duration, supporting prolonged Ca^{++} entry and muscle contraction during systole. This results in a prolonged period of channel inactivation during which the muscle is refractory (unresponsive) to restimulation. Such a long period is physiologically necessary because it allows the ventricles sufficient time to relax and refill before the next contraction.

There are different levels of refractoriness during the action potential of a myocyte, as illustrated in Figure 1-15. The degree of refractoriness primarily reflects the percentage of fast Na^+ channels that have recovered from their inactive state and are capable of reopening. As phase 3 of the action potential progresses, an increasing number of Na^+ channels recover from inactivated to resting states and can then open in response to the next depolarization. This, in turn, corresponds to an increasing probability that a stimulus will trigger an action potential and result in a propagated impulse.

The *absolute* refractory period refers to the time during which the cell is completely unexcitable to any new stimulation. The *effective* refractory period includes the absolute refractory period but extends beyond it to include a short interval of phase 3, during which stimulation produces a localized action potential that is not strong enough to propagate further. The *relative* refractory period is the interval during which stimulation triggers an action potential that is conducted, but the rate of rise of the action potential is lower during this period because some of the Na^+ channels are inactivated and some of the delayed rectifier K^+ channels remain activated, thus reducing the available net inward current. Following the relative refractory period, a short "supranormal" period is present in which a less-than-normal stimulus can trigger an action potential.

The refractory period of atrial cells is shorter than that of ventricular muscle cells, such that atrial rates can generally exceed ventricular rates during rapid arrhythmias (see Chapter 11).

Figure 1-15. Refractory periods (RPs) of the myocyte. During the absolute refractory period (ARP), the cell is unexcitable to stimulation. The effective refractory period includes a brief time beyond the ARP during which stimulation produces a localized depolarization that does not propagate (*curve 1*). During the relative refractory period, stimulation produces a weak action potential (AP) that propagates, but more slowly than usual (*curve 2*). During the supranormal period, a weaker-than-normal stimulus can trigger an AP (*curve 3*).

IMPULSE CONDUCTION

During depolarization, the electrical impulse spreads along each cardiac cell and rapidly from cell to cell because each myocyte is connected to its neighbors through low-resistance gap junctions. Gap junctions are a special type of ion channel that provide electrical and biochemical coupling between cardiac myocytes, allowing the action potential to spread rapidly through the myocardium. The speed of tissue depolarization (phase 0) and the conduction velocity along the cell depend on the net inward current (which is largely dependent on the number of sodium channels), on the value of the resting potential (which sets the degree of Na^+ channel inactivation), and on the resistance to current flow between cells though the gap junctions. Tissues with a high concentration of Na^+ channels, such as Purkinje fibers, have a large, fast inward current, which spreads quickly within and between cells to support rapid conduction. However, if the resting potential becomes less negative, the greater the fraction of fast sodium channels that are in the inactivated state and the less rapid the upstroke velocity (Fig. 1-16). Thus, alterations in the resting potential significantly impact the upstroke and conduction velocity of the action potential.

NORMAL SEQUENCE OF CARDIAC DEPOLARIZATION

Electrical activation of the heartbeat is normally initiated at the SA node (see Fig. 1-6). The impulse spreads to the surrounding atrial muscle through the intercellular gap junctions, providing electrical continuity between the cells. Ordinary atrial muscle fibers participate in the propagation of the impulse from the SA to the AV node, although in certain regions the fibers are more densely arranged, lowering intercellular resistance and thus facilitating conduction.

Figure 1-16. Dependence of speed of depolarization on resting potential. A. Normal resting potential (RP) and rapid rise of phase 0. **B.** Less negative RP results in slower rise of phase 0 and lower maximum amplitude of the action potential.

Fibrous tissue surrounds the tricuspid and mitral valves, such that there is no direct electrical connection between the atrial and ventricular chambers other than through the AV node. As the electrical impulse reaches the AV node, a delay in conduction (~ 0.1 seconds) is encountered. This delay occurs because the small-diameter fibers in this region conduct slowly, and the action potential is of the "slow" pacemaker type (recall that the fast sodium channels are permanently inactivated in pacemaker tissues, such that the upstroke velocity relies on the slower calcium channels). The pause in conduction at the AV node is actually beneficial because it allows the atria time to contract and fully empty their contents before ventricular stimulation. In addition, the delay allows the AV node to serve as a "gatekeeper" of conduction from atria to ventricles, which is critical for limiting the rate of ventricular stimulation during abnormally rapid atrial rhythms.

After traversing the AV node, the cardiac action potential spreads into the rapidly conducting bundle of His and Purkinje fibers, which distribute the electrical impulses to the bulk of the ventricular muscle cells, in a spatially synchronized manner. This allows for precisely timed stimulation and organized contraction of the ventricular myocytes, optimizing the volume of blood ejected by the heart.

EXCITATION-CONTRACTION COUPLING

This section reviews how the electrical action potential leads to physical contraction of cardiac muscle cells, a process known as excitation-contraction coupling. During this process, chemical energy in the form of high-energy phosphate compounds is translated into the mechanical energy of myocyte contraction.

CONTRACTILE PROTEINS IN THE MYOCYTE

Several distinct proteins are responsible for cardiac muscle cell contraction (Fig. 1-17). Of the major proteins, actin and myosin are the chief contractile elements. Two other proteins, tropomyosin and troponin, serve regulatory functions.

Myosin is arranged in thick filaments, each composed of lengthwise stacks of ~ 300 molecules. The myosin filament exhibits globular heads that are evenly spaced along its length and contain myosin ATPase, an enzyme that is necessary for contraction to occur. **Actin**, a smaller molecule, is arranged in thin filaments as an α-helix consisting of two strands that interdigitate between the thick myosin filaments (see Fig. 1-8). **Titin** (also termed connectin) is a very large protein that helps tether myosin to the Z line of the sarcomere and provides elasticity to the contractile process.

Tropomyosin is a double helix that lies in the grooves between the actin filaments and, in the resting state, inhibits the interaction between myosin heads and actin, thus preventing contraction. **Troponin** sits at regular intervals along the actin strands and is composed

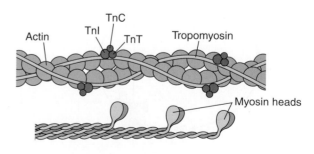

Figure 1-17. Schematic diagram of the main contractile proteins of the myocyte, actin, and myosin. Tropomyosin and troponin (components TnI, TnC, and TnT) are regulatory proteins.

of three subunits. The troponin T (TnT) subunit links the troponin complex to the actin and tropomyosin molecules. The troponin I (TnI) subunit inhibits the ATPase activity of the actin-myosin interaction. The troponin C (TnC) subunit is responsible for binding calcium ions that regulate the contractile process.

CALCIUM-INDUCED CALCIUM RELEASE AND THE CONTRACTILE CYCLE

The sensitivity of TnC to calcium establishes a crucial role for intracellular Ca^{++} ions in cellular contraction. The cycling of calcium in and out of the cytosol during each action potential effectively couples electrical excitation to physical contraction.

Recall that during phase 2 of the action potential, activation of L-type Ca^{++} channels results in an influx of Ca^{++} ions into the myocyte. The small amount of calcium that enters the cell in this fashion is not sufficient to cause contraction of the myofibrils, but it triggers a much greater Ca^{++} release from the SR, as follows: The T-tubule invaginations of the sarcolemmal membrane bring the L-type channels into close apposition with specialized Ca^{++} release receptors in the SR, known as **ryanodine receptors** (Fig. 1-18). When calcium enters the cell and binds to the ryanodine receptor, the receptor changes to an open conformation, which results in a much greater release of Ca^{++} into the cytosol from the abundant stores in the terminal cisternae of the SR. Thus, the initial L-type Ca^{++} channel influx is amplified by this mechanism, known as **calcium-induced calcium release (CICR)**, and the cytosolic calcium concentration dramatically increases.

As calcium ions bind to TnC, the activity of TnI is inhibited, which induces a conformational change in tropomyosin. The latter event exposes the active site between actin and myosin, enabling contraction to proceed.

Contraction ensues as myosin heads bind to actin filaments and "flex," thus causing the interdigitating thick and thin filaments to move past each other in an ATP-dependent reaction (Fig. 1-19). The first step in this process is activation of the myosin head by hydrolysis of ATP, following which the myosin head binds to actin and forms a cross bridge. The interaction

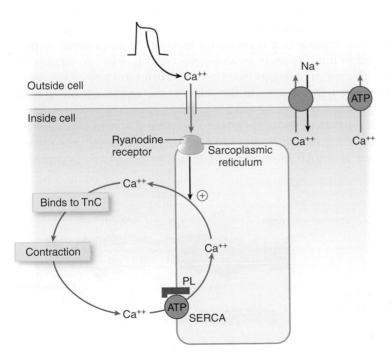

Figure 1-18. Calcium ion movements during excitation and contraction in cardiac muscle cells. Ca^{++} enters the cell through calcium channels during phase 2 of the action potential, triggering a much larger calcium release from the sarcoplasmic reticulum (SR) via the ryanodine receptor complex. The binding of cytosolic Ca^{++} to troponin C (TnC) allows contraction to ensue. Relaxation occurs as Ca^{++} is returned to the SR by sarco(endo)plasmic reticulum calcium ATPase (SERCA). Phospholamban (PL) is a major regulator of this pump, inhibiting Ca^{++} uptake in its dephosphorylated state. Excess intracellular calcium is returned to the extracellular environment by sodium-calcium exchange and to a smaller degree by the sarcolemmal Ca^{++}-ATPase.

Figure 1-19. The contractile process. A. Myosin head is activated by hydrolysis of ATP. **B.** During cellular depolarization, cytoplasmic calcium concentration increases and removes the troponin-tropomyosin inhibition, such that a cross bridge is formed between actin and myosin. **C.** Inorganic phosphate (P_i) is released and a conformational change in the myosin head draws the actin filament inward. **D.** ADP is released and replaced by ATP, causing the myosin head to dissociate from the actin filament. As the process repeats, the muscle fiber shortens. The cycle continues until cytosolic calcium concentration decreases at the end of phase 2 of the action potential.

between the myosin head and actin results in a conformational change in the head, causing it to pull the actin filament inward.

Next, while the myosin head and actin are still attached, ADP is released, and a new molecule of ATP then binds to the myosin head, causing it to release the actin filament. The cycle can then repeat. Progressive coupling and uncoupling of actin and myosin cause the muscle fiber to shorten by increasing the overlap between the myofilaments within each sarcomere. In the presence of ATP, this process continues for as long as the cytosolic calcium concentration remains sufficiently high to inhibit the troponin-tropomyosin blocking action.

Myocyte relaxation, like contraction, is synchronized with the electrical activity of the cell. Toward the end of phase 2 of the action potential, L-type channels inactivate, arresting the influx of Ca^{++} into the cell and abolishing the trigger for CICR. Concurrently, calcium is pumped back into the SR and out of the cell. Calcium is sequestered back into the SR primarily by **sarco(endo)plasmic reticulum Ca^{++} ATPase** (SERCA), as shown in Figure 1-18. The small amount of Ca^{++} that entered the cell through L-type calcium channels is removed via the sarcolemmal Na^+-Ca^{++} exchanger and to a lesser extent by the ATP-consuming calcium pump, sarcolemmal Ca^{++}-ATPase (see Fig. 1-10).

As the cytosolic Ca^{++} concentration falls and calcium ions dissociate from TnC, tropomyosin once again inhibits the actin-myosin interaction, leading to relaxation of the contracted cell. The contraction-relaxation cycle can then repeat with the next action potential.

INTRODUCTION TO CARDIAC SIGNALING SYSTEMS

β-Adrenergic and Cholinergic Signaling

There is substantial evidence that the concentration of Ca^{++} within the cytosol is the major determinant of the force of cardiac contraction with each heartbeat. Mechanisms that raise intracellular Ca^{++} concentration enhance force development, whereas factors that lower Ca^{++} concentration reduce the contractile force.

β-*Adrenergic stimulation* is one mechanism that enhances calcium fluxes in the myocyte and thereby strengthens the force of ventricular contraction (Fig. 1-20). Catecholamines (eg, norepinephrine) bind to the myocyte $β_1$-adrenergic receptor, which is coupled to and activates the G protein system (G_s) attached to the inner surface of the cell membrane. G_s in turn stimulates membrane-bound adenylate cyclase to produce cyclic AMP (cAMP) from ATP. cAMP then activates specific intracellular protein kinases (PKAs), which phosphorylate cellular proteins, including the L-type calcium channels within the cell membrane. Phosphorylation of the calcium channel augments Ca^{++} influx, which triggers a corresponding increase in Ca^{++} release from the SR, thereby enhancing the force of contraction.

β-Adrenergic stimulation of the myocyte also enhances myocyte *relaxation*. The return of Ca^{++} from the cytosol to the SR is regulated by **phospholamban (PL)**, a low molecu-

Figure 1-20. Effects of β-adrenergic and cholinergic stimulation on cardiac cellular signaling and calcium ion movement. The binding of a ligand (eg, norepinephrine) to the $β_1$-adrenergic receptor induces G protein–mediated stimulation of adenylate cyclase and formation of cyclic AMP (cAMP). The latter activates protein kinases, which phosphorylate cellular proteins, including ion channels. Phosphorylation of the slow Ca^{++} channel enhances calcium movement into the cell and therefore strengthens the force of contraction. Protein kinases also phosphorylate phospholamban (PL), reducing the latter's inhibition of Ca^{++} uptake by the sarcoplasmic reticulum. The enhanced removal of Ca^{++} from the cytosol facilitates relaxation of the myocyte. Cholinergic signaling, triggered by acetylcholine binding to the muscarinic receptor, activates inhibitory G proteins that reduce adenylate cyclase activity and cAMP production, thus antagonizing the effects of β-adrenergic stimulation.

lar weight protein in the SR membrane. In its dephosphorylated state, PL inhibits Ca^{++} uptake by SERCA (see Fig. 1-18). However, β-adrenergic activation of PKAs causes PL to become phosphorylated, an action that blunts PL's inhibitory effect (see Fig. 1-20). The subsequently greater uptake of calcium ions by the SR hastens Ca^{++} removal from the cytosol, promoting myocyte relaxation. The increased cAMP activity also results in phosphorylation of TnI, an action that inhibits actin-myosin interactions and therefore further enhances relaxation of the cell.

Cholinergic signaling via parasympathetic inputs (mainly from the vagus nerve) opposes the effects of β-adrenergic stimulation (see Fig. 1-20). Acetylcholine released from parasympathetic nerve terminals binds to the muscarinic M_2 receptor on cardiac cells. This receptor also activates G proteins, but in distinction to the β-adrenergic receptor, it is coupled to G_i, an inhibitory G protein system. G_i associated with cholinergic stimulation *inhibits* adenylate cyclase activity and reduces cAMP formation. At the sinus node, these actions of cholinergic stimulation serve to reduce heart rate. In the myocardium, the effect is to counteract the force of contraction induced by β-adrenergic stimulation. It should be noted that ventricular cells are much less sensitive to this cholinergic effect than atrial cells, likely reflecting different degrees of G protein coupling.

Thus, physiologic or pharmacologic catecholamine stimulation of the myocyte β_1-adrenergic receptor enhances contraction of the cell, while cholinergic stimulation opposes that enhancement. We will return to these important properties in later chapters.

Summary

This chapter has reviewed basic cardiac anatomy and cellular composition, the cardiac conduction system, excitation-contraction coupling, and cardiac signaling systems. The physiology of myocyte contraction will be described in Chapter 9. Each of these complex pieces integrate together to form an organ system that functions in an organized fashion, is robust to errors, and operates reliably over many decades. As a result, the heart is capable of purposeful stimulation billions of times during the life span of a normal person. With each contraction cycle, the heart receives and propagates blood through the circulation to provide nutrients to and remove waste products from the body's tissues. The remainder of this book explores what can go wrong with this remarkable system.

Review Questions

1. Which of the following anatomic descriptions is correct?

   a. There are two papillary muscles in the right ventricle.
   b. The mitral valve consists of three leaflets.
   c. The pulmonic valve lies anterior to the aortic valve.
   d. The ascending aorta crosses over the left pulmonary artery and becomes the aortic arch.

2. A 63-year-old man presents to the hospital with an acute myocardial infarction (heart attack) affecting the lateral wall of the left ventricle. Obstruction within which of the following coronary arteries is likely responsible?

a. A branch of the left anterior descending coronary artery
b. A branch of the circumflex coronary artery
c. A branch of the right coronary artery
d. A branch of the posterior descending coronary artery

3. Which of the following statements regarding cardiac action potentials is correct?

a. In the resting state, prior to depolarization, the cardiac myocyte cell membrane is more permeable to sodium than to potassium ions.
b. The phase 0 upstroke of pacemaker cells is most dependent on a rapid inward sodium current.
c. The plateau during phase 2 of a nonpacemaker cell action potential is due to a balance between an inward calcium current and outward potassium currents.
d. Calcium ions that enter the myocyte during depolarization are removed from the cell exclusively by an ATP-energized calcium pump (sarcolemmal Ca^{++}-ATPase).

Answers to Review Questions

1. Choice c is correct. The pulmonic valve is positioned anterior to the aortic valve (see Figs. 1-3 and 1-4). The left ventricle contains two papillary muscles, but the right ventricle contains three. The mitral valve consists of two leaflets; all of the other cardiac valves normally have three leaflets. The ascending aorta crosses over the *right* pulmonary artery as it becomes the aortic arch (see Fig. 1-2).

2. Choice b is correct. Obtuse marginal branches of the circumflex coronary artery supply lateral and posterior regions of the left ventricle (see Fig. 1-7). Branches of the left anterior descending coronary artery supply the anterior wall and anterior septum. Branches of the right coronary artery supply the right ventricle, and the posterior descending artery provides blood flow to inferior and posterior walls of the ventricles and the posterior septum.

3. Choice c is correct. The plateau of phase 2 of the action potential is due to a balance between the inward calcium current and outward potassium currents (see Fig. 1-13). In the resting state, the cardiac myocyte cell membrane is much more permeable to potassium than to other ions. The phase 0 upstroke of pacemaker cells relies solely on *calcium* influx, in distinction to nonpacemaker cells, in which a rapid sodium current is responsible instead. Calcium ions are removed from the myocyte primarily by the sarcolemmal Na^+-Ca^{++} exchanger and to a lesser extent by the ATP-energized calcium pump.

Acknowledgments

Contributors to previous editions of this chapter were Jacob E. Lemieux, MD; Ken Young Lin, MD; Vivek Iyer, MD; Kirsten Greineder, MD; Stephanie Harper, MD; Scott Hyver, MD; Paul Kim, MD; Rajeev Malhotra, MD; Laurence Rhines, MD; James D. Marsh, MD; and Gary R. Strichartz, PhD.

Additional Reading

Courneya C, Parker MJ. *Cardiovascular Physiology. A Clinical Approach.* Baltimore, MD: Lippincott Williams & Wilkins; 2011.

Eisner DA, Caldwell JL, Kistamas K, et al. Calcium and excitation-contraction coupling in the heart. *Circ Res.* 2017;121:181-195.

Grant AO. Cardiac ion channels. *Circ Arrhythm Electrophysiol.* 2009;2:185-194.

Katz AM. *Physiology of the Heart.* 5th ed. Philadelphia, PA: Lippincott Williams & Wilkins; 2010.

Moore KL, Dalley AF, Agur AMR. *Clinically Oriented Anatomy.* 8th ed. Philadelphia, PA: Lippincott Williams & Wilkins; 2018.

Murphy C, Lazzara R. Current concepts of anatomy and electrophysiology of the sinus node. *J Interv Card Electrophysiol.* 2016;46:9-18.

Zipes DP, Jalife J, Sevenson WG, eds. *Cardiac Electrophysiology: From Cell to Bedside.* 7th ed. Philadelphia, PA: Elsevier; 2017.

2 The Cardiac Cycle: Mechanisms of Heart Sounds and Murmurs

Vivek T. Kulkarni | Leonard S. Lilly

Each heartbeat is generated by electrical and mechanical events that result in rhythmic contraction and relaxation of the atria and ventricles. These actions generate heart sounds that can be auscultated at the bedside using a stethoscope. Cardiac diseases often cause abnormalities of the physical examination, including pathologic heart sounds and murmurs, and proper interpretation of such findings is essential in diagnosis and disease management. This chapter first describes the events that result in normal heart sounds and then focuses on the origins of pathologic heart sounds and murmurs.

Many cardiac diseases are mentioned briefly in this chapter as examples of abnormal heart sounds and murmurs. Each of these conditions is described in greater detail later in the book, so it is neither necessary nor desirable to memorize the examples presented here. Rather, the goal of this chapter is to explain the mechanisms by which the abnormal sounds are produced, so that their descriptions will make sense in later chapters.

CARDIAC CYCLE

The cardiac cycle represents the sequence of electrical and mechanical events that occur with each heartbeat. For example, Figure 2-1 displays the pressure relationships between the left-sided cardiac chambers during a normal cardiac cycle and serves as a platform for describing key events. **Systole** refers to the phase of ventricular contraction and **diastole** to the phase of ventricular relaxation and filling. Throughout the cardiac cycle, the right and left atria accept blood returning to the heart from the systemic veins and from the pulmonary veins, respectively. During diastole, blood passes from the atria into the ventricles across the open tricuspid and mitral valves, causing a gradual increase in ventricular diastolic pressures. In late diastole, spontaneous depolarization of the sinoatrial node spreads to atrial myocytes and triggers atrial contraction, propelling a final bolus of blood into each ventricle. This action, known as the "atrial kick," produces a brief further rise in atrial and ventricular pressures, labeled the "a" wave in Figure 2-1.

After a brief pause at the AV node, electrical depolarization and contraction of the ventricles follows, signaling the onset of ventricular systole. As the ventricles contract, the generated pressures rapidly exceed the pressures in the atria. This results in the forced closure of the tricuspid and mitral valves, producing the first heart sound, termed S_1. This sound has two nearly superimposed parts: the mitral component slightly precedes the tricuspid component because of the earlier electrical activation of the left ventricle (as described in Chapter 4).

As the right and left ventricular pressures rapidly rise further, they soon exceed the diastolic pressures within the pulmonary artery and aorta, forcing the pulmonic and aortic valves to open, and blood is ejected into the pulmonary artery and aorta. The ventricular pressures continue to increase during the initial portion of this ejection phase and then decline as ventricular relaxation commences. Since the pulmonic and aortic valves are open during this phase, the aortic and pulmonary artery pressures rise and fall in parallel to those of the corresponding ventricles.

At the conclusion of ventricular ejection, the ventricular pressures decline below those of the pulmonary artery and aorta (the pulmonary artery and aorta are elastic structures that dissipate pressure more gradually than do the ventricles), such that the pulmonic and aortic valves are forced to close, producing the second heart sound, S_2. Like the first heart sound (S_1), this sound consists of two parts: the aortic (A_2) component normally precedes the pulmonic (P_2) because the diastolic pressure gradient between the aorta and left ventricle is greater than that between the pulmonary artery and the right ventricle (RV), forcing the aortic valve to

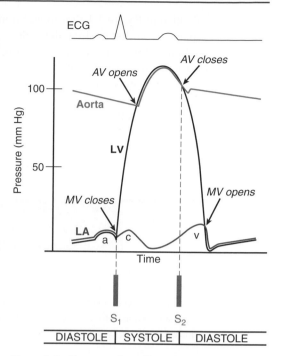

Figure 2-1. The normal cardiac cycle, showing pressure relationships between the left-sided heart chambers. During diastole, the mitral valve (MV) is open, so that the left atrial (LA) and left ventricular (LV) pressures are equal. In late diastole, LA contraction ("atrial kick") causes a small rise in LA and LV pressure (the *a* wave). During systolic contraction, the LV pressure rises; when it exceeds the LA pressure, the MV closes, contributing to the first heart sound (S_1). As LV pressure rises above the aortic pressure, the aortic valve (AV) opens, which is a silent event, and blood is ejected into the aorta. As the ventricle begins to relax and its pressure falls below that of the aorta, the AV closes, contributing to the second heart sound (S_2). As LV pressure falls further, below that of the LA, the MV opens, which is silent in the normal heart. In addition to the *a* wave, the LA pressure curve displays two other positive deflections: the *c* wave represents a small rise in LA pressure as the MV closes and bulges into the atrium, and the *v* wave is the result of passive filling of the LA from the pulmonary veins during systole, when the MV is closed.

shut more readily. The ventricular pressures fall rapidly during the subsequent relaxation phase. As they drop below the pressures in the right and left atria, the tricuspid and mitral valves open, allowing blood to flow from the atria into the ventricles through the remainder of diastole, completing the cardiac cycle, which then repeats with the next heartbeat.

At the bedside, systole can be approximated as the period from S_1 to S_2, and diastole from S_2 to the next S_1. Although the duration of systole remains constant from beat to beat, the length of diastole varies with the heart rate: the faster the heart rate, the shorter the diastolic phase. The main sounds, S_1 and S_2, provide a framework from which all other heart sounds and murmurs can be timed.

Notice in Figure 2-1 that in addition to the *a* wave, the atrial pressure curve (in red color) displays two other positive deflections during the cardiac cycle: the *c* wave represents a small rise in atrial pressure at the beginning of systole as the increasing ventricular pressure forces the tricuspid and mitral valves to close and to briefly bulge into their respective atria. The *v* wave represents the rise in pressure due to passive filling of the atria from the systemic and pulmonary veins during the phase of ventricular contraction, a period during which blood accumulates in the atria because the tricuspid and mitral valves are closed.

The pressure relationships and events depicted in Figure 2-1 are those that occur in the left side of the heart. Equivalent events occur simultaneously in the right side of the heart in the right atrium, RV, and pulmonary artery. At the bedside, clues to right heart function can be ascertained

Box 2-1	Jugular Venous Pulsations and Assessment of Right Heart Function

Bedside observation of jugular venous pulsations in the neck is a vital part of the cardiovascular examination. With no structures impeding blood flow between the internal jugular (IJ) veins and the superior vena cava and right atrium (RA), the height of the IJ venous column (termed the "jugular venous pressure" or JVP) is an accurate representation of the RA pressure. Thus, the JVP provides an easily obtainable measure of right heart function.

Technique of Measurement

The JVP is measured as the maximum vertical height of the internal jugular vein (in cm) above the center of the right atrium and in a normal person is ≤9 cm. Because the sternal angle is located ~5 cm above the center of the RA, the JVP is calculated at the bedside by adding 5 cm to the vertical height of the top of the IJ venous column above the sternal angle (see figure).

The right-sided IJ vein is usually the easiest to evaluate because it extends directly upward from the RA and superior vena cava. First, observe the pulsations in the skin overlying the IJ with the patient supine and the head of the bed at about a 45-degree angle. Shining a light obliquely across the neck helps to visualize the pulsations. Be sure to examine the IJ, not the external jugular vein. The former is medial to, or behind, the sternocleidomastoid muscle, whereas the external jugular is usually more lateral. Although the external jugular is typically easier to see, it does not always accurately reflect RA pressure because it contains valves that interfere with venous return to the heart. Additionally, it can sometimes be difficult to distinguish jugular venous pulsations from the neighboring carotid artery.

Unlike the carotid, the JVP is usually not pulsatile to palpation, it has a double or triple upstroke rather than a single one, and it declines in most patients by assuming the seated position or during inspiration.

If the top of the IJ column is not visible at 45 degrees, the column of blood is either too low (below the clavicle) or too high (above the jaw) to be measured in that position. In such situations, the head of the bed must be lowered or raised, respectively, so that the top of the column becomes visible. As long as the top can be ascertained, the vertical height of the JVP above or below the sternal angle will accurately reflect RA pressure, no matter the angle of the head of the bed.

Careful inspection of the JVP during the cardiac cycle reveals cyclical waveform components, as shown in the figure (notice the similarity of the deflections to the atrial pressure tracing in Fig. 2-1). There are two major upward components, the *a* and *v* waves, followed by two descents, termed *x* and *y*. The *x* descent, which represents the pressure decline following the *a* wave, may be interrupted by a small third upward deflection (the *c* wave) at the time of tricuspid valve closure, but that is often not distinguishable. The *a* wave represents transient venous distension caused by back pressure from RA contraction. The *v* wave corresponds to passive filling of the RA from the systemic veins during systole, when the tricuspid valve is closed. Opening of the tricuspid valve in early diastole allows blood to rapidly empty from the RA into the right ventricle; that fall in RA pressure corresponds to the *y* descent.

Conditions that abnormally raise right-sided cardiac pressures (eg, heart failure, tricuspid valve disease, pulmonic stenosis, pericardial diseases) elevate the JVP, while reduced intravascular volume (eg, dehydration) decreases it. In addition, specific disease states can influence the individual components of the JVP, examples of which are listed here for reference and explained in subsequent chapters:

Prominent *a*: right ventricular hypertrophy, tricuspid stenosis
Prominent *v*: tricuspid regurgitation
Prominent *y*: constrictive pericarditis

by examining the internal jugular vein pulsations in the neck, which mimic the right atrial pressure tracing shown in Figure 2-1, as these structures are continuous with each other (see Box 2-1).

HEART SOUNDS

One type of commonly used stethoscope contains two chest pieces for auscultation of the heart. The concave "bell" chest piece, meant to be applied lightly to the skin, accentuates low-frequency sounds. Conversely, the flat "diaphragm" chest piece is designed to be pressed firmly against the skin to eliminate low frequencies, and it therefore accentuates high-frequency sounds and murmurs. Another type of modern stethoscope incorporates both the bell and diaphragm functions into a single chest piece; in these models, placing the piece lightly on the skin brings out the low-frequency sounds, while firm pressure accentuates the high-frequency ones. Both types of stethoscopes are equally effective, and selection of which to use is a matter of personal choice. The sections below describe when, and where on the chest, to listen for high- vs low-frequency sounds.

First Heart Sound (S₁)

S₁ is produced by the closure of the mitral and tricuspid valves in early systole and is loudest near the apex of the heart (Fig. 2-2). It is a high-frequency sound, best heard with the diaphragm of the stethoscope. Although mitral closure usually precedes tricuspid closure, they are separated by only about 0.01 seconds, such that the human ear appreciates only a single sound. An exception occurs in patients with right bundle-branch block (see Chapter 4), in whom these components *may* be audibly split because of delayed right ventricular contraction and late closure of the tricuspid valve.

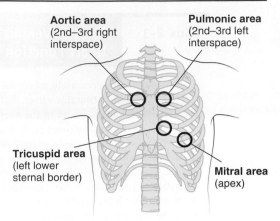

Figure 2-2. Standard positions of stethoscope placement for cardiac auscultation. The mitral area localizes to the cardiac *apex* while the aortic and pulmonic regions represent the cardiac *base*.

Three factors determine the intensity of S₁: (1) the distance separating the leaflets of the open valves at the onset of ventricular contraction, (2) the mobility of the mitral and tricuspid leaflets (normal or rigid because of stenosis), and (3) the rate of rise of ventricular pressure (Table 2-1).

The distance between the open valve leaflets at the onset of ventricular contraction relates to the electrocardiographic PR interval (see Chapter 4), the period between the onset of atrial and ventricular activation. Atrial contraction at the end of diastole forces the tricuspid and mitral valve leaflets apart. They start to passively drift back together, but once ventricular contraction causes the ventricular pressure to exceed that in the atrium, the leaflets are forced to close from whatever positions they occupy at that moment. An *accentuated* S₁ results when the PR interval is shorter than normal, because the valve leaflets have less time to drift back together and are therefore forced shut from a relatively wide distance.

Similarly, in *mild* mitral stenosis (see Chapter 8), impeded flow through the mitral valve causes a prolonged diastolic pressure gradient between the left atrium and ventricle, which keeps the mobile portions of the mitral leaflets farther apart than normal during late diastole. Because the leaflets are relatively wide apart at the onset of systole, they are forced shut loudly when the left ventricle contracts.

S₁ may also be accentuated when the heart rate is more rapid than normal (ie, tachycardia) because diastole is shortened and the leaflets have less time to drift back together before the ventricles contract.

TABLE 2-1 Causes of Altered Intensity of the First Heart Sound (S₁)

Accentuated S₁

1. Shortened PR interval
2. Mild mitral stenosis
3. High cardiac output states or tachycardia (eg, exercise)

Diminished S₁

1. Lengthened PR interval: first-degree AV nodal block
2. Mitral regurgitation
3. Severe mitral stenosis
4. "Stiff" left ventricle (eg, left ventricular hypertrophy due to systemic hypertension)

Conditions that *reduce* the intensity of S_1 are also listed in Table 2-1. In first-degree atrioventricular (AV) block (see Chapter 12), a diminished S_1 results from an abnormally prolonged PR interval, which delays the onset of ventricular contraction. Consequently, following atrial contraction, the mitral and tricuspid valves have *additional* time to float back together so that the leaflets are forced closed from only a small distance apart and the sound is softened.

In patients with mitral regurgitation (see Chapter 8), S_1 is often diminished in intensity because the mitral leaflets may not come into full contact with one another as they close. In *severe* mitral stenosis, the leaflets are nearly fixed in position throughout the cardiac cycle, and that reduced movement also lessens the intensity of S_1.

In patients with a stiffened left ventricle (eg, a hypertrophied chamber), atrial contraction generates a higher-than-normal ventricular pressure at the end of diastole. This greater pressure causes the mitral leaflets to drift together more rapidly, so that they are forced closed from a smaller-than-normal distance when ventricular contraction begins, thus reducing the intensity of S_1.

Second Heart Sound (S_2)

The second heart sound results from the closure of the aortic and pulmonic valves and therefore has aortic (A_2) and pulmonic (P_2) components. Unlike S_1, which is usually heard only as a single sound, the components of S_2 vary with the respiratory cycle: they are normally fused as one sound during expiration but become audibly separated during inspiration, a situation termed normal or **physiologic splitting** (Fig. 2-3).

One factor that contributes to normal splitting of S_2 is that expansion of the chest during inspiration causes the intrathoracic pressure to become more negative. The negative pressure transiently increases the capacitance (and reduces the impedance) of the intrathoracic pulmonary vessels. As a result, there is a temporary delay in the diastolic "back pressure" in the pulmonary artery responsible for the closure of the pulmonic valve. Another factor is that the negative intrathoracic pressure generated by inspiration enhances blood flow from the systemic veins into the chest, increasing venous return to the right atrium and RV. The increased filling of the RV augments the stroke volume during the next systolic contraction and therefore lengthens the time required for RV emptying before the pulmonic valve closes. As a result of these mechanisms, P_2 is delayed; that is, it occurs *later* during inspiration than during expiration.

Inspiration has the opposite effect on aortic valve closure. Because the negative intrathoracic pressure generated by inspiration increases the capacitance of the intrathoracic pulmonary veins, venous return to the left atrium and ventricle temporarily decreases. Reduced filling of the LV diminishes the stroke volume during the next systolic contraction and therefore shortens the time required for LV emptying. Therefore, aortic valve closure (A_2) occurs slightly *earlier* in inspiration than during expiration. The combination of an earlier A_2 and delayed P_2 during inspiration causes audible separation of the two components. Since these components are high-frequency sounds, they are best heard with the diaphragm of the stethoscope, and splitting of S_2 is usually most easily appreciated near the second left intercostal space next to the sternum (the pulmonic area in Fig. 2-2).

Abnormalities of S_2 include alterations in its intensity and changes in the pattern of splitting. The intensity of S_2 depends on the velocity of blood coursing back toward the valves from the aorta and pulmonary artery after the completion of ventricular contraction, and the suddenness with which that backward surge is arrested by the closing valves. In systemic hypertension or pulmonary arterial hypertension, the diastolic pressure in the respective great artery is higher than normal, such that the velocity of the blood surging toward the valve is augmented and S_2 is accentuated. Conversely, in *severe* aortic or pulmonic valve stenosis, the valve commissures are nearly fixed in position, such that the contribution of the stenotic valve to S_2 is diminished.

There are three types of abnormal splitting patterns of S_2: widened, fixed, and paradoxical. **Widened splitting** of S_2 refers to an increase in the time interval between A_2 and P_2, such that

Figure 2-3. Splitting patterns of the second heart sound (S2). A_2, aortic component; P_2, pulmonic component of S_2; S_1, first heart sound.

the two components are audibly separated *even during expiration* and become more widely separated in inspiration (see Fig. 2-3). This pattern is usually the result of delayed closure of the pulmonic valve, which occurs in right bundle-branch block (described in Chapter 4) and sometimes in pulmonic valve stenosis (see Chapter 16).

Fixed splitting of S_2 also represents an abnormally lengthened interval between A_2 and P_2, but in distinction to widened splitting, the widening persists unchanged through the respiratory cycle (see Fig. 2-3). The most common abnormality that causes fixed splitting of S_2 is an atrial septal defect (an abnormal communication between the right and left atria; see Chapter 16). In that condition, chronic volume overload of the right-sided circulation results in a high-capacitance, low-resistance pulmonary vascular system. This alteration in pulmonary artery hemodynamics delays the back pressure responsible for the closure of the pulmonic valve. Thus, P_2 occurs later than normal, even during expiration, such that there is wider-than-normal separation of A_2 and P_2. The pattern of splitting does not change (ie, it is fixed) during the respiratory cycle because (1) inspiration does not substantially increase further the already elevated pulmonary vascular capacitance and (2) augmented filling of the right atrium from the systemic veins during inspiration is counterbalanced by a reciprocal decrease in the left-to-right transatrial shunt, eliminating respiratory variations in right ventricular filling.

Paradoxical splitting (also termed "reversed" splitting) refers to audible separation of A_2 and P_2 during *expiration* that fuses into a single sound on *inspiration*, the opposite of the normal situation. It reflects an abnormal delay in the closure of the aortic valve such that P_2 *precedes* A_2. In adults, the most common cause is left bundle-branch block (LBBB). In LBBB, described in Chapter 4, the spread of electrical activity through the left ventricle is impaired, resulting in delayed left ventricular contraction and late closure of the aortic valve, causing A_2 to abnormally follow P_2 with wide separation between them. Then, during inspiration, as in the normal case, the pulmonic valve closure sound becomes delayed, and the aortic valve closure sound moves earlier. This results in narrowing, and often super-imposition, of the two sounds; thus, there is no apparent split at the height of inspiration (see Fig. 2-3). In addition to LBBB, paradoxical splitting may be observed under circumstances in which left ventricular ejection is prolonged, such as in some patients with aortic stenosis.

EXTRA SYSTOLIC HEART SOUNDS

Extra systolic heart sounds may occur in early, mid, or late systole.

Early Extra Systolic Heart Sounds

Abnormal early systolic sounds, or *ejection clicks*, occur shortly after S_1 and coincide with the opening of the aortic or pulmonic valves (Fig. 2-4). These sounds have a sharp, high-pitched quality, so they are heard best with the diaphragm of the stethoscope placed over the aortic and pulmonic areas (see Fig. 2-2). Ejection clicks indicate the presence of aortic or pulmonic valve stenosis or dilatation of the pulmonary artery or aorta. In stenosis of the aortic or pulmonic valve, the sound occurs as the deformed valve leaflets reach their maximal level of ascent into the great artery, just prior to blood ejection. At that moment, the rapidly ascending valve reaches its elastic limit and decelerates abruptly, an action thought to result in the sound generation. In dilatation of the root of the aorta or pulmonary artery, the sound is associated with sudden tensing of the aortic or pulmonic root with

Figure 2-4. Timing of extra systolic and diastolic heart sounds. S_4 is produced by atrial contraction into a "stiff" left ventricle (LV). An ejection click follows the opening of the aortic or pulmonic valve in cases of valve stenosis or dilatation of the corresponding great artery. S_3 occurs during the period of rapid ventricular filling; it is normal in young people, but its presence in adults implies LV contractile dysfunction. The timing of an opening snap (OS) in a patient with mitral stenosis is placed for comparison. It is not likely that more than one or two of these extra sounds would appear in the same person. LA, left atrium; MV, mitral valve.

the onset of blood flow into the vessel. The *aortic ejection click* is heard at both the base (represented by the aortic and pulmonary regions in Fig. 2-2) and the apex of the heart and does not vary with respiration. In contrast, the *pulmonic ejection click* is heard only at the base, and its intensity diminishes during inspiration (see Chapter 16).

Mid or Late Extra Systolic Heart Sounds

Clicks occurring in mid or late systole are usually the result of systolic prolapse of the mitral or tricuspid valves, in which the leaflets bulge abnormally from the ventricular side of the AV junction into the atrium during ventricular contraction, often accompanied by valvular regurgitation (described in Chapter 8). They are loudest over the mitral or tricuspid auscultatory regions, respectively.

Extra Diastolic Heart Sounds

Extra heart sounds in diastole include the opening snap (OS), the third heart sound (S_3), the fourth heart sound (S_4), and the pericardial knock.

Opening Snap

Opening of the mitral and tricuspid valves is normally silent, but mitral or tricuspid valvular stenosis (usually the result of rheumatic heart disease; see Chapter 8) produces a sound, termed a *snap*, when the affected valve opens. It is a sharp, high-pitched sound, and its timing does not vary significantly with respiration. In mitral stenosis (which is more common than tricuspid valve stenosis), the OS is heard best between the apex and the left sternal border, just after the aortic closure sound (A_2), when the left ventricular pressure falls below that of the left atrium (see Fig. 2-4).

Because of its proximity to A_2, the A_2-OS sequence can be confused with a widely split second heart sound. However, careful auscultation at the pulmonic area during inspiration reveals three sounds occurring in rapid succession (Fig. 2-5), which correspond to aortic closure (A_2), pulmonic closure (P_2), and then the OS. The three sounds become two on expiration when A_2 and P_2 normally fuse.

The severity of mitral stenosis can be approximated by the time interval between A_2 and the OS: the more advanced the stenosis, the shorter the interval. This occurs because the degree of left atrial pressure elevation corresponds to the severity of mitral stenosis. When the ventricle relaxes in diastole, the greater the left atrial pressure, the earlier the mitral valve opens. Compared with severe stenosis, mild disease is marked by a less elevated left atrial pressure, lengthening the time it takes for the left ventricular pressure to fall below that of the atrium. Therefore, in mild mitral stenosis, the OS is widely separated from A_2, whereas in more severe stenosis, the A_2-OS interval is narrower.

Figure 2-5. Timing of the opening snap (OS) in mitral stenosis does not change with respiration. On inspiration, normal splitting of the second heart sound (S_2) is observed so that three sounds are heard. A_2, aortic component; P_2, pulmonic component of S_2; S_1, first heart sound.

Third Heart Sound (S_3)

When present, an S_3 occurs in early diastole, following the opening of the AV valves, during the ventricular rapid filling phase (see Fig. 2-4). It is a dull, low-pitched sound best heard with the bell of the stethoscope. A left-sided S_3 is typically loudest over the cardiac apex while the patient lies in the left lateral decubitus position. A right-sided S_3 is better appreciated at the lower left sternal border. Production of the S_3 appears to result from tensing of the chordae tendineae during rapid filling and expansion of the ventricle.

An S_3 is a normal finding in children and young adults. In these groups, an S_3 implies the presence of a supple ventricle capable of normal rapid expansion in early diastole. Conversely, when heard in middle-aged or older adults, an S_3 is a sign of disease resulting from a dilated ventricle (eg, a patient with heart failure due to impaired systolic contraction, as described in Chapter 9) or from the increased transvalvular flow that accompanies advanced mitral or tricuspid regurgitation (described in Chapter 8). A pathologic S_3 is sometimes referred to as a **ventricular gallop.**

Fourth Heart Sound (S_4)

When an S_4 is present, it occurs in late diastole and coincides with contraction of the atria (see Fig. 2-4). This sound is generated by the left (or right) atrium ejecting blood into a stiffened ventricle. Thus, an S_4 usually indicates the presence of cardiac disease—specifically, a decrease in ventricular compliance typically resulting from ventricular hypertrophy or myocardial ischemia. Like an S_3, the S_4 is a dull, low-pitched sound and is best heard with the bell of the stethoscope. In the case of the more common left-sided S_4, the sound is loudest at the apex, with the patient lying in the left lateral decubitus position. S_4 is sometimes referred to as an **atrial gallop.**

Quadruple Rhythm or Summation Gallop

In a patient with both an S_3 and S_4, those sounds, in conjunction with S_1 and S_2, produce a quadruple beat. If a patient with a quadruple rhythm develops tachycardia, diastole becomes shorter in duration, the S_3 and S_4 coalesce, and a **summation gallop** results. The summation of S_3 and S_4 is heard as a long middiastolic, low-pitched sound, often louder than S_1 and S_2.

Pericardial Knock

A pericardial knock is an uncommon, high-pitched sound that occurs in patients with severe constrictive pericarditis (see Chapter 14). It appears early in diastole soon after S_2 and can be confused with an OS or an S_3. However, the knock appears slightly later in diastole than the timing of an OS and is louder and occurs earlier than does a ventricular gallop. It results from the abrupt cessation of ventricular filling that occurs when the expanding ventricle meets a rigid pericardium in early diastole, which is the hallmark of constrictive pericarditis.

MURMURS

A murmur is the sound generated by turbulent blood flow. Under normal conditions, the movement of blood through the vasculature is laminar, smooth, and silent. However, as a result of hemodynamic and/or structural changes, laminar flow can become disturbed and produce an audible noise. Murmurs result from any of the following mechanisms:

1. Flow across a partial obstruction (eg, aortic stenosis)
2. Increased flow through normal structures (eg, aortic systolic murmur associated with a high-output state, such as anemia)
3. Ejection into a dilated chamber (eg, aortic systolic murmur associated with aneurysmal dilatation of the aorta)
4. Regurgitant flow across an incompetent valve (eg, mitral regurgitation)
5. Abnormal shunting of blood from one vascular chamber to a lower-pressure chamber (eg, ventricular septal defect [VSD])

Murmurs are described by their timing, intensity, pitch, shape, location, radiation, and response to maneuvers. *Timing* refers to whether the murmur occurs during systole or diastole or is continuous (ie, begins in systole and continues into diastole). The *intensity* of the murmur is typically quantified by a grading system. In the case of *systolic murmurs*:

Grade 1/6 (or I/VI)	Barely audible (ie, requires a quiet room and a sharp ear!)
Grade 2/6 (or II/VI)	Faint but immediately audible
Grade 3/6 (or III/VI)	Easily heard
Grade 4/6 (or IV/VI)	Easily heard and associated with a palpable thrill (vibration)
Grade 5/6 (or V/VI)	Very loud; heard with the stethoscope lightly on the chest
Grade 6/6 (or VI/VI)	Audible without the stethoscope directly on the chest wall

And in the case of *diastolic murmurs*:

Grade 1/4 (or I/IV)	Barely audible
Grade 2/4 (or II/IV)	Faint but immediately audible
Grade 3/4 (or III/IV)	Easily heard
Grade 4/4 (or IV/IV)	Very loud

Pitch refers to the frequency of the murmur, ranging from high to low. High-frequency murmurs are caused by large pressure gradients between chambers (eg, aortic stenosis) and are best appreciated using the diaphragm of the stethoscope. Low-frequency murmurs imply less of a pressure gradient between chambers (eg, mitral stenosis) and are best heard using the stethoscope's bell piece.

Shape describes how the murmur changes in intensity from its onset to its completion. For example, a *crescendo-decrescendo* (or "diamond-shaped") murmur first rises and then falls off in intensity. Other shapes include *decrescendo* (ie, the murmur begins at its maximum intensity then becomes softer) and *uniform* (the intensity of the murmur does not change).

Location refers to the murmur's region of maximum intensity and is usually described in terms of specific auscultatory areas (see Fig. 2-2):

Aortic area	Second to third right intercostal spaces, next to the sternum
Pulmonic area	Second to third left intercostal spaces, next to the sternum
Tricuspid area	Lower left sternal border
Mitral area	Cardiac apex

From their primary locations, murmurs are often heard to *radiate* to other areas of the chest, and such patterns of transmission relate to the direction of the turbulent flow. Finally, similar types of murmurs can be distinguished from one another by simple bedside *maneuvers*, such as standing from a supine or seated position, Valsalva (forceful expiration against a closed airway), or strong hand grip, each of which alters the heart's loading conditions and can affect the intensity of many murmurs. Examples of the effects of maneuvers on specific murmurs are presented in Chapter 8.

When reporting a murmur, some or all of these descriptors are mentioned. For example, you might describe a particular patient's murmur of aortic stenosis as "A grade III/VI high-pitched, crescendo-decrescendo systolic murmur that is loudest at the upper right sternal border and radiates to the neck."

Examples

A. Ejection type

• Aortic stenosis
• Pulmonary stenosis

S_1 S_2

B. Pansystolic (holosystolic)

• Mitral regurgitation
• Tricuspid regurgitation
• Ventricular septal defect

S_1 S_2

C. Late systolic

• Mitral valve prolapse

S_1 Click S_2

Figure 2-6. Classification of systolic murmurs. Ejection murmurs are crescendo-decrescendo in configuration **(A)**, whereas pansystolic murmurs are uniform throughout systole **(B)**. A late systolic murmur often follows a midsystolic click and suggests mitral (or tricuspid) valve prolapse **(C)**.

Systolic Murmurs

Systolic murmurs are subdivided into systolic ejection murmurs, pansystolic murmurs, and late systolic murmurs (Fig. 2-6). A **systolic ejection murmur** is typical of aortic or pulmonic valve stenosis. It begins after the first heart sound and terminates before or during S_2, depending on its severity and whether the obstruction is of the aortic or pulmonic valve. The shape of the murmur is of the crescendo-decrescendo type (ie, its intensity rises and then falls).

The ejection murmur of *aortic stenosis* begins in systole after S_1, from which it is separated by a short audible gap (Fig. 2-7). This gap corresponds to the period of isovolumetric contraction of the left ventricle (the period after the mitral valve has closed but before the aortic valve has opened). The murmur becomes more intense as flow increases across the aortic valve during the rise in left ventricular pressure (crescendo). Then, as the ventricle relaxes, forward flow decreases, and the murmur lessens in intensity (decrescendo) and finally ends prior to the aortic component of S_2. The murmur may be immediately preceded by an ejection click, especially in mild forms of aortic stenosis.

Although the intensity of the murmur does not correlate well with the severity of aortic stenosis, other features do. For example, the more severe the stenosis, the longer it takes to force blood across the valve, and the later the murmur peaks in systole (Fig. 2-8). Also, as shown in Figure 2-8, as the severity of stenosis increases, the aortic component of S_2 softens because the leaflets become more rigidly fixed in place.

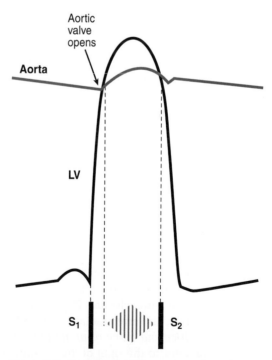

Figure 2-7. Systolic ejection murmur of aortic stenosis. There is a short delay between the first heart sound (S_1) and the onset of the murmur (*first dashed line*). LV, left ventricle; S_2, second heart sound.

Aortic stenosis causes a high-frequency murmur, reflecting the often sizable pressure gradient across the valve. It is best heard in the "aortic area" at the second and third right intercostal spaces close to the sternum (see Fig. 2-2). The murmur typically radiates toward the neck (the direction of turbulent blood flow) but often can be heard in a wide distribution, including the cardiac apex.

The murmur of *pulmonic stenosis* also begins after S_1. It may be preceded by an ejection click, but unlike aortic stenosis, it may extend beyond the A_2 sound. That is, if the stenosis is severe, it will result in a very prolonged right ventricular ejection time, elongating the murmur, which will continue beyond the closure of the aortic valve and end just before the closure of the pulmonic valve (P_2). Pulmonic stenosis is usually loudest at the second to third left intercostal spaces close to the sternum. It does not radiate as widely as aortic stenosis, but sometimes it is transmitted to the neck or left shoulder.

Young adults often have *benign systolic ejection murmurs* (also termed "innocent murmurs") resulting from increased systolic flow across normal aortic and pulmonic valves. This type of murmur often becomes softer or disappears when the patient sits upright.

Pansystolic (also termed **holosystolic**) murmurs are caused by regurgitation of blood across an incompetent mitral or tricuspid valve or through a VSD (see Chapter 16). These murmurs are characterized by a uniform intensity throughout systole (Fig. 2-6). In mitral and tricuspid valve regurgitation, as soon as ventricular systolic pressure exceeds atrial pressure (ie, when S_1 occurs), there is immediate retrograde flow across the regurgitant valve. Thus, there is no gap between S_1 and the onset of these pansystolic murmurs, in contrast to the systolic ejection murmurs discussed earlier. Similarly, there is no significant gap between S_1 and the onset of the systolic murmur of a VSD, because left ventricular systolic pressure exceeds right ventricular systolic pressure (and flow occurs) quickly after the onset of contraction.

A. Mild

B. Moderate

C. Severe

Figure 2-8. The severity of aortic stenosis affects the shape of the systolic murmur and the heart sounds. A. In mild stenosis, an ejection click (EJ) is often present, followed by an early peaking crescendo-decrescendo murmur and a normal aortic component of S_2 (A_2). **B.** As stenosis becomes more severe, the peak of the murmur becomes more delayed in systole and the intensity of A_2 lessens. The prolonged ventricular ejection time delays A_2 so that it merges with or occurs after the pulmonic component of S_2 (P_2); the ejection click may not be heard. **C.** In severe stenosis, the murmur peaks very late in systole, and A_2 is usually absent because of immobility of the valve leaflets. S_1, first heart sound; S_2, second heart sound.

The pansystolic murmur of advanced *mitral regurgitation* continues through the aortic closure sound because left ventricular pressure remains greater than that in the left atrium at the time of aortic closure. The murmur is heard best at the apex, is high pitched and "blowing" in quality, and often radiates toward the left axilla; its intensity does not change with respiration.

Tricuspid valve regurgitation is best heard along the left lower sternal border. It generally radiates to the right of the sternum and is high pitched and blowing in quality. The intensity of the murmur increases with inspiration because the negative intrathoracic pressure induced during inspiration enhances venous return to the heart. The latter augments right ventricular stroke volume, thereby increasing the amount of regurgitated blood.

The murmur of a *VSD* is heard best at the fourth to sixth left intercostal spaces, is high pitched, and may be associated with a palpable thrill (vibration). The intensity of the murmur does not increase with inspiration, nor does it radiate to the axilla, which helps distinguish it from tricuspid and mitral regurgitation, respectively. Of note, the *smaller* the VSD, the greater the turbulence of blood flow between the left and RVs and the *louder* the murmur. Some of the loudest murmurs ever heard are those associated with small VSDs.

Late systolic murmurs begin in mid-to-late systole and continue to the end of systole (see Fig. 2-6). The most common example is mitral regurgitation caused by *mitral valve prolapse*— bowing of abnormally redundant and elongated valve leaflets into the left atrium during ventricular contraction. This murmur is usually preceded by a midsystolic click and is described in Chapter 8.

DIASTOLIC MURMURS

Diastolic murmurs are divided into early decrescendo murmurs and mid-to-late rumbling murmurs (Fig. 2-9). **Early diastolic murmurs** result from regurgitant flow through either the aortic or pulmonic valve, with the former being much more common in adults. If produced by *aortic valve regurgitation*, the murmur begins at A_2, has a decrescendo shape, and terminates before the next S_1. Because diastolic relaxation of the left ventricle is rapid, a pressure gradient develops immediately between the aorta and lower-pressured left ventricle in patients with aortic regurgitation, and the murmur therefore displays its maximum intensity at its onset. Thereafter in diastole, as the aortic pressure falls and the LV pressure increases (as blood regurgitates into the ventricle), the gradient between the two chambers diminishes and the murmur decreases in intensity. Aortic regurgitation is a high-pitched murmur, typically best heard using the diaphragm of the stethoscope along the left sternal border with the patient sitting, leaning forward, and exhaling.

Pulmonic regurgitation in adults is usually due to pulmonary arterial hypertension. It is an early diastolic decrescendo murmur similar to that of aortic regurgitation, but it is best heard in the pulmonic area (Fig. 2-2), and its intensity may increase with inspiration.

Mid-to-late diastolic murmurs result from either turbulent flow across a *stenotic mitral or tricuspid valve* or less commonly from abnormally increased flow across a normal mitral or tricuspid valve (see Fig. 2-9). If resulting from stenosis, the murmur begins after S_2 and is preceded by an OS. The shape of this murmur is unique. Following valvular opening (and the OS), the murmur is at its loudest because the pressure gradient between the atrium and ventricle is at its maximum. The murmur then decrescendos or disappears during diastole as the transvalvular gradient decreases. The degree to which the murmur fades depends on the severity of the stenosis. If the stenosis is severe, the murmur is prolonged; if the stenosis is mild, the murmur disappears in mid-to-late diastole. Whether the stenosis is mild or severe, the murmur intensifies at the end of diastole in patients in normal sinus rhythm, when atrial contraction augments flow (and turbulence) across the valve (see Fig. 2-9). Since the pressure gradient across a stenotic mitral valve tends to be fairly low, the murmur of mitral stenosis is low pitched and is heard best with the bell of the stethoscope at the apex, while the patient lies in the left lateral decubitus position. The much less common murmur of tricuspid stenosis is better auscultated at the lower sternum, near the xiphoid process.

Hyperdynamic states such as fever, anemia, hyperthyroidism, and exercise increase flow across normal tricuspid and mitral valves and can therefore result in turbulence and a diastolic murmur. Similarly, in patients with advanced mitral regurgitation, the expected systolic murmur can be accompanied by an additional diastolic murmur owing to the increased volume of blood that must return across the valve to the left ventricle in diastole. Likewise, patients with either tricuspid regurgitation or an atrial septal defect (see Chapter 16) have increased flow across the tricuspid valve and may therefore display a diastolic flow murmur from that site.

Figure 2-9. Classification of diastolic murmurs. A. An early diastolic decrescendo murmur is typical of aortic or pulmonic valve regurgitation. **B.** Mid-to-late low-frequency rumbling murmurs are usually the result of mitral or tricuspid valve stenosis and follow a sharp opening snap (OS). Presystolic accentuation of the murmur occurs in patients in normal sinus rhythm because of the rise in atrial pressure during atrial contraction. **C.** In more severe mitral or tricuspid valve stenosis, the opening snap and diastolic murmur commence earlier, and the murmur is prolonged. S_1, first heart sound; S_2, second heart sound.

CONTINUOUS MURMURS

Continuous murmurs are heard throughout the cardiac cycle. Such murmurs result from conditions in which there is a persistent pressure gradient between two structures during both systole and diastole. An example is the murmur of *patent ductus arteriosus*, in which there is an abnormal congenital communication between the aorta and the pulmonary artery (see Chapter 16). During systole, blood flows from the high-pressure ascending aorta through the ductus into the lower-pressure pulmonary artery. During diastole, the aortic pressure remains greater than that in the pulmonary artery and the flow continues across the ductus. This murmur begins in early systole, crescendos to its maximum at S_2, and then decrescendos until the next S_1 (Fig. 2-10).

The "to-and-fro" combined murmur in a patient with both aortic stenosis and aortic regurgitation could be mistaken for a continuous murmur (see Fig. 2-10). During systole, there is a diamond-shaped ejection murmur and during diastole, a decrescendo murmur. However, in the case of a to-and-fro murmur, the sound does not extend through S_2 because it has discrete systolic and diastolic components.

Figure 2-10. A continuous murmur peaks at, and extends through, the second heart sound (S2). A to-and-fro murmur is not continuous; rather, there is a systolic component and a distinct diastolic component, separated by S_2. S_1, first heart sound.

Summary

- **Systole** refers to the phase of ventricular contraction, and **diastole** refers to the phase of ventricular relaxation and filling.

- The normal **cardiac cycle** consists of the following (left-sided events are described; equivalent events occur simultaneously in the right side of the heart): (1) during diastole, the mitral valve (MV) is open, so that the left atrial (LA) and left ventricular (LV) pressures are equal; (2) in late diastole, LA contraction causes a small rise in pressure in both the LA and LV; (3) after a short delay, ventricular contraction causes the LV pressure to rise, and when the LV pressure exceeds the LA pressure, the MV closes, contributing to the **first heart sound (S$_1$)**; (4) as LV pressure rises above the aortic pressure, the aortic valve (AV) opens, a silent event in a normal heart; (5) after contraction, as the LV relaxes and its pressure falls below that of the aorta, the AV closes, contributing to the **second heart sound (S$_2$)**; and (6) when the LV pressure declines below that of the LA, the mitral valve opens, the ventricle fills during diastole, and the cycle then repeats.

- **Extra systolic sounds** include ejection clicks, indicating aortic or pulmonic stenosis or dilatation of the aortic root or pulmonary artery, and mid-to-late clicks, indicating mitral or tricuspid valve prolapse.

- **Extra diastolic sounds** include the OS (eg, mitral stenosis), the S$_3$ sound (indicating heart failure or a volume overload state in older adults; an S$_3$ is a normal sound in children and young adults), and the S$_4$ sound (indicating atrial contraction into a ventricle with reduced compliance).

- Common murmurs include **systolic ejection murmurs** from aortic or pulmonic stenosis, **pansystolic murmurs** from mitral or tricuspid regurgitation, **late systolic murmurs** from mitral valve prolapse, **early diastolic murmurs** from aortic or pulmonic regurgitation, and **mid-to-late diastolic murmurs** from mitral stenosis.

- Tables 2-2 and 2-3 and Figure 2-11 summarize features of the heart sounds and murmurs described in this chapter.

TABLE 2-2 Common Heart Sounds

Sound	Location	Pitch	Significance
S$_1$	Apex	High	Normal closure of mitral and tricuspid valves
S$_2$	Base	High	Normal closure of aortic (A$_2$) and pulmonic (P$_2$) valves
Extra systolic sounds			
Ejection clicks	*Aortic:* apex and base	High	Aortic or pulmonic stenosis or dilatation of aortic root or pulmonary artery
	Pulmonic: base	High	
Mid-to-late click	*Mitral:* apex	High	Mitral or tricuspid valve prolapse
	Tricuspid: LLSB	High	
Extra diastolic sounds			
Opening snap	Apex	High	Mitral stenosis
S$_3$	*Left-sided:* apex	Low	Normal in children
			Abnormal in adults: indicates heart failure or volume overload state
S$_4$	*Left-sided:* apex	Low	Reduced ventricular compliance

LLSB, lower left sternal border.

TABLE 2-3	Common Murmurs	
Murmur Type	**Example**	**Location and Radiation**
Systolic ejection S₁ S₂	Aortic stenosis	Second right intercostal space → neck (but may radiate widely)
	Pulmonic stenosis	Second to third left intercostal spaces
Pansystolic S₁ S₂	Mitral regurgitation	Apex → axilla
	Tricuspid regurgitation	Left lower sternal border → right lower sternal border
Late systolic S₂ S₂	Mitral valve prolapse	Apex → axilla (note: if posterior mitral leaflet prolapses, may radiate to the base instead)
Early diastolic S₂ S₁	Aortic regurgitation	Along left side of the sternum
	Pulmonic regurgitation	Upper left side of the sternum
Mid-to-late diastolic S₂ S₁	Mitral stenosis	Apex

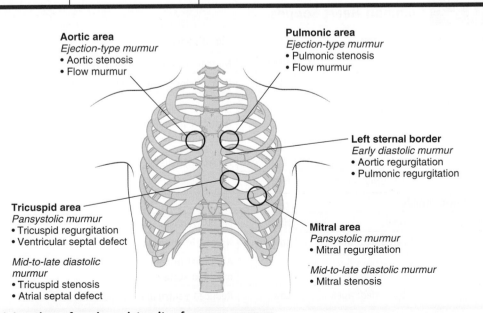

Aortic area
Ejection-type murmur
• Aortic stenosis
• Flow murmur

Pulmonic area
Ejection-type murmur
• Pulmonic stenosis
• Flow murmur

Left sternal border
Early diastolic murmur
• Aortic regurgitation
• Pulmonic regurgitation

Tricuspid area
Pansystolic murmur
• Tricuspid regurgitation
• Ventricular septal defect

Mid-to-late diastolic murmur
• Tricuspid stenosis
• Atrial septal defect

Mitral area
Pansystolic murmur
• Mitral regurgitation

Mid-to-late diastolic murmur
• Mitral stenosis

Figure 2-11 Locations of maximum intensity of common murmurs.

Review Questions

1. During which of the following periods is the left ventricle contracting?

   a. Between the closure of the aortic valve and the opening of the mitral valve
   b. Between the closure of the mitral valve and the opening of the aortic valve
   c. Immediately after the opening of the mitral valve
   d. Immediately before the closure of the aortic valve

2. A patient who normally has a heart rate of 60 beats per minute (bpm) suddenly develops an abnormal heart rhythm at a constant rate of 170 bpm. How does this rapid rate affect filling of the left ventricle?

   a. LV filling decreases due to restricted opening of the mitral valve leaflets.
   b. LV filling decreases due to a shorter diastolic phase of the cardiac cycle.
   c. LV filling decreases due to loss of atrial contraction.
   d. LV filling increases owing to abruptly shortened ventricular contraction.

3. Which of the following valvular lesions typically causes a pansystolic murmur?

   a. Aortic stenosis
   b. Pulmonic stenosis
   c. Aortic regurgitation
   d. Tricuspid regurgitation

Answers to Review Questions

1. Choice b is correct. Closure of the mitral valve occurs shortly after the onset of ventricular contraction. As ventricular contraction continues and ventricular pressure exceeds aortic pressure, the aortic valve opens. All of the other listed events occur during the period of ventricular relaxation.

2. Choice b is correct. As heart rate rises, the duration of systole remains essentially constant, but the diastolic phase of the cardiac cycle shortens. A shorter diastole allows less time for ventricular filling, so the amount of blood that accumulates in the LV decreases.

3. Choice d is correct. A pansystolic (also termed holosystolic) murmur represents uniform turbulent flow that lasts throughout systole. Such a murmur is typical of mitral regurgitation, tricuspid regurgitation, and ventricular septal defects. Aortic and pulmonic stenosis commonly result in crescendo-decrescendo systolic murmurs. Aortic regurgitation causes an early diastolic decrescendo murmur. You will learn more about these valvular abnormalities in Chapter 8.

Acknowledgments

Contributors to the previous editions of this chapter were David B. Fischer, MD; Henry Jung, MD; Nicole Martin, MD; Oscar Benavidez, MD; Bradley S. Marino, MD; and Allan Goldblatt, MD.

Additional Reading

Bickley LS. *Bates' Guide to Physical Examination and History Taking.* 12th ed. Philadelphia, PA: Wolters Kluwer/Lippincott Williams & Wilkins; 2017.
Constant J. *Essentials of Bedside Cardiology.* 2nd ed. Totowa, NJ: Humana Press; 2003.
LeBlond RF, Brown DD, Suneja M, Szot JF. *DeGowin's Diagnostic Examination.* 10th ed. New York, NY: McGraw-Hill; 2015.
Orient JM. *Sapira's Art and Science of Bedside Diagnosis.* 5th ed. Philadelphia, PA: Wolters Kluwer/Lippincott Williams & Wilkins; 2019.
Simel DL, Rennie D. *The Rational Clinical Examination: Evidence-Based Clinical Diagnosis.* New York, NY: McGraw-Hill; 2009.

3

Cardiac Imaging and Hemodynamic Assessment

Sanjay Divakaran | Ron Blankstein

Imaging plays a central role in the assessment of cardiac function and pathology. Traditional modalities such as chest radiography, echocardiography, cardiac catheterization with angiography, and nuclear imaging are fundamental in the diagnosis and management of cardiovascular diseases. These procedures are increasingly supplemented by newer techniques, including computed tomography (CT) and magnetic resonance imaging (MRI). In addition, cardiac catheterization and other techniques summarized in this chapter quantify intracardiac pressures and many aspects of cardiac function.

On first reading of this chapter, it would be beneficial to familiarize yourself with the information but not to memorize the details. The presented information is meant as a reference for diagnosis of conditions that will be explained in more detail in subsequent chapters.

CARDIAC RADIOGRAPHY

The extent of penetration of x-rays through the body is inversely proportional to tissue density. Air-filled tissues, such as the lung, absorb few x-rays and expose the underlying film or electronic recording sensor, causing it to appear black. In contrast, dense materials, such as bone, absorb more radiation and appear white (radiopaque). For a boundary to show between two structures, they must differ in density. Myocardium, valves, and other intracardiac structures have densities similar to that of adjacent blood; consequently, radiography cannot delineate these structures unless they happen to be calcified. Conversely, heart borders adjacent to a lung are depicted clearly because the heart and an air-filled lung have different densities.

Frontal and lateral radiographs are routinely used to assess the heart and lungs (Fig. 3-1). The *frontal* view is usually a posterior–anterior image in which the x-rays are transmitted from behind (ie, posterior to) the patient, pass through the body, and are then captured by the film (or electronic sensor) placed against the anterior chest. This positioning places the heart close to the x-ray recording film plate so that its image is only minimally distorted, allowing for an accurate assessment of size. In the standard *lateral* view, the patient's left side is placed against the film plate and the x-rays pass through the body from right to left. The frontal radiograph is useful for assessing the size of the left ventricle, left atrial appendage, pulmonary artery, aorta, and superior vena cava; the lateral view evaluates right ventricular size, posterior borders of the left atrium and ventricle, and the anteroposterior diameter of the thorax.

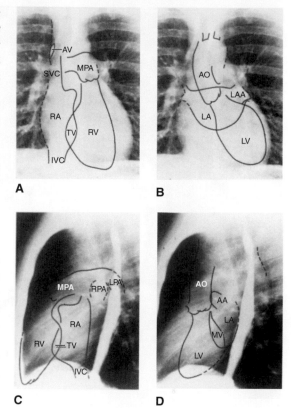

CARDIAC SILHOUETTE

Chest radiographs are useful to evaluate the size of heart chambers and the pulmonary consequences of cardiac disease. Alterations in chamber size are reflected by changes in the cardiac silhouette. In the frontal view of adults, an enlarged heart is identified by a **cardiothoracic ratio** (the maximum width of the heart divided by the maximum internal diameter of the thoracic cage) of >50%.

In certain situations, the cardiac silhouette inaccurately reflects heart size. For example, an elevated diaphragm, or narrow chest anteroposterior diameter, may cause the silhouette to expand transversely such that the heart appears larger than its actual dimensions. Therefore, the chest anteroposterior diameter should be assessed on the lateral view before concluding the heart is truly

Figure 3-1. Posteroanterior (A and B) and lateral (C and D) chest radiographs of a person without cardiopulmonary disease, illustrating cardiac chambers and valves. AO, aorta; AV, azygos vein; IVC, inferior vena cava; LA, left atrium; LAA, left atrial appendage; LPA, left pulmonary artery; LV, left ventricle; MPA, main pulmonary artery; MV, mitral valve; RA, right atrium; RPA, right pulmonary artery; RV, right ventricle; SVC, superior vena cava; TV, tricuspid valve. (Reprinted from Come PC, ed. *Diagnostic Cardiology: Noninvasive Imaging Techniques.* Philadelphia, PA: J.B. Lippincott; 1985, with permission.)

enlarged. The presence of a pericardial effusion around the heart can also widen the cardiac silhouette because fluid and myocardial tissue affect x-ray penetration similarly.

Radiographs can depict dilatation of individual cardiac chambers. Major causes of chamber and great vessel dilatation include heart failure, valvular lesions, abnormal intracardiac and extracardiac communications (shunts), and certain pulmonary disorders. Because dilatation takes time to develop, recent lesions, such as acute mitral valve insufficiency, may present without apparent cardiac enlargement. Of note, concentric ventricular hypertrophy alone (ie, without dilatation) may not result in radiographic abnormalities, because it generally occurs at the expense of the cavity's internal volume and produces little or no change in overall cardiac size.

The pattern of chamber enlargement may suggest specific disease entities. For example, dilatation of the left atrium and right ventricle, accompanied by signs of pulmonary hypertension, suggests mitral stenosis (Fig. 3-2). In contrast, dilatation of the pulmonary artery and right heart chambers, but without enlargement of the left-sided heart dimensions, can

Figure 3-2. Posteroanterior chest radiograph of a patient with severe mitral stenosis and secondary pulmonary vascular congestion. The radiograph shows a prominent left atrial appendage (*arrowheads*) with consequent straightening of the left heart border and suggestion of a double density right cardiac border (*arrows*) produced by the enlarged left atrium. The aortic silhouette is small, which suggests chronic low cardiac output. Radiographic signs of pulmonary vascular congestion include increased caliber of upper-zone pulmonary vessel markings and decreased caliber of lower-zone vessels.

be seen in patients with pulmonary vascular obstruction, in those with increased pulmonary artery blood flow (eg, due to an atrial septal defect), or in those with pulmonary hypertension of diverse causes (Fig. 3-3).

Chest radiographs can also detect dilatation of the aorta. Causes of aortic enlargement include aneurysm, dissection, and aortic valve disease (Fig. 3-4). Normal aging and atherosclerosis may also cause the aorta to become dilated and tortuous.

PULMONARY MANIFESTATIONS OF HEART DISEASE

The appearance of the pulmonary vasculature reflects abnormalities of pulmonary arterial and venous pressures and pulmonary blood flow. High pulmonary venous pressure, as occurs in left heart failure, causes increased vascular markings, redistribution of blood flow from the bases to the apices of the lungs (termed *cephalization* of vessels), interstitial edema, and alveolar edema (Fig. 3-5). Cephalization appears as an increase in the number or width of vascular markings at the apex (Fig. 3-5A). Interstitial edema occurs as pulmonary congestion progresses, and the connective tissue spaces become thickened with fluid (Fig. 3-5B). **Kerley B lines** (short horizontal parallel lines at the periphery of the lungs adjacent to the pleura, most often at the lung bases) depict fluid in interlobular spaces that results from interstitial edema (Fig. 3-5C). When fluid accumulates in the air spaces, alveolar forms of pulmonary edema produce opacity radiating from the hilar region bilaterally (known as a "butterfly" pattern), and air bronchograms may be seen (Fig. 3-5D). Fluid accumulation in the pleural spaces in heart failure (ie, pleural effusions) is manifest by blunting of the costophrenic angles (the angle between the ribs and the diaphragm).

Figure 3-3. Posteroanterior chest radiograph of a patient with pulmonary hypertension resulting from an atrial septal defect. Radiographic signs of pulmonary hypertension include pulmonary artery dilatation (*black arrows*; compare with the appearance of left atrial appendage dilatation in Fig. 3-2) and large central pulmonary arteries (*white arrows*) associated with small peripheral vessels (a pattern known as peripheral pruning).

Changes in pulmonary blood flow may also alter the appearance of the pulmonary vessels. For example, focal oligemia (reduction in the size of blood vessels due to decreased blood flow) is occasionally observed distal to a pulmonary embolism (termed the *Westermark sign*). The finding of enlarged central pulmonary arteries, but small peripheral vessels (termed *peripheral pruning*), suggests pulmonary hypertension (see Fig. 3-3).

Figure 3-4. Posteroanterior chest radiograph of a patient with aortic stenosis and insufficiency secondary to a bicuspid aortic valve. In addition to poststenotic dilatation of the ascending aorta (*black arrows*), the transverse aorta (*white arrow*) is prominent.

Figure 3-5. Posteroanterior radiographs of patients with heart failure (HF). A. Early manifestations of HF include upper-zone redistribution (cephalization) of vessels (*green arrows*); cardiomegaly is present. **B.** More pronounced manifestations of HF include interstitial edema with pulmonary vascular markings throughout the lung fields owing to edematous interlobular septae. Fluid-associated thickening of bronchial walls is visualized as peribronchiolar cuffing (*red arrow*). **C.** Enlarged view of Kerley B lines (*yellow arrows*) at the periphery of the lower left lung field. **D.** Severe HF manifest by diffuse alveolar edema. Air bronchograms (*blue arrows*) occur when the radiolucent bronchial tree is contrasted with opaque edematous tissue. Patients with HF often have a combination of interstitial and alveolar edema. (Courtesy of Gillian Lieberman, MD, Beth Israel Deaconess Medical Center, Boston, MA.)

Table 3-1 summarizes the major radiographic findings in common forms of cardiac disease.

ECHOCARDIOGRAPHY

Echocardiography plays an essential role in the diagnosis and serial evaluation of many cardiac disorders. It is safe, noninvasive, and relatively inexpensive. High-frequency (ultrasonic) waves generated by a piezoelectric element within a transducer travel

TABLE 3-1	Chest Radiography of Common Cardiac Disorders
Disorder	**Findings**
Congestive heart failure	• Cephalization of vessels • Interstitial edema (peribronchial cuffing, Kerley B lines) • Alveolar edema (air bronchograms) • Pleural effusions
Pulmonic valve stenosis	• Poststenotic dilatation of pulmonary artery
Aortic valve stenosis	• Poststenotic dilatation of ascending aorta
Aortic regurgitation	• Left ventricular dilatation • Dilated aorta
Mitral stenosis	• Left atrial dilatation • Signs of pulmonary venous congestion
Mitral regurgitation	• Left atrial dilatation • Left ventricular dilatation • Signs of pulmonary venous congestion in acute mitral regurgitation (see Chapter 8)

through the body and are reflected at interfaces where there are differences in the acoustic impedance of adjacent tissues. The reflected waves return to the transducer and are recorded. The machine measures the time elapsed between the initiation and reception of the sound waves, allowing it to calculate the distance between the transducer and each anatomic reflecting surface. Images are then constructed from these calculations.

Three types of imaging are routinely performed during an echocardiographic examination: M-mode, two-dimensional (2D), and Doppler. Each type of imaging can be performed from various body locations. Most commonly, *transthoracic* studies are performed, in which images are obtained by placing the transducer on the surface of the chest. When greater structural detail is required, *transesophageal* imaging is performed.

M-mode echocardiography, the oldest form of cardiac ultrasonography, provides data from only one ultrasonic beam and is now rarely used by itself. It supplements the other modalities to provide accurate measurements of wall thicknesses and timing of valve movements.

In **2D echocardiography**, multiple ultrasonic beams are transmitted from the transducer through a wide arc. The returning signals are integrated to produce 2D video images of the heart. As a result, this technique depicts anatomic relationships and defines the movement of cardiac structures relative to one another. Wall and valve motion abnormalities, and many types of intracardiac masses (eg, vegetations, thrombi, tumors), can be depicted.

Each 2D plane (Fig. 3-6) delineates only part of a given cardiac structure. Optimal evaluation of the entire heart is achieved by using combinations of views. In transthoracic echocardiography (TTE), in which the transducer is placed against the patient's skin, these include the parasternal long axis, parasternal short axis, apical views, and subcostal views. The *parasternal long-axis* view is recorded with the transducer in the third or fourth intercostal space to the left of the sternum. This view is particularly useful for evaluation of the left atrium, mitral valve, left ventricle, and left ventricular outflow tract (LVOT), which includes the aortic valve and adjacent interventricular septum. To obtain *parasternal short-axis* views, the transducer is rotated 90 degrees from its position for the long-axis view. The short-axis images depict transverse planes of the heart. Several different levels are imaged to assess the aortic valve, mitral valve, and left ventricular wall motion.

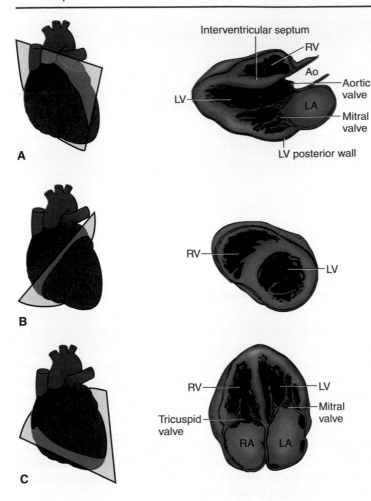

Interventricular septum

RV

Ao

Aortic valve

LV

LA

Mitral valve

LV posterior wall

A

RV

LV

B

RV

LV

Tricuspid valve

Mitral valve

RA   LA

C

Figure 3-6. Transthoracic two-dimensional echocardiographic views. A. Parasternal long-axis view. **B.** Parasternal short-axis view. Notice that the left ventricle appears circular in this view, while the right ventricle is crescent shaped. **C.** Apical four-chamber view. Ao, aorta; LA, left atrium; LV, left ventricle; RA, right atrium; RV, right ventricle. (Modified from Sahn DJ, Anderson F. *Two-Dimensional Anatomy of the Heart*. New York, NY: John Wiley & Sons; 1982.)

Apical TTE views are produced when the transducer is placed at the point of maximal apical impulse. The *apical four-chamber* view evaluates the mitral and tricuspid valves as well as the atrial and ventricular chambers, including the motion of the lateral, septal, and apical left ventricular walls. The *apical two-chamber* view shows only the left side of the heart, and it depicts movement of the anterior, inferior, and apical walls.

In some patients, such as those with obstructive airway disease, the parasternal and apical views do not adequately show cardiac structures because the excessive underlying air attenuates the acoustic signal. In such patients, the *subcostal* view, in which the transducer is placed inferior to the rib cage, may provide a better ultrasonic window.

Doppler imaging depicts blood flow direction and velocity and identifies regions of vascular turbulence. Additionally, it permits estimation of pressure gradients within the heart and great vessels. Doppler studies are based on the physical principle that waves reflected from a moving object undergo a frequency shift according to the moving object's velocity relative to the source of the waves. Color flow mapping converts the Doppler signals to a scale of colors that represent direction, velocity, and turbulence of blood flow in a semiquantitative way. The colors are superimposed on 2D images and show the location of stenotic and regurgitant valvular lesions and of abnormal communications within the heart and great vessels. For example, Doppler echocardiography in a patient with mitral regurgitation shows a jet of retrograde flow into the left atrium during systole (Fig. 3-7).

Sound frequency shifts are converted by the echo machine into blood flow velocity measurements by the following relationship:

$$v = \frac{fs \cdot c}{2f_0 (\cos\theta)}$$

in which v equals the blood flow velocity (m/sec); fs, the Doppler frequency shift (kHz); c, the velocity of sound in body tissue (m/sec); f_0, the frequency of the sound pulse emitted from the transducer (MHz); and θ, the angle between the transmitted sound pulse and the mean axis of the blood flow being assessed.

Transesophageal echocardiography (TEE) uses a miniaturized transducer mounted at the end of a modified endoscope to transmit and receive ultrasound waves from within the esophagus, thus producing very clear images of the neighboring cardiac structures (Fig. 3-8) and much of the thoracic aorta. Modern probes permit multiplanar imaging and Doppler interrogation. TEE is particularly helpful in the assessment of aortic and atrial abnormalities, conditions that are less well visualized by conventional transthoracic echo imaging. For example, TEE is more sensitive than transthoracic echo for the detection of thrombus within the left atrial appendage (Fig. 3-9). The proximity of the esophagus to the heart makes TEE imaging particularly advantageous in patients for whom transthoracic echo images are unsatisfactory (eg, those with chronic obstructive lung disease).

TEE is also advantageous in the evaluation of patients with prosthetic heart valves. During standard transthoracic imaging, artificial mechanical valves reflect a large portion of ultrasound waves, thus interfering with visualization of more posterior structures (termed *acoustic shadowing*). TEE aids visualization in such patients and is therefore the most sensitive noninvasive

Figure 3-7. Doppler color flow mapping of mitral regurgitation (MR). The color Doppler image, recorded in systole, is superimposed on an apical four-chamber view. The color Doppler signal filling the left atrium (LA) indicates retrograde flow of MR from the left ventricle (LV) across the mitral valve (*arrow*). RA, right atrium; RV, right ventricle.

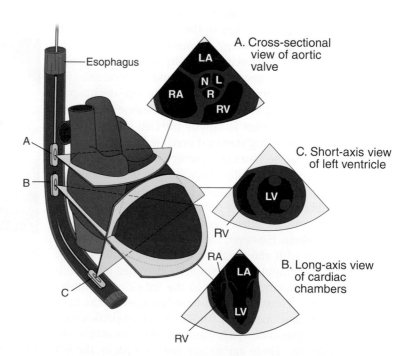

Figure 3-8. Transesophageal echocardiographic views. LA, left atrium; LV, left ventricle; RA, right atrium; RV, right ventricle; N, noncoronary cusp of aortic valve; L, left coronary cusp of aortic valve; R, right coronary cusp of aortic valve.

A. Cross-sectional view of aortic valve

C. Short-axis view of left ventricle

B. Long-axis view of cardiac chambers

Figure 3-9. Echocardiographic imaging of an intracardiac thrombus. A. Transesophageal echocardiographic image demonstrates thrombus within the left atrial appendage. (Courtesy of Scott Streckenbach, MD, Massachusetts General Hospital, Boston, MA.) **B.** Schematic drawing of same image. LA, left atrium; LAA, left atrial appendage.

technique for evaluating perivalvular leaks. In addition, TEE is more sensitive than TTE for detecting features of endocarditis, such as vegetations and myocardial abscesses.

TEE is commonly used to evaluate patients with cerebral ischemic events (ie, strokes) of unexplained etiology, because it can identify cardiovascular sources of embolism with high sensitivity. These etiologies include intracardiac thrombi or tumors, atherosclerotic debris within the aorta, and valvular vegetations. TEE is also highly sensitive and specific for the detection of aortic dissection.

In the operating room, TEE permits immediate evaluation after surgical repair of cardiac lesions. In addition, imaging of ventricular wall motion can identify periods of myocardial ischemia during surgery.

Newer ultrasound modalities include **3D echocardiography and intracardiac echocardiography**. The spatial reconstructions afforded by 3D echo are of particular benefit in the assessment of valvular defects (Fig. 3-10), intracardiac masses, and congenital malformations. Intracardiac echo utilizes a transducer mounted on a catheter to provide imaging during interventional procedures in the cardiac catheterization and electrophysiology laboratories.

Contrast echocardiography is sometimes used to improve imaging detail and to evaluate for abnormal intracardiac shunts. In one technique, called a "bubble study," agitated saline containing air microbubbles is rapidly injected into a peripheral vein. Using standard imaging, an echocontrast effect can be visualized passing through the cardiac chambers. Normally, there is rapid opacification of the right-sided chambers, but because the air microbubbles are filtered out (harmlessly) in the lungs, the contrast effect does not reach the left-sided chambers. However, the presence of an intracardiac shunt with abnormal right-to-left heart blood flow, or an intrapulmonary shunt, is identified when bubbles of contrast appear in the left-sided chambers as well. Newer inert gas-based contrast agents have been developed with sufficiently small particle size to intentionally pass through the pulmonary circulation. These agents are used to opacify the left

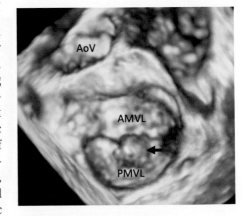

Figure 3-10. Three-dimensional transesophageal echocardiogram demonstrating systolic prolapse of the posterior mitral valve leaflet (*arrow*). AoV, aortic valve; AMVL, anterior mitral valve leaflet; PMVL, posterior mitral valve leaflet. (Courtesy of Yee-Ping Sun, MD, Brigham and Women's Hospital, Boston, MA.)

ventricular cavity to improve visualization of endocardial borders for better assessment of ventricular contraction.

Echocardiographic techniques can identify valvular lesions, complications of coronary artery disease (CAD), septal defects, intracardiac masses, cardiomyopathy, ventricular hypertrophy, pericardial disease, aortic disease, and congenital heart disease. Typical evaluation includes assessment of cardiac chamber sizes, wall thicknesses, wall motion, valvular function, blood flow, and intracardiac hemodynamics. A few of these topics are highlighted here.

VENTRICULAR ASSESSMENT

Echocardiography is commonly used for measurement of ventricular wall thickness and mass and calculation of the **ejection fraction**, a measure of contractile function (see Chapter 9). Furthermore, 2D echocardiography depicts regional ventricular wall motion abnormalities, a sign of CAD, and also allows assessment of right ventricular function.

Diastolic dysfunction (eg, caused by ischemic disease, ventricular hypertrophy, or restrictive cardiomyopathy; see Chapter 9) can be evaluated by Doppler techniques. For example, **Doppler tissue imaging** is a modality that can readily record the maximum velocity of mitral annular movement in early diastole, an indicator of the left ventricle's ability to relax normally. Doppler measurement of flow velocity across the mitral valve in early, compared with late, diastole also provides information about diastolic function.

VALVULAR LESIONS

Echocardiography can determine underlying causes of valvular abnormalities, and Doppler imaging quantitates the degree of valvular stenosis and regurgitation. The pressure gradient across a stenotic valve can be calculated from the maximum blood flow velocity (v) measured distal to the valve, using the simplified *Bernoulli equation*:

$$\text{Pressure gradient} = 4 \times v^2$$

As an example, if the peak velocity recorded distal to a stenotic aortic valve is 5 m/s, then the calculated peak pressure gradient across the valve $= 4 \times 5^2 = 100$ mm Hg.

Other calculations permit noninvasive determination of the cross-sectional area of stenotic valves. The *continuity equation* is often used to calculate aortic valve area. This equation assumes that blood flow (*F*, expressed in cc/sec) is the same at the aortic valve orifice (AV) as at a neighboring position along the flow stream (eg, in the LVOT):

$$F_{\text{LVOT}} = F_{\text{AV}}$$

As shown in Figure 3-11, blood flow at any position along a flow stream can also be expressed as the product of the Doppler velocity (*V*, in cm/s) and cross-sectional area (*A*, in cm^2) at that level. If location 1 in Figure 3-11 represents a position in the LVOT and location 2 represents the aortic valve, then

$$A_{\text{LVOT}} \times V_{\text{LVOT}} = A_{\text{AV}} \times V_{\text{AV}}$$

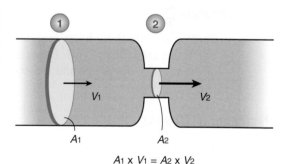

Figure 3-11. The continuity equation. Within a closed flow stream, the volume rate of flow at any point (calculated as the cross-sectional area at that site multiplied by the flow velocity at the same location) is equal to the volume rate of flow at sequential points. Thus, cross-sectional area and velocity at any location are inversely proportional to one another. Here, location 2 is narrower than location 1. Therefore, the velocity at location 2 must be greater for the same volume to pass per unit time.

The cross-sectional area of the LVOT (A_{LVOT}) is calculated simply as $\pi(d/2)^2$, where d represents the LVOT diameter, measured from the parasternal long-axis view. The velocities (V_{LVOT} and V_{AV}) are measured by Doppler interrogation, from the apical four-chamber view. The equation can then be solved for the aortic valve area (A_{AV}):

$$A_{AV} = \frac{A_{LVOT} \times V_{LVOT}}{V_{AV}}$$

Color Doppler analysis provides a qualitative assessment of the severity of regurgitant valve lesions. In mitral regurgitation (see Fig. 3-7), for example, the ratio of the regurgitant jet color Doppler area to the entire left atrial area has traditionally been used to classify the regurgitation as mild, moderate, or severe. More quantitative evaluation of mitral regurgitation can be performed by what is known as the proximal isovelocity surface area (PISA) method. This technique uses advanced color Doppler techniques to calculate the regurgitant volume and effective regurgitant orifice area, two values that predict clinical outcomes in patients with chronic mitral regurgitation.

CORONARY ARTERY DISEASE

Echocardiography demonstrates ventricular wall motion abnormalities associated with infarcted or ischemic myocardium. The location and degree of abnormal systolic contraction and decreased systolic wall thickening indicate the extent of an infarction and implicate the responsible coronary artery. Echocardiography also detects complications of infarction including thrombus formation, papillary muscle rupture, ventricular septal rupture, and aneurysm.

Although echocardiography can depict those *consequences* of CAD, transthoracic echo resolution in adults is insufficient to satisfactorily image the coronary arteries themselves. However, **stress echocardiography** is a technique that aids in the diagnosis of CAD. This technique visualizes left ventricular regional wall motion abnormalities that are induced by exercise, or the infusion of specific pharmacologic agents (eg, dobutamine), as a sign of myocardial ischemia (see Chapter 6).

CARDIOMYOPATHY

Cardiomyopathies are heart muscle disorders that include dilated, hypertrophic, and restrictive forms (see Chapter 10). Echocardiography can distinguish these and permits assessment of the severity of systolic and diastolic dysfunction.

PERICARDIAL DISEASE

Two-dimensional echocardiography can identify abnormalities in the pericardial cavity (eg, excessive pericardial fluid and tumor). Tamponade and constrictive pericarditis, the main complications of pericardial disease (see Chapter 14), are associated with particular echocardiographic abnormalities. In tamponade, the increased intrapericardial pressure compresses the cardiac chambers and results in cyclical "collapse" of the right atrium and right ventricle (Fig. 3-12). Constrictive pericarditis is associated with increased thickness of the pericardial echo (though pericardial thickness is better evaluated by CT or MR imaging, described later), abnormal patterns of diastolic left ventricular wall motion, alterations in pulmonary and hepatic venous flow patterns, and exaggerated changes in mitral and tricuspid valve inflow velocities during respiration.

Table 3-2 summarizes the echocardiographic features of common cardiac diseases.

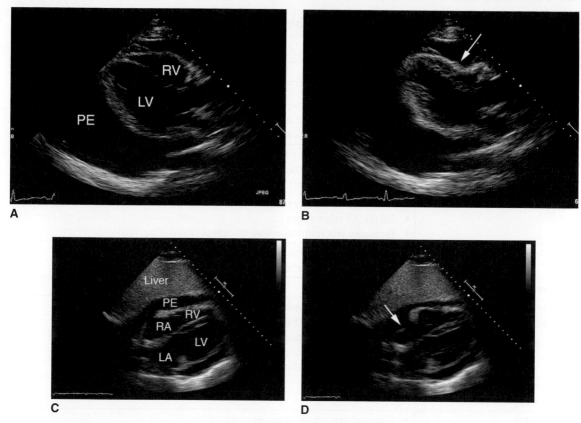

Figure 3-12. Echocardiogram of a patient with a pericardial effusion causing cardiac tamponade. A. Parasternal long-axis image showing a large pericardial effusion (PE) surrounding the heart. This frame was obtained in systole and shows normal appearance of the left (LV) and right (RV) ventricles. **B.** Same image as **(A)**, but this frame was obtained in early diastole and shows collapse of the RV free wall (*arrow*) due to compression by the effusion. **C.** Subcostal view, obtained in systole, demonstrating the PE surrounding the right atrium (RA), RV, left atrium (LA), and LV. **D.** Same image as **(C)**, obtained during diastole, showing inward collapse of the RA (*arrow*).

CARDIAC CATHETERIZATION

Intravascular catheters can be percutaneously inserted and maneuvered to the heart to measure intracardiac pressures, to determine cardiac output and vascular resistances, to inject radiopaque material to examine heart structures and blood flow, and to treat a number of cardiovascular disorders. In 1929, Werner Forssmann performed the first cardiac catheterization, *on himself*, thus ushering in the era of invasive cardiology. Much of what is known about the pathophysiology of cardiovascular disorders comes from decades of subsequent hemodynamic research utilizing cardiac catheterization.

MEASUREMENT OF PRESSURE

Before catheterization of an artery or vein, the patient is mildly sedated, and a local anesthetic is used to numb the skin site of catheter entry. The catheter, attached to a pressure transducer outside the body, is then introduced into the appropriate blood vessel. To measure pressures in the right atrium, right ventricle, and pulmonary artery, a catheter is inserted into a femoral, brachial, or jugular *vein*. Pressures in the aorta and left ventricle are measured via catheters inserted into a radial, brachial, or femoral *artery*. Once in the blood vessel, the catheter is

TABLE 3-2	Echocardiography in Common Cardiac Disorders
Disorder	**Findings**
Valvular lesions	
Mitral stenosis	• Enlarged left atrium • Thickened mitral valve leaflets • Decreased movement and separation of mitral valve leaflets • Decreased mitral valve orifice
Mitral regurgitation	• Enlarged left atrium (if chronic) • Enlarged left ventricle (if chronic) • Systolic flow from left ventricle into left atrium by Doppler
Aortic stenosis	• Thickened aortic valve cusps • Decreased valve orifice • Increased left ventricular wall thickness
Aortic regurgitation	• Enlarged left ventricle • Abnormalities of aortic valve or aortic root
Left ventricular function	
Myocardial infarction and complications	• Abnormal regional ventricular wall motion • Thrombus within left ventricle • Aneurysm of ventricular wall • Septal rupture (abnormal Doppler flow) • Papillary muscle rupture
Cardiomyopathies (described in Chapter 10)	
Dilated	• Enlarged ventricular chamber sizes • Decreased systolic contraction
Hypertrophic	• Normal or decreased ventricular chamber sizes • Increased ventricular wall thickness • Diastolic dysfunction (assessed by Doppler)
Restrictive	• Normal or decreased ventricular chamber sizes • Increased ventricular wall thickness common • Ventricular contractile function may be abnormal • Diastolic dysfunction (assessed by Doppler) • Enlarged atria (often marked enlargement)

guided by fluoroscopy (continuous x-ray images) to the area of study, where pressure measurements are made. Figure 3-13 depicts normal intracardiac and intravascular pressures.

The measurement of right heart pressures is performed with a specialized balloon-tipped catheter (a common version of which is known as the Swan-Ganz catheter) that is advanced through the right side of the heart with the aid of normal blood flow and into the pulmonary artery. As it travels through the right side of the heart, recorded pressure measurements identify the catheter tip's position (see Box 3-1).

Right Atrial Pressure

Right atrial pressure is equal to the central venous pressure (estimated by the jugular venous pressure on physical examination) because no obstructing valves impede blood return from the central veins into the right atrium. Similarly, right atrial pressure normally equals right ventricular pressure during diastole because the right heart functions as a "common chamber" when the tricuspid valve is open. The mean right atrial pressure is *reduced* when there

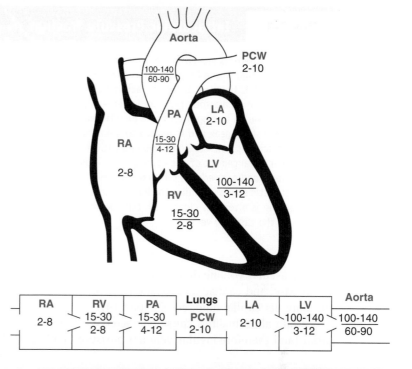

Figure 3-13. Diagrams indicating normal pressures in the cardiac chambers and great vessels. The **top** figure shows the normal anatomic relationship of the cardiac chambers and great vessels, whereas the figure on the **bottom** shows a simplified schematic to clarify the pressure relationships. Numbers indicate pressures in mm Hg. LA, left atrial mean pressure; LV, left ventricular pressure; PA, pulmonary artery pressure; PCW, pulmonary capillary wedge mean pressure; RA, right atrial mean pressure; RV, right ventricular pressure.

RA	RV	PA	Lungs	LA	LV	Aorta
2-8	15-30 / 2-8	15-30 / 4-12	PCW 2-10	2-10	100-140 / 3-12	100-140 / 60-90

Box 3-1	Intracardiac Pressure Tracings

When a catheter is inserted into a systemic vein and advanced into the right side of the heart, each cardiac chamber produces a characteristic pressure curve.

The normal *right atrial (RA)* pressure demonstrates three positive deflections (see the figure in Box 2-1 for an enlarged view): the *a* wave reflects RA contraction at the end of diastole, the *c* wave results from bulging of the tricuspid valve toward the right atrium as it closes in early systole, and the *v* wave represents passive filling of the right atrium from the systemic veins during systole, when the tricuspid valve is closed. The downward deflection that follows the *c* wave is known as the *x* descent, and the downward deflection after the *v* wave is called the *y* descent. Often the *a* and *c* waves merge so that only two major positive deflections are seen. In patients with atrial fibrillation, the *a* wave is absent because there is no organized left atrial contraction.

As the catheter is advanced into the *right ventricle (RV)*, a dramatic increase in systolic pressure is seen. The RV systolic waveform is characterized by a rapid upstroke and downstroke. In diastole, there is a gradual continuous increase in RV pressure as the chamber fills with blood.

(Continued)

Box 3-1	Intracardiac Pressure Tracings (continued)

As the catheter is moved forward into the *pulmonary artery (PA)*, the systolic pressure remains the same as that in the RV (as long as there is no obstruction to RV outflow, such as pulmonic valve stenosis). However, three characteristics of the recording indicate entry into the pulmonary artery: (1) the PA diastolic pressure is higher than that of the RV; (2) the descending systolic portion of the PA tracing inscribes a dicrotic wave, a small transient pressure increase that occurs after the systolic peak and is related to pulmonic valve closure; and (3) the diastolic portion of the PA tracing is downsloping compared with the upsloping RV diastolic pressure.

Further advancement of the catheter into a branch of the pulmonary artery results in the *pulmonary capillary wedge (PCW)* tracing, which reflects the left atrial pressure (Fig. 3-14). Its characteristic shape is similar to the RA tracing, but the pressure values are usually higher, and the tracing is often less clear (with the *c* wave not observed) because of damped transmission through the capillary vessels.

is intravascular volume depletion. It is *elevated* in right ventricular failure, right-sided valvular disease, and cardiac tamponade (in which the cardiac chambers are surrounded by high-pressure pericardial fluid; see Chapter 14).

Certain abnormalities cause characteristic changes in individual components of the right atrial (and therefore jugular venous) pressure (Table 3-3). For example, a prominent *a* wave

TABLE 3-3   Causes of Increased Intracardiac Pressures

Chamber and Measurement	Causes
Right atrial pressure	• Right ventricular failure • Cardiac tamponade
a wave	• Tricuspid stenosis • Right ventricular hypertrophy • Atrioventricular dissociation
v wave	• Tricuspid regurgitation
Right ventricular pressure	
Systolic	• Pulmonic stenosis • Pulmonary hypertension
Diastolic	• Right ventricular failure • Cardiac tamponade • Right ventricular hypertrophy
Pulmonary artery pressure	

Systolic and diastolic	• Pulmonary hypertension
	  • Left-sided heart failure
	  • Chronic lung disease
	  • Pulmonary vascular disease

Systolic only	• Increased flow (left-to-right shunt)
Pulmonary artery wedge pressure	• Left-sided heart failure • Mitral stenosis or regurgitation • Cardiac tamponade
a wave	• Left ventricular hypertrophy
v wave	• Mitral regurgitation • Ventricular septal defect

is seen in tricuspid stenosis and right ventricular hypertrophy. In these conditions, the right atrium contracts vigorously against the obstructing tricuspid valve or stiffened right ventricle, respectively, generating a prominent pressure wave. Similarly, amplified "cannon" *a* waves may be produced by conditions of atrioventricular dissociation (see Chapter 12), when the right atrium contracts against a closed tricuspid valve. A prominent *v* wave is observed in tricuspid regurgitation because normal right atrial filling is augmented by the regurgitated blood in systole.

Right Ventricular Pressure

Right ventricular systolic pressure is increased by pulmonic valve stenosis or pulmonary hypertension. Right ventricular diastolic pressure increases when the right ventricle is subjected to pressure or volume overload and may be a sign of right heart failure.

Pulmonary Artery Pressure

Elevation of systolic and diastolic pulmonary artery pressures occurs in three conditions: (1) *left*-sided heart failure, (2) parenchymal lung disease (eg, chronic bronchitis or end-stage emphysema), and (3) pulmonary vascular disease (eg, pulmonary embolism). Normally, the pulmonary artery diastolic pressure is equivalent to the left atrial pressure because of the low resistance of the pulmonary vasculature that separates them. If the left atrial pressure rises because of left-sided heart failure, both systolic and diastolic pulmonary artery pressures increase in an obligatory manner to maintain forward flow through the lungs. This situation leads to "passive" pulmonary hypertension.

In certain conditions, however, pulmonary vascular resistance becomes abnormally high, causing pulmonary artery diastolic pressure to be elevated compared with left atrial pressure. For example, pulmonary vascular obstructive disease may develop as a complication of a chronic left-to-right cardiac shunt, such as an atrial or ventricular septal defect (see Chapter 16).

Pulmonary Artery Wedge Pressure

If a catheter is advanced into the right or left pulmonary artery, its tip will ultimately reach one of the small pulmonary artery branches and temporarily occlude forward blood flow beyond it. During that time, a column of stagnant blood stands between the catheter tip and the portions of the pulmonary capillary and pulmonary venous segments distal to it (Fig. 3-14). That column of blood acts as an extension of the catheter, and the pressure recorded through

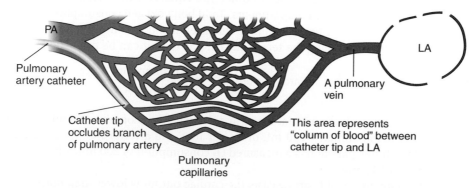

Figure 3-14 Diagram of a pulmonary artery catheter inserted into a branch of the pulmonary artery (PA). Flow is occluded in the arterial, arteriolar, and capillary vessels beyond the catheter; thus, these vessels act as a conduit that transmits the left atrial (LA) pressure to the catheter tip.

the catheter reflects that of the downstream chamber—namely, the left atrium. Such a pressure measurement is termed the *pulmonary artery wedge pressure* or *pulmonary capillary wedge pressure (PCW)* and closely matches the left atrial pressure in most individuals. Furthermore, while the mitral valve is open during diastole, the pulmonary venous bed, left atrium, and left ventricle normally share the same pressures. Thus, the PCW can be used to estimate the left ventricular diastolic pressure, a measurement of ventricular preload (see Chapter 9). As a result, measurement of PCW may be useful in managing certain critically ill patients in the intensive care unit.

Elevation of the mean PCW is seen in left-sided heart failure and in mitral stenosis or regurgitation. The individual components of the PCW tracing can also become abnormally high. The *a* wave may be increased in conditions of decreased left ventricular compliance, such as left ventricular hypertrophy or acute myocardial ischemia, and in mitral stenosis. The *v* wave is greater than normal when there is increased left atrial filling during ventricular contraction, as in mitral regurgitation.

MEASUREMENT OF BLOOD FLOW

Cardiac output is measured by either the thermodilution method or the Fick technique. In the **thermodilution method**, saline of a known temperature is injected rapidly through a catheter side port into the right side of the heart, at a specific distance from the distal tip of the catheter. The catheter tip, positioned in the pulmonary artery, contains a thermistor that registers the change in temperature induced by the injected saline. The cardiac output is proportional to the rate of the temperature change and is automatically calculated by the equipment.

The **Fick method** relies on the principle that the quantity of oxygen consumed by tissues is related to the amount of O_2 content removed from blood as it flows through the tissue capillary bed:

$$O_2 \text{ consumption} = O_2 \text{ content removed} \times \text{Flow}$$

$$\frac{mL\ O_2}{min} \qquad \frac{mL\ O_2}{mL\ blood} \qquad \frac{mL\ blood}{min}$$

Or, in more applicable terms:

$$O_2 \text{ consumption} = AVO_2 \text{ difference} \times \text{Cardiac output}$$

where the arteriovenous O_2 (AVO_2) difference equals the difference in oxygen content between the arterial and venous compartments. Total body oxygen consumption can be determined by analyzing expired air from the lungs, and arterial and venous O_2 content is measured in blood samples. By rearranging the terms, the cardiac output can be calculated:

$$\text{Cardiac output} = \frac{O_2 \text{ consumption}}{AVO_2 \text{ difference}}$$

For example, if the arterial blood in a normal adult contains 190 mL of O_2 per liter and the venous blood contains 150 mL of O_2 per liter, the arteriovenous difference is 40 mL of O_2 per liter. If this patient has a measured O_2 consumption of 200 mL/min, the calculated cardiac output is 5 L/min.

In many forms of heart disease, the cardiac output is lower than normal. In that situation, the total body oxygen consumption does not change significantly; however, a greater percentage of O_2 is extracted per volume of circulating blood by the metabolizing tissues. The result is a lower-than-normal venous O_2 content and therefore an increased AVO_2 difference. In our example, if the patient's venous blood O_2 content fell to 100 mL/L, the AVO_2 difference would increase to 90 mL/L, and the calculated cardiac output would be reduced to 2.2 L/min.

Because the normal range of cardiac output varies with a patient's size, it is common to report the **cardiac index**, which is equal to the cardiac output divided by the patient's body surface area (normal range of cardiac index = 2.6–4.2 L/min/m²).

CALCULATION OF VASCULAR RESISTANCE

Once pressures and cardiac output have been determined, pulmonary and systemic vascular resistances can be calculated, based on the principle that the pressure difference across a vascular bed is proportional to the product of flow and resistance. The calculations are:

$$PVR = \frac{MPAP - LAP}{CO} \times 80$$

PVR, pulmonary vascular resistance (dynes-sec-cm⁻⁵)
MPAP, mean pulmonary artery pressure (mm Hg)
LAP, mean left atrial pressure (mm Hg)
CO, cardiac output (L/min)

$$SVR = \frac{MAP - RAP}{CO} \times 80$$

SVR, systemic vascular resistance (dynes-sec-cm⁻⁵)
MAP, mean arterial pressure (mm Hg)
RAP, mean right atrial pressure (mm Hg)
CO, cardiac output (L/min)

The normal PVR ranges from 20 to 130 dynes-sec-cm⁻⁵. The normal SVR is 700-1600 dynes-sec-cm⁻⁵.

CONTRAST ANGIOGRAPHY

This technique uses radiopaque contrast to visualize regions of the cardiovascular system. A catheter is introduced into an appropriate vessel and guided under fluoroscopy to the site of injection. Following administration of the contrast agent, x-rays are transmitted through the area of interest. A continuous series of x-ray exposures is recorded to produce a motion picture cineangiogram (often simply called a "cine" or "angiogram").

Selective injection of contrast into specific heart chambers can be used to identify valvular insufficiency, intracardiac shunts, thrombi within the heart, and congenital malformations and to measure ventricular contractile function (Fig. 3-15). However, the noninvasive techniques described in this chapter (eg, echocardiography) have largely supplanted the need for invasive contrast angiography for these purposes.

An important application of contrast injection is **coronary artery angiography**, to examine the location and severity of coronary atherosclerotic lesions. To maximize the test's sensitivity and reproducibility, each patient is imaged in several standard views. When necessary, angioplasty and stent placement can be performed (Figs. 3-16 and 3-17; see Chapter 6).

Complications of catheterization and contrast angiography are uncommon and include myocardial perforation by the catheter, precipitation of arrhythmias and conduction blocks, damage to vessel walls, hemorrhage, dislodgement of atherosclerotic plaques, pericardial

A

B

Figure 3-15. Left ventriculogram, in diastole (A) and systole (B) in the right anterior oblique projection, from a patient with normal ventricular contractility. A catheter (*black arrow*) is used to inject contrast into the left ventricle (LV). The catheter can also be seen in the descending aorta (*white arrowhead*). AO, aortic root.

tamponade (see Chapter 14), and infection. The contrast medium itself can potentially cause anaphylaxis and renal toxicity in susceptible patients.

Table 3-4 summarizes the catheterization findings in common cardiac abnormalities. Therapeutic interventional catheterization techniques are described in Chapters 6 and 8.

A

B

Figure 3-16. Cardiac catheterization and stenting of a proximal left anterior descending artery (LAD) stenosis, shown in an anteroposterior cranial projection. A. When contrast agent is injected into the left main coronary artery (LM), the left circumflex artery (LCX) fills normally, but the LAD is almost completely occluded at its origin (*white arrow*). **B.** After the stenosis is successfully stented, the LAD and its branches fill robustly.

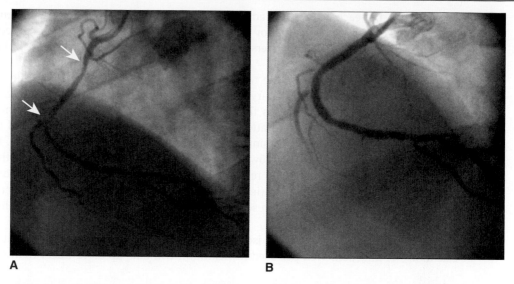

Figure 3-17. Cardiac catheterization and stenting of right coronary artery (RCA) stenoses. Both images are obtained in the left anterior oblique (LAO) projection. **A.** The stenotic segment is located between the *white arrows*. **B.** After stenting, the caliber of the vessel and flow have improved.

NUCLEAR IMAGING

Heart function can be evaluated using injected, radioactively labeled tracers and γ-camera detectors. The resulting images reflect the distribution of the tracers within the cardiovascular system. Nuclear techniques are used to assess myocardial perfusion, to image blood passing through the heart and great vessels, to localize and quantify myocardial ischemia and infarction, and to assess myocardial metabolism.

ASSESSMENT OF MYOCARDIAL PERFUSION

Ischemia and infarction resulting from CAD can be detected by myocardial perfusion imaging using various radioisotopes, including compounds labeled with thallium-201 (^{201}Tl) and technetium-99m (^{99m}Tc). Of the latter, ^{99m}Tc-sestamibi and ^{99m}Tc-tetrofosmin are commonly used. Both ^{201}Tl- and ^{99m}Tc-labeled compounds are sensitive for the detection of ischemic or scarred

TABLE 3-4	Cardiac Catheterization and Angiography in Cardiac Disorders
Disorder	**Finding**
Coronary artery disease	• Identification of atherosclerotic lesions
Mitral regurgitation	• Large systolic *v* wave in left atrial pressure tracing
Mitral stenosis	• Abnormally high pressure gradient between the left atrium and left ventricle in diastole
Tricuspid insufficiency	• Large systolic *v* wave in the right atrial pressure tracing
Aortic stenosis	• Systolic pressure gradient between the left ventricle and aorta
Heart failure	• Reduced ejection fraction (see Chapter 9) if systolic dysfunction • Elevated diastolic pressure with normal ejection fraction if diastolic dysfunction

myocardium, but each has distinct advantages. For example, the ^{99m}Tc-labeled agents provide better image quality and are superior for detailed single photon emission computed tomography (SPECT, as in Fig. 3-18). Conversely, enhanced detection of myocardial cellular viability is possible with ^{201}Tl imaging.

In the case of ^{201}Tl imaging, the radioisotope is injected intravenously while the patient exercises on a treadmill or stationary bicycle. Because thallium is a potassium analogue, it enters normal myocytes, a process thought to be partially governed by sodium-potassium ATPase. The intracellular concentration of thallium, estimated by the density of the image, depends on vascular supply (perfusion) and membrane function (tissue viability). In the normal heart, the radionuclide scan shows a homogenous distribution of thallium in the myocardial tissue. Conversely, myocardial regions that are scarred (by previous infarction) or have reduced perfusion during exercise (ie, transient myocardial ischemia) do not accumulate as much thallium as normal heart muscle. Consequently, these areas appear on the thallium scan as light or "cold" spots.

When evaluating for myocardial ischemia, an initial set of images is taken right after exercise and ^{201}Tl injection. Well-perfused myocardium will take up more tracer than ischemic or

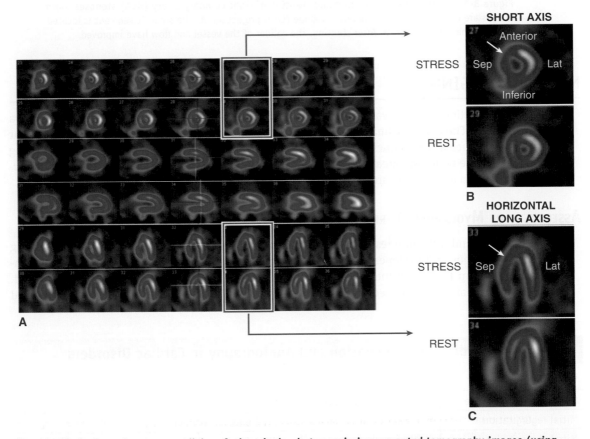

Figure 3-18. Stress and rest myocardial perfusion single photon emission computed tomography images (using 99mTc-tetrofosmin) of a patient with a high-grade stenosis within the proximal left anterior descending coronary artery. A. Miniaturized reproduction of the complete scan showing tomographic images in each of the three views (from *top* to *bottom*: short axis, vertical long axis, and horizontal long axis). The *first*, *third*, and *fifth* rows demonstrate images during stress, and the *second*, *fourth*, and *sixth* rows are matching images acquired at rest. **B, C.** Enlarged selected panels from **(A)** showing stress and rest images in the short-axis and horizontal long-axis views. The *arrows* indicate regions of decreased perfusion during stress but normal perfusion on the matching resting scans, consistent with inducible ischemia. Lat, lateral wall of the LV; Sep, septal wall. (Courtesy of Marcelo Di Carli, MD, Brigham and Women's Hospital, Boston, MA.)

infarcted myocardium at this time. Delayed images are acquired several hours later, because ^{201}Tl accumulation does not remain fixed in myocytes. Rather, continuous redistribution of the isotope occurs across the cell membrane. After 3-4 hours of redistribution, when additional images are obtained, all viable myocytes will have equal concentrations of ^{201}Tl. Consequently, any uptake abnormalities on the initial exercise scan that were caused by myocardial *ischemia* will have resolved (ie, filled in) on the delayed scan (and are therefore termed "reversible" defects), and those representing *infarcted* or scarred myocardium will persist as cold spots ("fixed" defects).

Of note, some myocardial segments that demonstrate persistent ^{201}Tl defects on both stress and redistribution imaging are falsely characterized as nonviable, scarred tissue. Sometimes, these areas represent ischemic, noncontractile, but metabolically active areas that have the potential to regain function if an adequate blood supply is restored. For example, such areas may represent **hibernating myocardium**, segments that demonstrate diminished contractile function owing to chronic reduction of coronary blood flow (see Chapter 6). This viable state (in which the affected cells can be predicted to regain function following coronary revascularization) can often be differentiated from irreversibly scarred myocardium by repeat imaging at rest after the injection of additional ^{201}Tl to enhance uptake by viable cells.

^{99m}Tc-sestamibi (commonly referred to as MIBI) is an example of a widely used ^{99m}Tc-labeled compound. This agent is a large lipophilic molecule that, like thallium, is taken up in the myocardium in proportion to blood flow. The uptake mechanism differs in that the compound crosses the myocyte membrane passively, driven by the negative membrane potential. Once inside the cell, it further accumulates in mitochondria, driven by that organelle's even more negative membrane potential. The myocardial distribution of MIBI reflects perfusion at the moment of injection, and in contrast to thallium, it remains fixed intracellularly, that is, it *redistributes only minimally over time*. Consequently, performing a MIBI procedure is more flexible, as images can be obtained up to 4-6 hours after injection and repeated as necessary. In a typical MIBI study, injection of a small tracer dose and imaging are initially performed at rest. Later, a larger tracer dose is administered after exercise, and imaging is repeated to assess for ischemic zones.

Stress nuclear imaging studies with either ^{201}Tl- or ^{99m}Tc-labeled compounds have greater sensitivity and specificity than standard exercise electrocardiography for the detection of ischemia but are more expensive and should be ordered judiciously. Nuclear imaging is particularly appropriate for patients with baseline electrocardiogram (ECG) abnormalities of the ST segment that preclude accurate interpretation of a standard exercise test. Examples include patients with electronic pacemaker rhythms, those with left bundle branch block, those with ST abnormalities due to left ventricular hypertrophy, and those who take certain medications that alter the ST segment, such as digoxin. Nuclear scans also provide more accurate anatomic localization of the ischemic segment(s) and quantification of the extent of ischemia compared with standard exercise testing. In addition, electronic synchronizing (gating) of nuclear images to the ECG cycle permits ventricular wall motion analysis.

Patients with orthopedic or neurologic conditions, as well as those with severe physical deconditioning or chronic lung disease, may be unable to perform an adequate exercise test on a treadmill or bicycle. In such patients, stress images can be obtained instead by administering pharmacologic agents, such as adenosine, regadenoson, or dipyridamole. These agents induce diffuse coronary vasodilation, augmenting blood flow to myocardium perfused by healthy coronary arteries. Since ischemic regions are already maximally dilated (because of local metabolite accumulation), the drug-induced vasodilation causes a "steal" phenomenon, *reducing* isotope uptake in regions distal to significant coronary stenoses (see Chapter 6). Alternatively, the inotrope dobutamine (see Chapter 17) can be infused intravenously to increase myocardial oxygen demand, followed by nuclear imaging, as a means to assess for ischemia.

RADIONUCLIDE VENTRICULOGRAPHY

Radionuclide ventriculography (RVG, also known as blood pool imaging) is occasionally used to analyze right and left ventricular function. A radioisotope (usually ^{99m}Tc) is bound to red blood cells or to human serum albumin and then injected as a bolus. Nuclear images are obtained at fixed time intervals as the labeled material passes through the heart and great vessels. Multiple images are displayed sequentially to produce a dynamic picture of blood flow. Calculations, such as determination of the ejection fraction, are based on the difference between radioactive counts present in the ventricle at the end of diastole and at the end of systole. Therefore, measurements are largely independent of any assumptions of ventricular geometry and are highly reproducible.

RVG has been used historically to assess baseline cardiac function in patients scheduled to undergo potentially cardiotoxic chemotherapy and to follow cardiac function over time in such patients. However, echocardiography is easier to perform, does not expose the patient to ionizing radiation, and now commonly serves this role instead.

ASSESSMENT OF MYOCARDIAL METABOLISM

Positron emission tomography (PET) is a specialized nuclear imaging technique used to assess myocardial perfusion and viability. PET imaging employs positron-emitting isotopes attached to metabolic or flow tracers. Sensitive detectors measure positron emission from the tracer molecules.

Myocardial perfusion is commonly assessed using nitrogen-13–labeled ammonia or rubidium-82. Both are taken up by myocytes in proportion to blood flow. *Myocardial viability* can be determined by PET by assessing glucose utilization in myocardial tissue. In normal myocardium under fasting conditions, glucose is used for ~20% of energy production, with free fatty acids providing the remaining 80%. In ischemic conditions, however, metabolism shifts toward glucose use, and the more ischemic the myocardial tissue, the stronger the reliance on glucose. Fluoro-18 deoxyglucose (^{18}FDG) is used to study glucose uptake. This substance competes with glucose both for transport into myocytes and for subsequent phosphorylation. Unlike glucose, however, ^{18}FDG is not metabolized and becomes trapped within the myocyte.

Combined evaluation of perfusion and ^{18}FDG metabolism allows assessment of both regional blood flow and glucose uptake, respectively. PET scanning thus helps determine whether areas of ventricular contractile dysfunction with decreased flow represent irreversibly damaged scar tissue or whether the region is still viable (eg, hibernating myocardium). In scar tissue, both blood flow to the affected area and ^{18}FDG uptake are decreased. Because the myocytes in this region are permanently damaged, such tissue is not likely to benefit from revascularization. Hibernating myocardium, in contrast, shows decreased blood flow but normal or elevated ^{18}FDG uptake. Such tissue may benefit from revascularization procedures (see Chapter 6).

^{18}FDG PET imaging is also useful for the diagnosis, and assessment of response to therapy, in inflammatory cardiomyopathies such as sarcoidosis (see Chapter 10).

Table 3-5 summarizes the radionuclide imaging abnormalities associated with common cardiac conditions.

COMPUTED TOMOGRAPHY

CT uses a series of thin x-rays to generate cross-sectional images of the heart and vasculature. An x-ray device is programmed to rotate around the patient and the generated beams are partially absorbed by body tissues. The remaining beams emerge and are captured by electronic

TABLE 3-5	Nuclear Imaging in Cardiac Disorders
Disorder	**Findings**
Myocardial ischemia	
Stress-delayed reinjection ^{201}Tl	• Low uptake during stress with complete or partial fill-in with delayed or reinjection images
Rest-stress ^{99m}Tc-labeled compounds	• Normal uptake at rest with decreased uptake during stress
PET (N-13 ammonia/^{18}FDG)	• Decreased flow with normal or increased ^{18}FDG uptake during stress
Myocardial infarction	
Stress-delayed reinjection ^{201}Tl	• Low uptake during stress and low uptake after reinjection
Rest-stress ^{99m}Tc-labeled compounds	• Low uptake in rest and stress images
PET (N-13 ammonia/^{18}FDG)	• Decreased flow and decreased ^{18}FDG uptake at rest
Hibernating myocardium	
Rest-delayed ^{201}Tl	Complete or partial fill-in of defects after reinjection
PET (N-13 ammonia/^{18}FDG)	Decreased flow and normal or increased ^{18}FDG uptake at rest

^{18}FDG, fluoro-18 deoxyglucose; N-13, nitrogen-13; PET, positron emission tomography; ^{99m}Tc, technetium-99m; ^{201}Tl, thallium-201.

detectors, which relay information to a computer for image composition. CT scanning typically requires administration of an intravenous contrast agent to distinguish intravascular contents (ie, blood) from neighboring soft tissue structures (eg, myocardium).

Applications of CT in cardiac imaging include assessment of the great vessels, pericardium, myocardium, and coronary arteries. CT is used to diagnose aortic dissection and aneurysms (Fig. 3-19). It can identify abnormal pericardial fluid, thickening, and calcification. Myocardial abnormalities, such as regional hypertrophy or ventricular aneurysms, and intracardiac thrombus formation can be distinctly visualized by CT. A limitation of conventional CT techniques is the artifact generated by patient motion (ie, breathing) during image acquisition. Modern **spiral CT** (also called helical CT) imaging allows more rapid image acquisition, often during a single breath-hold, at relatively lower radiation doses than conventional CT. This technique is particularly important in the diagnosis of pulmonary embolism. When an intravenous iodine-based contrast agent is administered, emboli create the appearance of "filling defects" in otherwise contrast-enhanced pulmonary vessels (Fig. 3-20).

Electron beam computed tomography (EBCT) uses a direct electron beam to acquire images in a matter of milliseconds. A rapid succession of images depicts cardiac structures at multiple instances during a single cardiac cycle. Displaying these images in a cine format can provide estimates of left ventricular volumes and ejection fraction. Capable of detecting coronary artery calcification, EBCT has been used primarily to screen for CAD. Because calcified coronary artery plaques have a radiodensity similar to that of bone, they appear attenuated (white) on CT. The coronary artery calcium score (*Agatston score*), a measure of total coronary calcium, correlates well with atherosclerotic plaque burden and predicts the risk of coronary events, independently of other cardiac risk factors.

Newer CT technology can characterize atherosclerotic stenoses in great detail. **Multidetector row CT** scanners acquire as many as 320 anatomic sections with each rotation, providing excellent spatial resolution. Administration of intravenous contrast and computer reformatting allows visualization of the arterial lumen and regions of coronary narrowings (Fig. 3-21). Because image acquisition is timed with the cardiac cycle, a relatively low heart rate is desirable, such that a β-blocker is often administered prior to scanning.

Figure 3-19. Computed tomography (CT) imaging of aortic dissection. A, B. Axial images demonstrate an intimal flap (*blue arrowheads*) separating the true and false lumens of the descending thoracic and abdominal aorta. **C.** CT angiography (CTA) with three-dimensional reconstructions. In this left anterior oblique view, the origin of the dissection (*blue arrowhead*) is apparent in the distal portion of the aortic arch. The dissection continues to the level of the renal arteries (*white arrowhead*) and beyond. **D.** In this CTA left posterior oblique view, the dissection extends to the infrarenal aorta (*white arrowhead*) and involves the left common and external iliac arteries (*blue arrowhead*). AA, ascending aorta; LCI, left common iliac artery; LEI, left external iliac artery; LK, left kidney; PA, main pulmonary artery; RCI, right common iliac artery; RK, right kidney. (Courtesy of Suhny Abbara, MD, Massachusetts General Hospital, Boston, MA.)

Figure 3-20. Spiral (helical) computed tomography image demonstrating a massive pulmonary embolism. The *white arrows* point to a large thrombus within the right pulmonary artery. It appears as a filling defect within the otherwise contrast-enhanced pulmonary vasculature. AA, ascending aorta; DA, descending aorta; LPA, left pulmonary artery; PA, main pulmonary artery; RPA, right pulmonary artery; SVC, superior vena cava.

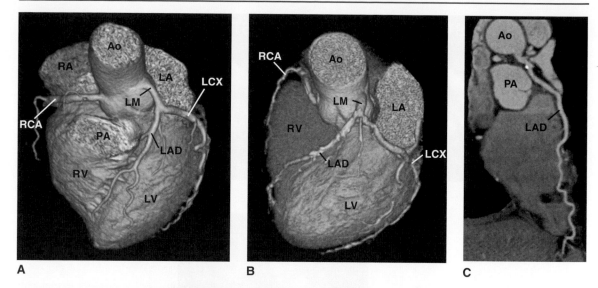

A   **B**   **C**

Figure 3-21. Computed tomography (CT) coronary angiography. After a patient is imaged in a high-resolution axial CT scanner, three-dimensional reconstructions (termed *volume renderings*) are generated. **A.** Volume rendering of a normal CT angiogram. **B.** Volume rendering of a CT angiogram that demonstrates diffuse coronary artery disease. Notice that the caliber of each vessel is irregular along its length. **C.** This curved reformat of the left anterior descending artery (LAD) depicts the entire course of the vessel in a single, flat image, making it easier to detect stenoses. None are present here. Ao, aorta; LA, left atrium; LCX, left circumflex artery; LM, left main coronary artery; LV, left ventricle; PA, pulmonary artery; RA, right atrium; RCA, right coronary artery; RV, right ventricle. (Courtesy of Suhny Abbara, MD, Massachusetts General Hospital, Boston, MA.)

CT is not as sensitive as conventional angiography for the detection of coronary lesions, and it cannot adequately evaluate stenosis within coronary artery stents. However, CT is rapid, relatively inexpensive, and less invasive than conventional angiography. Its role in assessing patients with symptoms suggestive of CAD and for following the progression of known coronary disease is under active evaluation.

MAGNETIC RESONANCE IMAGING

MRI uses a powerful magnetic field to obtain detailed images of internal structures. This technique is based on the magnetic polarity of hydrogen nuclei, which align themselves with an applied magnetic field. Radiofrequency excitation causes the nuclei to move out of alignment momentarily. As they return to their resting states, the nuclei emit the absorbed energy into signals that are translated into computer-generated images. Therefore, unlike CT imaging, MRI requires no ionized radiation. Among all the imaging modalities, MRI is best at differentiating tissue contrasts (blood, fluid, fat, and myocardium) and can often do so even without the use of contrast agents.

The detail of soft tissue structures is often exquisitely demonstrated in magnetic resonance images (Fig. 3-22). Cardiac MRI (CMR) has an established role in evaluating congenital anomalies, such as shunts, and diseases of the aorta, including aneurysm and dissection. It is also used to assess left and right ventricular mass and volume, intravascular thrombus, cardiomyopathies, pericardial disease, and neoplastic disease (Fig. 3-23). ECG-gated and cine MRI techniques capture images at discrete times in the cardiac cycle, allowing for the evaluation of valvular and ventricular function.

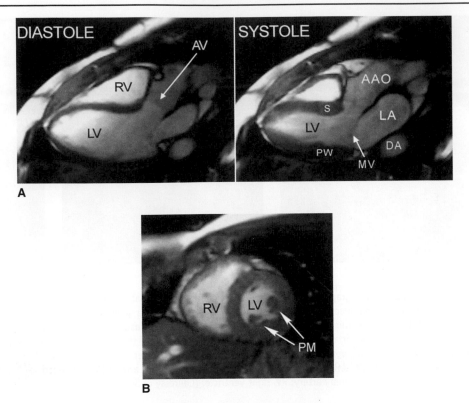

Figure 3-22. Cardiac magnetic resonance images of a normal person. A. Three-chamber long-axis view of the heart in diastole and systole showing the left ventricle (LV), right ventricle (RV), and left atrium (LA). The mitral valve (MV), aortic valve (AV), ascending aorta (AAO), and descending aorta (DA) are also imaged. **B.** Midventricular short-axis view demonstrating the LV, RV, and left ventricular papillary muscles (PMs). PW, posterior wall; S, septum. (Courtesy of Raymond Y. Kwong, MD, Brigham and Women's Hospital, Boston, MA.)

Two applications of CMR deserve special mention. **Coronary magnetic resonance angiography (coronary MRA)** is a noninvasive, contrast-free angiographic imaging modality. Laminar blood flow appears as bright signal intensity, whereas turbulent blood flow, at the site of stenosis, results in less bright or absent signal intensity. This technique has shown high sensitivity and accuracy for the detection of important CAD in the left main coronary artery and in the proximal and midportions of the three major coronary vessels. Coronary MRA is also useful in delineating coronary artery congenital anomalies.

In **contrast-enhanced MRI**, a gadolinium-based agent is administered intravenously to identify infarcted (irreversibly damaged) myocardium and to differentiate it from impaired (but viable) muscle segments. This technique is based on the fact that gadolinium is excluded from viable cells with intact cell membranes but can permeate and concentrate in infarcted zones, producing "hyperenhancement" on the image (Fig. 3-24). Owing to the high spatial resolution of this technique, the transmural extent of myocardial scar can be depicted, and the pattern of infarcting tissue can be differentiated from that of acute myocarditis, a condition that may present with similar clinical features. The use of late-enhancing gadolinium imaging also allows for the identification of poorly contractile "hibernating" myocardium, tissue that is chronically ischemic, but would be expected to recover function if adequate blood perfusion is restored, as described in the nuclear imaging section.

A   **B**

Figure 3-23. Magnetic resonance imaging of an intracardiac mass. Both images are apical four-chamber views.
A. Before a gadolinium-based contrast agent is administered, an abnormal left atrial mass (indicated by the *oval*)
demonstrates diminished signal relative to the surrounding tissue. In this respect, it resembles a nonvascular thrombus.
B. After contrast injection, the mass enhances similar to the surrounding tissue, indicating that it is vascularized. Biopsy
revealed a spindle cell carcinoma. LA, left atrium; LV, left ventricle; RA, right atrium; RV, right ventricle. (Courtesy of
Raymond Y. Kwong, MD, Brigham and Women's Hospital, Boston, MA.)

A   **B**

**Figure 3-24. Gadolinium-enhanced magnetic resonance images demonstrating a region of nonviable myocardium.
Both images are short-axis views. A.** Imaging before administration of gadolinium demonstrates thinning of the
anterior and anteroseptal myocardium (*blue arrow*) suggestive of infarcted tissue (compared to short-axis view of healthy
myocardial wall in Fig. 3.22-B). **B.** After contrast injection, the subendocardial regions of the anterior and anteroseptal
segments of the left ventricle selectively enhance (*white arrows*), indicating that scar tissue is present. Because more than
half the thickness of the ventricular wall is scarred, coronary revascularization would have a low likelihood of improving
contractile function of these myocardial segments. LV, left ventricle; RV, right ventricle. (Courtesy of Raymond Y. Kwong,
MD, Brigham and Women's Hospital, Boston, MA.)

INTEGRATION

This chapter has presented an overview of imaging and catheterization techniques available to assess cardiac structure and function. Many of these tools are expensive and yield similar information. For example, estimates of ventricular contractile function can be made by echocardiography, nuclear imaging, contrast angiography, gated CT, or MRI. Myocardial viability can be assessed using nuclear imaging studies, gadolinium MRI, or dobutamine echocardiography.

Determining the single best test for any given patient depends on a number of factors. One is the ease by which images may be obtained. In a critically ill patient, bedside echocardiography provides a readily acquired measure of left ventricular systolic function. Conversely, obtaining similar information from a nuclear or magnetic resonance study would require a trip to the respective scanner. Other factors to consider include the magnitude of radiation exposure and the invasiveness of a given imaging technique. Expense, available equipment, and institutional expertise also play roles in selecting an imaging approach. When used appropriately, each of these tools can provide important information to guide the diagnosis and management of cardiovascular disorders.

Summary

- Imaging and catheterization techniques provide important information to guide the diagnosis and management of cardiovascular disorders; key uses are summarized here and in Table 3-6.

- **Chest radiography** can detect chamber dilatation and visualize pulmonary signs of heart failure.

- **Transthoracic echocardiography** can assess ventricular systolic and diastolic dysfunction, identify valvular abnormalities and vegetations, diagnose consequences of myocardial infarction, and demonstrate pericardial and congenital abnormalities.

- **Transesophageal echocardiography** is used to visualize intracardiac thrombus, evaluate prosthetic valve dysfunction, identify valvular vegetations and myocardial abscess in endocarditis, and diagnose aortic dissection.

- Diagnostic **cardiac catheterization** is the "gold standard" to assess intracardiac pressures and to identify and grade coronary artery stenoses.

- **Nuclear imaging** can diagnose myocardial ischemia and distinguish viable myocardium from scar tissue.

- **Positron emission tomography** is used to assess for ischemia and can distinguish viable myocardium from scar tissue.

- **Computed tomography** is sensitive for the diagnosis of aortic dissection and pulmonary embolism, can assess pericardial conditions, and detect coronary artery calcification and stenoses.

- **Magnetic resonance imaging** demonstrates great detail of soft tissue structures and is used to define the specific conditions listed in Table 3-6.

TABLE 3-6	Summary of Cardiac Imaging Techniques

Imaging Technique	Findings	Examples of Clinical Uses
Chest radiography	• Cardiac and mediastinal contours • Pulmonary vascular markings	• Detect chamber dilatation • Identify consequences of stenotic and regurgitant valve lesions and intracardiac shunts • Visualize pulmonary signs of heart failure
Transthoracic echocardiography (TTE)	• Wall thickness, chamber dimensions • Anatomic relationships and motion of cardiac structures • Flow direction, turbulence, and velocity measurements • Echo contrast studies • Stress echocardiography	• Assess global and segmental ventricular contraction • Identify valvular abnormalities and vegetations • Diagnose consequences of myocardial infarction (eg, ventricular aneurysm, papillary muscle rupture, intraventricular thrombus) • Identify myocardial, pericardial, and congenital abnormalities
Transesophageal echocardiography (TEE)	• Similar to TTE but higher resolution	• Visualize intracardiac thrombus • Evaluate prosthetic valves and perivalvular leaks • Identify valvular vegetations and myocardial abscess in endocarditis • Diagnose aortic dissection
Cardiac catheterization	• Pressure measurement • Contrast angiography	• Evaluate intracardiac pressures (eg, in valvular disease, heart failure, pericardial disease) • Visualize ventricular contractile function, regurgitant valve lesions • Identify coronary anatomy and severity of stenoses
Nuclear SPECT imaging (using ^{99m}Tc-labeled compounds or ^{201}Tl)	• Regional myocardial perfusion • Myocardial viability	• Detect, quantify, and localize myocardial ischemia • Perform stress testing in patients with baseline ECG abnormalities • Distinguish viable myocardium from scar tissue
Radionuclide ventriculography	• Ventricular contractile function	• Calculate ventricular ejection fraction and quantitate intracardiac shunts
Positron emission tomography (PET)	• Myocardial perfusion and metabolism	• Evaluate contractile function • Distinguish viable myocardium from scar tissue
Computed tomography (CT)	• Anatomy and structural relationships	• Diagnose abnormalities of the great vessels (aortic dissection, pulmonary embolism) • Assess pericardial disease and myocardial abnormalities • Detect coronary artery calcification and stenoses
Magnetic resonance imaging (MRI)	• Detailed soft tissue anatomy	• Assess myocardial structure and function (eg, ventricular mass and volume, neoplastic disease, intracardiac thrombus, cardiomyopathies) • Diagnose aortic and pericardial disease • Detect areas of ischemic vs infarcted myocardium

ECG, electrocardiogram; SPECT, single photon emission computed tomography; ^{99m}Tc, technetium-99m; ^{201}Tl, thallium-201.

Review Questions

1. Which of the following chest radiograph findings is *not* typically associated with heart failure?

   a. Cephalization of vessels
   b. Peripheral pruning of vessels
   c. Kerley B lines
   d. Butterfly pattern

2. A 62-year-old woman presents with a 6-month history of shortness of breath during exertion. She undergoes cardiac catheterization and the following pressure measurements and calculations are made:

	Value	Normal Range
Right atrial pressure (RAP)	15 mm Hg	2-8 mm Hg
Mean pulmonary artery pressure (MPAP)	50 mm Hg	9-19 mm Hg
Left atrial pressure (LAP)	8 mm Hg	2-10 mm Hg
Mean arterial pressure (MAP)	90 mm Hg	70-105 mm Hg
Cardiac output (CO)	5.2 L/min	4.0-8.0 L/min

   What is the systemic vascular resistance?

   a. 646 dynes-sec-cm^{-5}
   b. 980 dynes-sec-cm^{-5}
   c. 1154 dynes-sec-cm^{-5}
   d. 2850 dynes-sec-cm^{-5}

   What is the pulmonary vascular resistance?

   a. 646 dynes-sec-cm^{-5}
   b. 980 dynes-sec-cm^{-5}
   c. 1154 dynes-sec-cm^{-5}
   d. 2850 dynes-sec-cm^{-5}

3. Which of the following statements regarding cardiac imaging is correct?

   a. Pericardial thickness is more accurately measured by echocardiography than by magnetic resonance imaging (MRI).
   b. Gadolinium enhancement is a contrast technique used with cardiac computed tomography (CT) imaging to identify prior myocardial infarction.
   c. During nuclear imaging, technetium-99m–labeled compounds such as ^{99m}Tc-sestamibi are taken up by regions of infarcted tissue but not healthy myocardium.
   d. Cardiac MRI can distinguish between blood, fat, and myocardium without the administration of contrast agents.

Answers to Review Questions

1. **Choice b is correct.** Peripheral pruning of vessels (enlarged central pulmonary arteries but small peripheral vessels) is typical of pulmonary hypertension, not heart failure. The many features of heart failure on chest radiographs include cephalization of vessels

(increased pulmonary venous pressure causes redistribution of blood flow from the bases to the apices of the lungs), interstitial edema, Kerley B lines (short horizontal parallel lines at the lung periphery due to fluid in interlobular spaces), and alveolar edema producing a "butterfly" pattern.

2. **For systemic vascular resistance, choice c is correct. For pulmonary vascular resistance, choice a is correct.** The patient's right heart catheterization reveals normal left atrial pressure, mean arterial pressure, and cardiac output but elevated mean pulmonary artery pressure and right atrial pressure.

The systemic vascular resistance (SVR) is calculated by the formula on page 63:

$$SVR = \frac{MAP - RAP}{CO} \times 80$$
$$= \frac{90 - 15}{5.2} \times 80$$
$$= 1154 \ dynes\text{-}sec\text{-}cm^{-5}$$

The pulmonary vascular resistance (PVR) is calculated by the formula on page 63:

$$PVR = \frac{MPAP - LAP}{CO} \times 80$$
$$= \frac{50 - 8}{5.2} \times 80$$
$$= 646 \ dynes\text{-}sec\text{-}cm^{-5}$$

In this patient, the SVR is normal (normal range: 700-1600 dynes-sec-cm^{-5}), but the PVR is elevated (normal range: 20-130 dynes-sec-cm^{-5}). That, in combination with the normal left atrial pressure, indicates that the elevated right atrial and pulmonary artery pressures are due to disease in the pulmonary parenchyma or pulmonary vasculature, rather than from left-sided heart disease.

3. **Choice d is correct.** Of available imaging modalities, cardiac MR is best at differentiating tissue contrasts such as blood, fluids, fat, and myocardium. The resolution of echocardiography is not sufficient to accurately measure pericardial thickness; CT and MRI are much better suited to accurately do so. Gadolinium enhancement is a technique used with cardiac MRI, not CT imaging. In nuclear imaging, ^{99m}Tc-sestamibi is taken up by healthy myocardium in proportion to blood flow; perfusion *defects* are present in regions of infarction.

Acknowledgments

Contributors to previous editions of this chapter were Diana M. López, MD; David B. Fischer, MD; Henry Jung, MD; Ken Young Lin, MD; Nicole Martin, MD; Deborah Bucino, MD; Sharon Horesh, MD; Shona Pendse, MD; Albert S. Tu, MD; Patrick Yachimski, MD; and Patricia Come, MD.

Additional Reading

Doherty JU, Kort S, Mehran R, et al. ACC/AATS/AHA/ASE/ASNC/HRS/SCAI/SCCT/SCMR/STS 2017 appropriate use criteria for multimodality imaging in valvular heart disease. *J Am Coll Cardiol.* 2017;70:1647-1672.

Doherty JU, Kort S, Mehran R, et al. ACC/AATS/AHA/ASE/ASNC/HRS/SCAI/SCCT/SCMR/STS 2019 appropriate use criteria for multimodality imaging in the assessment of cardiac structure and function in nonvalvular heart disease. *J Am Coll Cardiol.* 2019;73:488-516.

Mangla A, Oliveros E, Williams KA Sr, et al. Cardiac imaging in the diagnosis of coronary artery disease. *Curr Probl Cardiol.* 2017;42:316-366.

Motwani M, Swoboda PP, Plein S, et al. Role of cardiovascular magnetic resonance in the management of patients with stable coronary artery disease. *Heart.* 2018;104:888-894.

Murthy VL, Bateman TM, Beanlands RS, et al. Clinical quantification of myocardial blood flow using PET: joint position paper of the SNMMI cardiovascular council and the ASNC. *J Nucl Cardiol.* 2018;25:269-297.

Otto CM. *Textbook of Clinical Echocardiography.* 6th ed. Philadelphia, PA: Elsevier Saunders; 2018.

Wamil M, Newton JD, Rana BS, et al. Transoesophageal echocardiography: what the general cardiologist needs to know. *Heart.* 2017;10:629-640.

The Electrocardiogram

Daniel C. Pipilas | Bruce A. Koplan | Leonard S. Lilly

Cardiac contraction relies on the organized flow of electrical impulses through the heart. The electrocardiogram (ECG) is an easily obtained recording of that activity and provides a wealth of information about cardiac structure and function. This chapter presents the electrical basis of the ECG in health and disease and leads the reader through the basics of interpretation. To practice using these principles and to become skillful at interpreting ECG tracings of your patients, you should also familiarize yourself with a complete electrocardiographic manual, examples of which are listed at the end of this chapter.

ELECTRICAL MEASUREMENT—SINGLE-CELL MODEL

This section begins by observing the propagation of an electrical impulse along a single cardiac muscle cell, illustrated in Figure 4-1. On the right side of the diagram, a voltmeter records the electrical potential at the cell's surface on graph paper. In the resting state, the cell is polarized; that is, the entire outside of the cell is electrically positive with respect to the inside, because of the ionic distribution across the cell membrane, as described in Chapter 1. In this resting state, the voltmeter electrodes, which are placed on opposite outside surfaces of the cell, do not record any electrical activity, because there is no electrical potential difference between them (the myocyte surface is homogeneously charged).

This equilibrium is disturbed, however, when the cell is stimulated (see Fig. 4-1B). During the action potential, cations rush across the sarcolemma into the cell and the polarity at the stimulated region transiently reverses such that the outside becomes negatively charged with respect to the inside; that is, the region **depolarizes**. At that moment, an electrical potential is created on the cell surface between the depolarized area (negatively charged surface) and the still-polarized (positively charged surface) portions of the cell. As a result, an electrical current begins to flow between these two regions.

By convention, the direction of an electrical current is said to flow from areas that are negatively charged to those that are positively charged. When a depolarization current is directed toward the (+) electrode of the voltmeter, an *upward* deflection is recorded. Conversely, if it is directed away from the (+) electrode, a *downward* deflection is recorded. Because the

Figure 4-1. Depolarization of a single cardiac muscle cell. A. In the resting state, the surface of the cell is positively charged relative to the inside. Because the surface is homogeneously charged, the voltmeter electrodes outside the cell do not record any electrical potential difference ("flat line" recording). **B.** Stimulation of the cell initiates depolarization (*blue shaded area*); the outside of the depolarized region becomes negatively charged relative to the inside. Because the current of depolarization is directed toward the (+) electrode of the voltmeter, an upward deflection is recorded. **C.** Depolarization spreads, creating a greater upward deflection by the recording electrode. **D.** The cell has become fully depolarized. The surface of the cell is now completely negatively charged compared with the inside. Because the surface is again homogeneously charged, a flat line is recorded by the voltmeter. **E.** Notice that if the position of the voltmeter electrodes had been reversed, the electrical current would have been directed away from the (+) electrode, causing the deflection to be downward.

depolarization current in this example proceeds from left to right—that is, toward the (+) electrode—an upward deflection is recorded by the voltmeter. As the wave of depolarization propagates rightward along the cell, additional electrical forces directed toward the (+) electrode record an even greater upward deflection (see Fig. 4-1C). Once the cell has become fully depolarized (see Fig. 4-1D), its outside is completely negatively charged with respect to the inside, the opposite of the initial resting condition. However, because the surface charge is homogeneous once again, the external electrodes measure a potential difference of zero, and the voltmeter records a neutral "flat line" at this time.

Note that in Figure 4-1E, if the voltmeter electrode positions had been reversed, such that the (+) pole was placed to the *left* of the cell, then as the wave of depolarization proceeds toward the right, the current would be directed *away* from the (+) electrode, and the recorded deflection would be *downward*. This relationship should be kept in mind when the polarity of ECG leads is described below.

Depolarization initiates myocyte contraction and is then followed by **repolarization**, the process by which the cellular charges return to the resting state. In Figure 4-2, as the left side of the cardiac muscle cell in our example begins to repolarize, its surface charge becomes positive once again. An electrical potential is therefore generated, and current flows from the still negatively charged surface toward the positively charged region. Since this current is directed away from the voltmeter's (+) electrode, a downward deflection is recorded, opposite to that which was observed during the process of depolarization.

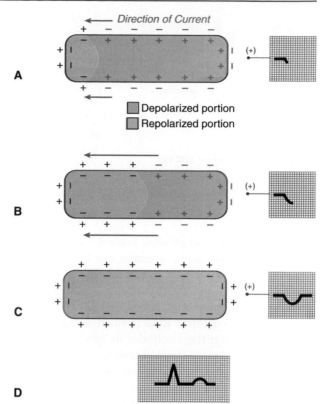

Figure 4-2. Sequence of repolarization of a single cardiac muscle cell. A. As repolarization commences, the surface of the cell at that site becomes positively charged, and a current is generated from the still negatively charged surface areas to the repolarized region (*blue arrows*). Because the current is directed away from the (+) electrode of the voltmeter, a downward deflection is recorded. **B.** Repolarization progresses. **C.** Repolarization is complete, and the outside surface of the cell is once again homogeneously charged, so that no further electrical potential is detected (flat line once again). **D.** Sequence of cardiac depolarization and repolarization as measured by an ECG machine at the skin surface. As described in the text, repolarization actually proceeds in the direction *opposite* to that of depolarization in the intact heart, such that the deflections of repolarization are inverted compared to the schematics presented in parts **A-C** of this figure. Therefore, *the deflections of depolarization and repolarization of the normal heart are oriented in the same direction*. Note that the wave of repolarization is more prolonged and of lower amplitude than that of depolarization.

Repolarization is a slower process than depolarization, so the inscribed deflection of repolarization is usually wider and of lower magnitude. Once the cell has returned to the resting state, the surface charges are once again homogeneous and no further electrical potential is detected, resulting in a neutral flat line on the voltmeter recording (Fig. 4-2C).

The depolarization and repolarization of a single cardiac muscle cell have been considered here. As a wave of depolarization spreads through the entire heart, each cell generates electrical forces, and it is the sum of these forces, measured at the skin's surface, that is recorded by the ECG machine.

It is important to note that in the intact heart, the sequence by which regions repolarize is actually *opposite* to that of their depolarization. This occurs because myocardial action potential durations are more prolonged in cells near the inner endocardium (the first cells stimulated by Purkinje fibers) than in myocytes near the outer epicardium (the last cells to depolarize). Thus, the cells close to the endocardium are the first to depolarize but are the last to repolarize. As a result, the direction of repolarization recorded by the ECG machine is usually the *inverse* of what was presented in the single-cell example in Figure 4-2. That is, unlike the single-cell model, the electrical deflections of depolarization and repolarization in the intact heart are usually oriented in the *same* direction on the ECG tracing (see Fig. 4-2D).

The direction and magnitude of the deflections on an ECG recording depend on how the generated electrical forces are aligned to a set of specific reference axes, known as ECG leads, as described in the next section.

ELECTROCARDIOGRAPHIC LEAD REFERENCE SYSTEM

Current ECG technology utilizes thin, flexible electrodes placed on the skin, held in place by adhesive tabs, on each of the four limbs and on the chest in the standard arrangement as shown in Figure 4-3. The right leg electrode is not used for measurement but serves as

Figure 4-3. Placement of electrocardiogram (ECG) electrodes.
A. Standard positions. **B.** Close-up view of chest electrode placement, at the standard positions listed in Table 4-1.

an electrical ground. Table 4-1 lists the standard locations of the chest electrodes. Note that incorrect lead placement can be a source of error in clinical practice. For example, accidentally switching the right and left arm leads, or placing a chest lead in the wrong location, can cause the calculated electrical axis to be inaccurate or create the incorrect appearance of prior myocardial infarction.

A complete ECG (termed a "12-lead ECG") is produced by recording electrical activity between the electrodes in specific patterns. This results in six reference axes in the body's frontal plane (termed *limb leads*) plus six in the transverse plane (termed *chest leads*). Figure 4-4 demonstrates the orientation of the six limb leads, which are electronically constructed as described in the following paragraphs.

The ECG machine records lead **aVR** by selecting the right arm electrode as the (+) pole with respect to the other electrodes. This is known as a **unipolar** lead, because though there is a (+) pole, there is no single (−) pole; rather, the other limb electrodes are averaged to create a composite (−) reference. When the instantaneous electrical activity of the heart points in the direction of the right arm, an upward deflection is recorded in lead aVR. Conversely, when electrical forces are directed away from the right arm, the ECG inscribes a downward deflection in aVR.

Similarly, lead **aVF** is recorded by setting the left leg as the (+) pole, such that a positive deflection is recorded when forces are directed toward the feet. Lead **aVL** is selected when the left arm electrode made the (+) pole, and it records an upward deflection when electrical activity is aimed in that direction.

In addition to these three unipolar leads, three **bipolar** limb leads are part of the standard ECG recording (Fig. 4-4). Bipolar indicates that one limb electrode is the (+) pole and another single electrode provides the (−) reference. In this case, the ECG machine inscribes an upward deflection if electrical forces are heading toward the (+) electrode and records a downward

TABLE 4-1	Positions of ECG Chest Electrodes
V_1	4th ICS, 2 cm to the right of the sternum
V_2	4th ICS, 2 cm to the left of the sternum
V_3	Midway between V_2 and V_4
V_4	5th ICS, left midclavicular line
V_5	Same level as V_4, left anterior axillary line
V_6	Same level as V_4, left midaxillary line

ICS, intercostal space.

Figure 4-4. The six limb leads are derived from the electrodes placed on the arms and left leg. Top. Each unipolar lead has a single (+) designated electrode; the (−) pole is an average of the other electrodes. **Bottom.** Each bipolar lead has specific (−) and (+) designated electrodes. Although these illustrations show outstretched arms to depict the location of the electrodes, such positioning is not necessary when acquiring a patient's ECG recording. Even in the natural position of the arms by the patient's sides, directionality of the leads is maintained.

deflection if the forces are heading toward the (−) electrode. A simple mnemonic to remember the orientation of the bipolar leads is that the lead name indicates the number of *l*'s in the placement sites. For example, lead I connects the *l*eft arm to the right arm, lead II connects the right arm to the *l*eft *l*eg, and lead III connects the *l*eft arm to the *l*eft *l*eg. Table 4-2 summarizes how the six limb leads are derived.

TABLE 4-2	Limb Leads		
Lead		**(+) Electrode**	**(−) Electrode**
Bipolar leads			
I		LA	RA
II		LL	RA
III		LL	LA
Unipolar leads			
aVR		RA	a
aVL		LA	a
aVF		LL	a

aThe (−) electrode for this lead is constructed by combining the other limb electrodes.
LA, left arm; LL, left leg; RA, right arm.

By overlaying these six limb leads, an axial reference system is established (Fig. 4-5). In the figure, each lead is presented with its (+) pole designated by an arrowhead and the (−) aspect by dashed lines. Note that each 30-degree sector of the circle falls along the (+) or (−) pole of one of the standard six ECG limb leads. Also note that the (+) pole of lead I points to 0 degrees and that, by convention, measurement of the angles proceeds clockwise from 0 degrees as +30 degrees, +60 degrees, and so forth. The complete ECG recording provides a simultaneous "snapshot" of the heart's electrical activity, taken from the perspective of each of these lead reference axes.

Figure 4-5. The axial reference system is created by combining the six limb leads shown in Figure 4-4. Each lead has a (+) region indicated by the *arrowhead* and a (−) region indicated by the *dashed line*.

Figure 4-6 demonstrates how the magnitude and direction of electrical activity are represented by the ECG recording in each lead. This figure should be studied until the following four points are clear:

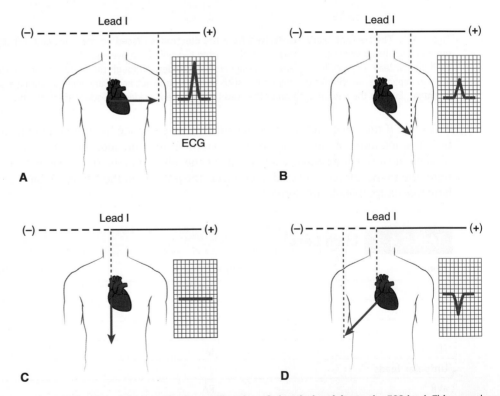

Figure 4-6. Relationship of the magnitude and direction of electrical activity to the ECG lead. This example uses lead I, but the same principles apply to all leads. **A.** Example in which the electrical vector is oriented parallel to lead I and is directed toward the (+) electrode; therefore, a tall upward deflection is recorded by the lead. **B.** Example of a vector that is still oriented toward the (+) electrode of lead I but not parallel to the lead, so that only a component of the force is recorded. Thus, the recorded deflection is still upward but of lower amplitude compared with that shown in **(A). C.** The electrical vector in this example is perpendicular to lead I so that no deflection is generated. **D.** The vector is directed toward the (−) region of lead I, causing the ECG to record a downward deflection.

1. An electrical force directed toward the (+) pole of a lead results in an upward deflection on the ECG recording of that lead.
2. Forces that head away from the (+) electrode result in a downward deflection in that lead.
3. The magnitude of the deflection, either upward or downward, reflects how parallel the electrical force is to the axis of the lead being examined. The more parallel the electrical force is to the lead, the greater the magnitude of the deflection.

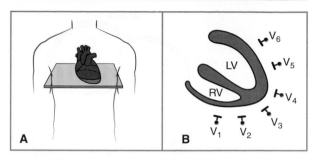

Figure 4-7. The chest (precordial) leads. A. The cross-sectional plane of the chest. **B.** Arrangement of the six chest electrodes shown in the cross-sectional plane. Note that the right ventricle is anterior to the left ventricle.

4. An electrical force directed perpendicular to an electrocardiographic lead does not register any activity by that lead (a flat line on the recording).

The six standard limb leads examine the electrical forces in the frontal plane of the body. However, because electrical activity travels in three dimensions, recordings from a perpendicular plane are also essential (Fig. 4-7). This is accomplished by the use of the six electrodes placed on the anterior and left lateral aspect of the chest (see Fig. 4-3B), creating the chest (also termed "precordial") leads. The orientation of these leads around the heart in the cross-sectional plane is shown in Figure 4-7B. These are unipolar leads, and, as with the unipolar limb leads, electrical forces directed *toward* these individual (+) electrodes result in an upward deflection on the recording of that lead, and forces heading *away* record a downward deflection.

A complete ECG records samples from each of the six limb leads and each of the six chest leads in a standard order, examples of which are presented later in this chapter (see Figs. 4-28-4-36).

SEQUENCE OF NORMAL CARDIAC ACTIVATION

Conduction of electrical impulses through the heart is an orderly process. The normal beat begins at the sinoatrial node, located at the junction of the right atrium and the superior vena cava (Fig. 4-8). The wave of depolarization spreads rapidly through the right and left atria and then reaches the atrioventricular (AV) node, where it encounters an expected delay. The impulse then travels rapidly through the bundle of His and into the right and left bundle branches. The latter divide into the Purkinje fibers, which radiate toward the myocardial fibers, stimulating them to depolarize and contract.

Each heartbeat is represented on the ECG by three major deflections that record the sequence of electrical propagation (see Fig. 4-8B). The **P wave** represents depolarization of the atria. Following the P wave, the tracing returns to its baseline as a result of the conduction delay at the AV node. The second main deflection of the ECG, the **QRS complex,** represents depolarization of the ventricular muscle cells. After the QRS complex, the tracing returns to baseline once again, and after a brief delay, repolarization of the ventricular cells is signaled by the **T wave.** Occasionally, an additional small deflection follows the T wave (the **U wave, see Fig. 4-8C**), which is believed to represent late phases of ventricular repolarization.

The QRS complex may take one of several shapes but can always be subdivided into individual components (Fig. 4-9). If the first deflection of the QRS complex is *downward*, it is known as a Q wave. However, if the initial deflection is upward, then that particular complex *does not have a Q wave.* The R wave is defined as the first *upward* deflection, whether or not a Q wave is present. Any downward deflection *following* the R wave is known as an S wave.

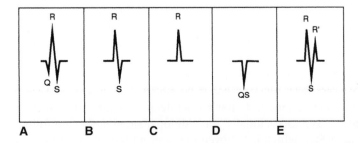

Figure 4-8. Cardiac conduction pathway.
A. The electrical impulse begins at the sinoatrial (SA) node (*1*) then traverses the atria (*2*). After a delay at the AV node (*3*), conduction continues through the bundle of His and into the right and left bundle branches (*4*). The latter divide into Purkinje fibers, which stimulate contraction of the myocardial cells. **B.** Corresponding waveforms on the ECG recording: (*1*) the SA node discharges (too small to generate any deflection on ECG), (*2*) P wave inscribed by depolarization of the atria, (*3*) delay at the AV node, and (*4*) depolarization of the ventricles (QRS complex). The T wave represents ventricular repolarization. **C.** On some ECG recordings, an additional wave of repolarization follows the T wave, termed a U wave.

Figure 4-9 demonstrates several common variations of the QRS complex. In certain pathologic states, such as bundle-branch blocks, additional deflections may be inscribed, as shown in the figure. Please study Figure 4-9 until you can confidently differentiate a Q from an S wave.

Figure 4-10 illustrates the course of normal ventricular depolarization as it is recorded in the frontal plane by two of the ECG leads: aVF and aVL. The recording in aVF represents electrical activity from the perspective of the inferior (ie, underside) aspect of the heart, and aVL records from the perspective of the left lateral side. Recall that in the resting state, the surfaces of myocardial cells are homogeneously charged such that no electrical activity is detected by the external ECG leads and the machine records zero voltage.

The initial portion of ventricular myocardium that is stimulated to depolarize with each cardiac cycle is the midportion of the interventricular septum, on the left side. Because depolarization reverses the cellular charge, the surface of that region becomes negative with respect to the inside,

Figure 4-9. **Examples of QRS complexes. A.** The first deflection is downward (Q wave), followed by an upward deflection (R wave), and then another downward wave (S wave). **B.** Because the first deflection is upward, this complex does *not* have a Q wave; rather, the downward deflection *after* the R wave is an S wave. **C.** A QRS complex without downward deflections lacks Q and S waves. **D.** QRS composed of only a downward deflection; this is simply a Q wave but is often referred to as a QS complex. **E.** A second upward deflection (seen in bundle-branch blocks) is referred to as R'.

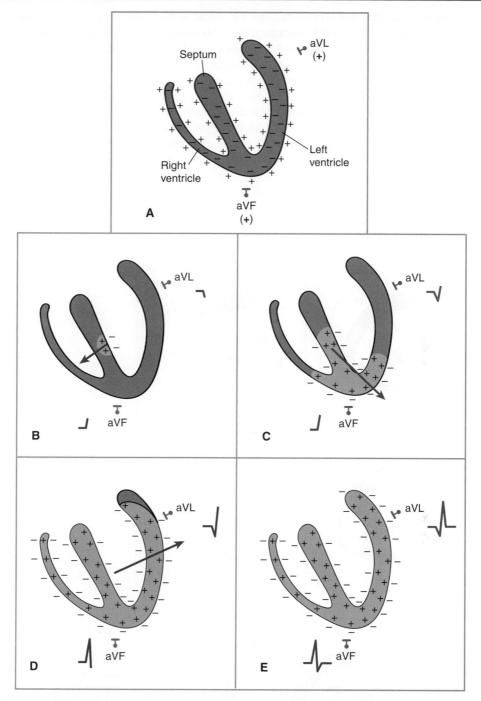

Figure 4-10. Normal ventricular depolarization in the frontal plane as recorded by leads aVL and aVF. A. In the resting state, the surface is homogeneously charged so that the leads do not record any electrical potential. **B.** The first area to depolarize is the left side of the ventricular septum. This results in forces heading away from aVL (downward deflection on aVL recording) but toward the (+) region of aVF, such that an upward deflection is recorded by that lead. **C, D.** Depolarization continues; the forces from the thicker-walled left ventricle outweigh those of the right, such that the electrical vector swings leftward and posteriorly toward aVL (upward deflection) and away from aVF. **E.** At the completion of depolarization, the surface is again homogeneously charged, and no further electrical forces are recorded.

and an electrical potential is generated (see Fig. 4-10B, arrow). The initial current is directed toward the right ventricle and inferiorly. Because the force is directed *away* from the (+) pole region of lead aVL, an initial *downward* deflection is recorded in that lead. At the same time, the electrical force is directed *toward* the (+) pole region of lead aVF, causing an initial *upward* deflection to be recorded there. As the wave of depolarization spreads through the ventricular myocardium, the progression of net electrical vectors is depicted by the series of arrows in Figure 4-10.

As the lateral walls of the ventricles are depolarized, the electrical forces of the thicker left side outweigh those of the right. Therefore, the arrow's orientation is increasingly directed toward the left ventricle (leftward and posteriorly). At the completion of depolarization, the myocytes are again homogeneously charged, no further net electrical force is generated, and the ECG voltage recording returns to baseline in both leads. Thus, in this example of depolarization in a normal heart, lead aVL inscribes an initial small Q wave followed by a tall R wave. Conversely, in lead aVF, there is an initial upward deflection (R wave) followed by a downward S wave.

The sequence of ventricular depolarization can similarly be examined in the transverse (horizontal) plane of the body from the six chest (precordial) leads (Fig. 4-11). Once again,

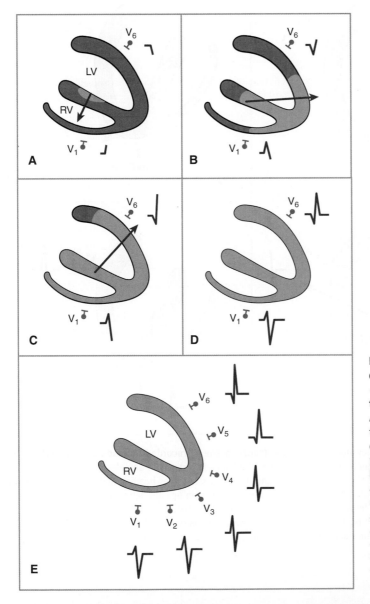

Figure 4-11. Sequence of depolarization in the transverse (horizontal) plane recorded by the chest (precordial) leads. **A-D.** Depolarization begins at the left side of the septum. The electrical vector then progresses posteriorly toward the thick-walled left ventricle. Thus, V_1, which is an anterior lead, records an initial upward deflection followed by a downward wave, whereas V_6, a posterior lead, inscribes the opposite. **E.** In the normal pattern of the QRS from V_1 to V_6, the R wave becomes progressively taller as the S wave becomes less deep.

the first region to depolarize is the midportion of the interventricular septum on the left side. Depolarization proceeds from there toward the right ventricle (which is anterior to the left ventricle), then toward the cardiac apex, and finally around the lateral walls of both ventricles. Because the initial forces are directed anteriorly—that is, toward the ($+$) pole of V_1—the initial deflection recorded by lead V_1 is upward. These same initial forces are directed away from V_6 (which overlies the lateral wall of the left ventricle), so an initial downward deflection is recorded there. As the wave of depolarization spreads, the electrical forces of the left ventricle outweigh those of the right, and the vector swings posteriorly toward the bulk of the left ventricular muscle. As the forces swing away from lead V_1, the deflection there becomes *downward*, whereas it becomes more *upright* in lead V_6. Leads V_2 through V_5 record intermediate steps in this process, such that the R wave becomes progressively taller from lead V_1 through lead V_6 (see Fig. 4-11E), a pattern known as "R-wave progression." Typically, the height of the R wave becomes greater than the depth of the S wave in lead V_3 or V_4; the lead in which this occurs is termed the "transition" lead.

INTERPRETATION OF THE ELECTROCARDIOGRAM

From a technical standpoint, the ECG is recorded on a special grid divided into lines spaced 1 mm apart in both the horizontal and the vertical directions. Each fifth line is made heavier to facilitate measurement. On the vertical axis, voltage is measured in millivolts (mV), and in the standard case, each 1-mm line separation represents 0.1 mV. The horizontal axis represents time. Because the standard recording speed is 25 mm/s, each 1 mm division represents 0.04 seconds and each heavy line (5 mm) represents 0.2 seconds (Fig. 4-12).

Figure 4-12. Enlarged view of an ECG strip. A standard ECG is recorded at 25 mm/s, so that each 1 mm on the horizontal axis represents 0.04 seconds. Each 1 mm on the vertical axis represents 0.1 mV. Measurements in this example are as follows: PR interval (from the beginning of the P wave to the beginning of the QRS) = 4 small boxes = 0.16 seconds; QRS duration (from the beginning to the end of the QRS complex) = 1.75 small boxes = 0.07 seconds; and QT interval (from the beginning of the QRS to the end of the T wave) = 8 small boxes = 0.32 seconds. The corrected QT interval $= \dfrac{QT}{\sqrt{R\text{-}R}}$. Because the RR interval = 15 small boxes (0.6 seconds), the corrected QT interval $= \dfrac{0.32}{\sqrt{0.6}} = 0.41$ seconds.

Many cardiac disorders alter the ECG recording in a diagnostically useful way, and it is important to interpret each tracing in a standard fashion to avoid missing subtle abnormalities. Here is a commonly followed sequence of analysis, followed by a description of each:

1. Check voltage calibration
2. Heart rhythm
3. Heart rate
4. Intervals (PR, QRS, QT)
5. Mean QRS axis
6. Abnormalities of the P wave
7. Abnormalities of the QRS (hypertrophy, bundle-branch block, infarction)
8. Abnormalities of the ST segment and T wave

CALIBRATION

ECG machines routinely inscribe a 1.0-mV vertical signal at the beginning or end of each 12-lead tracing to document the voltage calibration of the machine. In the normal case, each 1-mm vertical box on the ECG represents 0.1 mV, so that the calibration signal records a 10-mm deflection (eg, as shown later in Fig. 4-28). However, in patients with markedly increased voltage of the QRS complex (eg, some patients with left ventricular hypertrophy or bundle-branch blocks), the very large deflections do not fit on the standard tracing. To facilitate interpretation in such a case, the recording is often purposely made at half the standard voltage (ie, each 1-mm box = 0.2 mV), and this is indicated on the ECG tracing by a change in the height of the 1.0-mV calibration signal (at half the standard voltage, the signal would be 5 mm tall). It is important to check the height of the calibration signal on each ECG to ensure that the voltage criteria used to define specific abnormalities are applicable.

HEART RHYTHM

Classifying a patient's heart rhythm requires identification of the P wave and QRS complex and the relationship between them. The normal cardiac rhythm, initiated by depolarization of the sinus node, is known as **sinus rhythm**. An ECG tracing shows sinus rhythm if the following criteria are met: (1) each P wave is followed by a QRS; (2) each QRS is preceded by a P wave; (3) the P wave is upright in leads I, II, and III; and (4) the PR interval is 0.12 seconds or greater (three small boxes).

If the heart rate in sinus rhythm is between 60 and 100 bpm, then **normal sinus rhythm** is present. If <60 bpm, the rhythm is **sinus bradycardia;** if >100 bpm, the rhythm is **sinus tachycardia.** Other abnormal rhythms (termed *arrhythmias* or *dysrhythmias*) are described in Chapters 11 and 12.

HEART RATE

There are several methods for determining the heart rate from an ECG. Three of the most commonly used are presented in Figure 4-13. The standard ECG recording paper speed is 25 mm/s. Using this fact, the heart rate can be calculated exactly by method 1 in Figure 4-13.

It is rarely necessary, however, to determine the *exact* heart rate, and a more rapid estimation can be made with just a bit of memorization. Simply "count off" the number of large boxes between two consecutive QRS complexes, using the sequence

$$300 - 150 - 100 - 75 - 60 - 50$$

which corresponds to the heart rate in beats per minute, as illustrated in Figure 4-13 (method 2).

Method 1   First, count the number of small boxes (1 mm each) between two adjacent QRS complexes (ie, between 2 "beats"). Then, since the standard paper speed is 25 mm/s:

$$\frac{\text{Heart Rate}}{\text{(beats/min)}} = \frac{(25\ \text{mm/s} \times 60\ \text{s/min})}{\text{Number of mm between beats}} = \frac{1500}{\text{number of mm between beats}}$$

In this example, there are 23 mm between the first 2 beats.

23 mm between beats

Therefore, the heart rate $= \dfrac{1500}{23} = 65$ bpm

Method 1 is particularly helpful for measuring fast heart rates (>100 bpm)

Method 2   The "count-off" method requires memorizing the sequence:

300—150—100—75—60—50

Then use this sequence to count the number of large boxes between two consecutive beats:

Start here   300   100   60   150   75   50

The second QRS falls between 75 and 60 bpm; therefore, the heart rate is approximately midway between them ~67 bpm. Knowing that the heart rate is ~60-70 bpm is certainly close enough.

Method 3   ECG recording paper often indicates 3-second time markers at the top or bottom of the tracing:

marker   3 s   marker

To calculate the heart rate, count the number of QRS complexes between the 3-second markers (=6 beats in this example) and multiply by 20. Thus, the heart rate here is ~120 bpm.

It's even easier (and more accurate) to count the number of complexes between the first and third markers on the strip (representing 6 second of the recording) and then multiply by 10 to determine the heart rate.

Method 3 is particularly helpful for measuring irregular heart rates.

Figure 4-13. Methods to calculate heart rate.

When the rhythm is *irregular*, methods 1 and 2 cannot be easily applied, so the heart rate in such a case may be better approximated by counting the number of complexes during 6 seconds of the recording and multiplying that number by 10. ECG paper usually has time markers, spaced 3 seconds apart, printed at the top or bottom of the tracing that facilitates this measurement (see Fig. 4-13, method 3).

INTERVALS (PR, QRS, QT)

The PR interval, QRS interval, and QT interval are measured as demonstrated in Figure 4-12. For each of these, it is appropriate to take the measurement in the lead in which the interval is the longest in duration (the intervals can vary a bit in each lead). The **PR interval** is measured from the onset of the P wave to the onset of the QRS. The **QRS interval** is measured from the beginning to the end of the QRS complex. The **QT interval** is measured from the beginning of the QRS to the end of the T wave. The normal ranges of the intervals are listed in Table 4-3, along with conditions associated with abnormal values.

Because the QT interval varies with heart rate (the faster the heart rate, the shorter the QT), the **corrected QT interval** (QTc) is determined by dividing the measured QT by the square root of the RR interval (see Fig. 4-12). This is also shown at the bottom of Table 4-3 and is known as the Bazett formula. More simply, when the heart rate is in the normal range (60-100 bpm), a rapid rule can be applied: if the QT interval is visually less than half the interval between two consecutive QRS complexes, then the QT interval is within the normal range.

MEAN QRS AXIS

The mean QRS axis represents the average of the instantaneous electrical forces generated during the sequence of ventricular depolarization as measured in the frontal plane. The normal range is defined as between −30 degrees and +90 degrees (Fig. 4-14). A mean axis that is more negative than −30 degrees implies **left axis deviation**, whereas an axis greater than +90 degrees represents **right axis deviation**. The mean axis can be determined precisely by plotting the QRS complexes of different leads on the axial reference diagram for the limb leads (see Fig. 4-5), but this is tedious and is not necessary. The following rapid approach to axis determination generally provides sufficient accuracy.

First, recall from Figure 4-5 that each ECG lead has a (+) region and a (−) region. Electrical activity directed toward the (+) half results in an upward deflection, whereas activity toward the (−) half results in a downward deflection on the ECG recording of that lead. To determine whether the axis is normal or abnormal, examine the QRS complexes in limb leads I and II. As illustrated in Figure 4-15, if the QRS is primarily positive in both of these leads

TABLE 4-3	Electrocardiographic Intervals		
Interval	Normal	Decreased Interval	Increased Interval
PR	0.12-0.20 s (3-5 small boxes)	• Preexcitation syndrome • Junctional rhythm	• First-degree AV block
QRS	≤0.10 s (≤2.5 small boxes)		• Bundle-branch blocks • Ventricular ectopic beat • Toxic drug effect (eg, certain antiarrhythmic drugs—see Chapter 17) • Severe hyperkalemia
QT	Corrected QT[a] ≤0.44 s	• Hypercalcemia • Tachycardia	• Hypocalcemia • Hypokalemia (↑ QU interval owing to ↑ U wave) • Hypomagnesemia • Myocardial ischemia • Congenital prolongation of QT • Toxic drug effect

[a] Corrected QT $= \dfrac{QT}{\sqrt{R\text{-}R}}$.

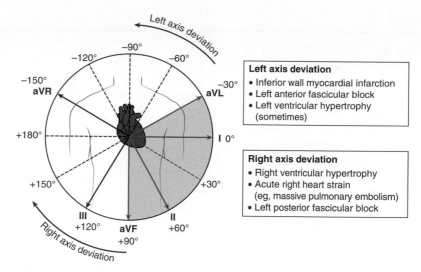

Left axis deviation
• Inferior wall myocardial infarction
• Left anterior fascicular block
• Left ventricular hypertrophy
  (sometimes)

Right axis deviation
• Right ventricular hypertrophy
• Acute right heart strain
  (eg, massive pulmonary embolism)
• Left posterior fascicular block

Figure 4-14. A normal mean QRS axis falls within the shaded area (between −30 degrees and +90 degrees).
A mean axis more negative than −30 degrees is termed *left axis deviation*, whereas an axis more positive than +90 degrees is *right axis deviation*. The figure shows common conditions that result in axis deviation.

If the QRS complex is mainly upward (positive) in limb lead I, then the mean axis falls within the "+" region of that lead, shown as the blue half of the circle below.

Similarly, if the QRS is predominantly upward in limb lead II, then the mean axis falls within the "+" half of lead II, shown as the red half here.

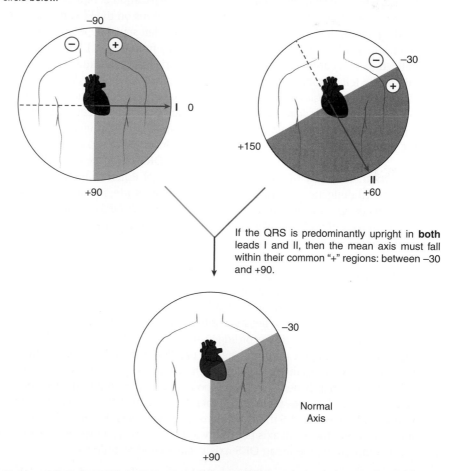

If the QRS is predominantly upright in **both** leads I and II, then the mean axis must fall within their common "+" regions: between −30 and +90.

Figure 4-15. The mean axis is within the normal range if the QRS complex is predominantly upright in limb leads I and II.

(ie, the upward deflection is greater than the downward deflection in each of them), then the mean vector falls within the normal range, and no further calculation is necessary. However, if the QRS in *either* lead I or II is not primarily upward, then the axis is *abnormal*, and the approximate axis should then be determined by the more precise method described in the following paragraphs. Please be aware that some ECG teaching resources recommend examining leads I and aVF, rather than leads I and II, to determine whether the mean axis falls in the normal range. However, using leads I and aVF for this purpose would erroneously classify a mean axis between 0 degrees and −30 degrees as being abnormal, as lead aVF would record a primarily downward deflection in that case. Examining leads I and II instead avoids that error.

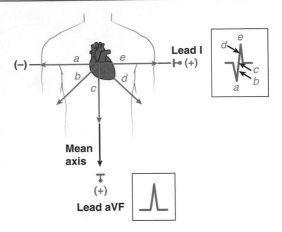

Figure 4-16. Example of the sequence of ventricular depolarization when the mean axis is +90 degrees. Because the mean axis is perpendicular to limb lead I, an isoelectric QRS complex (height of upward deflection = height of downward deflection) is recorded by that lead (see text for details).

To understand how to determine the mean axis with greater precision when necessary, first consider the special example demonstrated in Figure 4-16. The sequence of a ventricular depolarization is represented in this figure by vectors *a* through *e*, along with the corresponding deflections on the ECG recording of lead I. In this particular patient, the initial deflection (representing left septal depolarization) points to the patient's right side. Because it is directed completely away from the (+) pole of lead I, a strong downward deflection is recorded by the lead. As depolarization continues, the arrow swings downward and to the left, resulting in less negative deflections in lead I. After arrow *c*, the electrical vector swings into the positive region of lead I, so that upward deflections are recorded.

Note that in this special example, in which electrical forces begin exactly opposite lead I's (+) electrode and terminate when pointed directly at that electrode, the mean electrical vector points straight downward (in the direction of arrow *c*), *perpendicular* to the lead I axis. Also note the configuration of the inscribed QRS complex in lead I. There is a downward deflection, followed by an upward deflection of equal magnitude (when the upward and downward deflections of a QRS are of equal magnitude, it is termed an **isoelectric complex**). Thus, *when an ECG limb lead inscribes an isoelectric QRS complex, it indicates that the mean electrical axis of the ventricles is perpendicular to that particular lead.*

Therefore, an easy way to determine the mean QRS axis is to glance at the six limb lead recordings and observe which one has the most isoelectric-appearing complex: the mean axis is simply perpendicular to it. One step remains. When the mean axis is perpendicular to a lead, it could be perpendicular in either a clockwise *or* a counterclockwise direction. In the example of Figure 4-16, the isoelectric complex appears in lead I, such that the mean vector could be at +90 degrees *or* it could be at −90 degrees, because both are perpendicular. To determine which of these is correct requires inspecting the recording of the ECG lead that is perpendicular to the one inscribing the isoelectric complex (and is therefore parallel to the mean axis). If the QRS is predominantly upright in that perpendicular lead, then the mean vector points toward the (+) pole of that lead. If it is predominantly negative, then it points away from the lead's (+) pole. In the example, the isoelectric complex appears in lead I; therefore, the next step is to inspect the perpendicular lead, which is aVF (see Fig. 4-5 if this relationship is not clear). Because the QRS complex in aVF is primarily upward, the mean axis points toward its (+) pole, which is in fact located at +90 degrees.

To summarize, the mean QRS axis is calculated as follows:

1. Inspect limb leads I and II. If the QRS is primarily upward in both, then the axis is normal and you are done. If not, then proceed to the next step.

2. Inspect the six limb leads and determine which one contains the QRS that is most isoelectric. The mean axis is perpendicular to that lead.

3. Inspect the lead that is perpendicular to the lead containing the isoelectric complex. If the QRS in that perpendicular lead is primarily upward, then the mean axis points to the (+) pole of that lead. If primarily negative, then the mean QRS points to the (−) pole of that lead.

Conditions that result in left or right axis deviation are listed in Figure 4-14. In addition, the vertical position of the heart in many normal children and adolescents may result in a mean axis that is slightly rightward (greater than +90 degrees).

In some patients, isoelectric complexes are inscribed in *all* the limb leads. That situation arises when the heart is tilted, so that the mean QRS points straight forward or back from the frontal plane, as it may be in patients with chronic obstructive lung disease; in such a case, the mean axis is said to be *indeterminate.*

ABNORMALITIES OF THE **P** WAVE

The P wave represents depolarization of the right atrium followed quickly by the depolarization of the left atrium; the two components are nearly superimposed on one another (Fig. 4-17). The P wave is usually best visualized in lead II, the lead that is most parallel to the flow of electrical current through the atria from the sinoatrial to the AV node. When the *right* atrium is enlarged, the initial component of the P wave is larger than normal (the P is taller than 2.5 mm in lead II).

Left atrial enlargement is best observed in lead V_1. Normally, V_1 inscribes a P wave with an initial positive deflection reflecting right atrial depolarization (directed anteriorly), followed by a negative deflection, owing to the left atrial forces oriented posteriorly (see Fig. 1-2 for anatomic relationships). Left atrial enlargement is therefore manifested by a greater-than-normal negative deflection (at least 1 mm wide and 1 mm deep) in lead V_1 (see Fig. 4-17).

ABNORMALITIES OF THE **QRS** COMPLEX

Ventricular Hypertrophy

Hypertrophy of the left or right ventricle causes the affected chamber to generate greater-than-normal electrical activity. Ordinarily, the thicker-walled left ventricle produces forces that are more prominent than those of the right. However, in **right ventricular hypertrophy** (RVH), the augmented right-sided forces may outweigh those of the left. Therefore, chest leads V_1 and V_2, which overlie the right ventricle, record greater-than-normal upward deflections: the R wave becomes taller than the S wave in those leads, the opposite of the normal situation

Figure 4-17. The P wave represents superimposition of right atrial (RA) and left atrial (LA) depolarization. RA depolarization occurs slightly earlier than LA depolarization, because of the proximity of the RA to the sinoatrial node. In RA enlargement, the initial component of the P wave is prominent (>2.5 mm tall) in lead II. In LA enlargement, there is a large terminal downward deflection in lead V_1 (>1 mm wide and >1 mm deep).

	Lead II	Lead V_1
Normal	RA·····⌒····· LA·····⌒····· Combined	····⌒···· ····⌣····
RA enlargement (P height > 2.5 mm in lead II)	RA⌒LA	RA⌒LA
LA enlargement (Negative P in V_1 >1 mm wide and >1 mm deep)	RA⌒LA	RA⌣LA

Figure 4-18. Ventricular hypertrophy. The *arrows* indicate the sequence of average electrical forces during ventricular depolarization. **A.** Right ventricular (RV) hypertrophy. The RV forces outweigh those of the left, resulting in tall R waves in leads V_1 and V_2 and a deep S wave in lead V_6 (compare to normal QRS complexes in Fig. 4-11E). **B.** Left ventricular (LV) hypertrophy exaggerates the normal pattern of depolarization, with greater-than-normal forces directed toward the LV, resulting in a tall R wave in V_6 and a deep S wave in lead V_1.

(Fig. 4-18). In addition, the increased right ventricular mass shifts the mean axis of the heart, resulting in right axis deviation (mean axis greater than +90 degrees).

In **left ventricular hypertrophy**, greater-than-normal forces are generated by that chamber, which simply exaggerates the normal situation. Leads that directly overlie the left ventricle (chest leads V_5 and V_6 and limb leads I and aVL) show taller-than-normal R waves. Leads on the other side of the heart (V_1 and V_2) demonstrate the opposite: deeper-than-normal S waves. Many different criteria are used for the diagnosis of left ventricular hypertrophy by ECG. Three of the most helpful criteria are listed in Figure 4-18.

Bundle-Branch Blocks

Interruption of conduction through the right or left bundle branches may develop from ischemic or degenerative damage. As a result, the affected ventricle does not depolarize in the normal sequence. Rather than rapid uniform stimulation by the Purkinje fibers, the cells of that ventricle must rely on relatively slow myocyte-to-myocyte spread of electrical activity traveling from the unaffected ventricle. This delayed process prolongs depolarization and widens the QRS complex. A normal QRS duration is ≤0.10 seconds (≤2.5 small boxes). When a bundle-branch block widens the QRS duration to 0.10-0.12 seconds (2.5-3.0 small boxes), an *incomplete* bundle-branch block is present. If the QRS duration is >0.12 seconds (3.0 small boxes), *complete* bundle-branch block is identified.

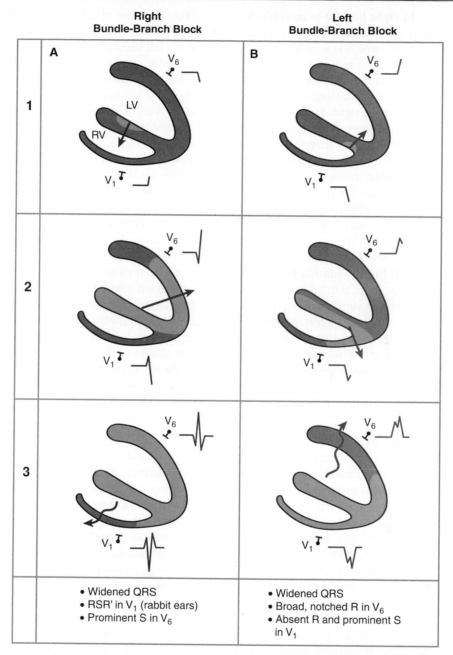

Figure 4-19. Bundle-branch blocks. Schematic view of the ventricles in the horizontal plane showing that · interruption of conduction through the right or left bundles results in delayed, slowed activation of the respective ventricle and widening of the QRS complex. The *blue color* shows progressive depolarization of the ventricles, and the *red arrows* show the sequence of electrical vectors that result. **A.** In **right bundle-branch block**, normal initial activation of the septum (*1*) is followed by depolarization of the left ventricle (*2*). Slow cell-to-cell spread activates the right ventricle (RV) *after* the left ventricle (LV) has nearly fully depolarized (*3*), so that the late forces generated by the RV are unopposed. Therefore, V_1 records an abnormal terminal upward deflection (R'), and V_6 records an abnormal, terminal deep S wave, as shown in panel *3*. **B.** In **left bundle-branch block**, the initial septal depolarization is blocked, such that the first forces are oriented from right to left. Thus, the normal initial R wave in V_1 and Q wave in V_6 are absent (*1*). After the RV depolarizes (*2*), late, slow activation of the LV results in a terminal upward deflection in V_6 and downward deflection in V_1 (*3*).

In **right bundle-branch block** (RBBB) (Fig. 4-19; see also Fig. 4-29), normal depolarization of the right ventricle is interrupted. In this case, initial depolarization of the ventricular septum (which is stimulated by a branch of the left bundle) is unaffected so that the normal small R wave in lead V_1 and small Q wave in lead V_6 are recorded. As the wave of depolarization spreads down the septum and into the left ventricular free wall, the sequence of depolarization is indistinguishable from normal, because left ventricular forces *normally* outweigh those of the right. However, by the time the left ventricle has almost fully depolarized, slow cell-to-cell spread has finally reached the "blocked" right ventricle and depolarization of that chamber begins, unopposed by left ventricular activity (because that chamber has nearly fully depolarized). This prolonged depolarization process widens the QRS complex and produces a late depolarization current in the direction of the anteriorly situated right ventricle. Since the terminal portion of the QRS complex in RBBB represents these right ventricular forces acting alone, the ECG records an abnormal terminal *upward* deflection (known as an R′ wave) over the right ventricle in lead V_1 and a downward deflection (S wave) in V_6 on the opposite side of the heart. The appearance of the QRS complex in lead V_1 in RBBB (upward R, downward S, then upward R′) is often described as having the appearance of "rabbit ears."

Left bundle-branch block (LBBB) produces even more prominent QRS abnormalities. In this situation, normal initial depolarization of the left septum does *not* occur; rather, the right side of the ventricular septum is first to depolarize, through branches of the right bundle. Thus, the initial forces of depolarization are directed toward the left ventricle instead of the right (see Fig. 4-19B; see also Fig. 4-30). Therefore, an initial *downward* deflection is recorded in V_1, and the normal small Q wave in V_6 is absent. Only after depolarization of the right ventricle does slow cell-to-cell spread reach the left ventricular myocytes. These slowly conducted forces inscribe a widened QRS complex with abnormal terminally upward deflections in the leads overlying the left ventricle (eg, V_5 and V_6), as shown in Figure 4-19B.

Fascicular Blocks

Recall from Chapter 1 that the left bundle branch subdivides into two main divisions, termed fascicles: the left anterior fascicle and the left posterior fascicle. Although LBBB implies that conduction is blocked in the entire left bundle branch, impairment can also occur in just one of the two fascicles, resulting in left anterior or left posterior fascicular blocks (also termed *hemiblocks*). The main significance of fascicular blocks in ECG interpretation is that they can markedly alter the mean QRS axis.

Anatomically, the anterior fascicle of the left bundle runs along the front of the left ventricle toward the anterior papillary muscle (which is located in the anterior and superior portion of the chamber), whereas the posterior fascicle travels to the posterior papillary muscle (which is located in the posterior, inferior, and medial aspect of the left ventricle). Under normal conditions, conduction via the left anterior and left posterior fascicles proceeds simultaneously, such that electrical activation of the left ventricle is uniform, spreading outward from the bases of the two papillary muscles. However, if conduction is blocked in one of the two divisions, then initial LV depolarization arises exclusively from the unaffected fascicle (Fig. 4-20).

In the case of **left anterior fascicular block (LAFB)**, left ventricular activation begins via the left posterior fascicle alone, at the posterior papillary muscle, and then spreads to the rest of the ventricle. Because the left posterior fascicle first activates the posterior, inferior, medial region of the left ventricle, the initial impulses are directed downward (ie, toward the feet) and toward the patient's right side (see Fig. 4-20). This results in a positive deflection (initial small R wave) in the inferior leads (leads II, III, and aVF) and a negative deflection (small Q wave) in the left lateral leads, I and aVL. As depolarization then spreads upward and to the left, toward the "blocked" anterior, superior, and lateral regions of the left ventricle, a positive deflection (R wave) is inscribed in leads I and aVL, while a negative deflection (S wave) develops in the inferior leads. The predominance of these leftward forces, resulting from the abnormal activation of the anterior superior left ventricular wall, results in *left axis deviation*. A complete 12-lead ECG demonstrating the pattern of LAFB is shown later (see Fig. 4-34).

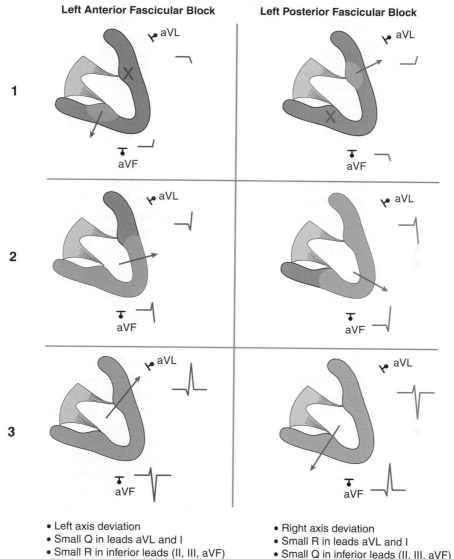

- Left axis deviation
- Small Q in leads aVL and I
- Small R in inferior leads (II, III, aVF)

- Right axis deviation
- Small R in leads aVL and I
- Small Q in inferior leads (II, III, aVF)

Figure 4-20. Left anterior and left posterior fascicular blocks and their patterns in the ECG limb leads. The schematic at the top of the figure shows the left ventricle (LV) in the frontal plane. The mitral valve (MV) chordae tendineae insert into the anterior (A) and posterior (P) papillary muscles, which are important landmarks: the anterior fascicle of the left bundle branch courses toward the anterior papillary muscle, whereas the posterior fascicle travels to the posterior papillary muscle (the fascicles are not shown). Notice that the anterior papillary muscle is *superior* to the posterior papillary muscle. **Left side of the figure.** In left anterior fascicular block, activation begins solely in the region of the posterior papillary muscle (*1*) because initial conduction to the anterior papillary muscle is blocked (denoted by the *red X*). As a result, the initial forces of depolarization are directed downward toward the feet, producing an initial positive deflection (R wave) in lead aVF and a negative deflection (Q wave) in lead aVL. As the wave of depolarization spreads toward the left side and superiorly, aVF begins to register a negative deflection, and aVL starts to record a positive deflection (*2*). Panel *3* shows the complete QRS complexes at the end of depolarization. **Right side of the figure.** In left posterior fascicular block (denoted by the *red X*), LV activation begins solely in the region of the anterior papillary muscle (*1*). Thus, the initial forces are directed upward and toward the patient's left side, producing an initial R wave in aVL and a Q wave in aVF. Panels *2* and *3* show how the spread of depolarization travels in the direction opposite that of LAFB.

Left posterior fascicular block (LPFB) is less common than LAFB. In LPFB, ventricular activation begins via the left anterior fascicle alone at the base of the anterior papillary muscle (see Fig. 4-20). As that anterosuperior left ventricular region depolarizes, the initial forces are directed upward and to the patient's left (creating a positive R wave in leads I and aVL and a negative Q wave in the inferior leads). As the impulse then spreads downward and to the right toward the initially blocked region, an S wave is inscribed in leads I and aVL, while an R wave is recorded in leads II, III, and aVF. Because the bulk of these delayed forces head toward the patient's right side, *right axis deviation* of the QRS mean axis occurs (see Fig. 4-36).

In contrast to RBBBs and LBBBs, LAFB and LPFB do not result in significant widening of the QRS because rapidly conducting Purkinje fibers bridge the territories served by the anterior and posterior fascicles. Therefore, although the sequence of conduction is altered, the total time required for depolarization is usually only slightly prolonged. Also note that although LBBBs and RBBBs are most easily recognized by analyzing the patterns of depolarization in the precordial (chest) leads, in the case of LAFB and LPFB, it is the recordings in the limb leads (as in Fig. 4-20) that are most helpful.

A   Normal Q waves

B   Pathologic Q waves

Figure 4-21. Normal vs pathologic Q waves. Compared with the small Q waves generated during normal depolarization (**A**, *blue arrow*), pathologic Q waves are more prominent with a width ≥1 mm (1 small box) or depth >25% of the height of the QRS complex (**B**, *green arrow*).

Pathologic Q Waves in Myocardial Infarction

As you will learn in Chapter 7, sudden complete occlusion of a coronary artery typically results in a syndrome known as *acute ST-segment elevation myocardial infarction* (STEMI). When this occurs, a sequence of abnormalities of the ST segment and T wave evolves over a period of hours, as described in the next section. Unless reperfusion of the occluded artery is quickly achieved, irreversible necrosis of the heart muscle served by that vessel ensues and is marked by the formation of **pathologic Q waves** as part of the electrocardiographic QRS complex.

Recall that it is normal for small initial Q waves to appear in some of the ECG leads. For example, initial septal depolarization routinely inscribes small Q waves in leads V_6 and aVL. Such physiologic Q waves are of short duration (≤0.04 seconds or 1 small box) and of low magnitude (<25% of the QRS total height). In distinction, pathologic Q waves are more prominent (Fig. 4-21; also see Fig. 4-29), typically having a width ≥1 small box in duration or a depth >25% of the total height of the QRS. The ECG lead groupings in which pathologic Q waves appear reflect the anatomic site of the infarction (Table 4-4; also see Fig. 4-23).

Pathologic Q waves develop in the leads overlying infarcted tissue because necrotic muscle does not generate electrical forces (Fig. 4-22). This results in an imbalance whereby electrical

TABLE 4-4   Localization of Myocardial Infarction

Anatomic Site	Leads With Abnormal ECG Complexes[a]	Coronary Artery Most Often Responsible
Inferior	II, III, aVF	RCA
Anteroseptal	V_1-V_2	LAD
Anteroapical	V_3-V_4	LAD (distal)
Anterolateral	V_5-V_6, I, aVL	CFX
Posterior	V_1-V_2 (tall R wave, not Q wave)	RCA

[a]Pathologic Q waves in all of leads V_1-V_6 implies an "extensive anterior MI" usually associated with a proximal left coronary artery occlusion.
CFX, left circumflex coronary artery; LAD, left anterior descending coronary artery; RCA, right coronary artery.

forces generated by other regions of healthy myocardium become abnormally unopposed. Thus, the ECG electrode over the infarcted region detects electrical currents from the healthy tissue on opposite regions of the ventricle, which are directed *away* from the infarct and the recording electrode, thus inscribing the downward deflection. Q waves are permanent evidence of an ST-elevation type of myocardial infarction with tissue necrosis; only rarely do they disappear over time.

Notice in Table 4-4 that in the case of a posterior wall myocardial infarction (see Fig. 4-23A), it is not pathologic Q waves that are evident on the ECG. Because standard electrodes are not typically placed on the patient's back overlying the posterior wall, other leads must be relied on to indirectly identify the presence of such an infarction. Chest leads V_1 and V_2, which are directly opposite the posterior wall, record the *inverse* of what leads placed on the back would demonstrate. Therefore, *taller-than-normal R waves in leads V_1 and V_2* are the equivalent of pathologic Q waves in the diagnosis of a posterior wall MI. It may be recalled that RVH also produces tall R waves in leads V_1 and V_2. These conditions can be distinguished, however, as RVH causes right axis deviation, which is not a feature of posterior wall MI.

It is important to note that if a Q wave appears in only a single ECG lead, it is not diagnostic of an infarction. True pathologic Q waves should appear in the groupings listed in Table 4-4 and Figure 4-23. For example, if a pathologic Q wave is present in lead III but not in II or aVF, it likely does not indicate an infarction. Also, Q waves are *disregarded* in lead aVR because electrical forces are *normally* directed away from the right arm. In the presence of LBBB, Q waves are usually not helpful in the diagnosis of MI because of the markedly abnormal pattern of depolarization in that condition.

ST-SEGMENT AND T-WAVE ABNORMALITIES

Transient Myocardial Ischemia

Among the most important abnormalities of the ST segments and T waves are those related to coronary artery disease. Because ventricular repolarization is very sensitive to myocardial perfusion, reversible deviations of the ST segments and T waves (usually depression of the ST segment and/or inversion of the T wave) are common during transient episodes of myocardial ischemia, as will be explained in Chapter 6.

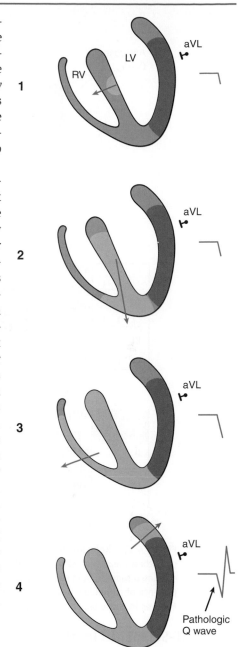

Figure 4-22. Sequence of depolarization recorded by lead aVL, overlying a lateral wall infarction (*dark shaded region*). A pathologic Q wave is recorded because the necrotic muscle does not generate electrical forces; rather, at the time when the lateral wall *should* be depolarizing (panel *3*), the activation of the healthy muscle on the *opposite* side of the heart is unopposed, such that net forces are directed away from aVL. The terminal R wave recorded by aVL reflects depolarization of the remaining viable myocardium beyond the infarct.

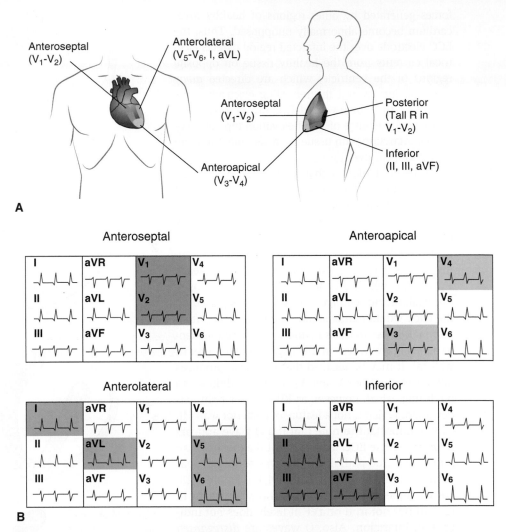

Figure 4-23. Relationship between ECG leads and cardiac anatomic regions. A. The lead groupings listed in parentheses represent each region. **B.** Miniaturized 12-lead ECG schematic drawings showing the standard orientation of printed samples from each lead. The major anatomic groupings are colored and labeled in each drawing. While the presence of pathologic Q waves in leads V_1 and V_2 are indicative of anteroseptal infarction, be aware that *tall initial R waves* in those leads can indicate a posterior wall infarction (not shown in part **B**), as described in the text.

Acute ST-Segment Elevation MI

As described in the previous section, pathologic Q waves can develop following one major type of myocardial infarction (STEMI) but do not differentiate between an acute event and an MI that occurred weeks or years earlier. However, an *acute* STEMI results in a temporal sequence of ST and T-wave abnormalities that permits this distinction (Fig. 4-24). The initial abnormality is elevation of the ST segment, often with a peaked appearance of the T wave. At this early stage, myocardial cells are still viable and Q waves have not yet developed. In patients who achieve successful acute coronary reperfusion (by fibrinolytic therapy or percutaneous coronary intervention, as described in Chapter 7), the ST segments return to baseline, and the sequence of changes described in the next paragraph do not occur.

In patients who *do not* achieve successful acute reperfusion, within several hours myocyte death leads to loss of the amplitude of the R wave and pathologic Q waves begin to be inscribed by the ECG leads positioned over the infarction territory. During the first 1-2 days following infarction, the ST segments remain elevated, the T wave inverts, and the Q wave

Normal   Acute   Hours   Day 1-2   Days   Weeks
                                                       later   later

- ST elevation   • ST elevation   • T-wave inversion • ST normalizes   • ST & T normal
                  • ↓R wave   • Q wave deeper   • T wave inverted   • Q wave persists
                  • Q wave begins

Figure 4-24. ECG evolution during acute ST-elevation myocardial infarction. However, as described in Chapter 7, if successful early reperfusion of the coronary occlusion is achieved, the initially elevated ST segment returns to baseline without subsequent T-wave inversion or Q-wave development.

deepens (see Fig. 4-24). Several days later, the ST-segment elevation returns to baseline, but the T waves remain inverted. Weeks or months following the infarct, the ST segment and T waves have usually returned to normal, but the pathologic Q waves persist, a permanent marker of the MI. If the ST segment *remains* elevated several weeks later, it is likely that a bulging fibrotic scar (ventricular aneurysm) has developed at the site of infarction.

These evolutionary changes of the QRS, ST, and T waves are recorded by the leads overlying the zone of infarction (see Table 4-4 and Fig. 4-23). Typically, *reciprocal* changes are observed in leads opposite that site. For example, in acute anteroseptal MI, ST-segment elevation is expected in chest leads V_1 and V_2; simultaneously, however, reciprocal changes (ST *depression*) may be inscribed by the leads overlying the opposite (inferior) region, namely in leads II, III, and aVF. An example of reciprocal ST changes is shown later in Figure 4-32.

The mechanism by which ST-segment deviations develop during acute MI has not been established with certainty. It is believed, however, that the abnormality results from injured myocardial cells immediately adjacent to the infarct zone producing abnormal diastolic or systolic currents. One explanation, the *diastolic current theory*, contends that these damaged cells are capable of depolarization but are abnormally "leaky," allowing ionic flow that prevents the cells from fully repolarizing (Fig. 4-25). Because the surface of such partially depolarized cells in the resting state would be relatively negatively charged compared with normal fully repolarized zones, an electrical current is generated between the two regions. This current is directed away from the more negatively charged ischemic area, causing the baseline of the ECG leads overlying that region to *shift downward*. Because the ECG machine records only *relative* position, rather than absolute voltages, the downward deviation of the baseline is not apparent. Following ventricular depolarization (indicated by the QRS complex), after *all* the myocardial cells have fully depolarized (including those of the injured zone), the net electrical potential surrounding the heart is *true zero*. However, compared with the abnormally displaced downward baseline, the ST segment *appears* elevated (see Fig. 4-25). As the myocytes then repolarize, the injured cells return to the abnormal state of diastolic ion leak, and the ECG again inscribes the abnormally depressed baseline. Thus, ST elevation in acute STEMI may in part reflect an abnormal shift of the recording baseline.

The *systolic current theory* of ST segment shifts contends that in addition to altering the resting membrane potential, ischemic injury shortens the action potential duration of affected cells. As a result, the ischemic cells repolarize faster than neighboring normal myocytes. Since the positive surface charge of the damaged myocytes is restored earlier than that of the normal cells, a voltage gradient develops between the two zones, creating an electrical current directed *toward* the ischemic area. This gradient occurs during the ST interval of the ECG, resulting in ST elevation in the leads overlying the ischemic region (Fig. 4-26).

Acute Non–ST-Segment Elevation MI

As described in Chapter 7, not all acute myocardial infarctions result in ST-segment elevation and potential Q-wave development. A more limited type of infarction, known as acute *non–ST-elevation MI* (NSTEMI), typically results from an acute *partially* occlusive coronary

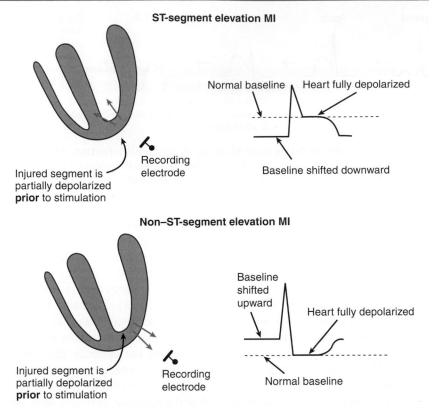

Figure 4-25. ST deviations in acute MI: diastolic injury current. Top. Ionic leak results in partial depolarization of injured myocardium in diastole, prior to electrical stimulation, which produces forces heading away from that site and shifts the ECG baseline downward. This is not noticeable on the ECG because only relative, not absolute, voltages are recorded. Following stimulation, when the entire myocardium has fully depolarized, the voltage is true zero but gives the appearance of ST elevation compared with the abnormally depressed baseline. **Bottom.** In non–ST-segment elevation MI, the process is similar, but the ionic leak typically arises from the subendocardial tissue. As a result, the partial depolarization before stimulation results in electrical forces directed *toward* the recording electrode; hence, the baseline is shifted *upward*. When fully depolarized, the voltage is true zero, but the ST segment *appears* depressed compared with the shifted baseline.

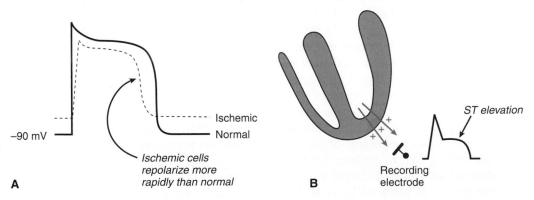

Figure 4-26. ST deviation in acute ST-segment elevation MI: systolic injury current. A. Compared with normal myocytes (*solid line*), ischemic myocytes (*dashed line*) display a reduced resting membrane potential and repolarize more rapidly. **B.** More rapid repolarization causes the surface of the ischemic zone to be relatively positively charged at the time the ST segment is inscribed. The associated electrical current (*arrows*) is directed *toward* the recording electrode overlying that site, so that the ST segment is abnormally elevated.

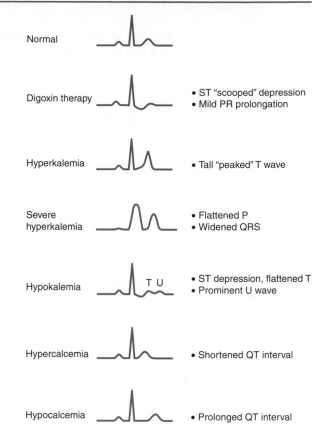

Normal

Digoxin therapy
- ST "scooped" depression
- Mild PR prolongation

Hyperkalemia
- Tall "peaked" T wave

Severe hyperkalemia
- Flattened P
- Widened QRS

Hypokalemia   T U
- ST depression, flattened T
- Prominent U wave

Hypercalcemia
- Shortened QT interval

Figure 4-27. Conditions that alter repolarization of myocytes and result in ST-segment and T-wave abnormalities.

Hypocalcemia
- Prolonged QT interval

thrombus. In such infarctions, it is ST-segment depression and/or T-wave inversion, rather than ST elevation, that appears in the leads overlying the infarcting myocardium.

The extent of myocardial damage with this form of infarction is less than in STEMI, often involving only the subendocardial layers of the myocardium. As a result, pathologic Q waves do not develop, because the remaining viable cells are able to generate some electrical activity.

In NSTEMI, the diastolic current theory maintains that diastolic ionic leak of injured cells adjacent to the subendocardial infarct zone generates electrical forces directed from the inner endocardium to the outer epicardium and therefore toward the overlying ECG electrode. Thus, the baseline of the ECG is shifted *upward* (see Fig. 4-25, bottom). Following full cardiac depolarization, the electrical potential of the heart returns to true zero but, relative to the abnormal baseline, gives the appearance of ST-segment *depression*.

In addition to myocardial ischemia and infarction, there are several other causes of ST-segment and T-wave abnormalities that result from alterations in myocyte repolarization. The most commonly encountered of these are illustrated in Figure 4-27.

Summary

- The electrocardiogram (ECG) depicts the sequence of electrical impulses through the heart.
- A complete ECG (12-lead ECG) is produced by recording electrical activity between the electrodes in specific patterns, which results in six **reference axes** in the body's frontal plane (limb leads) plus six in the transverse plane (chest leads).
- Each heartbeat is represented on the ECG by three major deflections that record the sequence of electrical propagation: (1) the **P wave** represents depolarization of the

atria, (2) the **QRS complex** records depolarization of the ventricular muscle cells, and (3) the **T wave** indicates repolarization of the ventricular cells.

- Many cardiac disorders alter the ECG recording in a diagnostically useful way, and it is important to interpret each tracing in a consistent fashion to avoid missing subtle abnormalities: (1) check **voltage calibration**, (2) **heart rhythm**, (3) **heart rate**, (4) **intervals** (PR, QRS, QT), (5) **mean QRS axis**, (6) abnormalities of the **P wave**, (7) abnormalities of the **QRS** (hypertrophy, bundle-branch block, pathologic Q waves), and (8) abnormalities of the **ST segment and T wave** (Table 4-5).

- **Examples of normal and abnormal ECGs** are presented in 4-28-4-36. Using Table 4-5 as a guide, try to systematically assess the findings in these tracings before looking at the complete interpretations in the figure legends. For more extensive practice, the reader is referred to any of the complete ECG texts and guides listed under "Additional Reading."

TABLE 4-5 Summary of Sequence of ECG Interpretation

1. **Calibration**
   - Check 1.0-mV vertical box inscription (normal standard = 10 mm)
2. **Rhythm**
   - Sinus rhythm is present if:
     - Each P wave is followed by a QRS complex
     - Each QRS is preceded by a P wave
     - P wave is upright in leads I, II, and III
     - PR interval is >0.12 s (3 small boxes)
   - If these criteria are not met, determine type of arrhythmia (see Chapter 12)
3. **Heart rate**
   - Use one of three methods:
     - 1500/(number of mm between beats)
     - Count-off method: 300—150—100—75—60—50
     - Number of beats in 6 s × 10
   - Normal rate = 60-100 bpm (bradycardia <60, tachycardia >100)
4. **Intervals**
   - Normal PR = 0.12-0.20 s (3-5 small boxes)
   - Normal QRS ≤ 0.10 s (≤2.5 small boxes)
   - Normal QT ≤ half the RR interval, if heart rate is normal
5. **Mean QRS axis**
   - Normal if QRS is primarily upright in leads I and II (+90 degrees to −30 degrees)
   - Otherwise, determine axis by isoelectric/perpendicular method
6. **P-wave abnormalities**
   - Inspect P in leads II and V_1 for left and right atrial enlargement
7. **QRS wave abnormalities**
   - Inspect for left and right ventricular hypertrophy
   - Inspect for bundle-branch blocks
   - Inspect for pathologic Q waves: What anatomic distribution?
8. **ST-segment or T-wave abnormalities**
   - Inspect for ST elevations:
     - ST-segment elevation MI
     - Pericarditis (see Chapter 14)
   - Inspect for ST depressions or T-wave inversions:
     - Myocardial ischemia or non–ST-elevation MI
     - Typically accompany ventricular hypertrophy or bundle-branch blocks
     - Metabolic or chemical abnormalities (see Fig. 4-27)
9. **Compare with patient's previous ECGs**

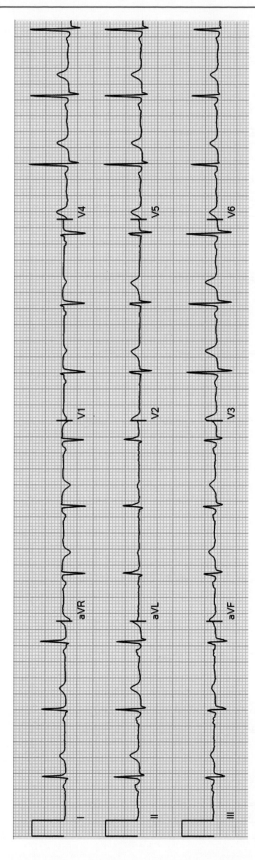

Figure 4-28. 12-lead ECG (normal). The rectangular upward deflection at the beginning of each line is the voltage calibration signal (1 mV). *Rhythm:* normal sinus. *Rate:* 70 bpm. *Intervals:* PR, 0.15; QRS, 0.08; QT, 0.39 seconds. *Axis:* +30 degrees (QRS is isoelectric in lead III). The P wave, QRS complex, ST segment, and T waves are normal.

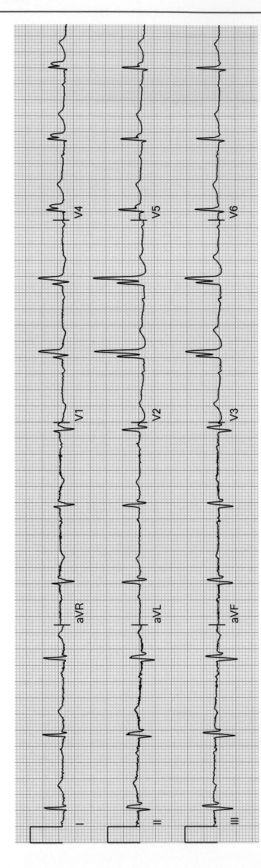

Figure 4-29. 12-lead ECG (abnormal). *Rhythm:* normal sinus. *Rate:* 65 bpm. *Intervals:* PR, 0.19; QRS, 0.15; QT, 0.43 seconds. *Axis:* –20 degrees. *P wave:* normal. *QRS:* widened with RSR' in lead V₁ consistent with right bundle-branch block (RBBB). Also, pathologic Q waves are in leads II, III, and aVF, consistent with inferior wall myocardial infarction (an old one, because the ST segments do not demonstrate an acute injury pattern).

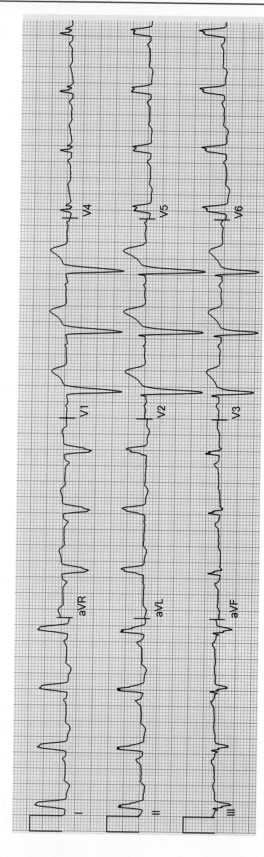

Figure 4-30. 12-lead ECG (abnormal). *Rhythm:* normal sinus. *Rate:* 80 bpm. *Intervals:* PR, 0.16; QRS, 0.14; QT, 0.40 seconds. *Axis:* +15 degrees. *P wave:* normal. *QRS:* widened with RR' in leads V_4–V_6 consistent with left bundle–branch block (LBBB). The ST-segment and T-wave abnormalities are secondary to LBBB.

Figure 4-31. 12-lead ECG (abnormal). *Rhythm:* normal sinus. *Rate:* 66 bpm. *Intervals:* PR, 0.16; QRS, 0.08; QT, 0.40 seconds. *Axis:* +10 degrees. *P wave:* normal. *QRS:* pathologic Q waves in leads V₁–V₄, consistent with anteroseptal and anteroapical myocardial infarction (MI). The *ST segment and T waves* do not demonstrate an acute injury pattern; thus, the MI is old.

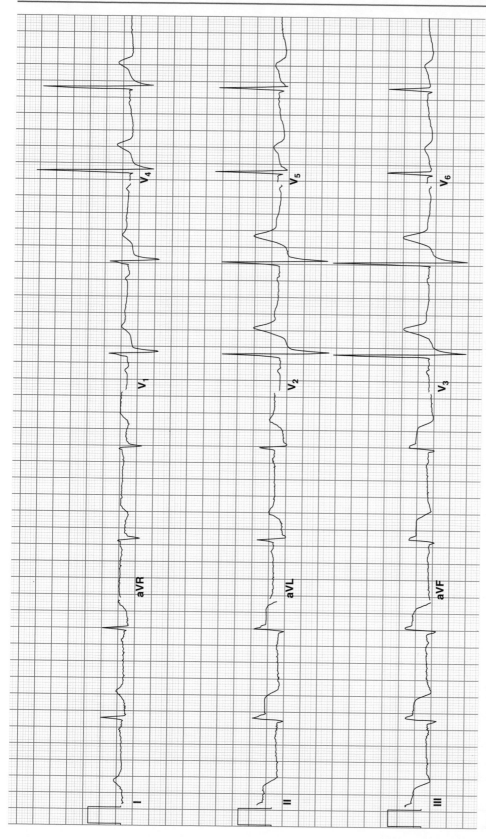

Figure 4-32. 12-lead ECG (abnormal). *Rhythm:* sinus bradycardia. *Rate:* 55 bpm. *Intervals:* PR, 0.20 (in aVF); QRS, 0.10; QT, 0.44 seconds. *Axis:* normal (QRS is predominantly upright in leads I and II). *P wave:* normal. *QRS:* voltage in chest leads is prominent but does not meet criteria for ventricular hypertrophy; pathologic Q waves are present in II, III, and aVF, indicating inferior wall MI, and the tall R wave in V₂ is suggestive of posterior MI involvement as well. Marked *ST-segment elevation* is apparent in II, III, and aVF, indicating that this is an *acute STEMI*. Note the reciprocal ST-segment depression in leads I and aVL.

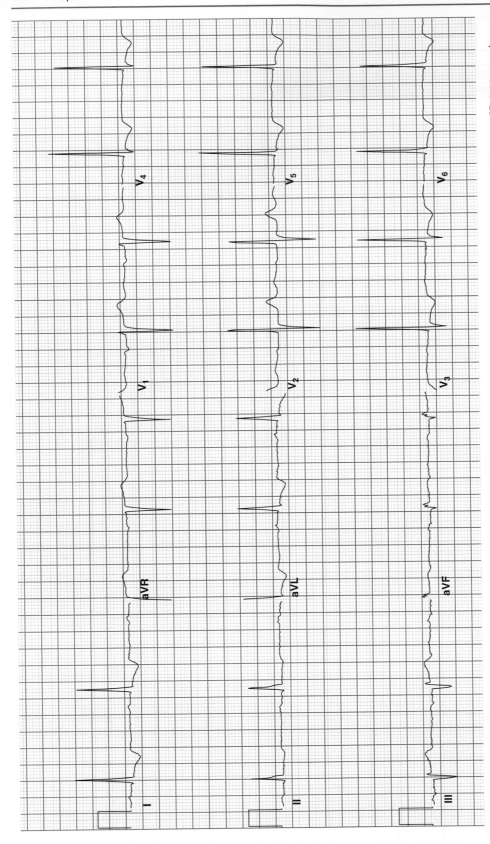

Figure 4-33. 12-lead ECG (abnormal). *Rhythm:* sinus bradycardia. *Rate:* 55 bpm. *Intervals:* PR, 0.24 (first-degree AV block; see Chapter 12); QRS, 0.09; QT, 0.44 seconds. *Axis:* 0 degrees. *P wave:* normal. *QRS:* left ventricular hypertrophy (LVH): S in V_1 (14 mm) + R in V_5 (22 mm) > 35 mm. Pathologic Q waves in leads III and aVF indicate an old inferior MI. The *ST-segment depression and T-wave inversion* are secondary to the abnormal repolarization resulting from LVH.

Figure 4-34. 12-lead ECG (abnormal). *Rhythm:* normal sinus. *Rate:* 68 bpm. *Intervals:* PR, 0.24 (first-degree AV block; see Chapter 12); QRS, 0.10; QT, 0.36 seconds. *Axis:* −45 degrees (left axis deviation). *P wave:* borderline left atrial enlargement (terminal deflection of P wave in V_1 is 1 mm wide and 1 mm deep—just barely). *QRS:* pattern of left anterior fascicular block (LAFB; see Fig. 4-20). The abnormally small R waves in leads V_2-V_4 are associated with LAFB resulting from the reduction of initial anterior forces. The *ST segment and T waves* are unremarkable.

Figure 4-35. 12-lead ECG (abnormal). *Rhythm:* normal sinus. *Rate:* 95 bpm. *Intervals:* PR, 0.20; QRS, 0.10; QT, 0.34 seconds. *Axis:* +160 degrees (right axis deviation [RAD]). *P wave:* right atrial enlargement (P wave in lead II is >2.5 mm tall). *QRS:* right ventricular hypertrophy (RVH): R greater than S in V$_1$ with RAD. The *T waves* are inverted in the anterior leads, at least in part reflecting abnormal repolarization resulting from RVH. At the bottom of the figure, the fourth row labeled "II" is a continuous rhythm strip of lead II.

Figure 4-36. 12-lead ECG (abnormal). *Rhythm:* normal sinus. *Rate:* 62 bpm. *Intervals:* PR, 0.14; QRS, 0.10; QT, 0.52 (corrected QT, 0.53, which is prolonged). *Axis:* +95 degrees (right axis deviation [RAD]). *QRS:* pattern of left posterior fascicular block (LPFB), with small R wave in leads I and aVL, small Q wave in leads II, III, and aVF, and RAD (see Fig. 4-20 for further description of LPFB). The prolonged QT interval in this patient is the result of antiarrhythmic medication.

Review Questions

1.

The figure shows a single lead from an ECG of a 58-year-old man who sustained an episode of syncope (loss of consciousness). What is the corrected QT interval?

a. 0.30 s
b. 0.40 s
c. 0.50 s
d. 0.60 s

2. Which of the following is a cause of left axis deviation?

a. Anterior ST-elevation MI
b. Left anterior fascicular block
c. Pulmonary hypertension
d. Right bundle-branch block

3. A 42-year-old patient's 12-lead ECG shows that the QRS complex is isoelectric (the R wave and S wave have the same amplitude) in lead II, and the QRS is primarily positive in lead aVL. What is the mean electrical axis?

    a. −120 degrees
    b. + 60 degrees
    c. + 150 degrees
    d. −30 degrees

4. Which of the following conditions would NOT be expected to abnormally reduce the amplitude of the QRS complexes on an ECG?

    a. Obesity
    b. Hypertension
    c. Chronic obstructive airways disease
    d. Pericardial effusion (fluid around the heart)

Answers to Review Questions

1. **Choice c is correct.** The QT interval is measured from the beginning of the QRS to the end of the T wave (see Fig. 4-12). In this tracing, the QT interval is 0.4 s (2 large boxes on the ECG grid, which is easiest to measure on the first beat in the figure since the start of the upstroke of that QRS happens to fall on a large box grid line). The *corrected* QT (QT_c) is calculated by dividing the QT interval by the square root of the R-R interval (eg, the interval from the peak of one QRS complex to the next). The R-R interval here is 0.64 s (3 large boxes plus 1 small box, easiest to measure on this tracing from the 5th to the 6th QRS, since the peak of the 5th QRS happens to fall on a large box grid line). Therefore,

$$\text{Corrected QT} = \frac{\text{QT}}{\sqrt{\text{R-R interval}}} = \frac{0.40}{\sqrt{0.64}} = 0.5 \,\text{s}$$

which is prolonged (normal corrected QT_c is ≤0.44 s in men). A prolonged QT_c interval can lead to ventricular arrhythmias and syncope, as will be described in Chapter 12. In this patient's case, the QT_c prolongation was a side effect of an antipsychotic medication.

2. **Choice b is correct.** Left axis deviation is defined as a mean electrical axis that is more negative than −30 degrees. As shown in Figure 4-14, the most common causes are left anterior fascicular block, prior inferior wall myocardial infarction, and left ventricular hypertrophy (note that only a minority of patients with LVH actually have left axis deviation).

3. **Choice d is correct.** The mean electrical axis is perpendicular to the lead that inscribes an isoelectric QRS complex (see Fig. 4-16). Since lead II lies at + 60 degrees (see Fig. 4-14) and the QRS is isoelectric in that lead, the mean axis is at either + 150 or −30 degrees (ie, + 60 degrees plus or minus 90 degrees). The next step is to inspect the lead that lies perpendicular to the lead with the isoelectric complex, which in this case is lead aVL (see Fig. 4-14, showing that aVL is perpendicular to lead II). Since you are told that the QRS is primarily positive in lead aVL, the mean QRS axis is directed toward the positive aspect of that lead, which is −30 degrees. If the QRS complex had been primarily downward in lead aVL instead, then the mean axis would be pointed away from that lead, at + 150 degrees (see Fig. 4-14).

4. **Choice b is correct.** Hypertension often results in left ventricular hypertrophy, which *increases* the QRS amplitude in many leads (see Fig. 4-18B). Each of the other conditions is associated with reduced amplitude of the QRS owing to impaired electrical transmission (because of abnormal air, fluid or tissue density) between the heart and the skin surface where the ECG leads are placed.

Acknowledgments

Contributors to previous editions of this chapter were David B. Fischer, MD; Stephen R. Pomedli, MD; Lilit Garibyan, MD; Kyle Low, MD; and Price Kerfoot, MD.

Additional Reading

Goldberger AL, Goldberger ZD, Shvilkin A. *Goldberger's Clinical Electrocardiography: A Simplified Approach*. 9th ed. Philadelphia, PA: Elsevier Saunders; 2017.

Nathanson LA, McClennen S, Safran C, Goldberger AL. *ECG Wave-Maven: Self-Assessment Program for Students and Clinicians*. 2001-2016. http://ecg.bidmc.harvard.edu

O'Keefe JH Jr, Hammill SC, Freed MS, et al. *The Complete Guide to ECGs*. 4th ed. Sudbury, MA: Jones and Bartlett Publishers; 2016.

Thaler MS. *The Only EKG Book You'll Ever Need*. 9th ed. Philadelphia, PA: Lippincott Williams & Wilkins; 2018.

Wagner GS, Strauss DG. *Marriott's Practical Electrocardiography*. 12th ed. Baltimore, MD: Lippincott Williams & Wilkins; 2014.

Atherosclerosis

Siddharth M. Patel | Peter Libby

Atherosclerosis is responsible for the majority of deaths in developed nations. Through its major manifestations of myocardial infarction and stroke, it has also become a major cause of mortality in the developing world. Commonly known as "hardening of the arteries," atherosclerosis derives its name from the Greek roots *athere-*, meaning "gruel," and *-skleros*, meaning "hardness." Recent evidence has demonstrated that chronic inflammation drives the atherosclerotic process and transduces traditional risk factors (such as elevated blood cholesterol) into altered behavior of vascular wall cells, contributing to the disease and its thrombotic complications. The course of atherogenesis can smolder throughout adulthood, punctuated by acute cardiovascular events.

This chapter consists of two sections. The first part describes the normal arterial wall, the pathogenesis of atherosclerotic plaque formation, and the complications that lead to clinical manifestations of the disease. The second section describes findings from population studies that have identified specific risk factors for atherosclerotic events, thereby offering opportunities for prevention and treatment.

VASCULAR BIOLOGY OF ATHEROSCLEROSIS

NORMAL ARTERIAL WALL

The arterial wall consists of three layers (Fig. 5-1): the **intima**, closest to the arterial lumen and therefore most "intimate" with the blood; the middle layer, known as the **media**; and the outer layer, the **adventitia**. A single layer of endothelial cells covers the surface of the intima and provides a biologically active barrier between circulating blood and the vessel wall. The media is the thickest layer of the normal artery. Boundaries of elastin, known as the *internal* and *external elastic laminae*, separate this middle layer from the intima and adventitia, respectively. The media consists of smooth muscle cells (SMCs) and extracellular matrix and serves the contractile and elastic functions of the vessel. The elastic component, more prominent in large arteries (eg, the aorta and its primary branches), stretches during the high pressure of systole and then recoils during diastole, propelling blood forward. The muscular component, more prominent in smaller arteries such as arterioles, constricts or relaxes to alter vessel resistance and therefore luminal blood flow (flow = pressure/resistance; see Chapter 6). The adventitia contains nerves, lymphatics, and blood vessels (vasa vasorum) that nourish the cells of the arterial wall.

Figure 5-1. Schematic diagram of the arterial wall. The intima, the innermost layer, overlies the muscular media demarcated by the internal elastic lamina. The external elastic lamina separates the media from the outer layer, the adventitia. (Modified from Lieberman M. *Marks' Basic Medical Biochemistry: A Clinical Approach.* 4th ed. Philadelphia, PA: Wolters Kluwer Health; 2013:649.)

Far from an inert conduit, the living arterial wall hosts dynamic interchanges between its cellular components—most importantly, endothelial cells, vascular SMCs, and their surrounding extracellular matrix. An understanding of the dysfunction that leads to atherosclerosis requires knowledge of the normal function of these components, as described in the following sections.

Endothelial Cells

In a healthy artery, the endothelium performs structural, metabolic, and signaling functions that maintain homeostasis of the vessel wall. The tightly adjoined endothelial cells form a barrier that contains blood within the lumen of the vessel and controls the passage of solutes and cells from the circulation into the subendothelial space. As blood traverses the vascular tree, it encounters antithrombotic molecules produced by the normal endothelium that prevent it from clotting or that promote fibrinolysis (the breakdown of fibrin clots). Some of these molecules reside on the endothelial surface (eg, heparan sulfate, thrombomodulin, and plasminogen activators; see Chapter 7), while other antithrombotic products of the endothelium enter the circulation (eg, prostacyclin and nitric oxide [NO]; see Chapter 6). Although a net anticoagulant state normally prevails, the endothelium can also produce prothrombotic and antifibrinolytic molecules when subjected to various stressors.

Furthermore, endothelial cells secrete substances that modulate contraction of SMCs in the underlying medial layer. These substances include vasodilators (eg, NO and prostacyclin) and vasoconstrictors (eg, endothelin) that alter the arteriolar resistance and therefore luminal blood flow. In a normal artery, the predominance of vasodilator substances results in net smooth muscle relaxation.

Endothelial cells can also modulate the immune response. In the absence of pathologic stimulation, healthy arterial endothelial cells resist leukocyte adhesion and thereby oppose local inflammation. However, endothelial cells respond to local injury or infection by expressing cell surface adhesion molecules, which attach mononuclear cells to the endothelium, and chemokines—substances that facilitate leukocyte recruitment to the site of injury. These effects result in part by activation of the transcription factor nuclear factor kappa B (NFκB).

In summary, the normal endothelium provides a protective, nonthrombogenic surface with homeostatic vasodilatory and anti-inflammatory properties (Fig. 5-2).

Vascular Smooth Muscle Cells

SMCs within the medial layer of normal muscular arteries have both contractile and synthetic capabilities. Various vasoactive substances modulate the *contractile* function, resulting in

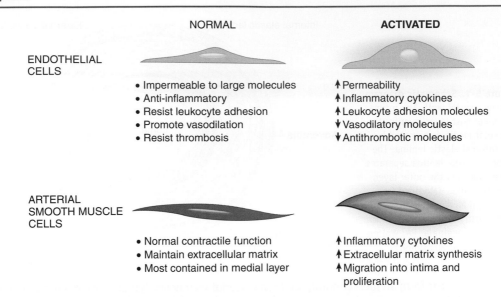

Figure 5-2. Endothelial and smooth muscle cell activation by inflammation. Normal endothelial and SMCs maintain the integrity and elasticity of the normal arterial wall while limiting immune cell infiltration. Inflammatory activation of these vascular cells corrupts their normal functions and favors proatherogenic mechanisms that drive plaque development.

vasoconstriction or vasodilation. Such agonists include circulating molecules (eg, angiotensin II), those released from local nerve terminals (eg, acetylcholine), and others originating from the overlying endothelium (eg, endothelin and NO). SMCs also *synthesize* the collagen, elastin, and proteoglycans that form the bulk of the vascular extracellular matrix (see Fig. 5-2). In addition, SMCs produce vasoactive and inflammatory mediators, including interleukin (IL)-1 and IL-6, and tumor necrosis factor (TNF).

In normal arteries, most SMCs reside in the medial layer, although human arteries also contain some SMCs in the intima, particularly in sites predisposed to atherosclerosis. During atherogenesis, medial SMCs can migrate into the intima, proliferate, and augment synthesis of extracellular matrix macromolecules while they dampen contractile protein content.

Extracellular Matrix

In healthy arteries, fibrillar collagen, elastin, and proteoglycans make up most of the extracellular matrix in the medial layer. Interstitial collagen fibrils, constructed from intertwining helical proteins, possess great biomechanical strength, while elastin provides flexibility. Together these components maintain the structural integrity of the vessel, despite the high pressure within the lumen. The extracellular matrix also regulates the growth of its resident cells. Native fibrillar collagen, in particular, can inhibit SMC proliferation in vitro. Furthermore, the matrix influences cellular responses to stimuli—matrix-bound cells respond in a specific manner to growth factors and resist apoptosis (programmed cell death).

Atherosclerotic Arterial Wall

The arterial wall is a dynamic and regulated structure, but certain stimuli can disturb normal homeostasis and pave the way for atherogenesis. For example, as described later, vascular endothelial cells, as well as SMCs, react readily to inflammatory mediators, such as IL-1 and TNF, and can *produce* them as well.

With the recognition that vascular wall cells respond to, and produce, proinflammatory agents, investigations into the role of "activated" endothelial and SMCs in atherogenesis

Figure 5-3. Schematic diagram of the evolution of atherosclerotic plaque. (*1*) Accumulation of lipoprotein particles in the intima. The darker color depicts modification of the lipoproteins (eg, by oxidation or glycation). (*2*) Oxidative stress, including constituents of modified LDL, induces local cytokine elaboration. (*3*) These cytokines promote increased expression of adhesion molecules that bind leukocytes and of chemoattractant molecules (eg, monocyte chemoattractant protein-1 [MCP-1]) that direct leukocyte migration into the intima. (*4*) After entering the artery wall in response to chemoattractants, blood monocytes encounter stimuli such as macrophage colony–stimulating factor (M-CSF) that augment their expression of scavenger receptors. (*5*) Scavenger receptors mediate the uptake of modified lipoprotein particles and promote the development of foam cells. Macrophage foam cells are a source of additional cytokines and effector molecules such as superoxide anion (O_2^-) and matrix metalloproteinases. (*6*) SMCs migrate into the intima from the media. Note the increasing intimal thickness. (*7*) Intimal SMCs divide and elaborate extracellular matrix, promoting matrix accumulation in the growing atherosclerotic plaque. In this manner, the fatty streak evolves into a fibrofatty lesion. (*8*) In later stages, calcification can occur (not depicted) and fibrosis continues, sometimes accompanied by smooth muscle cell death (including programmed cell death or apoptosis), yielding a relatively acellular fibrous capsule surrounding a lipid-rich core that may also contain dying or dead cells. IL-1, interleukin 1; LDL, low-density lipoprotein. (Modified from Libby PL, Zipes DP, eds. *Braunwald's Heart Disease: A Textbook of Cardiovascular Medicine*. 11th ed. Philadelphia, PA: Elsevier; 2019.)

burgeoned. As a consequence, vascular endothelium and SMCs joined classical inflammatory cells, such as mononuclear phagocytes and T lymphocytes, as key players in early atheroma formation and in advanced plaque progression. This fundamental research has identified several key components that contribute to the atherosclerotic inflammatory process, including endothelial dysfunction, accumulation of lipids within the intima, recruitment of leukocytes and SMCs to the vessel wall, formation of foam cells, and deposition of extracellular matrix (Fig. 5-3), as described in the following sections. The cells of atherosclerotic lesions continuously interact and modify each other's behavior, shaping the plaque over decades into one of many possible profiles. This section categorizes these mechanisms into three pathologic stages: the fatty streak, plaque progression, and plaque disruption (Fig. 5-4). In the arterial tree, lesions of all three stages can coexist, often side by side.

Fatty Streak

Fatty streaks represent the earliest visible lesions of atherosclerosis. On gross inspection, they appear as areas of yellow discoloration on the artery's inner surface, but they neither protrude substantially into the arterial lumen nor impede blood flow. Surprisingly, fatty streaks exist in the aorta and coronary arteries of most people by age 20. They do not cause symptoms and may regress over time. Although the precise initiation of fatty streak development is not known, observations in animals suggest that various stressors cause early endothelial dysfunction, as described in the next section. Such dysfunction allows entry, retention, and modification of lipids within the subendothelial space, where they serve as proinflammatory mediators that initiate leukocyte recruitment and foam cell formation—the pathologic hallmarks of the fatty streak (Fig. 5-3).

Endothelial Dysfunction

Abnormal function of the arterial endothelium represents a primary event in atherogenesis. The predisposition of certain regions of arteries (eg, branch points) to develop atheromata

FATTY STREAK

- Endothelial dysfunction
- Lipoprotein entry and modification
- Leukocyte recruitment
- Foam cell formation

A

PLAQUE PROGRESSION

- Smooth muscle cell migration
- Altered matrix synthesis and degradation
- Lipid core formation

B

PLAQUE DISRUPTION

- Disrupted plaque integrity
- Thrombus formation

C

Figure 5-4. Stages of plaque development. A. The fatty streak develops as a result of endothelial dysfunction, lipoprotein entry and modification, leukocyte recruitment, and foam cell formation. **B.** Plaque progression involves migration of SMCs into the intima, where they divide and secrete extracellular matrix. The fibrous cap contains a lipid core. **C.** Hemodynamic stresses and degradation of extracellular matrix increase the susceptibility of the fibrous cap to rupture, allowing superimposed thrombus formation. (Modified from Libby P, Ridker PM, Maseri A. Inflammation and atherosclerosis. *Circulation*. 2002;105:1136.)

supports the role of hydrodynamic conditions in regulating this process. In straight sections of arteries, the normal laminar (ie, smooth) shear forces favor the endothelial production of NO, an endogenous vasodilator, inhibitor of platelet aggregation, and anti-inflammatory substance (see Chapter 6). Moreover, laminar flow and high shear stress activates transcription factors such as Krüppel-like factor 2 (KLF2) that evokes an "atheroprotective" panel of endothelial functions and accentuates expression of the antioxidant enzyme superoxide dismutase, which protects against reactive oxygen species. Conversely, disturbed flow occurs near arterial branch points, causing low shear stress, which impairs these locally atheroprotective endothelial functions. Accordingly, arteries with few branches (eg, the internal mammary artery) show relative resistance to atherosclerosis, whereas branching vessels (eg, the common carotid and left coronary arteries) contain common sites for atheroma formation.

Endothelial dysfunction may also result from exposure to a "toxic" chemical environment. For example, tobacco smoking, elevated circulating lipid levels, and diabetes—all known risk factors for atherosclerosis—can promote endothelial dysfunction. Each of these stimuli increases endothelial production of reactive oxygen species—notably, superoxide anion—that interact with other intracellular molecules to influence endothelial function.

When physical and chemical stressors disrupt endothelial homeostasis, an activated state ensues manifested by impairment of the endothelium's role as a permeability barrier, the release of inflammatory cytokines, increased production of cell surface adhesion molecules that recruit leukocytes, altered release of vasoactive substances (eg, prostacyclin and NO), and interference with normal antithrombotic properties. These undesired effects of dysfunctional endothelium lay the groundwork for subsequent events in the development of atherosclerosis (see Figs. 5-2 and 5-3).

Lipoprotein Entry and Modification

The activated endothelium no longer serves as an effective barrier to the passage of circulating lipoproteins into the arterial wall. Increased endothelial permeability allows the entry of low-density lipoprotein (LDL) into the intima, a process facilitated by an elevated circulating LDL concentration in patients with hypercholesterolemia. In addition to high LDL concentrations from diet, several monogenic causes of elevated LDL exist, including mutations of the LDL receptor, of apolipoprotein B, and of proprotein convertase subtilisin-kexin type 9 (PCSK9), a protease involved in regulation of the LDL receptor. Once within the intima, LDL accumulates in the subendothelial space by binding to proteoglycans in the extracellular matrix. This "trapping" increases the residence time of LDL within the vessel wall, where the lipoprotein may undergo chemical modifications that may promote the development of atherosclerotic lesions. Hypertension, a major risk factor for atherosclerosis, may further promote retention of lipoproteins in the intima by accentuating the production of LDL-binding proteoglycans by SMCs.

Oxidation is one type of modification that befalls LDL trapped in the subendothelial space. It can result from the local action of reactive oxygen species and pro-oxidant enzymes derived from activated endothelial or SMC or from macrophages that penetrate the vessel wall. In addition, the microenvironment of the subendothelial space sequesters oxidized LDL from antioxidants in the plasma. In diabetic patients with sustained hyperglycemia, *glycation* of LDL can occur—a modification that may ultimately render LDL antigenic and proinflammatory. These biochemical alterations of LDL may contribute to the inflammation within plaques. In the fatty streak, and likely throughout plaque development, modified LDL (mLDL) promotes leukocyte recruitment and foam cell formation.

Leukocyte Recruitment

Recruitment of leukocytes (primarily monocytes and T lymphocytes) to the vessel wall is a key step in atherogenesis. The process depends on the expression of leukocyte adhesion molecules (LAMs) on the normally nonadherent endothelial luminal surface and on chemoattractant signals (eg, monocyte chemotactic protein-1 [MCP-1]) that direct diapedesis (passage of cells through the intact endothelial layer) and migration into the subintimal space. Two major subsets of LAM persist in the inflamed atherosclerotic plaque: the immunoglobulin gene superfamily (especially vascular cell adhesion molecule-1 [VCAM-1] and intercellular adhesion molecule-1 [ICAM-1]) and the selectins (particularly, E-selectin and P-selectin). These LAMs and chemoattractant signals direct mainly monocytes to the forming lesion. Hypercholesterolemia favors accumulation in blood of a subset of monocytes that is characterized the by expression of high levels of proinflammatory cytokines (eg, IL-1 and TNF), distinguished in mice by expression of the cell surface marker Ly6c. Although outnumbered by monocytes, T lymphocytes also localize within plaques and direct the adaptive immune response.

mLDL and proinflammatory cytokines can induce LAM and chemoattractant cytokine (chemokine) expression independently, but mLDL may also stimulate endothelial and SMC to *produce* proinflammatory cytokines, thereby reinforcing the direct action. This dual ability of mLDL to promote leukocyte recruitment and inflammation directly and indirectly persists throughout atherogenesis.

Foam Cell Formation

After monocytes adhere to and penetrate the intima (Figs. 5-3 and 5-4A), they differentiate into macrophages and imbibe lipoproteins to form foam cells. Foam cells do not arise from uptake of LDL cholesterol by the classic cell surface LDL receptor–mediated endocytosis as described in Box 5-1 (eg, as occurs in normal hepatocytes), because the high cholesterol content in these cells suppresses expression of that receptor. Furthermore, the classic LDL receptor does not recognize mLDL particles. Rather, macrophages rely on a family of "scavenger" receptors that preferentially bind and internalize mLDL. Unlike uptake via the classic LDL receptor, mLDL ingestion by scavenger receptors evades feedback inhibition and permits engorgement of the macrophages with cholesterol and cholesteryl ester, resulting in the typical appearance of foam cells. Although such uptake may initially provide benefit by sequestering potentially damaging mLDL particles, the impaired efflux of these cells as compared to the rate of influx, as well

Box 5-1 The Lipoprotein Transport System

Lipoproteins ferry water-insoluble fats through the bloodstream. These particles consist of a lipid core surrounded by more hydrophilic phospholipid, free cholesterol, and apolipoproteins (also called *apoproteins*). The apoproteins present on various classes of lipoprotein molecules serve as the "conductors" of the system, directing the lipoproteins to specific tissue receptors and mediating enzymatic reactions. Five major classes of lipoproteins exist, distinguished by their densities, lipid constituents, and associated apoproteins. In order of increasing density, they are **chylomicrons, very-low-density lipoproteins (VLDLs), intermediate-density lipoproteins (IDLs), low-density lipoproteins (LDLs)**, and **high-density lipoproteins (HDLs)**. The major steps in the lipoprotein pathways are labeled in the figure below and described as follows. The key apoproteins (apo) at each stage are indicated in the figure in parentheses.

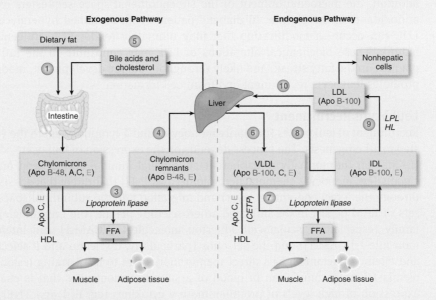

Exogenous (Intestinal) Pathway

1. Dietary fats are absorbed by the small intestine and repackaged as chylomicrons, accompanied by apo B-48. Chylomicrons are large particles, particularly rich in triglycerides, that enter the circulation via the lymphatic system.
2. Apo E and subtypes of apo C are transferred to chylomicrons from HDL particles in the bloodstream.
3. Apo C (subtype CII) enhances interactions of chylomicrons with *lipoprotein lipase* (*LPL*) on the endothelial surface of adipose and muscle tissue. This reaction hydrolyzes the triglycerides within chylomicrons into free fatty acids (FFAs), which are stored by adipose tissue or used for energy in cardiac and skeletal muscle.
4. Chylomicron remnants are removed from the circulation by the liver, mediated by apo E.
5. One fate of cholesterol in the liver is incorporation into bile acids, which are exported to the intestine, completing the exogenous pathway cycle.

Endogenous (Hepatic) Pathway

Because dietary fat availability is not constant, the endogenous pathway provides a reliable supply of triglycerides for tissue energy needs:

6. The liver packages cholesterol and triglycerides into VLDL particles, accompanied by apo B-100 and phospholipid. The triglyceride content of VLDL is much higher than that of cholesterol, but this is the main means by which the liver releases cholesterol into the circulation.

Box 5-1　　　**The Lipoprotein Transport System** (continued)

7. VLDL is catabolized by LPL (similar to chylomicrons, as described in step 3), releasing fatty acids to muscle and adipose tissue. During this process, VLDL also interacts with HDL, exchanging some of its triglyceride for apo C subtypes, apo E, and cholesteryl ester from HDL. The latter exchange (important in reverse cholesterol transport, as described in the next section) is mediated by cholesteryl ester transfer protein (CETP).
8. Approximately 50% of the VLDL remnants (termed intermediate-density lipoproteins [IDL]) are then cleared in the liver by hepatic receptors that recognize apo E.
9. The remaining IDL is catabolized further by LPL and hepatic lipase (HL), which remove additional triglyceride, apo E, and apo C, forming LDL particles.
10. Plasma clearance of LDL occurs primarily via LDL receptor–mediated endocytosis in the liver and peripheral cells, directed by LDLs apo B-100 and apo E.

Cholesterol Homeostasis and Reverse Cholesterol Transport

Intracellular cholesterol content is tightly maintained by *de novo* synthesis, cellular uptake, storage, and efflux from the cell. The enzyme *HMG-CoA reductase* is the rate-limiting element of cholesterol biosynthesis, and cellular uptake of cholesterol is controlled by receptor-mediated endocytosis of circulating LDL (see step 10). When intracellular cholesterol levels are low, the transcription factor *sterol regulatory element–binding protein (SREBP)* is released from the endoplasmic reticulum. The active fragment of SREBP enters the nucleus to increase transcription of HMG-CoA reductase and the LDL receptor—which, through their subsequent actions, tend to normalize the intracellular cholesterol content.

Under conditions of intracellular cholesterol excess (as in the figure above), peripheral cells increase the transcription of the ATP-binding cassette A1 and G1 genes (ABCA1 and ABCG1, respectively). The ABCA1 gene codes for a transmembrane protein transporter that initiates efflux of cholesterol from the cell to lipid-poor circulating apo A-I (which is synthesized by the liver and intestine), thus forming nascent (immature) HDL particles. ABCG1 facilitates further efflux of cholesterol to form more mature HDL particles. As free cholesterol is acquired by circulating HDL, it is esterified by *lecithin cholesterol acyltransferase (LCAT)*, an enzyme activated by apo A-I. The hydrophobic cholesteryl esters move into the particle's core. Most cholesteryl esters in HDL can then be exchanged for triglycerides in the circulation (via the enzyme CETP) with any of the apo B–containing lipoproteins (ie, VLDL, IDL, LDL), which deliver the cholesterol back to the liver. HDL can also transport cholesterol to the liver and steroid hormone–producing tissues via the SR-B1 scavenger receptor.

as local proliferation, leads to their accumulation in the plaque. This mitigates their protective role by fueling foam cell apoptosis and the release of proinflammatory cytokines that promote atherosclerotic plaque progression. During atherogenesis, the clearance of dead foam cells can become inefficient, thus promoting the accumulation of cellular debris and extracellular lipids, forming the lipid-rich center of a plaque (often termed the *necrotic core*).

Plaque Progression

Whereas endothelial cells play a central role in the formation of the fatty streak, SMCs in the intima promote plaque progression by producing extracellular matrix that traps lipoproteins and adds to the bulk of the lesion. During decades of development, the typical atherosclerotic plaque develops a thrombogenic lipid core that underlies a protective fibrous cap. Not all fatty streaks progress into fibrofatty lesions, and it is unknown why some evolve and others do not.

Early plaque growth typically involves a compensatory outward remodeling of the arterial wall that preserves the diameter of the lumen and permits plaque accumulation without limitation of blood flow, hence producing no ischemic symptoms. Lesions at this stage can thus evade detection by angiography and do not cause symptoms due to ischemia. Later plaque growth, however, can outstrip the compensatory arterial enlargement, restrict the vessel lumen, and impede perfusion. Such flow-limiting plaques can result in tissue ischemia, causing symptoms such as angina pectoris (see Chapter 6) or intermittent claudication of the extremities (see Chapter 15).

Many acute coronary syndromes (acute myocardial infarction and unstable angina pectoris) result when the fibrous cap of an atherosclerotic plaque ruptures, exposing prothrombotic molecules within the lipid core and precipitating an acute thrombus that suddenly occludes the arterial lumen. As described in this section, the extracellular matrix plays a pivotal role in fortifying the fibrous cap, isolating the thrombogenic plaque interior from coagulation substrates in the circulation.

Smooth Muscle Cell Migration

The transition from fatty streak to fibrous atheromatous plaque involves the migration of SMCs from the arterial media into the intima, proliferation of SMCs within the intima, and secretion of extracellular matrix macromolecules by SMCs. Foam cells, activated platelets entering through microfissures in the plaque surface, and endothelial cells can all elaborate substances that signal SMC migration and proliferation (Figs. 5-4B and 5-5).

Foam cells produce several factors that contribute to SMC recruitment. For example, they release platelet-derived growth factor (PDGF)—also released by platelets and endothelial cells—which likely stimulates the migration of SMCs across the internal elastic lamina and into the subintimal space, where they subsequently replicate. PDGF additionally stimulates the growth of resident SMCs in the intima. Foam cells also release cytokines and growth factors (eg, TNF, IL-1, fibroblast growth factor, and transforming growth factor-β [TGF-β]) that further incite SMC proliferation and/or the synthesis of extracellular matrix proteins. Furthermore, proinflammatory cytokines induce SMC and leukocyte activation, promoting further cytokine release, thus sustaining inflammation in the lesion.

According to the traditional concept, plaques grow gradually and continuously, but current evidence suggests subclinical events may punctuate this progression with bursts of smooth muscle replication. For example, morphologic evidence of resolved intraplaque hemorrhages indicates that breaches in plaque integrity can occur without clinical symptoms or signs. Such plaque disruptions expose tissue factor from foam cells to blood, which activates coagulation and microthrombus formation. Activated platelets within such microthrombi release additional stimuli—including PDGF—that can spur a local wave of SMC migration and proliferation.

Activated T cells also contribute to plaque evolution. Cells of the T helper 1 subtype (Th1) produce proinflammatory cytokines that promote plaque progression and instability,

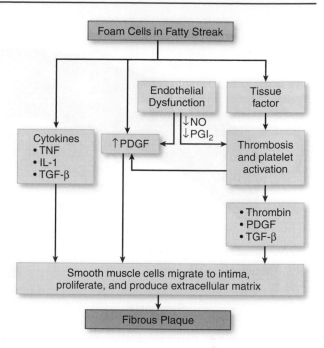

Figure 5-5. Progression from the fatty streak involves the migration and proliferation of SMCs. Substances released from foam cells, dysfunctional endothelial cells, and platelets contribute to this process. IL-1, interleukin-1; NO, nitric oxide; PDGF, platelet-derived growth factor; PGI_2, prostacyclin; TGF-β, transforming growth factor-β; TNF, tumor necrosis factor.

while lymphocytes of the T helper 2 subtype (Th2) and regulatory T cells (Treg) produce factors, including TGF-β and IL-10, which can *inhibit* SMC proliferation and potentially mitigate plaque growth.

Extracellular Matrix Metabolism

As the predominant collagen-synthesizing cell type, SMCs favor fortification of the fibrous cap. Net matrix deposition depends on the balance of its synthesis by SMCs and its degradation, mediated in part by a class of proteolytic enzymes known as matrix metalloproteinases (MMP). While PDGF and TGF-β stimulate production of interstitial collagens by SMCs, the Th1-derived cytokine interferon-γ (IFN-γ) *inhibits* SMC collagen synthesis. Furthermore, inflammatory cytokines stimulate local foam cells to secrete collagen- and elastin-degrading MMP, thereby weakening the fibrous cap and predisposing it to rupture (Fig. 5-6).

Plaque Disruption

Plaque Integrity

The tug-of-war between matrix synthesis and degradation continues over decades but not without consequences. Death of smooth muscle and foam cells, including by activation of apoptosis, liberates cellular contents, contributing to accumulation of lipids and cellular debris within the growing core. The size of the lipid core has biomechanical implications for the stability of the plaque. With increasing size and protrusion into the arterial lumen, mechanical stress focuses on the plaque border abutting normal tissue, called the shoulder region.

The structure of the fibrous cap contributes to plaque integrity. Whereas lesions with thick fibrous caps may cause pronounced arterial narrowing, they have less propensity to rupture. Conversely, plaques that have thinner caps (and often appear less obstructive by angiography) tend to be fragile and more likely to rupture and incite thrombosis (Fig. 5-4C). Current clinical terminology describes the extremes of the spectrum of integrity as "stable plaques" (marked by a thick fibrous cap and small lipid core) or "vulnerable plaques" (marked by a thin

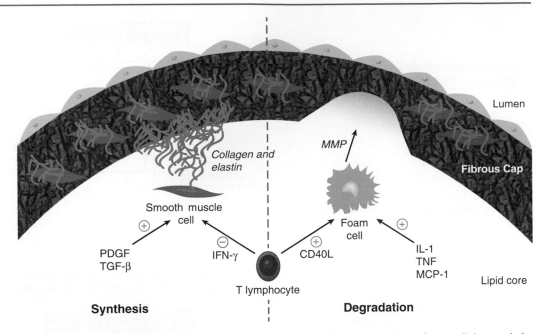

Figure 5-6. Matrix metabolism underlies fibrous cap integrity. The net deposition of extracellular matrix is the result of competing synthesis and degradation reactions. Smooth muscle cells synthesize the bulk of the fibrous cap constituents, such as collagen and elastin. Foam cells elaborate destructive proteolytic enzymes, such as the collagen-degrading matrix metalloproteinases (MMP) and the elastolytic cathepsins. T-lymphocyte–derived factors favor destruction of the fibrous cap. All plaque residents, however, contribute to the cytokine milieu of the plaque, providing multiple activating and inhibitory stimuli as shown. IFN-γ, interferon-γ; IL-1, interleukin-1; MCP-1, monocyte chemoattractant protein-1; PDGF, platelet-derived growth factor; TGF-β, transforming growth factor-β; TNF, tumor necrosis factor. (Modified from Libby P. The molecular bases of acute coronary syndromes. *Circulation*. 1995;91:2844-2850; Young JL, Libby P, Schönbeck U. Cytokines in the pathogenesis of atherosclerosis. *Thromb Haemost*. 2002;88:554-567.)

fibrous cap, rich lipid core, extensive macrophage infiltrate, and a paucity of SMCs; Fig. 5-7). Despite the common use of these terms, this distinction vastly oversimplifies the heterogeneity of plaques and may overestimate the ability to foresee a plaque's "clinical future" based on structural information. Most plaques with the so-called "vulnerable" morphology do not actually cause clinical events; hence, attempts to specifically identify such plaques may not direct therapy in an effective manner. Moreover, a substantial minority of fatal thrombi in coronary arteries arise from matrix-rich plaques with intact fibrous caps, a morphology that may arise from superficial erosion of the lesion by mechanisms that are not well understood.

The substrate of fibrous cap rupture vs. erosion appear to differ substantially. In contrast to the lipid-rich thin fibrous capped atheroma associated with rupture, lesions complicated by erosion tend to have abundant extracellular matrix, less lipid collection, and fewer macrophages (see Fig. 5-7). Yet, innate immune inflammatory pathways may participate in plaque erosion. Polymorphonuclear leukocytes and the neutrophil extracellular traps (NETs) that they can elaborate when dying may propagate endothelial erosion and the resultant thrombi that account for up to a third of acute coronary syndromes.

Thrombogenic Potential
Rupture of atherosclerotic plaque does not inevitably cause major clinical events such as myocardial infarction or stroke. As described in the previous section, small nonocclusive thrombi may incorporate into the plaque, stimulating further smooth muscle growth and extracellular matrix deposition (see Fig. 5-7). The balance between the thrombogenic and fibrinolytic potential of the

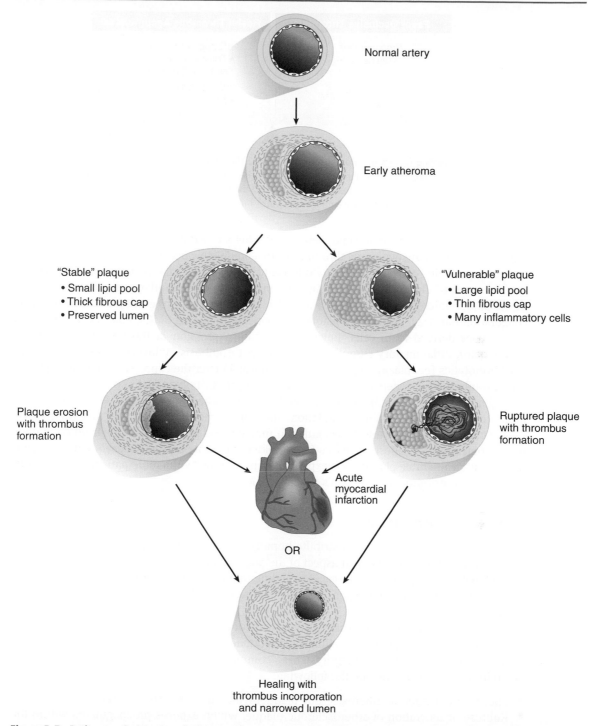

Figure 5-7. Pathways of plaque evolution. Stable plaque is characterized by a small lipid core and a thick fibrous cap, whereas vulnerable plaque tends to have a large lipid core and a relatively thin fibrous cap. The latter is subject to rupture, resulting in thrombosis. A resulting occlusive clot can cause an acute cardiac event, such as myocardial infarction. A lesser thrombus may resorb, but the wound-healing response stimulates smooth muscle cell proliferation and collagen production, leading to further narrowing the vessel lumen. Within stable plaques, superficial erosion can occur leading to coronary thrombosis driven by polymorphonuclear leukocytes and the NETs they elaborate when dying. This type of thrombosis often lacks prominent inflammatory infiltrates and is instead characterized by proteoglycan accumulation. Eroded plaques can also undergo wound healing by thrombus incorporation.

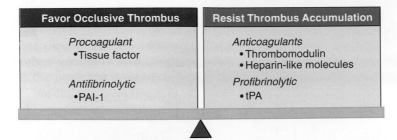

Figure 5-8. Competing factors in thrombus accumulation. The clinical manifestations of plaque disruption rely not only on the stability of the fibrous cap but also on the thrombogenic potential of the plaque core. The balance of physiologic mediators dictates the prominence of the thrombus, resulting in either luminal occlusion or resorption into the plaque. PAI-1, plasminogen activator inhibitor-1; tPA, tissue plasminogen activator.

plaque, and the fluid phase of blood, determines whether disruption of the fibrous cap leads to a transient, nonobstructive mural thrombus or to a completely occlusive clot.

The probability of a major thrombotic event reflects the balance between the competing processes of clot formation and dissolution by fibrinolysis. Inflammatory stimuli found in the plaque microenvironment (eg, CD40L) elicit tissue factor, the initiator of the extrinsic coagulation pathway, from many plaque components including SMCs, endothelial cells, and macrophage-derived foam cells. Beyond enhancing expression of the potent procoagulant tissue factor, inflammatory stimuli further support thrombosis by favoring the expression of antifibrinolytics (eg, plasminogen activator inhibitor-1) over the expression of anticoagulants (eg, thrombomodulin, heparin-like molecules) and profibrinolytic mediators (eg, tissue plasminogen activator; Fig. 5-8). Moreover, as described earlier, the activated endothelium also promotes thrombin formation, coagulation, and fibrin deposition at the vascular wall.

A person's propensity toward coagulation may depend on genetics, comorbid conditions (eg, diabetes), and/or lifestyle factors (eg, smoking, visceral obesity). Consequently, the concept of the "vulnerable plaque" has expanded to that of the "vulnerable patient," to acknowledge other contributors to a person's vascular risk.

COMPLICATIONS OF ATHEROSCLEROSIS

Atherosclerotic plaques do not distribute homogeneously throughout the vasculature. They usually develop first in the dorsal aspect of the abdominal aorta and proximal coronary arteries, followed by the popliteal arteries, descending thoracic aorta, internal carotid arteries, and renal arteries. Therefore, the regions perfused by these vessels most commonly suffer the consequences of atherosclerosis.

Complications of atherosclerotic plaques—including calcification, rupture, hemorrhage, and embolization—can have dire clinical consequences due to acute restriction of blood flow or alterations in vessel wall integrity. These complications, which are discussed in greater detail in later chapters, include the following:

- Spotty calcification of atherosclerotic plaque, which may increase its fragility.
- Rupture or ulceration of atherosclerotic plaque, which exposes procoagulants within the plaque to circulating blood, causing a thrombus to form at that site. Such thrombosis can occlude the vessel and result in infarction of the involved organ. Alternatively, the thrombus can organize, incorporate into the lesion, and add to the bulk of the plaque.
- Hemorrhage into the plaque owing to rupture of the fibrous cap or of the microvessels that form within the lesion. The resulting intramural hematoma may further narrow the vessel lumen.
- Embolization of fragments of disrupted atheroma to distal vascular sites.

- Weakening of the vessel wall: the fibrous plaque subjects the neighboring medial layer to increased pressure, which may provoke atrophy and loss of elastic tissue with subsequent expansion of the artery, forming an aneurysm.
- Microvessel growth within plaques, providing a source for intraplaque hemorrhage and further leukocyte trafficking.

The complications of atherosclerotic plaque may result in specific clinical consequences in different organ systems (Fig. 5-9). When lesion growth eventually outstrips the compensatory outward enlargement of the plaque, the lesion can narrow the vessel lumen and, in the case of the coronary arteries, cause intermittent chest discomfort on exertion (angina pectoris). In contrast, plaque that does not compromise the vessel lumen but has characteristics of vulnerability (eg, a thin fibrous cap, a large lipid core, spotty calcifications) can rupture, leading to acute thrombosis and myocardial infarction (see Chapter 7). Such nonstenotic plaques are often numerous and dispersed throughout the arterial tree, and because they do not limit arterial flow, they do not produce symptoms and often evade detection by exercise testing or angiography.

The description presented here of atherogenesis and its complications can explain the limitations of widely employed treatments. For example, percutaneous intervention (angioplasty and stent placement) of symptomatic coronary stenoses effectively relieves angina pectoris but does not necessarily prevent future myocardial infarction or prolong life, with

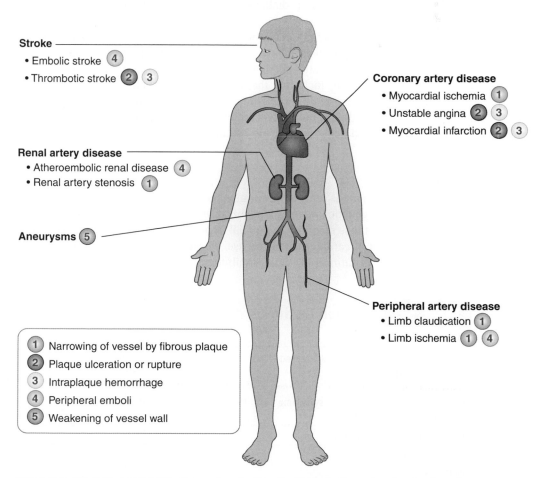

Figure 5-9. Clinical sequelae of atherosclerosis. Complications of atherosclerosis arise from the mechanisms listed in the figure.

the exception of patients in the early phase of an acute ST-elevation myocardial infarction, as described in Chapter 7. This disparity likely reflects the multiplicity of nonocclusive plaques at risk of precipitating thrombotic events. It follows that lifestyle modifications and drug therapies that curb the risk factors for plaque formation, and lessen features associated with "vulnerability," provide a critical foundation for preventing progression and complications of atherosclerosis.

ATHEROSCLEROSIS RISK FACTORS

In the early 20th century, most viewed atherosclerosis as an inevitable process of aging. But in 1948, the landmark Framingham Heart Study began to examine the relationship between specific attributes and cardiovascular disease, establishing the concept of atherosclerotic risk factors. Among later studies, the Multiple Risk Factor Intervention Trial (MRFIT) screened more than 325,000 men, offering an opportunity to correlate risk factors with subsequent cardiovascular disease and mortality. Of the major risk factors, those that are not modifiable include advanced age, male gender, and heredity—that is, a history of coronary heart disease among first-degree relatives at a young age (before age 55 for a male relative or before age 65 for a female relative). Risk factors for atherosclerosis amenable to modification include undesirable concentrations and composition of circulating lipids (dyslipidemia), tobacco smoking, hypertension, diabetes mellitus, and lack of physical activity and obesity (Table 5-1).

In addition to these standard predictors, certain biologic markers associated with the development of cardiovascular events have been undergoing rigorous evaluation as "novel" risk markers. These include elevated circulating levels of the lipoprotein particle Lp(a) and certain markers of inflammation, including the acute-phase reactant C-reactive protein (CRP). Furthermore, recent genome-wide association studies (GWAS) have sought to identify variants in genetic loci associated with increased cardiovascular risk.

The following sections address these risk factors and biologic markers.

GENETICS

Genetic predisposition, as reflected by family history, comprises a major risk factor for atherosclerosis. Previous genetic understanding of coronary artery disease was limited to monogenic mutations such as those resulting in familial hypercholesterolemia which conferred a severalfold increased risk of cardiovascular disease. These directly causative mutations spurred the development of the statins and PSCK9 inhibitors (see Chapter 17).

TABLE 5-1	Common Cardiovascular Risk Factors
Modifiable risk factors	
Dyslipidemia (elevated LDL, decreased HDL) Tobacco smoking Hypertension Diabetes mellitus, metabolic syndrome Lack of physical activity	
Nonmodifiable risk factors	
Advanced age Male sex Heredity	

However, recent large-scale GWAS have enabled polygenic risk assessment. While each of the many polygenic variations contributes less to overall cardiovascular risk than a single monogenic mutation, the summative effect of multiple such acquired mutations can have considerable impact on clinical risk. In the future, such clinical polygenic risk scores may aid the identification of individuals with a predisposition for atherosclerosis that traditional risk factors miss, signaling the need for early preventative therapy.

Furthermore, the recent identification of cardiovascular risk due to clonal hematopoiesis of indeterminate potential (CHIP), a precursor to hematologic malignancy, may contribute to our understanding of the mechanisms of atherosclerosis. With aging, somatic, acquired mutations in bone marrow stem cells can lead to clonal expansion of hematopoietic cells in peripheral blood without hematologic abnormalities. Patients who harbor these clones have increased all-cause mortality driven by primarily by cardiovascular events rather than by hematologic malignancy. Clonal hematopoiesis may serve as a novel risk marker, independent of classical risk factors, that helps to identify individuals who might benefit from targeted therapies.

INFLAMMATION

As discussed earlier, the pathogenesis of atherosclerosis involves inflammation at every stage, and immune cells play a key role in the modification of plaques. For example, plaque rupture preferentially occurs where the fibrous cap is thin and weakened. Immune cells abound at these sites and can produce numerous inflammatory cytokines (eg, IL-1 and IL-6) and proteolytic enzymes which work to weaken the fibrous cap, converting a stable plaque to a vulnerable plaque prone to rupture. These proinflammatory cytokines incite increased hepatic production of acute-phase reactants such as CRP, fibrinogen, and serum amyloid A.

Indeed, biomarkers of inflammation such as high-sensitivity CRP and IL-6 are associated with an increased risk of cardiovascular events. Large studies of apparently healthy men and women indicate that those with higher CRP levels have increased risk of adverse cardiovascular outcomes, independent of serum cholesterol concentrations and other traditional risk markers. Multiple prospective studies affirm that CRP measured by a highly sensitive assay (hsCRP) independently predicts myocardial infarction, stroke, peripheral artery disease, and sudden cardiac death. Although it serves as a marker of risk not captured by traditional algorithms, CRP itself does not mediate atherogenesis.

Data support the use of CRP levels to guide therapy. For example, the prospective JUPITER trial studied 17,800 healthy individuals with above-median levels of CRP who did not have elevated LDL and demonstrated a reduced incidence of major cardiovascular events in patients who were treated with a statin, compared to those who received a placebo.

The recently published CANTOS trial evaluating a monoclonal antibody targeting IL-1β, a cytokine upstream of IL-6, demonstrated a significant reduction in recurrent cardiovascular events independent of lipid lowering. This trial provided important support of the inflammatory hypothesis. Having demonstrated for the first time that an agent targeting inflammation and autoimmunity can provide clinical benefit outside of the traditional risk factors, the field is ripe for further investigation of novel anti-inflammatory agents that can provide clinical benefit.

TRADITIONAL RISK FACTORS

Dyslipidemia

A large and consistent body of evidence establishes abnormal circulating lipid levels as a major risk factor for atherosclerosis. Observational studies have consistently shown a relationship between hypercholesterolemia and coronary artery disease. The coronary risk rises approximately twofold for a person with a total cholesterol level of 240 mg/dL compared with a person whose cholesterol level is 200 mg/dL. In particular, elevated levels of circulating LDL correlate with an increased incidence of atherosclerosis and coronary artery disease. Thus, LDL is commonly known as "bad cholesterol." Elevated serum LDL may persist for many reasons, including a high-fat diet or abnormalities in the LDL receptor clearance mechanism. Patients with genetic defects in the LDL receptor, which leads to *familial hypercholesterolemia*, cannot remove LDL from the circulation efficiently. Heterozygotes with this condition have one normal and one defective gene coding for the receptor. They display high plasma LDL levels and develop premature atherosclerosis. Homozygotes who *completely* lack functional LDL receptors may experience vascular events, such as acute myocardial infarction, as early as the first decade of life.

In addition to LDL, another circulating lipoprotein that is associated with cardiovascular events is lipoprotein (a), referred to as Lp(a) and pronounced "L-P-little-a." Lp(a) is a variant of LDL whose major apolipoprotein (apo B-100) links by a disulfide bridge to another protein, apo(a). Apo(a) structurally resembles plasminogen, a plasma protein important in the endogenous lysis of fibrin clots (see Chapter 7). Thus, the detrimental effect attributed to Lp(a) may relate to competition with normal plasminogen activity.

Lp(a) levels in the population are skewed with trailing prevalence of the higher levels. Diet and exercise have little impact on Lp(a) concentration. Until recently, traditional lipid-lowering agents (with the exception of niacin) had little or no effect on Lp(a) reduction. PCSK9 inhibitors (described in Chapter 17) can lower Lp(a) by as much as 30%, but whether that effect of treatment independently translates into a reduction in ischemic events has not been determined.

Increasing evidence also implicates triglyceride-rich lipoproteins, such as VLDL and IDL, in the development of atherosclerosis. Current human genetic evidence strongly supports a causal role of triglyceride-rich lipoproteins in atherosclerotic events. Blood triglyceride concentrations serve as a biomarker of triglyceride-rich lipoproteins. It is likely that the cholesterol carried by these particles exerts the pathogenic effects.

Elevated HDL particles (termed "good cholesterol") are associated with protection against atherosclerosis, often attributed to HDL's ability to transport cholesterol away from the peripheral tissues back to the liver for disposal (termed "reverse cholesterol transport") and its putative antioxidative and anti-inflammatory properties. Yet, several lines of evidence cast doubt on HDL's protective role in atherosclerosis. The risk long attributed to low HDL may actually arise because of high concentrations of triglyceride-rich lipoproteins which tend to vary inversely with HDL levels. Of note, poorly controlled type 2 diabetes mellitus commonly associates with this combination of hypertriglyceridemia and low HDL levels.

Lipid-Altering Therapy

Strategies that improve abnormal lipid levels can limit the consequences of atherosclerosis. Many large studies of patients with coronary disease show that dietary or pharmacologic reduction of serum cholesterol can prevent cardiovascular events.

Lifestyle modifications that may be beneficial include maintenance of healthy diet and weight and augmented physical activity. However, even intensive lifestyle modification is rarely sufficient to prevent cardiovascular events in individuals with long established atherosclerotic risk factors. Hence, many individuals require pharmacologic agents to optimize cardiovascular outcomes. Major groups of lipid-altering agents in current clinical use (see Chapter 17) include HMG-CoA reductase inhibitors (also known as "statins"), intestinal cholesterol absorption inhibitors (eg, ezetimibe), and inhibitors of PCSK9. Of available classes of medication, the statins have emerged as the key LDL-lowering drugs that reduce cardiovascular events in a wide range of patients. These agents inhibit the rate-limiting enzyme responsible for cholesterol biosynthesis. The resulting reduction in intracellular cholesterol concentration promotes increased LDL receptor expression and thus augments clearance of LDL particles from the bloodstream. Statins also lower the rate of VLDL synthesis by the liver (thus lowering circulating triglyceride levels). Major clinical trials evaluating statins have demonstrated reductions in ischemic cardiac events, ischemic strokes, and mortality rates in individuals both with and without a history of prior atherosclerotic cardiovascular events. Statins have also earned an enviable safety record after decades of widespread use.

Recent genetic studies have identified gain-of-function mutations in the *PCSK9* gene as a cause of hypercholesterolemia. The PCSK9 protein normally chaperones LDL receptors into cytoplasmic lysosomes for degradation. Therapeutic monoclonal antibodies (administered subcutaneously) have been developed that inhibit PCSK9 and lower serum LDL levels by reducing degradation of LDL receptors, thus boosting LDL clearance from the circulation. Large randomized clinical trials have shown robust LDL reductions when PCSK9 inhibitors are added to statin therapy, and further reduction in cardiovascular event rates compared to statin therapy alone. Thus, these agents have become an important therapeutic option for patients with familial hypercholesterolemia, for those intolerant of statins, and for high-risk individuals with persistent hypercholesterolemia despite treatment with statins and ezetimibe.

Based on evidence from a large number of clinical trials that have affirmed that more intense LDL lowering yields greater clinical benefit ("lower is better"), the American College of Cardiology and the American Heart Association issued updated cholesterol guidelines in 2018 that focus on groups of patients most likely to benefit from lipid-lowering therapy (Table 5-2). Of note, pharmacologic lipid-altering therapy is recommended for all patients at highest risk, including those with established clinical atherosclerotic cardiovascular disease, individuals with baseline LDL cholesterol ≥190 mg/dL, and diabetics. In primary prevention, the use of pharmacologic therapy depends on the patient's calculated risk of a future cardiovascular event, as indicated in the table.

Older classes of drugs that lower LDL include niacin and bile acid sequestrants. However, these agents currently have very limited use as they have not demonstrated the magnitude of outcomes benefits and favorable risk/benefit balance as the statins, ezetimibe, or PCSK9 inhibitors.

Past clinical trials of pharmaceuticals that predominantly reduce blood triglycerides (fibrates, omega-3 fatty acids) have not shown mortality benefits and have fallen out of favor for cardiovascular use. These agents are now prescribed to lower severely elevated serum triglyceride levels (>500 mg/dL) to prevent pancreatitis. In contrast, the recent prospective randomized REDUCE-IT trial showed that oral high-dose icosapent ethyl, a highly purified omega-3 fatty acid ethyl ester preparation, reduced the risk of ischemic events (including cardiovascular death) in patients with hypertriglyceridemia receiving concomitant statin therapy.

Tobacco Smoking

Numerous studies have shown that tobacco smoking predisposes to atherosclerosis and ischemic heart disease. Even low-level smoking worsens outcomes, but the heaviest smokers have the greatest risk of cardiovascular events. Tobacco smoking potentially promotes atherosclerotic disease in several ways, including enhanced oxidative stress, endothelial dysfunction, increased platelet adhesiveness, inappropriate stimulation of the sympathetic nervous system by nicotine, and displacement of oxygen by carbon monoxide from hemoglobin. Extrapolation from animal experiments suggests that smoking not only accelerates atherogenesis but also increases the propensity for thrombosis—both components of the "vulnerable patient."

Fortunately, smoking cessation can reverse some of the adverse outcomes. People who stop smoking greatly reduce their likelihood of coronary heart disease, compared with those who continue to smoke. In one study, after 3 years of cessation, the risk of coronary artery disease for former smokers became similar to subjects who never smoked.

Hypertension

Elevated blood pressure (either systolic or diastolic) augments the risk of developing atherosclerosis, coronary heart disease, and stroke (see Chapter 13). The association of elevated

TABLE 5-2	Guideline Recommendations for Lipid-Altering Therapy
Patient Group	**Recommendation**
Clinical atherosclerotic disease (ASCVD) (Coronary artery disease, history of stroke, transient ischemic cerebral attack, peripheral vascular disease, or aortic aneurysm)	1. High-intensity statin[a] to achieve ≥50% LDL reduction 2. If LDL remains ≥70 mg/dL: Consider adding ezetimibe 3. If very high risk[b] and LDL still ≥70 mg/dL on maximally tolerated statin + ezetimibe: Consider adding PCSK9 inhibitor
LDL cholesterol ≥190 mg/dL at baseline	1. High-intensity statin[a] to achieve ≥50% LDL reduction 2. If <50% LDL reduction achieved or LDL remains ≥100 mg/dL: Consider adding ezetimibe 3. If LDL reduction still <50%: Consider adding bile acid sequestrant (see Chapter 17; do not add if triglycerides >300 mg/dL) 4. If pt has heterozygous familial hypercholesterolemia and LDL still ≥100 mg/dL (or if baseline LDL ≥ 220 mg/dL, age 40-75 and LDL still ≥130 mg/dL): Consider adding PCSK9 inhibitor
Diabetes	
Age 40-75	
• Regardless of ASCVD risk • Multiple ASCVD risk factors • 10-year ASCVD risk[d] ≥20%	*Moderate-intensity statin[c] to achieve ≥30% LDL reduction* High-intensity statin[a] to achieve ≥50% LDL reduction High-intensity statin[a] plus ezetimibe, if needed, to achieve LDL ≥ 50% reduction
Age > 75	Data are limited; statin therapy reasonable after discussion of benefits and risks
Age 20-39	Consider statin if diabetes of long duration, estimated GFR < 60 mL/min/1.73 m², or presence of albuminuria, retinopathy, neuropathy, or reduced ankle-brachial index (see Chapter 15)
Primary prevention (age 40-75, nondiabetic, LDL 70-189 mg/dL): Calculate 10-year risk of cardiovascular event[d]:	
• Low risk (<5%)	Lifestyle improvements
• Borderline risk (5%-7.5%)	If risk enhancers present[e]: Consider moderate-intensity statin[c]
• Intermediate risk (7.5%-20%)	Moderate-intensity statin,[c] especially if risk enhancers present,[e] to achieve ≥30% LDL reduction (if decision to treat uncertain, consider obtaining coronary calcium score[f]) If insufficient reduction of LDL due to statin intolerance, consider adding ezetimibe or bile acid sequestrant (see Chapter 17)
• High risk (≥20%)	Moderate-high intensity statin[a,c] to achieve ≥50% LDL reduction

[a]High-intensity statin: Atorvastatin 40-80 mg daily or rosuvastatin 20-40 mg daily; for age ≥75, or if statin adverse effects, consider moderate-intensity statin[c] instead.

[b]Very high-risk includes prior major ASCVD events (recent acute coronary syndrome, history of myocardial infarction, ischemic stroke, symptomatic peripheral vascular disease) or one major ASCVD event and multiple high-risk attributes (age ≥65, heterozygous familial hypercholesterolemia, prior coronary artery bypass graft surgery or percutaneous coronary intervention, diabetes, hypertension, current smoking, chronic kidney disease).

[c]Moderate-intensity statin: atorvastatin 10-20 mg daily, rosuvastatin 5-10 mg daily, or simvastatin 20-40 mg daily.

[d]10-year ASCVD risk can be estimated using the online calculator: http://my.americanheart.org/cvriskcalculator.

[e]ASCVD risk enhancers: Family history premature coronary artery disease (ie, before age 55 in male relatives or before age 65 in female relatives), persistently elevated LDL ≥ 160 mg/dL, chronic kidney disease, metabolic syndrome (defined as ≥3 of the following: increased waist circumference, hypertension, hyperglycemia, elevated triglycerides, low HDL), inflammatory diseases (rheumatoid arthritis, psoriasis, HIV), South Asian ancestry, premature menopause, elevated triglycerides (≥175 mg/dL), high-sensitivity C-reactive protein ≥2.0 mg/L, lipoprotein (a) >50 mg/dL, and ankle-brachial index <0.9.

[f]Coronary calcium quantification by CT imaging is described in Chapter 3; if score is 0, withhold statin; if score is ≥100, initiate statin; if score is 1-99 and age ≥55, initiate statin.

Derived from recommendations in Grundy SM, Stone NJ, Bailey AL, et al. 2018 Guideline on the management of blood cholesterol. *J Am Coll Cardiol.* 2019;73:3168-3209.

blood pressure with cardiovascular disease does not appear to have a specific threshold. Rather, risk increases continuously with progressively higher pressure.

Hypertension may accelerate atherosclerosis in several ways. Animal studies have shown that elevated blood pressure injures vascular endothelium and may increase the permeability of the vessel wall to lipoproteins. Cyclic circumferential strain, increased in hypertensive arteries, can enhance SMC production of proteoglycans that bind and retain LDL particles, promoting their accumulation in the intima and facilitating their oxidative modification. Angiotensin II, a mediator of hypertension (described in Chapter 13), acts not only as a vasoconstrictor but also as a stimulator of oxidative stress (through activation of NADPH oxidases, a source of superoxide anion, O_2^-) and as a proinflammatory cytokine. Thus, hypertension may also promote atherogenesis by contributing to a pro-oxidant and inflammatory state.

Antihypertensive Therapy

Like dyslipidemias, treatment of hypertension should start with lifestyle modifications but often requires pharmacologic intervention. The Dietary Approaches to Stop Hypertension (DASH) studies demonstrate that a diet high in fruits and vegetables, with low fat dairy products and an overall reduced sodium content, significantly improves systolic and diastolic blood pressures. Regular exercise can also reduce resting blood pressure levels. Many medications effectively lower blood pressure, as described in Chapters 13 and 17.

Diabetes Mellitus and the "Metabolic Syndrome"

Diabetes mellitus affects an estimated 170 million people worldwide, a prevalence projected to grow 40% worldwide by 2030. In the United States alone, 18.2 million people have diabetes, and projections suggest that one in every three children born in 2000 will eventually develop the condition. With a three- to fivefold increased risk of acute coronary events, 80% of diabetic patients succumb to atherosclerosis-related conditions, including coronary heart disease, stroke, and peripheral artery disease.

The predisposition of diabetic patients to atherosclerosis may relate in part to accompanying dyslipidemia, to nonenzymatic glycation of proteins, or to the associated prothrombotic tendency and antifibrinolytic state. Diabetics frequently have impaired endothelial function, gauged by the reduced bioavailability of NO, and increased leukocyte adhesion. Tight control of serum glucose levels in diabetic patients reduces the risk of *microvascular* complications, such as retinopathy and nephropathy. However, until recently, therapies for type 2 diabetes had not shown benefit on *macrovascular* outcomes, such as myocardial infarction and stroke. The mainstay of therapy had been the treatment of hypertension and dyslipidemia in diabetic patients to reduce the risk of cardiac and cerebrovascular complications. However, newer antihyperglycemic drugs, notably glucagon-like peptide-1 (GLP-1) receptor agonists and sodium-glucose cotransporter 2 (SGLT2) inhibitors, have recently been shown to reduce cardiovascular event rates in type 2 diabetics.

The **metabolic syndrome** (also known as the "insulin resistance syndrome") refers to a cluster of risk factors, including hypertension, hypertriglyceridemia, reduced HDL, hyperglycemia, and visceral obesity (excessive adipose tissue in the abdomen). This constellation associates with a high risk for atherosclerosis in both diabetic and nondiabetic patients, and using currently accepted criteria, 25% of Americans have this condition. The presence of insulin resistance in this syndrome appears to promote atherogenesis long before affected persons develop overt diabetes.

Lack of Physical Activity

Exercise may mitigate atherogenesis in several ways. In addition to its beneficial effects on the lipid profile and blood pressure, exercise enhances insulin sensitivity and endothelial production of NO. Observational studies of both men and women indicate that even modest activities, such as brisk walking, for as little as 30 minutes per day can protect against cardiovascular mortality.

Estrogen Status

Cardiovascular disease dominates other causes of mortality in women, including breast and other cancers. Before menopause, women have a lower incidence of coronary events than men. After menopause, however, men and women have similar rates. Such observations led to the conjecture that estrogen (the levels of which decline after menopause) exerts athero-protective properties. Physiologic estrogen levels in premenopausal women raise HDL and lower LDL. Experimentally, estrogen also exhibits potentially beneficial antioxidant and anti-platelet actions and improves endothelium-dependent vasodilation.

Observational studies suggested that hormone therapy reduced the risk of coronary artery disease in postmenopausal women, prompting many physicians to prescribe such medications for cardiovascular prevention purposes. However, the Heart and Estrogen/Progestin Replacement Study demonstrated an association between such hormone use and an early *increased* risk of vascular events in women with preexisting coronary disease. Subsequent randomized primary prevention studies from the Women's Health Initiative were terminated prematurely because estrogen-plus-progestin treatment increased cardiovascular risk by 24% overall, with a striking 81% higher risk during the first year of therapy. Because currently available clinical trial data do not show that gonadal hormone therapy lowers cardiovascular events and that it may actually be harmful, such therapy should not be commenced for the sole goal of reducing cardiovascular risk.

BIOMARKERS OF CARDIOVASCULAR RISK

Despite identification of the well-established risk factors just described, one out of five cardiovascular events occurs in patients lacking these attributes. In conjunction with growing knowledge about the pathogenesis of atherosclerosis, several novel markers of risk have emerged. These biomarkers serve three primary roles: (1) as a means to help stratify the risk of atherosclerotic disease and thus guide the choice of therapies, (2) as clinical measures to assess treatment effects, and (3) as potential targets of new therapeutic regimens. The use of high-sensitivity C-reactive protein (hsCRP), multicomponent genetic risk scores, coronary artery calcium scores (see Chapter 3), ankle-brachial index (see Chapter 15), and CHIP status may sharpen risk stratification beyond traditional algorithms. Yet, so far only guiding therapy by inflammatory status as gauged by hsCRP has proven capable of improving outcomes in prospective randomized clinical trials.

OUTLOOK

Despite accumulating knowledge of the pathogenesis of atherosclerosis and its clinical sequelae, this disease remains a major cause of death throughout the world. Although improvements in cardiovascular care have reduced age-adjusted mortality from this condition, it will continue to grow as a menace as the population ages and as developing countries adopt the adverse dietary and activity habits of a Western lifestyle. Ongoing research into the biology of atherosclerosis, as well as advances in therapeutic procedures and medications, will undoubtedly continue to further our abilities to combat this condition. Yet, we have not fully capitalized on what we already know—that much cardiovascular risk is modifiable. Effective control of the risk factors described earlier remains a critical component to tame this global scourge. It is here that the relationship between the patient and health care provider, and the role of medical professionals as community leaders advocating healthy lifestyles, remains of cardinal importance.

Summary

- Atherosclerosis is the **leading cause of mortality and morbidity** in developed nations and has become a major cause of death in the developing world.

- The arterial wall consists of the **intima** (closest to the arterial lumen), the **media** (the middle layer), and the **adventitia** (the outer layer).

- The **normal endothelium** provides a protective, nonthrombogenic surface with homeostatic vasodilatory and anti-inflammatory properties.

- Early in atherogenesis, injurious stimuli **activate endothelial and smooth muscle cells**, which recruit inflammatory cells to the vessel wall.

- Atherosclerotic plaques form over decades and can display features associated with clinical stability or a propensity to provoke thrombotic events (**"vulnerable" plaques**).

- Clinical atherosclerotic events result from **narrowing of the vessel lumen, aneurysm formation, or plaque disruption** with superimposed thrombus formation.

- Common manifestations of atherosclerosis include **angina pectoris, myocardial infarction, stroke, and peripheral artery disease.**

- **Modifiable risk factors** for atherosclerosis include dyslipidemia, smoking, hypertension, and diabetes.

- **Nonmodifiable risk factors** include advanced age, male sex, and a family history of premature coronary disease.

- Novel biomarkers, such as high-sensitivity **C-reactive protein (hsCRP)**, may prove useful in defining risk.

Review Questions

1. Which of the following statements about the vascular biology of atherosclerosis is correct?

   a. In normal arteries, the majority of smooth muscle cells reside in the intima.
   b. Foam cells arise from uptake of LDL via LDL receptor–mediated endocytosis.
   c. Foam cells elaborate matrix metalloproteinases that degrade collagen.
   d. Secretion of interferon-γ by T lymphocytes increases collagen synthesis by smooth muscle cells.

2. Which of the following blood measurements is NOT a risk factor for future cardiovascular events?

   a. Elevated LDL cholesterol
   b. Elevated Lp(a)
   c. Elevated high-sensitivity C-reactive protein
   d. Elevated HDL cholesterol

3. A 66-year-old man who sustained an anterior wall myocardial infarction 6 months ago is taking high-dose atorvastatin therapy (80 mg daily). A recent serum lipid panel shows that his LDL cholesterol is 110 mg/dL. What is the next appropriate step in lipid management?

  a. Prescribe a PCSK9 inhibitor.
  b. Add daily ezetimibe.
  c. Add a second statin drug.
  d. The LDL level is satisfactory; no further intervention needed.

Answers to Review Questions

1. **Choice c is correct.** In atherogenesis, after monocytes penetrate the intima, they differentiate into macrophages and internalize modified LDL by scavenger receptors (not LDL receptors), in an unregulated fashion, to form foam cells. Inflammatory cytokines then stimulate local foam cells to secrete metalloproteinases which degrade collagen and elastin, thus weakening the fibrous cap (see Fig. 5-6). Interferon-γ secreted by T lymphocytes *inhibits* collagen synthesis by smooth muscle cells, also weakening the fibrous cap and predisposing it to rupture. In contrast, platelet-derived growth factor (PDGF) and transforming growth factor-β (TGF-β) *promote* collagen synthesis by smooth muscle cells and contribute to the integrity of the fibrous cap. In normal arteries, the majority of smooth muscles cells reside in the *media*.

2. **Choice d is correct.** Elevated blood levels of LDL cholesterol, Lp(a), and high-sensitivity CRP are all associated with increased risk of cardiovascular events. In contrast, elevated levels of HDL are generally associated with protection against atherosclerosis.

3. **Choice b is correct.** This patient has clinical atherosclerotic disease and is at high risk, having sustained a myocardial infarction 6 months ago, such that his target LDL is <70 mg/dL (see Table 5-2). His current high-intensity statin therapy and lifestyle improvements are appropriate as initial therapy, but his LDL remains >70 mg/dL. The next step in management should be the addition of ezetimibe, an intestinal cholesterol-absorption inhibitor (Table 5-2). If the LDL still remains >70 mg/dL on this combination, a PCSK9 inhibitor should then be considered in addition. Addition of a second statin would likely have little impact on LDL but would increase the risk of adverse events.

Acknowledgments

Contributors to the previous editions of this chapter were Sarrah Shahawy, MD; Jordan B. Strom, MD; James L. Young, MD; Mary Beth Gordon, MD; Rushika Fernandopulle, MD; Gopa Bhattacharyya, MD; and Joseph Loscalzo, MD, PhD.

Additional Reading

Bhatt DL, Steg PG, Miller M, et al. Cardiovascular risk reduction with icosapent ethyl for hypertriglyceridemia. *N Engl J Med.* 2019;380:11-22.

Cholesterol Treatment Trialists' (CTT) Collaborators. Efficacy and safety of LDL-lowering therapy among men and women: meta-analysis of individual data from 174,000 participants in 27 randomised trials. *Lancet.* 2015;385:1397-1405.

Ference BA, Ginsberg HN, Graham I, et al. Low-density lipoproteins cause atherosclerotic cardiovascular disease. 1. Evidence from genetic, epidemiologic, and clinical studies. A consensus statement from the European Atherosclerosis Society Consensus Panel. *Eur Heart J.* 2017;38:2459-2472.

Gimbrone MA Jr, Garcia-Cardena G. Endothelial cell dysfunction and the pathobiology of atherosclerosis. *Circ Res*. 2016;118: 620-636.

Grundy SM, Stone NJ, Bailey AL, et al. 2018 AHA/ACC/AACVPR/AAPA/ABC/ACPM/ADA/AGS/APhA/ASPC/NLA/PCNA Guideline on the management of blood cholesterol: executive summary: A report of the American College of Cardiology/ American Heart Association Task Force on Clinical Practice Guidelines. *J Am Coll Cardiol*. 2019;73:3168-3209.

Jaiswal S, Natarajan P, Silver AJ, et al. Clonal hematopoiesis and risk of atherosclerotic cardiovascular disease. *N Engl J Med*. 2017;377:111-121.

Libby P, Loscalzo J, Ridker PM, et al. Inflammation, immunity, and infection in atherothrombosis. *J Am Coll Cardiol*. 2018;72:2071-2081.

Libby P, Pasterkamp G, Crea F, et al. Reassessing the mechanisms of acute coronary syndromes. *Circ Res*. 2019;124:150-160.

Lupsa BC, Inzucchi SE. Diabetes medications and cardiovascular disease: at long last progress. *Curr Opin Endocrinol Diabetes Obes*. 2018;25:87-93.

Moore KJ, Koplev S, Fisher EA, et al. Macrophage trafficking, inflammatory resolution, and genomics in atherosclerosis: JACC Macrophage in CVD Series (Part 2). *J Am Coll Cardiol*. 2018;72:2181-2197.

Natarajan P, Young R, Stitziel NO, et al. Polygenic risk score identifies subgroup with higher burden of atherosclerosis and greater relative benefit from statin therapy in the primary prevention setting. *Circulation*. 2017;135:2091-2101.

Paré G, Çaku A, McQueen M, et al. Lipoprotein(a) levels and the risk of myocardial infarction among 7 ethnic groups. *Circulation*. 2019;139:1472-1482.

Ridker PM, Everett BM, Thuren T, et al. Antiinflammatory therapy with canakinumab for atherosclerotic disease. *N Engl J Med*. 2017;377:1119-1131.

Sabatine MS, Giugliano RP, Keech AC, et al. Evolocumab and clinical outcomes in patients with cardiovascular disease. *N Engl J Med*. 2017;376:1713-1722.

Schwartz GG, Steg PG, Szarek M, et al. Alirocumab and cardiovascular outcomes after acute coronary syndrome. *N Engl J Med*. 2018;379:2097-2107.

6

Ischemic Heart Disease

David D. Berg | Marc S. Sabatine | Leonard S. Lilly

In 1772, the British physician William Heberden reported a disorder in which patients developed an uncomfortable sensation in the chest when walking. Labeling it *angina pectoris*, Heberden noted that this discomfort would disappear soon after the patient stood still but would recur with similar activities. Although he did not know the cause, it is likely that he was the first to describe the symptoms of ischemic heart disease, a condition of imbalance between myocardial oxygen supply and demand, most often caused by atherosclerosis of the coronary arteries. Ischemic heart disease now afflicts millions of Americans and is the leading cause of death in industrialized nations.

The clinical presentation of ischemic heart disease can be highly variable and forms a spectrum of syndromes (Table 6-1). For example, ischemia may be accompanied by the same exertional symptoms described by Heberden. In other cases, it may occur without any clinical manifestations at all, a condition termed *silent ischemia*. This chapter describes the causes and consequences of chronic ischemic heart disease syndromes and provides a framework for the diagnosis and treatment of affected patients.

Angina pectoris remains the most common manifestation of ischemic heart disease and literally means "strangling in the chest." Although other conditions may lead to similar discomfort, *angina* refers specifically to the uncomfortable sensation in the chest and neighboring structures that arises from an imbalance between myocardial oxygen supply and demand.

TABLE 6-1	Clinical Definitions
Syndrome	**Description**
Ischemic heart disease	Condition in which imbalance between myocardial oxygen supply and demand results in myocardial hypoxia and accumulation of waste metabolites, most often caused by atherosclerotic disease of the coronary arteries (often termed *coronary artery disease*)
Angina pectoris	Uncomfortable sensation in the chest and neighboring anatomic structures produced by myocardial ischemia
Stable angina	Chronic pattern of transient angina pectoris, precipitated by physical activity or emotional upset, relieved by rest within a few minutes; episodes often associated with temporary depression of the ST segment, but permanent myocardial damage does not result
Variant angina	Typical anginal discomfort, usually *at rest*, which develops because of coronary artery spasm rather than an increase of myocardial oxygen demand; episodes often associated with transient shifts of the ST segment, usually ST elevation (also termed *Prinzmetal angina*)
Silent ischemia	Asymptomatic episodes of myocardial ischemia; can be detected by electrocardiogram and other laboratory techniques
Unstable angina	Pattern of increased frequency and duration of angina episodes produced by less exertion or at rest; high frequency of progression to myocardial infarction if untreated
Myocardial infarction	Region of myocardial necrosis usually caused by prolonged cessation of blood supply; most often results from acute thrombus at the site of coronary atherosclerotic stenosis; may be a first clinical manifestation of ischemic heart disease, or there may be a history of angina pectoris

DETERMINANTS OF MYOCARDIAL OXYGEN SUPPLY AND DEMAND

In the normal heart, the oxygen requirements of the myocardium are continuously matched by the coronary arterial supply. Even during vigorous exercise, when the metabolic needs of the heart increase, so does the delivery of oxygen to the myocardial cells so that the balance is maintained. The following sections describe the key determinants of myocardial oxygen supply and demand in a normal person (Fig. 6-1) and how they are altered by the presence of atherosclerotic coronary artery disease (CAD).

Figure 6-1. Major determinants of myocardial oxygen supply and demand. *P*, ventricular pressure; *r*, ventricular radius; *h*, ventricular wall thickness.

Myocardial Oxygen Supply

The supply of oxygen to the myocardium depends on the **oxygen content** of the blood and the rate of **coronary blood flow**. The oxygen content is determined by the hemoglobin concentration and the degree of systemic oxygenation. In the absence of severe anemia or lung disease, oxygen content remains fairly constant. In contrast, coronary blood flow is much more dynamic, and regulation of that flow is responsible for matching the oxygen supply with metabolic requirements.

As in all blood vessels, coronary artery flow (Q) is directly proportional to the vessel's perfusion pressure (P) and is inversely proportional to the coronary vascular resistance (R). That is,

$$Q \propto \frac{P}{R}$$

However, unlike other arterial systems in which the greatest blood flow occurs during systole, *the predominance of coronary perfusion from the aorta takes place during diastole.* The reason for this is that systolic flow is impaired by the compression of the small coronary branches as they course through the contracting myocardium. Coronary flow is unimpaired in diastole because the relaxed myocardium does not compress the coronary vasculature. Thus, in the case of the coronaries, **perfusion pressure** can be approximated by the aortic diastolic pressure (or more accurately, by the difference between the aortic diastolic pressure and the left ventricular diastolic pressure). Conditions that lower aortic diastolic pressure (such as hypotension or aortic valve regurgitation) reduce coronary artery perfusion pressure and may decrease myocardial oxygen supply.

Coronary vascular resistance is the other major determinant of coronary blood flow. In the normal artery, this resistance is dynamically modulated by (1) forces that externally compress the coronary arteries and (2) factors that alter intrinsic coronary tone.

External Compression

External compression is exerted on the coronary vessels during the cardiac cycle by contraction of the surrounding myocardium. The degree of compression is directly related to intramyocardial pressure and is therefore greatest during systole, as described in the previous section. Moreover, when the myocardium contracts, the subendocardium, adjacent to the high intraventricular pressure, is subjected to greater force than are the outer muscle layers. This is one reason that the subendocardium is the region most vulnerable to ischemic damage.

Intrinsic Control of Coronary Arterial Tone

Unlike most tissues, the heart cannot increase oxygen extraction on demand because in its basal state, it removes nearly as much oxygen as possible from its blood supply. Thus, *any additional oxygen requirement must be met by an increase in blood flow*, and autoregulation of coronary vascular resistance is the most important mediator of this process. Factors that participate in the regulation of coronary vascular resistance include the accumulation of local metabolites, endothelium-derived substances, and neural innervation.

Metabolic Factors

The accumulation of local metabolites significantly affects coronary vascular tone and acts to modulate myocardial oxygen supply to meet changing metabolic demands. During states of tissue hypoxia, aerobic metabolism and oxidative phosphorylation in the mitochondria are inhibited, and generation of high-energy phosphates, including adenosine triphosphate (ATP), is impaired. Consequently, adenosine diphosphate (ADP) and adenosine monophosphate (AMP) accumulate and are subsequently degraded to adenosine. Adenosine is a potent vasodilator and is thought to be the primary metabolic mediator of vascular tone. By binding to receptors on vascular smooth muscle, adenosine decreases calcium entry into cells, which leads to relaxation, vasodilatation, and increased coronary blood flow. Other metabolites that act locally as vasodilators include lactate, acetate, hydrogen ions, and carbon dioxide.

Endothelial Factors

Endothelial cells of the arterial wall produce numerous vasoactive substances that contribute to the regulation of vascular tone. *Vasodilators* produced by the endothelium include nitric oxide (NO), prostacyclin, and endothelium-derived hyperpolarizing factor (EDHF). Endothelin 1 is an example of an endothelium-derived *vasoconstrictor.*

The discovery and significance of **endothelium-derived NO** are highlighted in Box 6-1. In brief, NO regulates vascular tone by diffusing into and then relaxing neighboring arterial

Box 6-1	Endothelium-Derived Relaxing Factor, Nitric Oxide, and the Nobel Prize

Normal arterial endothelial cells synthesize potent vasodilator substances that contribute to the modulation of vascular tone. Among the first of these to be identified were prostacyclin (an arachidonic acid metabolite) and a substance termed endothelium-derived relaxing factor (EDRF).

EDRF was first studied in the 1970s. In experimental preparations, it was shown that ACh has two opposite actions on blood vessels. Its direct effect on vascular smooth muscle cells is to cause vasoconstriction, but when an intact endothelial lining overlies the smooth muscle cells, vasodilatation occurs instead. Subsequent experiments showed that ACh causes the endothelial cells to release a chemical mediator (that was termed EDRF), which quickly diffuses to the adjacent smooth muscle cells and results in their relaxation with subsequent vasodilatation of the vessel.

Further research demonstrated that the mysterious EDRF is actually the NO radical. Binding of ACh (or another endothelial-dependent vasodilator such as serotonin or histamine) to endothelial cells catalyzes the formation of NO from the amino acid L-arginine (see figure). NO then diffuses to the adjacent vascular smooth muscle, where it activates guanylyl cyclase (G-cyclase). G-cyclase in turn forms cGMP, which results in smooth muscle cell relaxation through mechanisms that involve a reduction in cytosolic Ca^{++}.

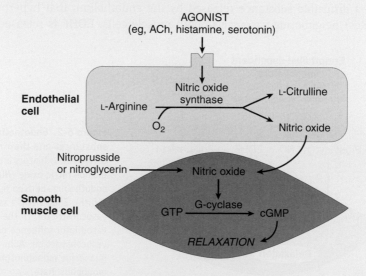

continued

Box 6-1 **Endothelium-Derived Relaxing Factor, Nitric Oxide, and the Nobel Prize (continued)**

In contrast to the endothelial-dependent vasodilators, some agents cause smooth muscle relaxation *independent* of the presence of endothelial cells. For example, the drugs sodium nitroprusside and nitroglycerin result in vasodilatation by providing an exogenous source of NO to vascular smooth muscle cells, thereby activating G-cyclase and forming cGMP without endothelial cell participation.

In the cardiac catheterization laboratory, the intracoronary administration of ACh in a normal person causes vasodilatation of the vessel, presumably through the release of NO. However, in conditions of endothelial dysfunction, such as atherosclerosis, intracoronary ACh administration results in paradoxical *vasoconstriction* instead. This likely reflects reduced production of NO by the dysfunctional endothelial cells, resulting in unopposed direct vasoconstriction of the smooth muscle by ACh. Of particular interest is that the loss of vasodilatory response to infused ACh is evident in persons with certain cardiac risk factors (eg, elevated LDL cholesterol, hypertension, cigarette smoking) even before the physical appearance of atheromatous plaque. Thus, the impaired release of NO may be an early and sensitive predictor for the later development of atherosclerotic lesions.

The significance of these discoveries was highlighted in 1998, when the Nobel Prize in medicine was awarded to the scientists who discovered the critical role of NO as a cardiovascular signaling molecule.

smooth muscle by a cyclic guanosine monophosphate (cGMP)-dependent mechanism. The production of NO by normal endothelium occurs in the basal state and is additionally stimulated by many substances and conditions. For example, its release is augmented when the endothelium is exposed to acetylcholine (ACh), thrombin, products of aggregating platelets (eg, serotonin and ADP), or even the shear stress of blood flow. Although the *direct* effect of many of these substances on vascular smooth muscle is to cause *vasoconstriction*, the induced release of NO from the normal endothelium results in *vasodilatation* instead (Fig. 6-2).

Prostacyclin, an arachidonic acid metabolite, has vasodilator properties similar to those of NO (see Fig. 6-2). It is released from endothelial cells in response to many stimuli, including hypoxia, shear stress, ACh, and platelet products (eg, serotonin). It causes relaxation of vascular smooth muscle by a cyclic AMP–dependent mechanism.

EDHF also appears to have important vasodilatory properties. Like endothelial-derived NO, it is a diffusible substance released by the endothelium that hyperpolarizes (and therefore relaxes) neighboring vascular smooth muscle cells. EDHF is released by some of the same

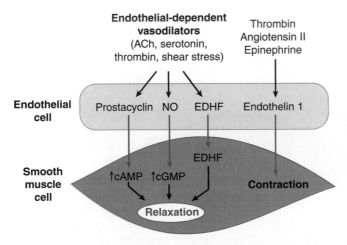

Figure 6-2. Endothelium-derived vasoactive substances and their regulators. Endothelium-derived vasodilators are shown on the *left* and include nitric oxide (NO), prostacyclin, and endothelium-derived hyperpolarizing factor (EDHF). Endothelin 1 is an endothelium-derived vasoconstrictor. In the normal state, the vasodilator influence predominates over that of vasoconstriction. ACh, acetylcholine; cGMP, cyclic guanosine monophosphate; cAMP, cyclic adenosine monophosphate.

factors that stimulate NO, including ACh and normal pulsatile blood flow. In the coronary circulation, EDHF appears to be more important in modulating relaxation in small arterioles than in the large conduit arteries.

Endothelin 1 is a potent vasoconstrictor produced by endothelial cells that partially counteracts the actions of the endothelial vasodilators. Its expression is stimulated by several factors, including thrombin, angiotensin II, epinephrine, and the shear stress of blood flow.

Under normal circumstances, the healthy endothelium promotes vascular smooth muscle *relaxation* (vasodilatation) through elaboration of substances such as NO and prostacyclin, the influences of which predominate over the endothelial vasoconstrictors (see Fig. 6-2). However, as described later in the chapter, the dysfunctional endothelium (eg, in atherosclerotic vessels) secretes reduced amounts of vasodilators, causing the balance to shift toward vasoconstriction instead.

Neural Factors

The neural control of vascular resistance has both sympathetic and parasympathetic components. Under normal circumstances, the contribution of the parasympathetic nervous system is relatively minor, but the sympathetic nervous system plays an important role. Coronary vessels contain both α-adrenergic and β_2-adrenergic receptors. Stimulation of α-adrenergic receptors results in vasoconstriction, whereas stimulation of β_2-receptors promotes vasodilatation.

It is the interplay among the metabolic, endothelial, and neural regulating factors that determines the net impact on coronary vascular tone. For example, catecholamine stimulation of the heart may initially cause coronary *vasoconstriction* via the α-adrenergic receptor neural effect. However, catecholamine stimulation also increases myocardial oxygen consumption through increased heart rate and contractility (β_1-adrenergic effect), and the resulting increased production of local metabolites may induce net coronary *vasodilatation* instead.

Myocardial Oxygen Demand

The three major determinants of myocardial oxygen demand are (1) ventricular wall stress, (2) heart rate, and (3) contractility (which is also termed the *inotropic state*). In addition, very small amounts of oxygen are consumed in providing energy for basal cardiac metabolism and electrical depolarization.

Ventricular **wall stress** (σ) is the tangential force acting on the myocardial fibers, tending to pull them apart, and energy is expended in opposing that force. Wall stress is related to intraventricular pressure (P), the radius of the ventricle (r), and ventricular wall thickness (h) and is approximated by Laplace's relationship:

$$\sigma = \frac{P \times r}{2h}$$

Thus, wall stress is directly proportional to systolic ventricular pressure. Circumstances that increase pressure in the left ventricle, such as aortic stenosis or hypertension, augment wall stress and myocardial oxygen consumption. Conditions that decrease ventricular pressure, such as antihypertensive therapy, reduce myocardial oxygen consumption.

Because wall stress is also directly proportional to the radius of the left ventricle, conditions that augment left ventricular (LV) filling (eg, mitral or aortic regurgitation) raise wall stress and oxygen consumption. Conversely, any physiologic or pharmacologic maneuver that decreases LV filling and size (eg, nitrate therapy) reduces wall stress and myocardial oxygen consumption.

Finally, wall stress is *inversely* proportional to ventricular wall thickness because the force is spread over a greater muscle mass. A hypertrophied heart has lower wall stress and oxygen consumption per gram of tissue than a thin-walled heart. Thus, when hypertrophy develops in conditions of chronic pressure overload, such as aortic stenosis, it serves a compensatory role in reducing oxygen consumption.

The second major determinant of myocardial oxygen demand is **heart rate**. If the heart rate accelerates—during physical exertion, for example—the number of contractions and the amount of ATP consumed per minute increases and oxygen requirements rise. Conversely, slowing the heart rate (eg, with a β-blocker drug) decreases ATP utilization and oxygen consumption.

The third major determinant of oxygen demand is myocardial **contractility**, a measure of the force of contraction (see Chapter 9). Circulating catecholamines, or the administration of positive inotropic drugs, directly augment the force of contraction, which increases oxygen consumption. Conversely, negative inotropic effectors, such as β-adrenergic–blocking drugs, decrease myocardial oxygen consumption.

In the normal state, autoregulatory mechanisms modulate coronary tone to match myocardial oxygen supply with oxygen requirements. In the absence of obstructive coronary disease, these mechanisms maintain a fairly constant rate of coronary flow, as long as the aortic perfusion pressure is ~ 60 mm Hg or greater. In the setting of advanced coronary atherosclerosis, however, the fall in perfusion pressure distal to the arterial stenosis, along with dysfunction of the endothelium of the involved segment, sets the stage for a mismatch between the available blood supply and myocardial metabolic demands.

PATHOPHYSIOLOGY OF ISCHEMIA

The traditional view has been that myocardial ischemia in CAD results from fixed atherosclerotic plaques that narrow the vessel's lumen and limit myocardial blood supply. However, research has demonstrated that the reduction of blood flow in this condition results from the *combination* of fixed vessel narrowing *and* abnormal vascular tone related to atherosclerosis-induced endothelial cell dysfunction.

FIXED VESSEL NARROWING

The hemodynamic significance of fixed atherosclerotic coronary artery stenoses relates to both the fluid mechanics and the anatomy of the vascular supply.

Fluid Mechanics

Poiseuille law states that for flow through a vessel,

$$Q = \frac{\Delta P \pi r^4}{8 \eta L}$$

in which Q is flow, ΔP is the pressure difference between the points being measured, r is the vessel radius, η is the fluid viscosity, and L is the vessel length. By analogy to Ohm law, flow is also equal to the pressure difference divided by the resistance (R) to flow:

$$Q = \frac{\Delta P}{R}$$

By combining these two formulas and rearranging, resistance to blood flow in a vessel can be expressed as

$$R = \frac{8 \eta L}{\pi r^4}$$

Thus, vascular resistance is governed, in part, by the geometric component L/r^4. That is, the hemodynamic significance of a stenotic lesion depends on its length and, far more importantly, on the degree of vessel narrowing (ie, the reduction of r) that it causes.

Anatomy

The coronary arteries consist of large, proximal epicardial segments and smaller, distal resistance vessels (arterioles). The proximal vessels are subject to overt atherosclerosis that results in stenotic plaques. The distal vessels are usually free of flow-limiting plaques and can adjust their vasomotor tone in response to metabolic needs. These resistance vessels serve as a reserve, increasing their diameter with exertion to meet increasing oxygen demand and dilating, even at rest, if a proximal stenosis is sufficiently severe.

The hemodynamic significance of a coronary artery stenosis depends on both the degree of narrowing of the epicardial portion of the vessel and the amount of *com-

Figure 6-3. Resting and maximal coronary blood flows are affected by the magnitude of proximal arterial stenosis (percent lesion diameter). The *dotted line* indicates resting blood flow, and the *solid line* represents maximal blood flow (ie, when there is full dilatation of the distal resistance vessels). Compromise of maximal blood flow is evident when the proximal stenosis reduces the coronary lumen diameter by more than ~70%. Resting flow may be compromised if the stenosis exceeds ~90%. (Modified from Gould KL, Lipscomb K. Effects of coronary stenoses on coronary flow reserve and resistance. *Am J Cardiol.* 1974;34:50.)

pensatory vasodilatation* the distal resistance vessels are able to achieve (Fig. 6-3). If a stenosis narrows the lumen diameter by <60%, the maximal potential blood flow through the artery is not significantly altered and, in response to exertion, the resistance vessels can dilate to provide adequate blood flow. When a stenosis narrows the diameter by more than ~70%, resting blood flow is normal, but maximal blood flow is reduced even with full dilatation of the resistance vessels. In this situation, when oxygen demand increases (eg, from the elevated heart rate and force of contraction during physical exertion), coronary flow reserve is inadequate, oxygen demand exceeds supply, and myocardial ischemia results. If the stenosis compromises the vessel lumen by more than ~90%, then even with maximal dilatation of the resistance vessels, blood flow may be inadequate to meet basal requirements and ischemia can develop *at rest.*

Although collateral connections (see Chapter 1) may become apparent between unobstructed coronaries and sites distal to atherosclerotic stenoses, and such flow can buffer the fall in myocardial oxygen supply, it is often not sufficient to prevent ischemia during exertion in critically narrowed vessels.

Endothelial Cell Dysfunction

In addition to fixed vessel narrowing, the other major contributor to reduced myocardial oxygen supply in chronic CAD is endothelial dysfunction. Abnormal endothelial cell function can contribute to the pathophysiology of ischemia in two ways: (1) by inappropriate vasoconstriction of coronary arteries and (2) through loss of normal antithrombotic properties.

Inappropriate Vasoconstriction

In normal persons, physical activity or mental stress results in measurable coronary artery *vasodilatation*. This effect is thought to be regulated by activation of the sympathetic nervous system, with increased blood flow and shear stress stimulating the release of endothelial-derived vasodilators, such as NO. It is postulated that in normal coronary arteries, the relaxation effect of NO outweighs the direct α-adrenergic vasoconstrictor effect of catecholamines on arterial smooth muscle, such that vasodilatation predominates. However, in patients with dysfunctional endothelium (eg, due to atherosclerosis), an *impaired release of endothelial vasodilators* leaves the direct catecholamine effect unopposed, such that relative vasoconstriction occurs instead. The resultant decrease in coronary blood flow contributes to ischemia. Even the vasodilatory effect of local metabolites (such as adenosine) is attenuated in patients with dysfunctional endothelium, further uncoupling the regulation of vascular tone from metabolic demands.

In patients with risk factors for CAD, such as hypercholesterolemia, diabetes mellitus, hypertension, and cigarette smoking, impaired endothelial-dependent vasodilatation is noted even *before* visible atherosclerotic lesions have developed. This suggests that endothelial dysfunction occurs very early in the atherosclerotic process.

Inappropriate vasoconstriction also appears to be important in acute coronary syndromes, such as unstable angina and myocardial infarction (MI). As described in Chapter 7, the usual cause of acute coronary syndromes is disruption of atherosclerotic plaque, with superimposed platelet aggregation and thrombus formation. Normally, the products of platelet aggregation in a developing clot (eg, serotonin and ADP) result in vasodilatation because they stimulate the endothelial release of NO. However, with dysfunctional endothelium, the direct *vasoconstricting* actions of platelet-derived products predominate (Fig. 6-4), further compromising flow through the arterial lumen.

Loss of Normal Antithrombotic Properties

In addition to their vasodilatory actions, factors released from endothelial cells (including NO and prostacyclin) also exert antithrombotic properties by interfering with platelet aggregation (see Fig. 6-4). However, in states of endothelial cell dysfunction, release of these substances is reduced and the antithrombotic effect is attenuated. Thus, in syndromes characterized by thrombosis (ie, the acute coronary syndromes described in Chapter 7), the impaired release of NO and prostacyclin allows platelets to aggregate and to secrete their potentially harmful procoagulants and vasoconstrictors.

OTHER CAUSES OF MYOCARDIAL ISCHEMIA

In addition to atherosclerotic CAD, other conditions may result in an imbalance between myocardial oxygen supply and demand and result in ischemia. Other common causes of decreased myocardial oxygen supply include (1) decreased perfusion pressure due to hypotension (eg, in a patient with hypovolemia or septic shock) and (2) a severely decreased blood oxygen content (eg, marked anemia or impaired oxygenation of blood by the lungs). For example, a patient with massive bleeding from the gastrointestinal tract may develop myocardial ischemia and angina pectoris, even in the absence of atherosclerotic coronary disease, because of reduced oxygen supply (ie, loss of hemoglobin and hypotension).

On the other side of the balance, a profound increase in myocardial oxygen demand can cause ischemia even in the absence of coronary atherosclerosis. This can occur, for example, with rapid tachycardias, acute hypertension, or severe aortic stenosis.

A

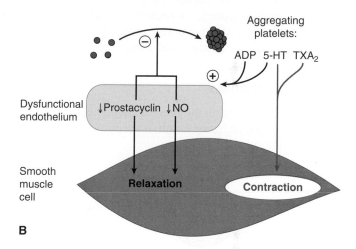

B

Figure 6-4. The interaction between platelets and endothelial cells. A. Normal endothelium. Aggregating platelets release thromboxane (TXA$_2$) and serotonin (5-HT), the direct vascular effects of which cause contraction of vascular smooth muscle and vasoconstriction. However, platelet products (eg, ADP and 5-HT) also stimulate the endothelial release of the potent vasodilators nitric oxide (NO) and prostacyclin, such that the net effect is smooth muscle relaxation instead. Endothelial production of NO and prostacyclin also serves antithrombotic roles, which limit further platelet aggregation. ADP, adenosine diphosphate. **B.** Dysfunctional endothelium demonstrates impaired release of the vasodilator substances, such that net smooth muscle *contraction* and *vasoconstriction* supervene. The reduced endothelial release of NO and prostacyclin diminishes their antiplatelet effect, such that thrombosis proceeds unchecked.

CONSEQUENCES OF ISCHEMIA

The consequences of ischemia reflect the inadequate myocardial oxygenation and local accumulation of metabolic waste products. For example, during ischemia, myocytes convert from aerobic to anaerobic metabolic pathways. The reduced generation of ATP impairs the interaction of the contractile proteins and results in a transient reduction of both ventricular systolic contraction and diastolic relaxation, as each is an energy-dependent process. The consequent elevation of LV pressure during diastole is transmitted (via the left atrium and pulmonary veins) to the pulmonary capillaries and can precipitate pulmonary congestion and the symptom of dyspnea (shortness of breath). In addition, metabolic products such as lactate, serotonin, and adenosine accumulate locally. It is suspected that one or more of these compounds activate peripheral pain receptors in the C7 through T4 distribution and may be the mechanism by which the discomfort of angina is produced. The accumulation of local metabolites and transient abnormalities of myocyte ion transport may also precipitate arrhythmias (see Chapter 11).

The ultimate fate of the myocardium subjected to ischemia depends on the severity and duration of the imbalance between oxygen supply and demand. It was previously thought that an ischemic cardiac episode results in either irreversible myocardial necrosis (ie, MI) or rapid and full recovery of myocyte function. It is now known that in addition to those outcomes, ischemic insults can sometimes result in a period of prolonged contractile dysfunction *without* myocyte necrosis, and recovery of normal function may ultimately follow.

For example, **stunned myocardium** refers to the tissue that, after suffering an episode of severe acute, transient ischemia (but not necrosis), demonstrates prolonged systolic dysfunction even after the return of normal myocardial blood flow. In this setting, the functional, biochemical, and structural abnormalities following ischemia are reversible, and contractile function gradually recovers. The mechanism responsible for this delayed recovery of function involves myocyte calcium overload and the accumulation of oxygen-derived free radicals during ischemia. In general, the magnitude of stunning is proportional to the degree of the preceding ischemia, and this state is likely the pathophysiologic response to an ischemic insult that falls short of causing irreversible necrosis.

In contrast, **hibernating myocardium** refers to tissue that manifests *chronic* ventricular contractile dysfunction due to a persistently reduced blood supply, usually because of multivessel CAD. In this situation, irreversible damage has not occurred, and ventricular function can promptly improve if appropriate blood flow is restored by percutaneous or surgical revascularization. Special "viability" imaging studies (eg, positron emission tomography or dobutamine echocardiography, as described in Chapter 3) of patients with CAD and contractile dysfunction can differentiate hibernating from infarcted myocardium. That distinction can help guide the decision of whether to undertake coronary revascularization, because hibernating myocardium would be expected to regain contractile function with restoration of blood flow, whereas infarcted myocardium would not.

ISCHEMIC SYNDROMES

Depending on the underlying pathophysiologic process and the timing and severity of a myocardial ischemic insult, a spectrum of distinct clinical syndromes may result, as illustrated in Figure 6-5.

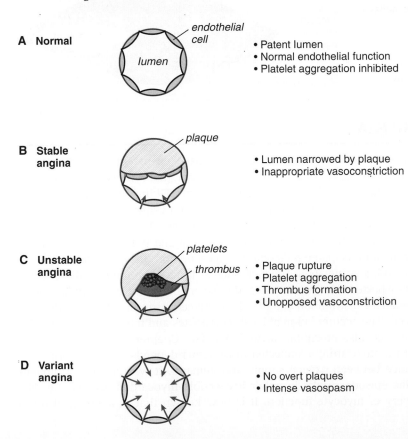

A Normal
- Patent lumen
- Normal endothelial function
- Platelet aggregation inhibited

B Stable angina
- Lumen narrowed by plaque
- Inappropriate vasoconstriction

C Unstable angina
- Plaque rupture
- Platelet aggregation
- Thrombus formation
- Unopposed vasoconstriction

D Variant angina
- No overt plaques
- Intense vasospasm

Figure 6-5. Pathophysiologic findings in anginal syndromes. **A.** Normal coronary arteries are widely patent, and the endothelium functions normally. **B.** In stable angina, atherosclerotic plaque and inappropriate vasoconstriction (caused by dysfunctional endothelium) reduce the vessel lumen's size and coronary blood flow. **C.** In unstable angina, disruption of the plaque triggers platelet aggregation, thrombus formation, and vasoconstriction, all of which contribute to reduced coronary blood supply. **D.** In variant angina, atherosclerotic plaques are absent; rather, ischemia is due to intense vasospasm that reduces myocardial oxygen supply.

Stable Angina

Chronic *stable angina* manifests as a pattern of predictable, transient chest discomfort during exertion or emotional stress. It is generally caused by fixed, obstructive atheromatous plaque in one or more coronary arteries (see Fig. 6-5B). The pattern of symptoms is usually related to the degree of stenosis. As described in the earlier section on pathophysiology, when atherosclerotic stenoses narrow a coronary artery lumen diameter by more than ~70%, the reduced flow capacity may be sufficient to meet the low myocardial oxygen needs at rest but insufficient to compensate for a significant increase in oxygen demand (see Fig. 6-3). During physical exertion, for example, activation of the sympathetic nervous system results in increased heart rate, blood pressure, and contractility, all of which augment myocardial oxygen consumption. During the period that oxygen demand exceeds available supply, myocardial ischemia results and is often accompanied by the chest discomfort of angina pectoris. The ischemia and symptoms persist until the increased demand is alleviated and oxygen balance is restored.

Potentially contributing to the inadequate oxygen supply in stable angina is inappropriate coronary vasoconstriction caused, at least in part, by atherosclerosis-associated endothelial dysfunction. Recall that normally, the high myocardial oxygen demand during exertion is balanced by an increased supply of blood as the accumulation of local metabolites induces vasodilatation. With endothelial cell dysfunction, however, vasodilatation is impaired and the vessels may instead paradoxically vasoconstrict in response to exercise-induced catecholamine stimulation of α-adrenergic receptors on the coronary artery smooth muscle cells.

As a result, the extent of coronary artery narrowing in patients with atherosclerosis is not necessarily constant. Rather, it can vary from moment to moment because of the changes in the superimposed coronary vascular tone. For some patients with stable angina, alterations in tone play a minimal role in the decreased myocardial oxygen supply, and the level of physical activity required to precipitate angina is fairly constant. These patients have *fixed-threshold angina.* In other cases, the degree of dynamic obstruction caused by vasoconstriction or vasospasm plays a more prominent role, and such patients may have *variable-threshold angina.* For example, on a given day, a patient with variable-threshold angina can exert herself or himself without chest discomfort, but on another day, the same degree of myocardial oxygen demand *does* produce symptoms. The difference reflects alterations in vascular tone over the sites of fixed stenosis. Other clinical features of chronic stable angina are described in greater detail later in the chapter.

Unstable Angina

A patient with chronic stable angina may experience a sudden increase in the tempo and duration of ischemic episodes, occurring with lesser degrees of exertion and even at rest. This acceleration of symptoms is known as *unstable angina*, which can be a precursor to an acute MI. Unstable angina and acute MI are also known as *acute coronary syndromes* and most commonly result from rupture of an unstable atherosclerotic plaque with subsequent platelet aggregation and thrombosis (see Fig. 6-5C). These syndromes are described in detail in Chapter 7.

Variant Angina

A small minority of patients manifest episodes of focal *coronary artery spasm* in the absence of overt atherosclerotic lesions, and this syndrome is known as *variant angina* or *Prinzmetal angina*. In this case, intense vasospasm alone reduces coronary oxygen supply and results in angina (see Fig. 6-5D). The mechanism by which such profound spasm develops is not completely understood but may involve increased sympathetic activity in combination with endothelial dysfunction. It is thought that many patients with variant angina may actually have early atherosclerosis manifested only by dysfunctional endothelium, because the response to endothelium-dependent vasodilators (eg, ACh and serotonin) is often abnormal.

Variant angina often occurs at rest because ischemia in this case results from transient reduction of the coronary oxygen supply rather than from an increase in myocardial oxygen demand.

Silent Ischemia

Episodes of cardiac ischemia sometimes occur in the absence of perceptible discomfort or pain, and such instances are referred to as *silent ischemia.* These asymptomatic episodes most commonly occur in patients who on other occasions experience typical *symptomatic* angina and have an estimated prevalence of 20%-50% in this population. Conversely, in some patients, silent ischemia may be the *only* manifestation of CAD. It may be difficult to diagnose silent ischemia on clinical grounds, but its presence can be detected by laboratory techniques such as continuous ambulatory electrocardiography or exercise stress testing, as described later in the chapter. When considering the importance of anginal discomfort as a physiologic warning signal, the asymptomatic nature of silent ischemia becomes all the more concerning.

The reason why some episodes of ischemia are silent whereas others are symptomatic has not been elucidated. The degree of ischemia cannot fully explain the disparity, because even MI may present without symptoms in some patients. Silent ischemia has been reported to be more common among diabetic patients (possibly due to impaired pain sensation from peripheral neuropathy), the elderly, and in women.

Microvascular Angina

Microvascular angina refers to the clinical syndrome of angina pectoris in the absence of significant atherosclerotic coronary stenoses on coronary angiography. Some patients with microvascular angina show laboratory signs of ischemia during exercise testing along with abnormal myocardial perfusion imaging (see Chapter 3). Although the pathogenesis of ischemia in this disorder remains incompletely understood, it is thought to be related to inadequate vasodilatory reserve of the coronary resistance vessels. Specifically, it is speculated that the resistance vessels (which are too small to be visualized by coronary angiography) may not dilate appropriately during periods of increased myocardial oxygen demand. Patients with microvascular angina have a better prognosis than those with overt atherosclerotic disease but a poorer prognosis than the general population.

CLINICAL FEATURES OF CHRONIC STABLE ANGINA

HISTORY

The most important part of the clinical evaluation of ischemic heart disease is the history described by the patient. Because chest pain is such a common complaint, it is important to focus on the characteristics that help distinguish myocardial ischemia from other causes of discomfort. From a diagnostic standpoint, it would be ideal to interview and examine a patient during an actual episode of angina, but most people are asymptomatic during routine clinic examinations. Therefore, a careful history probing several features of the discomfort should be elicited.

Quality

Angina is most often described as a "pressure," "discomfort," "tightness," "burning," or "heaviness" in the chest. It is rare that the sensation is actually described as a "pain," and often a patient will correct the medical professional who refers to the anginal symptom as such. Sometimes, a patient likens the sensation to "an elephant sitting on my chest." Anginal discomfort is neither sharp nor stabbing, and it does not vary significantly with inspiration or movement of the chest wall. It is a steady discomfort that lasts a few minutes, yet rarely >5-10 minutes. It *always* lasts more than a few seconds, and this helps to differentiate it from sharper and briefer musculoskeletal pains.

While describing angina, the patient may place a clenched fist over his or her sternum, referred to as the **Levine sign**, as if defining the constricting discomfort by that tight grip.

Location

Anginal discomfort is usually *diffuse* rather than localized to a single point. It is most often located in the retrosternal area or in the left precordium but may occur anywhere in the chest, back, arms, neck, lower face, or upper abdomen. It often radiates to the shoulders and inner aspect of the arms, especially on the left side.

Accompanying Symptoms

During the discomfort of an acute anginal attack, generalized sympathetic and parasympathetic stimulation may result in *tachycardia*, *diaphoresis*, and *nausea*. Ischemia also results in transient dysfunction of LV systolic contraction and diastolic relaxation. The resultant elevation of LV pressure during diastole is transmitted to the pulmonary vasculature, often causing *dyspnea*. Transient *fatigue* and *weakness* are also common, particularly in elderly patients. When such symptoms occur as a consequence of myocardial ischemia but are unaccompanied by typical chest discomfort, they are referred to as "anginal equivalents."

Precipitants

Angina, when not caused by pure vasospasm, is precipitated by conditions that increase myocardial oxygen demand (eg, increased heart rate, contractility, or wall stress). These include physical exertion, anger, and other emotional excitement. Additional factors that increase myocardial oxygen demand and can precipitate anginal discomfort in patients with CAD include a large meal or cold weather. The latter induces peripheral vasoconstriction, which in turn augments myocardial wall stress as the left ventricle contracts against the increased resistance.

Angina is generally relieved within minutes after the cessation of the activity that precipitated it and even more quickly (within 3-5 minutes) by sublingual nitroglycerin. This response can help differentiate myocardial ischemia from many of the other conditions that produce chest discomfort.

Patients who experience angina primarily due to increased coronary vascular tone or vasospasm often develop symptoms at rest, independent of activities that increase myocardial oxygen demand.

Frequency

Although the level of exertion necessary to precipitate angina may remain fairly constant, the frequency of episodes varies considerably because patients quickly learn which activities cause their discomfort and avoid them. It is therefore important to inquire about reductions in activities of daily living when taking the history.

Risk Factors

In addition to the description of chest discomfort, a careful history should uncover risk factors that predispose to atherosclerosis and CAD, including cigarette smoking, dyslipidemia, hypertension, diabetes, and a family history of premature coronary disease (see Chapter 5).

Differential Diagnosis

Several conditions can give rise to symptoms that mimic the transient chest discomfort of angina pectoris, including other cardiac causes (eg, pericarditis), gastrointestinal disorders (eg, gastroesophageal reflux, peptic ulcer disease, esophageal spasm, or biliary pain), and musculoskeletal conditions (including chest wall pain, spinal osteoarthritis, and cervical radiculitis). The history remains of paramount importance in distinguishing myocardial ischemia from these disorders. In contrast to angina pectoris, gastrointestinal causes of recurrent chest pain are often precipitated by certain foods and are unrelated to exertion. Musculoskeletal causes of chest discomfort tend to be more superficial or can be localized to a discrete location on the chest wall (ie, the patient can point to the pain with one finger) and often vary with changes in position. Similarly, the presence of pleuritic pain (sharp pain aggravated by respiratory movements) argues against angina as the cause; this symptom is more likely a result of pericarditis or an acute pulmonary condition such as pulmonary embolism or acute pneumothorax. Useful differentiating features of recurrent chest pain are listed in Table 6-2.

TABLE 6-2	Causes of Recurrent Chest Pain
Condition	**Differentiating Features**
Cardiac	
Myocardial ischemia	• Retrosternal tightness or pressure; typically radiates to the neck, jaw, or left shoulder and arm • Lasts a few minutes (usually <10) • Brought on by exertion, relieved by rest or nitroglycerin • ECG: transient ST depressions or elevations, or flattened or inverted T waves
Pericarditis	• Sharp, pleuritic pain that varies with position; friction rub may be present on auscultation • Can last for hours to days • ECG: diffuse ST elevations and PR deviation (see Chapter 14)
Gastrointestinal	
Gastroesophageal reflux	• Retrosternal burning • Precipitated by certain foods, worsened by supine position, unaffected by exertion • Relieved by antacids
Peptic ulcer disease	• Epigastric ache or burning • Occurs after meals, unaffected by exertion • Relieved by antacids, not by nitroglycerin
Esophageal spasm	• Retrosternal pain accompanied by dysphagia • Precipitated by meals, unaffected by exertion • May be relieved by nitroglycerin
Biliary colic	• Constant, deep pain in right upper quadrant; can last for hours • Brought on by fatty foods, unaffected by exertion • Not relieved by antacids or nitroglycerin
Musculoskeletal	
Costochondral syndrome	• Sternal pain worsened by chest movement • Costochondral junctions tender to palpation • Relieved by anti-inflammatory drugs, not by nitroglycerin
Cervical radiculitis	• Constant ache or shooting pains; may be in a dermatomal distribution • Worsened by neck motion

ECG, electrocardiogram.

PHYSICAL EXAMINATION

If it is possible to examine a patient *during* an anginal attack, several transient physical signs may be detected (Fig. 6-6). An increased heart rate and blood pressure are common because of the augmented sympathetic response. Myocardial ischemia may lead to papillary muscle dysfunction and therefore mitral regurgitation. Ischemia-induced regional ventricular contractile abnormalities can sometimes be detected as an abnormal bulging impulse on palpation of the left chest. Ischemia decreases ventricular compliance, producing a stiffened ventricle and therefore an S_4 gallop on physical examination during atrial contraction (see Chapter 2). However, if the patient is free of chest discomfort during the examination, there may be *no* abnormal cardiac physical findings.

Physical examination should also assess for signs of atherosclerotic disease in more accessible vascular beds. For example, carotid bruits may indicate the presence of cerebrovascular disease, whereas femoral artery bruits or diminished pulses in the lower extremities can be a clue to peripheral arterial disease (see Chapter 15).

DIAGNOSTIC STUDIES

Once angina is suspected, several diagnostic procedures may be helpful in confirming myocardial ischemia as the cause. Because many of these tests are costly, it is important to choose the appropriate studies for each patient.

Electrocardiogram

One of the most useful tools is an electrocardiogram (ECG) obtained during an anginal episode. Although this is easy to arrange when symptoms occur in hospitalized patients, it may not be possible to "catch" episodes in people seen on an outpatient basis. During myocardial ischemia, ST-segment and T-wave changes can appear (Fig. 6-7). Acute ischemia usually results in transient horizontal or downsloping ST-segment depressions and T-wave flattening or inversions. Occasionally, ST-segment *elevations* are seen, suggesting more severe transmural myocardial ischemia, and can also be observed during the intense vasospasm of variant angina. In contrast to the ECG of a patient with an acute MI, the ST deviations seen in patients with stable angina quickly normalize with resolution of the patient's symptoms. In

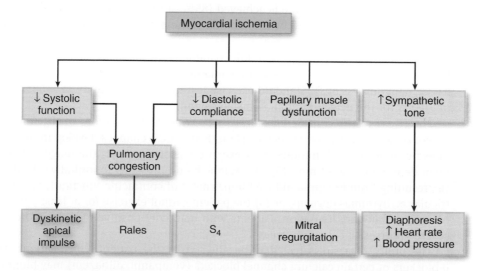

Figure 6-6. Pathophysiology of physical signs during acute myocardial ischemia.

Figure 6-7. Common transient ECG abnormalities during ischemia. Subendocardial ischemia causes ST-segment depressions and/or T-wave flattening or inversions. Severe transient transmural ischemia can result in ST-segment *elevations,* similar to the early changes in acute myocardial infarction. When transient ischemia resolves, so do the electrocardiographic changes.

fact, ECGs obtained during periods free of ischemia are completely normal in approximately half of patients with stable angina. In others, chronic "nondiagnostic" ST and T-wave deviations may be present. Evidence of a previous MI (eg, pathologic Q waves) on the ECG also points to the presence of underlying coronary disease.

Stress Testing

Because ECGs obtained during or between episodes of chest discomfort may be normal, such tracings do not rule out underlying ischemic heart disease. For this reason, provocative **exercise** or **pharmacologic stress tests** are valuable diagnostic and prognostic aids.

Standard Exercise Testing

For many patients suspected of having CAD, a standard exercise test is performed. During this test, the patient exercises on a treadmill or a stationary bicycle to progressively higher workloads and is observed for the development of chest discomfort or excessive dyspnea. The heart rate and ECG are continuously monitored, and blood pressure is checked at regular intervals. The test is continued until angina develops, signs of myocardial ischemia appear on the ECG, a target heart rate is achieved (85% of the maximal predicted heart rate [MHR]; the MHR is calculated as 220 beats/min minus the patient's age), or the patient becomes too fatigued to continue.

The test is considered *abnormal* if the patient's typical chest discomfort is reproduced or if ECG abnormalities consistent with ischemia develop (ie, >1 mm horizontal or downsloping ST-segment depressions). Standard exercise testing has a sensitivity of ~68% and specificity of ~77% for the detection of anatomically significant CAD.

The stress test is considered *markedly positive* if one or more of the following signs of severe ischemic heart disease occur: (1) ischemic ECG changes develop in the first 3 minutes of exercise or persist 5 minutes after exercise has stopped; (2) the magnitude of the ST-segment depressions is >2 mm; (3) the systolic blood pressure abnormally falls during exercise (ie, resulting from ischemia-induced impairment of contractile function); (4) high-grade ventricular arrhythmias develop; or (5) the patient cannot exercise for at least 2 minutes because of cardiopulmonary limitation. Patients with markedly positive tests are more likely to have severe multivessel coronary disease.

The utility of a stress test may be affected by the patient's medications. For example, β-blockers or certain calcium channel blockers (verapamil, diltiazem) may blunt the ability to achieve the target heart rate. In these situations, one must consider the purpose of the stress test. If it is to determine whether ischemic heart disease is present, then those medications are typically withheld for 24-48 hours before the test. On the other hand, if the patient has known ischemic heart disease and the purpose of the test is to assess the efficacy of the current medical regimen, testing should be performed while the patient takes his or her usual antianginal medications.

Nuclear Imaging Studies

Since a standard exercise test relies on ischemia-related changes on the ECG, the test is less useful in patients with baseline abnormalities of the ST segments (eg, as seen in left bundle branch block or LV hypertrophy). In addition, the standard exercise stress test sometimes yields equivocal results in patients for whom the clinical suspicion of ischemic heart disease is high. In these situations, radionuclide imaging can be combined with exercise testing to overcome these limitations and to increase the sensitivity and specificity of the study.

As described in Chapter 3, during such myocardial perfusion imaging, a radionuclide (commonly a technetium-99m–labeled compound) is injected intravenously at peak exercise, after which imaging is performed. The radionuclide accumulates in proportion to the degree of perfusion of viable myocardial cells. Therefore, areas of poor perfusion (ie, regions of ischemia) during exercise do not accumulate radionuclide and appear as "cold spots" on the image. Areas of irreversibly infarcted myocardium also do not take up the radionuclide, and they too will appear as cold spots. To differentiate between transient ischemia and infarcted tissue, imaging is also performed at rest (either before or several hours after the exercise portion of the test). If the cold spot fills in, a region of *transient ischemia* has been identified (see Fig. 3-18). If the cold spot remains unchanged, a region of irreversible *infarction* is likely.

Standard radionuclide exercise tests are ~85% sensitive and 70%-90% specific for the detection of clinically significant CAD. Positron emission tomography (PET; see Chapter 3), another form of nuclear stress imaging that is not as widely available, offers superior spatial and temporal resolution, with sensitivity and specificity of nearly 90%. Because these nuclear imaging techniques are expensive, their use in screening for CAD should be reserved for (1) patients in whom baseline ECG abnormalities preclude interpretation of a standard exercise test or for (2) improvement in test sensitivity when standard stress test results are discordant with the clinical suspicion of coronary disease.

Exercise Echocardiography

Exercise testing with *echocardiographic* imaging is another technique to diagnose myocardial ischemia in patients with baseline ST or T-wave abnormalities or in those with equivocal standard stress tests. In this procedure, LV contractile function is assessed by echocardiography at baseline and immediately after treadmill or bicycle exercise. The test indicates inducible myocardial ischemia if regions of ventricular contractile dysfunction develop with exertion, having sensitivity and specificity of 80%-90% for the detection of clinically significant CAD.

Pharmacologic Stress Tests

For patients unable to exercise (eg, those with hip or knee arthritis), *pharmacologic* stress testing can be performed instead using various agents, including vasodilators or inotropes. The most common approach is to use a coronary vasodilator such as adenosine, regadenoson, or dipyridamole. Adenosine and regadenoson bind to adenosine A_{2a} receptors on vascular smooth muscle cells, resulting in coronary vasodilatation. As ischemic regions are already maximally dilated (in compensation for the epicardial coronary stenoses), the vasodilatation induced by these agents increases flow to the myocardium perfused by healthy coronary arteries and thus "steals" blood away from the diseased segments. Dipyridamole causes a similar effect indirectly, as it blocks normal cellular uptake and destruction of adenosine, thereby increasing adenosine's circulating concentration and subsequent stimulation of the A_{2a} receptor. Administration of these pharmacologic agents is typically coupled with nuclear imaging, to reveal regions of impaired myocardial perfusion.

As an alternative to vasodilator agents, pharmacologic stress testing can also be performed using the inotrope *dobutamine*, which increases myocardial oxygen demand by augmenting heart rate and the force of contraction, thus simulating some of the effects of exercise. Accompanying imaging (typically nuclear imaging or echocardiography) reveals regions of drug-induced ischemia. Vasodilator pharmacologic stress testing is generally preferred over dobutamine testing for the assessment of ischemia, as the former produces greater incremental myocardial blood flow, and is technically easier and faster to perform. However, the vasodilator agents can cause bronchospasm in patients with reactive airway disease (by stimulating bronchiolar adenosine A_{2b} receptors), so dobutamine pharmacologic testing is preferred in that population. In addition, a vasodilator study cannot be performed successfully in a patient who has been exposed to methylxanthines (eg, caffeine or the bronchodilator theophylline) on the day of the study, as such agents competitively antagonize adenosine's interaction with its receptor and blunt its effect.

Coronary Angiography

The most direct means of identifying coronary artery stenoses is by coronary angiography, in which atherosclerotic lesions are visualized radiographically following the injection of radiopaque contrast material into the artery (Fig. 6-8; also see Chapter 3). Although generally safe, the procedure is associated with a small risk of complications directly related to its invasive nature. Therefore, coronary angiography is typically reserved for patients whose anginal symptoms do not respond adequately to pharmacologic therapy, for those with an unstable presentation, or when the results of noninvasive testing are so abnormal that severe CAD warranting revascularization is likely.

When the degree of stenosis of a region of intracoronary plaque, or its hemodynamic significance, is not clear, additional techniques can be applied in the cardiac catheterization laboratory. For example, **fractional flow reserve (FFR)** measurement is a technique that can assess the functional severity of a stenosis identified at angiography. A special manometer-tipped guidewire inserted through the catheter measures the pressure in the coronary artery distal to the stenosis during adenosine-induced vasodilatation. The FFR value is equal to the pressure distal to the stenosis (P_d) relative to the pressure proximal to the stenosis in the aorta (P_{ao}).

$$FFR = P_d / P_{ao}$$

A higher FFR value indicates a less severe stenosis. FFR values <0.80 identify severe stenoses that typically warrant mechanical

Figure 6-8. Example of coronary angiography. Injection of the right coronary artery demonstrates a stenosis in the midportion of the vessel, indicated by the *arrow*. (Courtesy of Pinak B. Shah, MD. Brigham and Women's Hospital, Boston, MA.)

intervention. An alternative measurement to FFR is the **instantaneous wave-free pressure ratio (iFR)**, which can be obtained directly from a manometer-tipped guidewire without having to administer a systemic vasodilator. Analogous to FFR values <0.80, iFR values <0.89 are suggestive of severe stenoses that generally warrant invasive coronary intervention.

Although coronary angiography is considered the "gold standard" for the diagnosis of CAD, it should be noted that it provides only anatomic information. The clinical significance of lesions detected by angiography depends on both the degree of narrowing and also on the pathophysiologic consequences. Therefore, treatment decisions should be based not only on the finding of severe stenoses but also by the functional consequences, manifested by the patient's symptoms, the viability of the myocardial segments served by stenotic vessels, and the degree of ventricular contractile dysfunction. Furthermore, standard arteriography does not reveal the composition of coronary atherosclerotic plaque or its vulnerability to rupture (see Chapter 5).

Noninvasive Imaging of Coronary Arteries

Diagnostic alternatives to coronary angiography have been developed to noninvasively visualize the coronary arteries. Coronary CT angiography (CCTA) performed with administration of intravenous contrast (see Fig. 3-21) can visualize stenoses of >50% of the coronary lumen with a sensitivity >90% and specificity of 80%-90%. CCTA is considered an alternative to stress testing to help exclude significant CAD in low- to intermediate-risk patients who present with undefined chest pain. The quality of images in CCTA is limited by cardiac motion, which can be reduced by slowing the heart rate with administration of a beta-blocker.

Cardiac CT without contrast administration can be used as a screening test to detect coronary artery calcification (CAC) as described in Chapter 3. CAC correlates with the extent of atherosclerosis and thus estimates plaque burden, but does not quantify individual coronary stenoses. Of note, the complete lack of CAC is a clinically useful finding as it strongly predicts the absence of CAD.

NATURAL HISTORY

The patient with chronic angina may show no change in a stable pattern of ischemia for many years. In some patients, however, the course may be punctuated by the occurrence of unstable angina, MI, or sudden cardiac death. These complications are often related to acute thrombosis at the site of disrupted atherosclerotic plaque (see Chapter 7). Why some patients, but not others, sustain these complications remains a subject of intense clinical and basic science investigation and may relate to the vulnerability of plaque to become disrupted.

The mortality associated with CAD has declined significantly in recent decades: the age-adjusted death rate has fallen by >50%. This is likely related to (1) atherosclerotic risk reduction through improved lifestyle changes (eg, less tobacco use, less dietary fat consumption, and more exercise); (2) improved therapeutic strategies and longevity following acute coronary syndromes (see Chapter 7); and (3) advances in therapies for chronic CAD.

TREATMENT

The goals of therapy in chronic ischemic heart disease are to decrease the frequency of anginal attacks, to prevent acute coronary syndromes such as MI, and to prolong survival. A long-term crucial step is to address the risk factors that led to the development of atherosclerotic coronary disease. Data convincingly demonstrate the benefit of smoking cessation, LDL cholesterol reduction, and blood pressure control in lowering the risk of coronary disease events (see Chapter 5). Attention to other risk factors for CAD (eg, obesity and physical inactivity) may also reduce the risk of adverse outcomes, though the benefits of these interventions are less well documented.

The following sections describe medical and surgical strategies to (1) reduce ischemia and its symptoms by restoring the balance between myocardial oxygen supply and demand and (2) prevent acute coronary syndromes and death in patients with chronic CAD.

MEDICAL TREATMENT OF AN ACUTE EPISODE OF STABLE ANGINA

When experiencing acute angina, the patient should cease physical activity. Sublingual nitroglycerin, an organic nitrate, is the drug of choice in this situation. Placed under the tongue, this medication produces a slight burning sensation as it is absorbed through the mucosa, and it begins to take effect in 1-2 minutes. Nitrates relieve ischemia primarily through vascular smooth muscle relaxation, particularly *venodilatation.* Venodilatation reduces venous return to the heart, with a subsequent decline in LV volume (a determinant of wall stress). The latter decreases myocardial oxygen consumption, thus helping to restore oxygen balance in the ischemic heart.

A second action of nitrates is to dilate the coronary vasculature, with subsequent augmentation of coronary blood flow. This effect may be of little value in patients with angina in whom maximal coronary dilatation has already resulted from the accumulation of local metabolites. However, when coronary vasospasm plays a role in the development of ischemia, nitrate-induced coronary vasodilatation may be particularly beneficial.

MEDICAL TREATMENT TO PREVENT RECURRENT ISCHEMIC EPISODES

Pharmacologic agents are also the first line of defense in the *prevention* of anginal attacks. The goal is to decrease the cardiac workload (ie, reduce myocardial oxygen demand) and to increase myocardial perfusion. The three classes of medications most commonly used are β-adrenergic blockers, organic nitrates, and calcium channel blockers (Table 6-3).

β-Blockers (see Chapter 17) exert their antianginal effect primarily by reducing myocardial oxygen demand. They are directed against β-adrenergic receptors, of which there are two classes: β_1-adrenergic receptors are restricted to the myocardium, whereas β_2-adrenergic receptors are located throughout the blood vessels and the bronchial tree. The stimulation of β_1-receptors by endogenous catecholamines and exogenous sympathomimetic drugs increases heart rate and contractility. Consequently, β-adrenergic *antagonists* decrease heart rate and the force of ventricular contraction, thereby relieving ischemia by reducing myocardial oxygen demand. In addition, slowing the heart rate may improve myocardial oxygen supply by augmenting the time spent in diastole, the phase when coronary perfusion primarily occurs.

In addition to suppressing angina, several studies have shown that β-blockers decrease the rates of recurrent infarction and mortality following an acute MI (see Chapter 7). Moreover, they have been shown to reduce the likelihood of an initial MI in patients with hypertension. Thus, β-blockers are first-line chronic therapy in the treatment of ischemic heart disease.

β-Blockers are generally well tolerated but have several potential side effects. For example, they may precipitate bronchospasm in patients with underlying asthma by antagonizing β_2-receptors in the bronchial tree. Although β_1-selective blockers are theoretically less likely to exacerbate bronchospasm in such patients, drug selectivity for the β_1-receptor is not complete, and in general, all β-blockers should be used cautiously, or avoided, in patients with significant obstructive airway disease.

β-Blockers are not used in patients with acutely *decompensated* LV dysfunction because they can intensify heart failure symptoms by further reducing inotropy. (However, as described

TABLE 6-3	Pharmacologic Agents Used in the Prevention and Treatment of Angina	
Drug Class	**Mechanism of Action**	**Adverse Effects**

Organic nitrates	↓ *Myocardial O_2 demand*
	   ↓ Preload (venodilatation)
	 ↑ *O_2 supply*
	   ↑ Coronary perfusion
	   ↓ Coronary vasospasm
		• Headache
		 • Hypotension
		 • Reflex tachycardia

β-Blockers	↓ *Myocardial O_2 demand*
	   ↓ Contractility
	   ↓ Heart rate
		• Excessive bradycardia
		 • ↓ LV contractile function
		 • Bronchoconstriction
		 • May mask hypoglycemic symptoms
		 • Fatigue

Calcium channel blockers (agent specific; see footnote)	↓ *Myocardial O_2 demand*
	   ↓ Preload (venodilatation)
	   ↓ Wall stress (↓BP)
	   ↓ Contractility (V, D)
	   ↓ Heart rate (V, D)
	 ↑ *O_2 supply*
	   ↑ Coronary perfusion
	   ↓ Coronary vasospasm
		• Headache, flushing
		 • ↓↓ LV contractility (V, D)
		 • Marked bradycardia (V, D)
		 • Edema (especially N, D)
		 • Constipation (especially V)

Ranolazine	↓ *Late phase inward sodium current*	• Dizziness, headache • Constipation, nausea

BP, blood pressure; D, diltiazem; LV, left ventricular; N, nifedipine and other dihydropyridine calcium channel antagonists; V, verapamil.

in Chapter 9, β-blockers actually *improve* outcomes in patients with stable chronic heart failure conditions.) β-Blockers are also relatively contraindicated in patients with marked bradycardia or certain types of heart block to avoid additional impairment of electrical conduction.

β-Blockers sometimes cause fatigue and sexual dysfunction. They should be used with caution in insulin-treated diabetic patients because they can mask tachycardia and other catecholamine-mediated responses that warn of hypoglycemia. One might also expect that β-blockers would decrease myocardial blood perfusion by blocking the vasodilating $β_2$-adrenergic receptors of the coronary arteries. However, this effect is usually attenuated by autoregulation and vasodilatation of the coronary vessels owing to the accumulation of local metabolites.

Organic nitrates (eg, nitroglycerin, isosorbide dinitrate, isosorbide mononitrate), as previously mentioned, relieve ischemia primarily through venodilatation (ie, lower wall stress results from a smaller ventricular radius) and possibly through coronary vasodilatation. The organic nitrates are the oldest of the antianginal drugs and come in several preparations (also described in Chapter 17). Sublingual nitroglycerin tablets or sprays are used in the treatment of acute attacks because of their rapid onset of action. In addition, when taken immediately before a person engages in activities known to provoke angina, these rapidly acting nitrates are useful as *prophylaxis* against anginal episodes.

Longer-acting anginal prevention can be achieved through a variety of nitrate preparations, including oral tablets of isosorbide dinitrate (or mononitrate) or a transdermal nitroglycerin patch, which is applied once a day. A limitation to chronic nitrate therapy is the development of drug tolerance (ie, decreased effectiveness of the drug during continued administration), which occurs to some degree in most patients. This undesired effect can be overcome by providing a nitrate-free interval for several hours each day, usually while the patient sleeps.

There is no evidence that nitrates improve survival or prevent infarctions in patients with chronic ischemic heart disease, and they are used purely for symptomatic relief. Common side effects include headache, light-headedness, and palpitations induced by vasodilatation and reflex sinus tachycardia. The latter can be prevented by combining a β-blocker with the nitrate regimen.

Calcium channel blockers (see Chapter 17) antagonize voltage-gated L-type calcium channels, but the actions of the individual drugs in this class vary. The dihydropyridines (eg, nifedipine and amlodipine) are potent vasodilators. They relieve myocardial ischemia by (1) decreasing oxygen demand (*venodilatation* reduces ventricular filling and size, *arterial dilatation* reduces the resistance against which the left ventricle contracts, and both actions reduce wall stress) and (2) increasing myocardial oxygen supply via coronary dilatation. By the latter mechanism, they are also potent agents for the relief of coronary artery vasospasm.

Nondihydropyridine calcium channel blockers (verapamil and diltiazem) also act as vasodilators but are not as potent in this regard as the dihydropyridines. However, these agents have additional beneficial antianginal effects stemming from their more potent cardiac depressant actions: they reduce the force of ventricular contraction (contractility) and slow the heart rate. Accordingly, verapamil and diltiazem also decrease myocardial oxygen demand by these mechanisms.

Questions have been raised about the safety of *short-acting* calcium channel blocking drugs in the treatment of ischemic heart disease. In meta-analyses of randomized trials, these drugs have been associated with an *increased* incidence of MI and mortality. The adverse effect may relate to the rapid hemodynamic effects and blood pressure swings induced by the short-acting agents. Therefore, only *long-acting* calcium channel blockers (ie, preparations taken once a day) are recommended in the treatment of chronic angina, generally as second-line drugs if symptoms are not controlled by β-blockers and nitrates.

The three standard groups of antianginal drugs described in this section can be used alone or in combination. However, care should be taken in combining a β-blocker with a nondihydropyridine calcium channel blocker (verapamil or diltiazem) because the additive negative chronotropic effect can cause excessive bradycardia and the combined negative inotropic effect can precipitate heart failure in patients with LV contractile dysfunction.

Ranolazine, a fourth type of anti-ischemic therapy, has been shown to decrease the frequency of anginal episodes and improve exercise capacity in patients with chronic CAD but differs from other anti-ischemic drugs in that it does not affect the heart rate or blood pressure. Although its mechanism of action has not been fully elucidated, it is believed to inhibit the late phase of the action potential's inward sodium current (I_{Na}^+) in ventricular myocytes. That late phase tends to be abnormally enhanced in ischemic myocardium, and the associated increased sodium influx results in higher-than-normal intracellular Ca^{++} (mediated by the trans-sarcolemmal Na^+-Ca^{++} exchanger; see Fig. 1-10). Such calcium overload is thought to result in impaired diastolic relaxation and contractile inefficiency. Inhibition of the late I_{Na}^+ by ranolazine counters these pathologic effects. Clinical studies have supported ranolazine's effectiveness in reducing angina, and its long-term safety, when used alone or in combination with other antianginal agents.

Although useful in controlling symptoms of angina, none of the antianginal drug groups has been shown to slow or reverse the atherosclerotic process responsible for the arterial lesions of chronic CAD. Moreover, although β-blockers have demonstrated mortality benefits in patients after MI, none of these agents has been shown to improve longevity in patients with chronic stable angina and preserved LV function.

MEDICAL TREATMENT TO PREVENT ACUTE CARDIAC EVENTS

Platelet aggregation and thrombosis are key elements in the pathophysiology of acute MI and unstable angina (see Chapter 7). **Antiplatelet therapy** reduces the risk of these acute coronary syndromes in patients with chronic angina and should be a standard part of the regimen used to treat CAD. For example, **aspirin** has antithrombotic actions through the inhibition of synthesis of thromboxane A_2, a mediator of platelet activation and aggregation, as well as anti-inflammatory properties that may be important in stabilizing atheromatous plaque. Unless contraindications are present (eg, allergy or gastric bleeding), aspirin should be continued indefinitely in all patients with CAD.

Platelet P2Y$_{12}$ ADP receptor antagonists (eg, clopidogrel, prasugrel, and ticagrelor) also prevent platelet activation and aggregation (see Chapter 17). They can be used as an antiplatelet substitute in patients who are allergic to aspirin. In addition, the combination of aspirin and a P2Y$_{12}$ inhibitor is superior to aspirin alone in reducing death and ischemic complications in patients with acute coronary syndromes, in those undergoing elective percutaneous coronary stenting, and in patients with a history of MI.

Recent clinical trial evidence shows that the combination of a **low-dose anticoagulant** (ie, rivaroxaban) plus aspirin further reduces the risk of death and ischemic complications in patients with chronic stable CAD compared with aspirin alone. Like P2Y$_{12}$ inhibitors, anticoagulants increase the risk of bleeding when added to aspirin, so this combination is generally reserved for patients at high cardiovascular risk who are at low risk for bleeding complications.

Lipid-lowering therapy is an important approach to reduce cardiovascular clinical events in patients with CAD. In particular, *HMG-CoA reductase inhibitors* (*statins*) lower MI and death rates in patients with established coronary disease and in those at risk of developing CAD. Randomized trials of statins have demonstrated a linear relationship between the magnitude of LDL cholesterol lowering and the relative reduction in cardiovascular risk. Thus, high-intensity lipid lowering (resulting in reduction of LDL cholesterol by >50%) is superior to less intense lipid-lowering therapy in preventing future ischemic events and cardiovascular death. The benefits of statin therapy may extend beyond LDL cholesterol reduction, because there is evidence that they also decrease vascular inflammation and improve endothelial dysfunction. Thus statins may help stabilize atherosclerotic plaques by multiple mechanisms.

In addition to statins, other specific drug classes (described further in Chapter 17) reduce serum LDL cholesterol and reduce cardiovascular event rates in patients with atherosclerotic disease. For example, *ezetimibe* is a selective inhibitor of cholesterol uptake at the brush border of small intestinal epithelial cells that lowers LDL cholesterol by 20%-25%. Monoclonal antibodies that target proprotein convertase subtilisin-kexin type 9 (PCSK9), termed *PCSK9 inhibitors*, are subcutaneously administered potent drugs that lower serum LDL cholesterol up to 60% in patients who are already on statin therapy. Ezetimibe and PCSK9 inhibitors each further reduce the risk of MI, stroke, and coronary revascularization when added to statin therapy. As a result, current guidelines recommend considering these therapies for high-risk patients whose LDL cholesterol remains >70 mg/dL despite high-intensity, or maximally tolerated, statin treatment. Finally, in CAD patients who have residual elevation of serum triglycerides despite statin therapy, the addition of a highly purified form of omega-3 fatty acid (ie, icosapent ethyl) reduces triglyceride levels and was shown to significantly lower cardiovascular event rates in a large clinical trial.

Certain **glucose-lowering therapies** (ie, sodium-glucose cotransporter 2 [SGLT2] inhibitors and glucagon-like peptide-1 [GLP-1] receptor agonists) decrease cardiovascular event rates in patients with type 2 diabetes and CAD and are important adjunctive therapies in that population.

Angiotensin-converting enzyme (ACE) inhibitors, beneficial in the treatment of hypertension (see Chapter 13), heart failure (see Chapter 9), and following MI (see Chapter 7), have also been studied as chronic therapy for patients with stable CAD not complicated by heart failure. Some (but not all) of these trials have shown reduced rates of death, MI, and stroke. Thus, many cardiologists recommend that an ACE inhibitor be included in the medical regimen of patients with chronic CAD.

REVASCULARIZATION

Many patients with chronic CAD and episodic angina become asymptomatic with pharmacologic therapy. However, coronary revascularization is pursued if (1) the patient's symptoms of angina do not respond adequately to antianginal drug therapy, (2) unacceptable side effects of medications occur, or (3) the patient is found to have high-risk coronary disease for which revascularization is known to improve survival (as described in the next section). The two techniques used to accomplish mechanical revascularization are percutaneous coronary intervention (PCI) and coronary artery bypass graft (CABG) surgery.

PCI includes **percutaneous transluminal coronary angioplasty (PTCA)**, a procedure performed under fluoroscopy in which a balloon-tipped catheter is inserted through a peripheral artery (usually a radial, femoral, or brachial artery) and maneuvered into the stenotic segment of a coronary vessel. The balloon at the end of the catheter is then inflated under high pressure to dilate the stenosis, after which the balloon is deflated and the catheter is removed from the body. The improvement in the size of the coronary lumen increases coronary perfusion and myocardial oxygen supply. Effective dilatation of the stenosis results from compression of the atherosclerotic plaque and often by creating a fracture within the lesion and stretching the underlying media. The risk of MI during the procedure is <1.5%, and mortality is <1%. Unfortunately, approximately one-third of patients who undergo balloon angioplasty develop recurrent symptoms within 6 months owing to restenosis of the dilated artery and require additional coronary interventions.

For this reason, **coronary stents** were developed for implantation at the time of PCI and have been shown to significantly reduce the rate of restenosis. Such stents are slender, cage-like metal support devices that in their collapsed configuration can be threaded into the region of stenosis by a catheter. Once in position, the stent is expanded into its open position by inflating a high-pressure balloon in its interior (Fig. 6-9). The balloon and attached catheter are then removed, but the stent is left permanently in place to serve as a scaffold to maintain

Figure 6-9. Placement of a coronary artery stent. A. A stent, in its original collapsed state, is advanced into the coronary stenosis on a balloon catheter. **B.** The balloon is inflated to expand the stent. **C.** The balloon is deflated, and the catheter is removed from the body, leaving the stent permanently in place.

arterial patency. Because stents are thrombogenic, a combination of oral antiplatelet agents (commonly, aspirin plus a platelet $P2Y_{12}$ receptor antagonist, such as clopidogrel) is crucial after stent implantation.

Compared with conventional balloon angioplasty, stent implantation decreases restenosis rates and reduces the need for repeat PCIs. Although restenosis resulting from vessel elastic recoil is greatly diminished by standard metal stent placement, neointimal proliferation (ie, migration of smooth muscle cells and production of extracellular matrix) remains an important cause of in-stent restenosis and recurrent anginal symptoms.

To address the problem of in-stent restenosis after PCI, **drug-eluting stents** were devised. These are fabricated with a polymer coat that incorporates an antiproliferative medication such as *sirolimus* (an immunosuppressive agent that inhibits T-cell activation), *everolimus* (an immunosuppressive similar to sirolimus), or *paclitaxel* (which interferes with cellular microtubule function). The medication is released from the stent over a period of 2-4 weeks, and this approach has shown great effect at preventing neointimal proliferation and reducing the need for repeat revascularization by more than half. However, just as neointimal proliferation is slowed, so too is protective endothelialization of the stent. The delay in endothelial cell coverage of the metal struts leaves patients at risk for thrombus formation within the stent should antiplatelet agents be discontinued prematurely. While this complication is uncommon with newer generation stents, it is potentially life-threatening, so patients are generally treated with a prolonged course of combination antiplatelet therapy (eg, aspirin plus a platelet $P2Y_{12}$ receptor antagonist for at least 12 months), followed by aspirin indefinitely, to mitigate the risk.

Although percutaneous revascularization techniques are generally superior to standard medical therapy for relief of angina, it is important to note that in the setting of stable coronary disease (ie, not an acute coronary syndrome), they have not been shown to reduce the risk of MI or death.

CABG surgery entails grafting portions of a patient's native blood vessels to bypass obstructed coronary arteries. Two types of surgical grafts are used (Fig. 6-10). The first employs native veins—typically, a section of the saphenous vein (a "superfluous" vessel removed from the leg) that is sutured from the base of the aorta to a coronary segment downstream from the region of stenosis. The second method uses arterial grafts—most commonly, an internal mammary artery (IMA, a "superfluous" branch of each subclavian artery)—that can be directly anastomosed distal to a stenotic coronary site. Vein grafts have a patency rate of up to 80% at 12 months but are vulnerable to accelerated atherosclerosis; 10 years after surgery, >50% have occluded. In contrast, IMA grafts are more resistant to atherosclerosis with a patency rate of 90% at 10 years. Therefore, IMA grafts are often used to perfuse sites of critical flow such as the left anterior descending artery. Clinical trial evidence supports the use of aggressive lipid-lowering drug therapy after CABG to improve the long-term patency rates of bypass grafts.

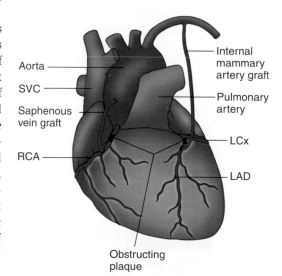

Figure 6-10. Coronary artery bypass surgery. Two types of bypasses are illustrated: (1) the left internal mammary artery originates from the left subclavian artery, and in this schematic, it is anastomosed to the left anterior descending (LAD) coronary artery distal to obstructing plaque; (2) one end of a saphenous vein graft is sutured to the proximal aorta and the other end to the right coronary artery (RCA) distal to a stenotic segment. SVC, superior vena cava; LCx, left circumflex artery.

In recent years, less invasive surgical alternatives to conventional CABG have been explored. These include "minimally invasive" operations with smaller incisions, the use of transcutaneous ports with videoscopic robotic assistance, and "off-pump" procedures, which avoid the use of cardiopulmonary bypass (heart-lung) machines. While there are theoretical advantages of avoiding the latter, studies examining off-pump procedures in comparison with standard CABG have shown comparable mortality benefit but poorer graft patency over time and an increased need for future revascularization. Additionally, there have been no major high-quality studies comparing benefits of minimally invasive operations to conventional CABG. In general, patient-specific risks and characteristics are considered by the surgeon when selecting which type of bypass procedure to undertake.

MEDICAL VS REVASCULARIZATION THERAPY

Many patients with chronic, stable angina can be successfully managed with pharmacologic therapy alone. However, if anginal symptoms prove refractory despite maximal pharmacologic therapy, or if intolerable drug side effects develop, coronary angiography is recommended for further therapeutic planning. Moreover, for patients whose angina *is* controlled by medications, it is standard to perform noninvasive testing (eg, exercise testing, echocardiography) to identify those with high-risk disease, because the long-term prognosis for such patients may be improved by coronary revascularization in some cases. Those with high-risk noninvasive test findings then typically proceed to coronary angiography.

In general, patients with severe LV systolic dysfunction, those with multivessel disease that includes a critical narrowing of the proximal left anterior descending artery (which threatens a large portion of the left ventricle), those with a high-grade ($\geq 50\%$) stenosis of the left main coronary artery, and those with diabetes (especially with multivessel disease) all achieve a survival benefit from coronary revascularization with CABG as compared with medical therapy. Studies comparing percutaneous coronary revascularization with CABG have consistently demonstrated improved survival with CABG in these clinical scenarios. However, for patients with less extensive disease (in whom the survival benefit of CABG over PCI has not been shown) or with very high surgical risk (eg, due to multiple comorbidities), PCI is a reasonable approach (Table 6-4).

Each of the described approaches for the treatment of coronary disease is benefiting from rapidly developing research advancements. New surgical techniques (increased use of various arterial grafts, less invasive operations), new drug-eluting stents (eg, incorporation of bioabsorbable/biodegradable polymers to decrease late stent thrombosis), novel adjuncts to stenting (potent antithrombotic drugs), and progress in pharmacologic management (eg, aggressive use of lipid-lowering and antithrombotic drugs) will likely further improve outcomes and better define the best therapeutic approaches for specific subsets of patients with chronic CAD.

TABLE 6-4	**Coronary Revascularization Procedures**
Percutaneous Coronary Interventions (PCI)	**Coronary Artery Bypass Graft Surgery (CABG)**
Less invasive than CABG	More effective for long-term relief of angina than PCI or pharmacologic therapy
Shorter hospital stay and easier recuperation than CABG	Most complete revascularization
Superior to pharmacologic therapy for relief of angina	Survival advantage in patients with • >50% left main coronary artery stenosis • Multivessel coronary disease, especially if LV contractile function is impaired

LV, left ventricle.

Summary

- **Cardiac ischemia results from an imbalance between myocardial oxygen supply and demand.**
- Determinants of **myocardial oxygen supply** are (1) the oxygen content of the blood and (2) coronary blood flow (which is dependent on the coronary perfusion pressure and coronary vascular resistance).
- Key regulators of **myocardial oxygen demand** include (1) the heart rate, (2) contractility, and (3) myocardial wall stress.
- In the presence of CAD, myocardial oxygen supply is compromised by **atherosclerotic plaques** that narrow the vascular lumen (reducing coronary blood flow) and by **endothelial cell dysfunction** that causes inappropriate vasoconstriction of coronary resistance vessels.
- **Angina pectoris** is the most frequent symptom of intermittent myocardial ischemia.
- The diagnosis of angina relies heavily on the patient's description of the discomfort and can be aided by laboratory studies (eg, **exercise or pharmacologic stress testing**).
- Angina may be accompanied by signs and symptoms of adrenergic stimulation, pulmonary congestion, and transient left ventricular systolic and diastolic dysfunction.
- Standard pharmacologic therapy for chronic angina includes agents to prevent ischemia and relieve symptoms (**β-blockers, nitrates, calcium channel antagonists**, alone or in combination) as well as agents that reduce the risk of acute coronary syndromes and death (eg, **aspirin, statins, angiotensin-converting enzyme inhibitors**).
- **Modifiable risk factors** for atherosclerosis (ie, dyslipidemia, smoking, hypertension, and diabetes) should be addressed.
- Revascularization with **PCI** or **CABG** surgery provides relief from ischemia in patients with chronic angina who are refractory to, or unable to tolerate, medical therapy. CABG confers improved survival rates to certain high-risk groups.

Review Questions

1. Which of the following is NOT a determinant of myocardial oxygen demand?

   a. Heart rate
   b. Contractility
   c. Coronary vascular resistance
   d. Ventricular wall thickness

2. A 72-year-old man with a history of coronary artery disease presents for office evaluation because of episodes of chest discomfort. His symptom occurs consistently during exercise and resolves with rest. There has been no recent change in the frequency or severity of these episodes. His current medications include aspirin, atorvastatin, metoprolol (a β-blocker), and isosorbide mononitrate (an organic nitrate). His heart rate is 95 beats/min and blood pressure is 146/78 mm Hg. His electrocardiogram is normal without any signs of acute myocardial ischemia. Which of the following would be the best next step in managing the patient's symptom?

a. Increase metoprolol dosage.
b. Add amlodipine (a calcium channel blocker).
c. Increase the aspirin dosage.
d. Refer for cardiac catheterization.

3. Which of the following developments during a standard exercise stress test is NOT suggestive of anatomically significant coronary artery disease?

a. 2-mm horizontal ST-segment depressions
b. Ventricular tachycardia
c. 30 mm Hg increase in systolic blood pressure at peak exercise
d. Inability to exercise due to cardiopulmonary limitation

Answers to Review Questions

1. Choice c is correct. In the normal heart, the oxygen requirements of the myocardium are continuously matched by the coronary arterial supply. When the metabolic demands of the heart increase, the delivery of oxygen to the myocardium must rise to maintain that balance. The primary determinants of myocardial oxygen demand are heart rate, contractility, and ventricular wall stress. Wall stress (σ) is approximated by Laplace's relationship: $\sigma = (P \times r)/2h$, in which P is intraventricular pressure, r the radius of the ventricle, and h is ventricular wall thickness. Coronary vascular resistance influences coronary blood flow, which is a major determinant of myocardial oxygen *supply*, not demand.

2. Choice a is correct. The clinical vignette describes a patient with chronic stable angina pectoris. Pharmacologic agents, including β-blockers, nitrates, calcium channel blockers, help restore the balance between myocardial oxygen demand and supply and are used for the treatment and prevention of anginal episodes. Among these, β-blockers are considered a first-line option. Although this patient is already on a β-blocker, his heart rate is in the high normal range and blood pressure is elevated, so the β-blocker dose could be increased before adding other pharmacologic agents. Coronary revascularization would be considered if the patient's anginal symptoms do not respond adequately to antianginal drug therapy.

3. Choice c is correct. An exercise stress test is abnormal if the patient develops typical chest discomfort in association with ECG abnormalities suggestive of myocardial ischemia (ie, >1 mm horizontal or downsloping ST-segment depressions). High-risk features, which increase the likelihood that the patient has severe multivessel coronary disease, include development of ECG abnormalities early in exercise, >2-mm ST-segment depressions, development of ventricular arrhythmias, and a *decline* in systolic blood pressure during exercise. In contrast, an increase in systolic blood pressure is an expected physiologic response to exercise.

Acknowledgments

Contributors to previous editions of this chapter were Jayme Wilder, MD; June-Wha Rhee, MD; Haley Naik, MD; Christopher P. Chiodo, MD; Carey Farquhar, MD; Anurag Gupta, MD; Rainu Kaushal, MD; William Carlson, MD; Michael E. Mendelsohn MD; and Patrick T. O'Gara, MD.

Additional Reading

Bhatt DL. Percutaneous coronary intervention in 2018. *JAMA*. 2018;319:2127-2128.

Bhatt DL, Steg G, Miller M, et al. Effects of icosapent ethyl on total ischemic events: from REDUCE-IT. *J Am Coll Cardiol*. 2019;73:2791-2802.

Doenst T, Haverich A, Serruys P, et al. PCI and CABG for treating stable coronary artery disease. *J Am Coll Cardiol*. 2019;73:964-976.

Eikelboom JW, Connolly SJ, Bosch J, et al. Rivaroxaban with or without aspirin in stable cardiovascular disease. *N Engl J Med*. 2017;377:1319-1330.

Fihn SD, Blankenship JC, Alexander KP, et al. 2014 ACC/AHA/AATS/PCNA/SCAI/STS focused updated on the guideline for the diagnosis and management of patients with stable ischemic heart disease: a report of the American College of Cardiology/American Heart Association Task Force on Clinical Practice Guidelines, and the American Association for Thoracic Surgery, Preventive Cardiovascular Nurses Association, Society for Cardiovascular Angiography and Interventions, and Society of Thoracic Surgeons. *Circulation*. 2014;130:1749-1767.

Grundy SM, Stone NJ, Bailey AL, et al. 2018 AHA/ACC/AACVPR/AAPA/ABC/ACPM/ADA/AGS/APhA/ASPC/NLA/PCNA Guideline on the Management of Blood Cholesterol: A Report of the American College of Cardiology/American Heart Association Task Force on Clinical Practice Guidelines. *Circulation*. 2019;139(25):e1082-e1143.

Gurbel PA, Fox KAA, Tantry US, et al. Combination antiplatelet and oral anticoagulant therapy in patients with coronary and peripheral artery disease. *Circulation*. 2019;139:2170-2185.

Levine GN, Bates ER, Bittl JA, et al. 2016 ACC/AHA guideline focused update on duration of dual antiplatelet therapy in patients with coronary artery disease: a report of the American College of Cardiology/American Heart Association Task Force on Clinical Practice Guidelines. *J Am Coll Cardiol*. 2016;68:1082-1115.

Sabatine MS, Giugliano RP, Keech AC, et al. Evolocumab and clinical outcomes in patients with cardiovascular disease. *N Engl J Med*. 2017;376:1713-1722.

Zelniker TA, Wiviott SD, Raz I, et al. SGLT2 inhibitors for primary and secondary prevention of cardiovascular and renal outcomes in type 2 diabetes: a systematic review and meta-analysis of cardiovascular outcomes trials. *Lancet*. 2019;393:31-39.

7

Acute Coronary Syndromes

David D. Berg | Marc S. Sabatine | Leonard S. Lilly

Acute coronary syndromes (ACSs) are life-threatening conditions that can punctuate the course of patients with coronary artery disease at any time. These syndromes form a continuum that ranges from an unstable pattern of angina pectoris to the development of a large acute myocardial infarction (MI), a condition of irreversible necrosis of heart muscle. All forms of ACS share a common pathophysiologic mechanism, as this chapter examines.

The frequency of ACS is staggering: more than 1.3 million people are admitted to hospitals in the United States each year with these conditions. Approximately 14% of people who experience an MI will die from it. Despite these sobering statistics, mortality associated with ACS has substantially declined in recent decades as a result of major therapeutic and preventive advances. This chapter considers the events that lead to an ACS, the pathologic and functional changes that follow, and therapeutic approaches that ameliorate the aberrant pathophysiology.

PATHOGENESIS OF ACUTE CORONARY SYNDROMES

Most ACSs result from disruption of atherosclerotic coronary plaque with subsequent platelet aggregation and formation of an intracoronary thrombus. The thrombus transforms a region of plaque narrowing to one of severe or complete occlusion, and the impaired blood flow causes a marked imbalance between myocardial oxygen supply and demand. The form of ACS that results depends on the degree of coronary obstruction and associated ischemia (Table 7-1). A *partially* occlusive thrombus is the typical cause of the closely related syndromes **unstable angina (UA)** and **non–ST-segment-elevation myocardial infarction** (**NSTEMI**), with the latter being distinguished from the former by the presence of myocardial necrosis. At the other end of the spectrum, if the thrombus *completely* obstructs the coronary artery, the result

TABLE 7-1	Spectrum of Acute Coronary Syndromes		
	Unstable Angina	**Non–ST-Elevation MI**	**ST-Elevation MI**
Usual coronary pathology	Partially occlusive thrombus	Partially occlusive thrombus	Completely occlusive thrombus
Myocyte necrosis	No	Yes	Yes

MI, myocardial infarction.

is more severe ischemia and a larger amount of necrosis, manifesting as an **ST-segment-elevation myocardial infarction** (**STEMI**).

The responsible thrombus in ACS is generated by interactions among atherosclerotic plaque, the coronary endothelium, circulating platelets, and the dynamic vasomotor tone of the vessel wall, which overwhelm the natural antithrombotic mechanisms described in the next section.

Normal Hemostasis

When a normal blood vessel is injured, the endothelial surface becomes disrupted and thrombogenic connective tissue is exposed. *Primary hemostasis* is the first line of defense against bleeding. This process begins within seconds of vessel injury and is mediated by circulating platelets, which adhere to collagen in the vascular subendothelium and aggregate to form a "platelet plug." While the primary hemostatic plug forms, the exposure of subendothelial tissue factor triggers the plasma coagulation cascade, initiating the process of *secondary hemostasis*. The plasma coagulation proteins involved in secondary hemostasis are sequentially activated at the site of injury and ultimately form a fibrin clot by the action of thrombin. The resulting clot stabilizes and strengthens the platelet plug.

The normal hemostatic system minimizes blood loss from injured vessels, but there is little difference between this physiologic response and the pathologic process of coronary thrombosis triggered by disruption of atherosclerotic plaques.

Endogenous Antithrombotic Mechanisms

Normal blood vessels, including the coronary arteries, are replete with safeguards that prevent spontaneous thrombosis and occlusion, some examples of which are shown in Figure 7-1.

Inactivation of Clotting Factors

Several natural inhibitors tightly regulate the coagulation process to oppose clot formation and maintain blood fluidity. The most important of these are antithrombin, proteins C and S, and tissue factor pathway inhibitor (TFPI).

Antithrombin is a plasma protein that irreversibly binds to thrombin and other clotting factors, inactivating them and facilitating their clearance from the circulation (see mechanism 1 in Fig. 7-1). The effectiveness of antithrombin is increased 1000-fold by binding to heparan sulfate, a heparin-like molecule normally present on the luminal surface of endothelial cells.

Protein C, **protein S**, and **thrombomodulin** form a natural anticoagulant system that inactivates the "acceleration" factors of the coagulation pathway (ie, factors Va and VIIIa). Protein C is synthesized in the liver and circulates in an inactive form. Thrombomodulin is a thrombin-binding receptor normally present on endothelial cells. Thrombin bound to thrombomodulin cannot convert fibrinogen to fibrin (the final reaction in clot formation). Instead, the thrombin-thrombomodulin complex activates protein C. Activated protein C degrades factors

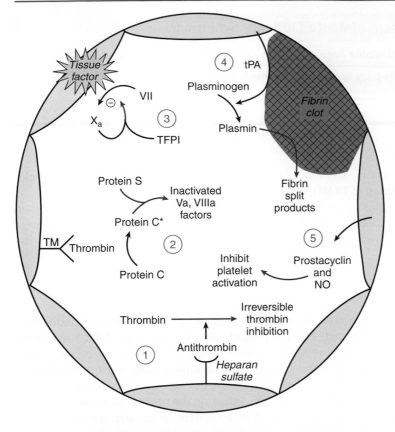

Figure 7-1. Endogenous protective mechanisms against thrombosis and vessel occlusion. (*1*) Inactivation of thrombin by antithrombin (AT), the effectiveness of which is enhanced by binding of AT to heparan sulfate. (*2*) Inactivation of clotting factors Va and VIIIa by activated protein C (protein C*), an action that is enhanced by protein S. Protein C is activated by the thrombomodulin (TM)-thrombin complex. (*3*) Inactivation of factor VII/ tissue factor complex by tissue factor pathway inhibitor (TFPI). (*4*) Lysis of fibrin clots by tissue plasminogen activator (tPA). (*5*) Inhibition of platelet activation by prostacyclin and nitric oxide (NO).

Va and VIIIa (see mechanism 2 in Fig. 7-1), thereby inhibiting coagulation. The presence of protein S in the circulation enhances the inhibitory function of protein C.

TFPI is a plasma serine protease inhibitor that is activated by coagulation factor Xa. The combined factor Xa-TFPI binds to and inactivates the complex of tissue factor with factor VIIa that normally triggers the extrinsic coagulation pathway (see mechanism 3 in Fig. 7-1). Thus, TFPI serves as a negative feedback inhibitor that interferes with coagulation.

Lysis of Fibrin Clots

Tissue plasminogen activator (tPA) is a protein secreted by endothelial cells in response to many triggers of clot formation. It cleaves the protein plasminogen to form active plasmin, which in turn enzymatically degrades fibrin clots (see mechanism 4 in Fig. 7-1). When tPA binds to fibrin in a forming clot, its ability to convert plasminogen to plasmin is greatly enhanced.

Endogenous Platelet Inhibition and Vasodilatation

Prostacyclin is synthesized and secreted by endothelial cells (see mechanism 5 in Fig. 7-1), as described in Chapter 6. Prostacyclin increases platelet levels of cyclic AMP and thereby strongly inhibits platelet activation and aggregation. It also *indirectly* inhibits coagulation via its potent vasodilating properties. Vasodilatation helps guard against thrombosis by augmenting blood flow (which minimizes contact between procoagulant factors) and by reducing shear stress (an inducer of platelet activation).

Nitric oxide (NO) is similarly secreted by endothelial cells, as described in Chapter 6. It acts locally to inhibit platelet activation, and it too serves as a potent vasodilator.

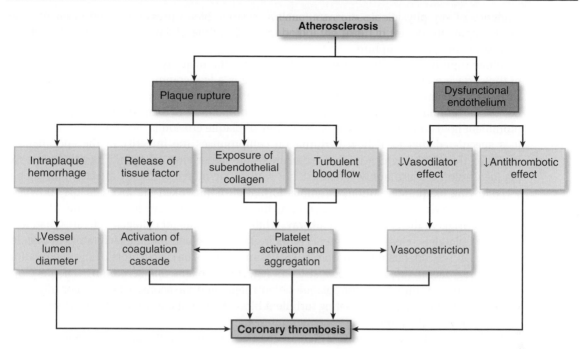

Figure 7-2. Mechanisms of coronary thrombus formation at atherosclerotic lesions. Factors that contribute to this process include plaque disruption (eg, rupture) and inappropriate vasoconstriction and loss of normal antithrombotic defenses because of dysfunctional endothelium.

PATHOGENESIS OF CORONARY THROMBOSIS

Normally, the mechanisms shown in Figure 7-1 serve to prevent spontaneous intravascular thrombus formation. However, abnormalities associated with atherosclerotic lesions may overwhelm these defenses and result in coronary thrombosis and vessel occlusion (Fig. 7-2). Atherosclerosis contributes to thrombus formation by (1) plaque rupture, which exposes the circulating blood elements to thrombogenic substances, and (2) endothelial dysfunction with the loss of normal protective antithrombotic and vasodilatory properties.

Atherosclerotic **plaque rupture** is considered the major trigger of coronary thrombosis. The underlying causes of plaque disruption are (1) chemical factors that destabilize atherosclerotic lesions and (2) physical stresses to which the lesions are subjected. As described in Chapter 5, atherosclerotic plaques consist of a lipid-laden core surrounded by a fibrous external cap. Substances released from inflammatory cells within the plaque can compromise the integrity of the fibrous cap. For example, T lymphocytes release interferon-γ (IFN-γ), which inhibits collagen synthesis by smooth muscle cells and thereby interferes with the usual strength of the cap. Additionally, cells within atherosclerotic lesions produce enzymes (eg, metalloproteinases) that degrade the interstitial matrix, further compromising plaque stability. A weakened or thin-capped plaque is subject to rupture, particularly in its "shoulder" region (the border with the normal arterial wall that is subjected to high circumferential stress) either spontaneously or by physical forces, such as intraluminal blood pressure and torsion from the beating myocardium.

ACSs sometimes occur in the setting of certain triggers, such as strenuous physical activity or emotional upset. The activation of the sympathetic nervous system in these situations increases blood pressure, heart rate, and the force of ventricular contraction—actions that may stress the atherosclerotic lesion, thereby causing the plaque to fissure or rupture. In addition, MI is most likely to occur in the early morning hours. This observation may relate to the tendency of key physiologic stressors (such as systolic blood pressure, blood viscosity, and plasma epinephrine levels) to be most elevated at that time of day, and these factors subject vulnerable plaques to rupture.

While rupture of the fibrous cap is responsible for the majority of ACSs, superficial *erosion* of the surface endothelium without plaque rupture is a less common, but increasingly recognized mechanism of plaque disruption and thrombus formation. Typically, "eroded" plaques have an accumulation of proteoglycans and other components of extracellular matrix without a prominent lipid core. Although the pathobiology of plaque erosion is incompletely understood, it is speculated that local flow perturbation compromises the integrity of the endothelium overlying the plaque, which leads to exposure of the underlying collagen. The risk factors for plaque erosion are also not well defined, but women are more commonly affected than men.

Following plaque disruption, thrombus formation is provoked via mechanisms shown in Figure 7-2. For example, with plaque rupture, the exposure of tissue factor from the atheromatous core triggers the coagulation pathway, while subendothelial collagen activates platelets. Activated platelets release the contents of their granules, which include facilitators of platelet aggregation (eg, adenosine diphosphate [ADP] and fibrinogen), activators of the coagulation cascade (eg, factor Va), and vasoconstrictors (eg, thromboxane and serotonin). The developing intracoronary thrombus, intraplaque hemorrhage, and vasoconstriction all contribute to narrowing the vessel lumen, creating turbulent blood flow that contributes to shear stress and further platelet activation.

Dysfunctional endothelium, which is apparent even in mild atherosclerotic coronary disease, also increases the likelihood of thrombus formation. In the setting of endothelial dysfunction, reduced amounts of vasodilators (eg, NO and prostacyclin) are released and inhibition of platelet aggregation by these factors is impaired, resulting in the loss of a key defense against thrombosis.

Not only is dysfunctional endothelium less equipped to prevent platelet aggregation, it is also less able to counteract the vasoconstricting products of platelets. During thrombus formation, vasoconstriction is promoted both by platelet products (thromboxane and serotonin) and by thrombin within the developing clot. The *normal* platelet-associated vascular response is vasodilatation, because platelet products stimulate endothelial NO and prostacyclin release, the influences of which predominate over direct platelet-derived vasoconstrictors (see Fig. 6-4). However, reduced secretion of endothelial vasodilators in atherosclerosis allows vasoconstriction to proceed unchecked. Similarly, thrombin in a forming clot is a potent vascular smooth muscle constrictor in the setting of dysfunctional endothelium. Vasoconstriction causes torsional stresses that can contribute to plaque rupture or can transiently occlude the stenotic vessel through heightened arterial tone. The reduction in coronary blood flow caused by vasoconstriction also reduces the washout of coagulation proteins, thereby enhancing thrombogenicity.

Significance of Coronary Thrombosis

The formation of an intracoronary thrombus results in one of the several potential outcomes (Fig. 7-3). For example, plaque rupture is sometimes superficial, minor, and self-limited, such that only a small, nonocclusive thrombus forms. In this case, the thrombus may simply become incorporated into the growing atheromatous lesion through fibrotic organization, or it may be lysed by natural fibrinolytic mechanisms. Recurrent asymptomatic plaque ruptures of this type may cause gradual progressive enlargement of the coronary stenosis.

However, deeper plaque rupture may result in greater exposure of subendothelial collagen and tissue factor, with formation of a larger thrombus that more substantially occludes the vessel's lumen. Such obstruction may cause prolonged severe ischemia and the development of an ACS. If the intraluminal thrombus at the site of plaque disruption *totally* occludes the vessel, blood flow beyond the obstruction will cease, prolonged ischemia will occur, and an MI (usually an ST-segment elevation MI) will result. Conversely, if the thrombus *partially*

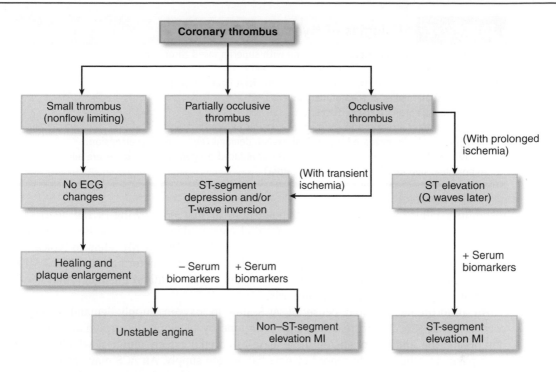

Figure 7-3. Consequences of coronary thrombosis. A small thrombus formed on superficial plaque rupture or erosion may not result in symptoms or electrocardiogram (ECG) abnormalities, but healing and fibrous organization may incorporate the thrombus into the plaque, causing the atherosclerotic lesion to enlarge. A partially occlusive thrombus narrows the arterial lumen, restricts blood flow, and can cause unstable angina or a non–ST-segment-elevation MI, either of which may result in ST-segment depression and/or T-wave inversion on the ECG. A totally occlusive thrombus with prolonged ischemia is the most common cause of ST-segment-elevation MI, in which the ECG initially shows ST-segment elevation, followed by Q-wave development if early reperfusion is not achieved. An occlusive thrombus that recanalizes, or one that develops in a region served by adequate collateral blood flow, may result in less prolonged ischemia and a non–ST-segment-elevation MI instead. Serum biomarkers of myocardial necrosis include cardiac-specific troponins and creatine kinase MB isoenzyme.

occludes the vessel (or if it totally occludes the vessel but only transiently because of spontaneous recanalization or by relief of superimposed vasospasm), the severity and duration of ischemia will be less, and a smaller NSTEMI or UA is the more likely outcome. The distinction between NSTEMI and UA is based on whether the event is severe enough to cause myocardial necrosis, indicated by the presence of certain serum biomarkers (see Fig. 7-3). Nonetheless, NSTEMI and UA act quite alike, and the management of these entities is similar.

Occasionally, an NSTEMI may result from total coronary occlusion. In this case, it is likely that a substantial collateral blood supply (see Chapter 1) limits the extent of necrosis, such that a larger STEMI is prevented.

Non-Atherothrombotic Causes of Acute Myocardial Infarction

Mechanisms other than plaque disruption and acute thrombus formation can precipitate an acute MI (Table 7-2). For example, coronary emboli from mechanical or infected cardiac valves may lodge in the coronary circulation, inflammation from acute vasculitis can initiate coronary occlusion, or patients with certain connective tissue disorders, or peripartum women, can on rare occasion experience a spontaneous coronary artery dissection (a tear in the vessel wall that may lead to coronary occlusion, as described in Chapter 15).

In addition, acute MI can occur in the absence of disrupted atherosclerotic plaque from any cause of a marked decline in oxygen supply (eg, intense coronary vasospasm, severe anemia,

TABLE 7-2	**Etiologies of Myocardial Infarction**

- Atherosclerotic plaque rupture or erosion with superimposed thrombus
- Vasculitic syndromes (see Chapter 15)
- Coronary embolism (eg, from endocarditis, artificial heart valves)
- Congenital anomalies of the coronary arteries
- Spontaneous coronary artery dissection
- Severe coronary artery spasm (primary or cocaine-induced)
- States of markedly increased myocardial oxygen demand (eg, severe hypertension, tachyarrhythmias, advanced aortic stenosis) or reduced oxygen supply (eg, severe anemia, hypoxemia, hypotension, marked bradycardia)

respiratory failure with hypoxemia, hypotension, or marked slowing of the heart rate) or because of a prominent increase in myocardial oxygen demand (eg, marked hypertension, rapid heart rhythms, or severe aortic stenosis). The label **Type 1 MI** refers to typical infarction due to disrupted atherosclerotic plaque with acute thrombus formation. **Type 2 MI** is the description for infarction resulting from an oxygen supply-demand mismatch that is not the result of plaque disruption and thrombosis.

An unfortunate potential cause of ACS due to oxygen supply-demand mismatch is cocaine abuse. Cocaine increases sympathetic tone by blocking the presynaptic reuptake of norepinephrine and by enhancing the release of adrenal catecholamines, which can lead to vasospasm and therefore decreased myocardial oxygen supply. An ACS may ensue because of increased myocardial oxygen demand resulting from cocaine-induced sympathetic myocardial stimulation (increased heart rate and blood pressure) in the face of the decreased oxygen supply.

PATHOLOGY AND PATHOPHYSIOLOGY

MI (either STEMI or NSTEMI) results when myocardial ischemia is sufficiently severe to cause myocyte necrosis. Although by definition UA does not result in necrosis, it may subsequently progress to MI if the underlying pathophysiology is not promptly corrected.

In addition to their clinical classifications, infarctions can be described pathologically by the extent of necrosis they produce within the myocardial wall. **Transmural infarcts** span the entire thickness of the myocardial wall and result from total, prolonged occlusion of an epicardial coronary artery. Conversely, **subendocardial infarcts** exclusively involve the innermost layers of the myocardium. The subendocardium is particularly susceptible to ischemia because it is the zone subjected to the highest pressure from the ventricular chamber, has few collateral connections that supply it, and is perfused by vessels that must pass through layers of contracting myocardium.

Infarction represents the culmination of a disastrous cascade of events, initiated by ischemia, that progresses from a potentially reversible phase to irreversible cell death. Myocardium that is supplied directly by an occluded vessel may die quickly. The adjacent tissue may not necrose immediately because it may be sufficiently perfused by nearby patent vessels. However, the neighboring cells may become increasingly ischemic over time, as demand for oxygen continues in the face of reduced oxygen supply. Thus, the region of infarction may subsequently extend outward. The amount of tissue that ultimately succumbs to infarction therefore relates to (1) the mass of myocardium perfused by the occluded vessel, (2) the magnitude and duration of impaired coronary blood flow, (3) the oxygen demand of the affected region, (4) the adequacy of collateral vessels that provide blood flow from neighboring nonoccluded coronary arteries, and (5) the degree of tissue response that modifies the ischemic process.

Pathologic Evolution of Infarction

The pathophysiologic alterations that transpire during MI occur in two stages: early changes at the time of acute infarction and late changes during myocardial healing and remodeling (Table 7-3).

Early Changes in Infarction

Early changes include the histologic evolution of the infarct and the functional impact of oxygen deprivation on myocardial contractility. These changes culminate in coagulative necrosis of the myocardium in 2-4 days.

As oxygen levels fall in the myocardium supplied by an abruptly occluded coronary vessel, there is a rapid shift from aerobic to anaerobic metabolism (Fig. 7-4). Because mitochondria can no longer oxidize fats or products of glycolysis, high-energy phosphate production drops dramatically and anaerobic glycolysis leads to the accumulation of lactic acid, resulting in a lowered pH.

Furthermore, the paucity of high-energy phosphates such as adenosine triphosphate (ATP) interferes with transmembrane Na^+–K^+-ATPase, with resultant elevation in the concentrations of intracellular Na^+ and extracellular K^+. Rising intracellular Na^+ contributes to cellular edema. Membrane leak and rising extracellular K^+ concentration contributes to alterations in the transmembrane electrical potential, predisposing the myocardium to lethal arrhythmias. Intracellular calcium accumulates in the damaged myocytes and is thought to contribute to the final common pathway of cell destruction through the activation of degradative lipases and proteases.

Collectively, these metabolic changes decrease myocardial function as early as 2 minutes following occlusive thrombosis. Without intervention, *irreversible* cell injury ensues in 20 minutes and is marked by the development of membrane defects. Proteolytic enzymes leak across the myocyte's altered membrane, damaging adjacent myocardium, and the release of certain macromolecules into the circulation serves as a clinical marker of acute infarction.

Early histologic changes include myocardial edema, wavy myofibers, and the presence of contraction bands (see Table 7-3). Edema of the myocardium develops within 4-12 hours, as vascular permeability increases and interstitial oncotic pressure rises (because of the leak of

TABLE 7-3	Pathologic Time Line in Transmural Infarction
Time	**Event**
Early changes	
1-2 min	ATP levels fall; cessation of contractility
10 min	50% depletion of ATP; cellular edema, decreased membrane potential, and susceptibility to arrhythmias
20-24 min	Irreversible cell injury
1-3 h	Wavy myofibers
4-12 h	Hemorrhage, edema, PMN infiltration begins
18-24 h	Coagulation necrosis (pyknotic nuclei with eosinophilic cytoplasm), edema
2-4 d	Total coagulation necrosis (no nuclei or striations, rimmed by hyperemic tissue); monocytes appear; PMN infiltration peaks
Late changes	
5-7 d	Yellow softening from resorption of dead tissue by macrophages
7+ d	Granulation tissue forms, ventricular remodeling
7 wk	Fibrosis and scarring complete

ATP, adenosine triphosphate; PMN, polymorphonuclear leukocyte.

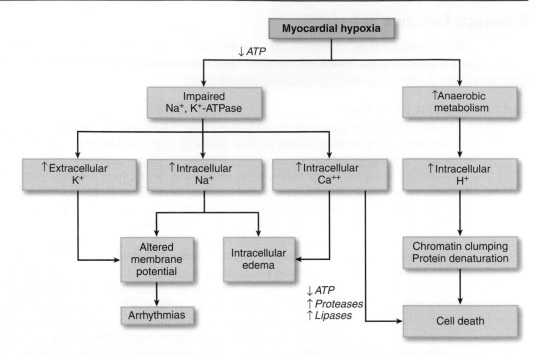

Figure 7-4. Mechanisms of cell death in myocardial infarction. Acute ischemia rapidly depletes the intracellular supply of adenosine triphosphate (ATP) as aerobic metabolism fails. Subsequent intracellular acidosis and impairment of ATP-dependent processes culminate in intracellular calcium accumulation, edema, and cell death.

intracellular proteins). **Wavy myofibers** appear as intercellular edema separates the myocardial cells that are tugged about by the surrounding, functional myocardium. **Contraction bands** can often be seen near the borders of the infarct: sarcomeres are contracted and consolidated and appear as bright eosinophilic belts (Fig. 7-5A).

An acute inflammatory response, with infiltration of neutrophils, begins after ~4 hours and incites further tissue damage. Within 18-24 hours, **coagulation necrosis** is evident on light microscopy (Fig. 7-5B) with pyknotic nuclei and bland eosinophilic cytoplasm.

Gross morphologic changes (dark, mottled discoloration of infarcted tissue) do not appear until 18-24 hours after coronary occlusion, although certain staining techniques (eg, tetrazolium) permit the pathologist to identify regions of infarction earlier.

Late Changes in Infarction

Late pathologic change in the course of an MI includes (1) the clearing of necrotic myocardium and (2) the deposition of collagen to form scar tissue.

Five to seven days after infarction, the process of wound healing progresses. Irreversibly injured myocytes do not regenerate; rather, the cells are replaced by fibrous tissue. Macrophages invade the inflamed myocardium shortly after neutrophil infiltration and remove necrotic tissue (Fig. 7-5C). This period of tissue resorption is termed **yellow softening** because connective tissue elements are destroyed and removed along with dead myocardial cells. The phagocytic clearing, combined with thinning and dilatation of the infarcted zone, results in structural weakness of the ventricular wall and the possibility of myocardial wall rupture at this stage.

Approximately 1 week after infarction, granulation tissue appears, representing the beginning of the scarring process (Fig. 7-5D). This is observed grossly as a red border at the edge of the infarct. **Fibrosis** subsequently ensues, and scarring is complete by 7 weeks after infarction (Fig. 7-5E).

Figure 7-5. Pathologic evolution in myocardial infarction. A. Acute infarct ~12 hours old showing contraction band necrosis, nuclear karyolysis, focal hemorrhage, and an absence of inflammation. **B.** Acute infarct ~24-48 hours old showing coagulation necrosis and dense infiltration of neutrophils. **C.** Healing infarct ~5 days old showing necrotic myocytes undergoing removal by macrophages, with the neutrophilic response having largely dissipated. **D.** Healing infarct ~10 days old showing granulation tissue with new blood vessels (neovascularization), mild chronic inflammation (macrophages and lymphocytes), fibroblasts, and early collagen deposition; viable myocardium is present at the upper left. **E.** Healed infarct ~1-2 months old showing dense fibrosis; the inflammation and new vessels have largely regressed; viable myocardium is present at the upper left. All images are hematoxylin and eosin–stained sections. (Courtesy of Robert Padera, MD, PhD, Brigham and Women's Hospital, Boston, MA.)

FUNCTIONAL ALTERATIONS

Impaired Contractility and Compliance

The destruction of functional myocardial cells in infarction quickly leads to impaired ventricular contraction (**systolic dysfunction**). Cardiac output is further compromised because *synchronous* contraction of myocytes is lost. Specific terms are used to describe the types of wall motion abnormalities that can result. A localized region of reduced contraction is termed *hypokinetic*, a segment that does not contract at all is called *akinetic*, and a *dyskinetic* region is one that bulges *outward* during contraction of the remaining functional portions of the ventricle.

During an ACS, the left ventricle is also adversely compromised by **diastolic dysfunction**. Ischemia and/or infarction impair diastolic relaxation (an energy-dependent process; see Chapter 1), which reduces ventricular compliance and contributes to elevated ventricular filling pressures.

Stunned Myocardium

Sometimes transient myocardial ischemia can result in a very prolonged, but gradually reversible, period of contractile dysfunction. As described in Chapter 6, **stunned myocardium** is tissue that demonstrates prolonged systolic dysfunction after a discrete episode of severe ischemia, despite restoration of adequate blood flow, and *gradually* regains contractile force days to weeks later. For example, stunning may occur following reperfusion therapy for acute STEMI, in which case prolonged contractile dysfunction of affected ventricular segments may simulate infarcted tissue. However, if the tissue is simply stunned rather than necrotic, its function will recover over time.

Ischemic Preconditioning

Brief ischemic insults to a region of myocardium may render that tissue more resistant to subsequent episodes, a phenomenon termed **ischemic preconditioning**. The clinical relevance is that patients who sustain an MI in the context of recent angina experience less morbidity and mortality than those without preceding ischemic episodes. The mechanism of this phenomenon is not fully understood but appears to involve multiple signaling pathways that involve both local and systemic mediators. Substances released during ischemia, including adenosine and bradykinin, are believed to be key triggers of these pathways.

Ventricular Remodeling

Following an MI, changes occur in the geometry of both infarcted and noninfarcted ventricular muscle. Such alterations in chamber size and wall thickness affect long-term cardiac function and prognosis.

In the early post-MI period, infarct *expansion* may occur, in which the affected ventricular segment enlarges without additional myocyte necrosis. Infarct expansion represents thinning and dilatation of the necrotic zone of tissue, likely because of "slippage" between the muscle fibers, resulting in a decreased volume of myocytes in the region. Infarct expansion can be detrimental because it increases ventricular size, which (1) augments wall stress, (2) impairs systolic contractile function, and (3) increases the likelihood of aneurysm formation.

In addition to early expansion of the infarcted territory, remodeling of the ventricle may also involve dilatation of the overworked *noninfarcted* segments, which are subjected to increased wall stress. This dilatation begins in the early postinfarct period and continues over the ensuing weeks and months. Initially, chamber dilatation serves a compensatory role because it increases cardiac output via the Frank–Starling mechanism (see Chapter 9), but progressive enlargement may ultimately lead to heart failure and predisposes to ventricular arrhythmias.

Adverse ventricular remodeling can be beneficially modified by certain interventions. At the time of infarction, for example, reperfusion therapies limit infarct size and therefore decrease the likelihood of infarct expansion. In addition, drugs that interfere with the renin-angiotensin-aldosterone system have been shown to attenuate progressive remodeling and to reduce short- and long-term mortality after infarction (as discussed later in the chapter).

CLINICAL FEATURES OF ACUTE CORONARY SYNDROMES

Because ACSs represent disorders along a continuum, their clinical features overlap. In general, the severity of symptoms and associated laboratory findings progress from UA on one side of the continuum, through NSTEMI, to STEMI on the other end of the continuum. Distinguishing among these syndromes is based on the clinical presentation, electrocardiographic findings, and serum biomarkers of myocardial damage. To institute appropriate immediate therapy, the most important distinction to make is between an ACS that causes ST-segment elevation on the electrocardiogram (STEMI) and those acute syndromes that do not (UA and NSTEMI).

CLINICAL PRESENTATION

Unstable Angina

UA presents as an acceleration of ischemic symptoms in one of the following three ways: (1) a crescendo pattern in which a patient with chronic stable angina experiences a sudden increase in the frequency, duration, and/or intensity of ischemic episodes; (2) episodes of angina that unexpectedly occur at rest, without provocation; or (3) the new onset of anginal episodes, described as severe, in a patient without previous symptoms of coronary artery disease. These presentations are different from the pattern of chronic stable angina, in which instances of chest discomfort are predictable, brief, and nonprogressive, occurring only during physical exertion or emotional stress. Patients with UA may progress further along the continuum of ACS and develop evidence of necrosis (ie, acute NSTEMI or STEMI) unless the condition is recognized and promptly treated.

Acute Myocardial Infarction

The symptoms and physical findings of acute MI (both STEMI and NSTEMI) can be predicted from the pathophysiology described earlier in this chapter and are summarized in Table 7-4. The discomfort experienced during an MI resembles angina pectoris qualitatively but is usually more severe, lasts longer, and may radiate more widely. Like angina, the sensation may result from the release of mediators such as adenosine and lactate from ischemic myocardial cells onto local nerve endings. Because ischemia in acute MI persists and proceeds to necrosis, these provocative substances continue to accumulate and activate afferent nerves for longer periods. The discomfort is often referred to other regions of the C7 through T4 dermatomes, including the neck, shoulders, and arms. Initial symptoms are usually rapid in onset and briskly crescendo to leave the patient with a profound "feeling of doom." Unlike a transient attack of angina, the discomfort does not wane with rest, and there may be little response to the administration of sublingual nitroglycerin.

The chest discomfort associated with an acute MI is often severe but not always. In fact, up to 25% of patients who sustain an MI are *asymptomatic* during the acute event, and the diagnosis is made only in retrospect. This is particularly common among diabetic patients who may not adequately sense pain because of associated neuropathy.

The combination of intense discomfort and baroreceptor unloading (if hypotension is present) may trigger a dramatic sympathetic nervous system response. Systemic signs of

TABLE 7-4	Signs and Symptoms of Myocardial Infarction
1. Characteristic pain	• Severe, persistent, typically substernal
2. Sympathetic effect	• Diaphoresis • Cool and clammy skin
3. Parasympathetic (vagal effect)	• Nausea, vomiting • Weakness
4. Inflammatory response	• Mild fever
5. Cardiac findings	• S₄ (and S₃ if systolic dysfunction present) gallop • Dyskinetic bulge (in anterior wall MI) • Systolic murmur (if mitral regurgitation or VSD)
6. Other	• Pulmonary rales (if heart failure present) • Jugular venous distention (if heart failure or right ventricular MI)

MI, myocardial infarction; S_3, third heart sound; S_4, fourth heart sound; VSD, ventricular septal defect.

subsequent catecholamine release include diaphoresis (sweating), tachycardia, and cool and clammy skin caused by vasoconstriction.

If the ischemia affects a sufficiently large amount of myocardium, left ventricular (LV) contractility can be reduced (systolic dysfunction), thereby decreasing the stroke volume and causing the diastolic volume and pressure within the LV to rise. The increase in LV pressure, compounded by the ischemia-induced stiffness of the chamber (diastolic dysfunction), is conveyed to the left atrium and pulmonary veins. The resultant pulmonary congestion decreases lung compliance and stimulates juxtacapillary receptors. These *J receptors* effect a reflex that results in rapid, shallow breathing and evokes the subjective feeling of dyspnea. Transudation of fluid into the alveoli exacerbates this symptom.

Physical findings during an acute MI depend on the location and extent of the infarct. An S_4 sound, indicative of atrial contraction into a noncompliant left ventricle, is frequently present (see Chapter 2). An S_3 sound, indicative of volume overload in the presence of failing LV systolic function, may also be heard. A systolic murmur may appear if ischemia-induced papillary muscle dysfunction causes mitral valvular insufficiency or if the infarct ruptures through the interventricular septum to create a ventricular septal defect (as discussed later in the chapter).

Myocardial necrosis also activates systemic responses to inflammation. Cytokines such as interleukin-1 (IL-1) and tumor necrosis factor (TNF) are released from macrophages and vascular endothelium in response to tissue injury. These mediators evoke an array of clinical responses, including low-grade fever.

Not all patients with severe chest discomfort are experiencing an MI or UA. Table 7-5 lists other common causes of acute chest discomfort and clinical, laboratory, and radiographic features to differentiate them from an ACS.

DIAGNOSIS OF ACUTE CORONARY SYNDROMES

The distinctions among the ACSs are made on the basis of (1) the patient's presenting symptoms, (2) acute ECG abnormalities, and (3) detection of specific serum biomarkers of myocardial necrosis (see Table 7-6; Fig. 7-3). Specifically, UA is a clinical diagnosis supported by the patient's symptoms, transient ST abnormalities on the ECG (usually ST depression and/or T-wave inversion), and the absence of serum biomarkers of myocardial necrosis. Non–ST-segment elevation MI is distinguished from UA by the detection of serum biomarkers of myocardial necrosis and often more persistent ST or T-wave abnormalities. The hallmark of ST-segment-elevation MI is an appropriate clinical history coupled with ST-segment elevations on the ECG plus detection of serum biomarkers of myocardial necrosis.

TABLE 7-5	Conditions That May Be Confused With Acute Coronary Syndromes
Condition	**Differentiating Features**
Cardiac	
Acute coronary syndrome	• Retrosternal pressure, radiating to the neck, jaw, or left shoulder and arm; more severe and lasts longer than previous anginal attacks • ECG: localized ST elevations or depressions
Pericarditis	• Sharp pleuritic pain (worsens with inspiration) • Pain varies with position (relieved by sitting forward) • Friction rub auscultated over precordium • ECG: diffuse ST elevations (see Chapter 14)
Aortic dissection	• Tearing, ripping pain that migrates over time (chest and back; see Chapter 15) • Possible asymmetry of arm blood pressures • Widened mediastinum on chest radiograph
Pulmonary	
Pulmonary embolism	• Localized pleuritic pain, accompanied by dyspnea • Pleural friction rub may be present • Predisposing conditions for venous thrombosis
Pneumonia	• Pleuritic chest pain • Cough and sputum production • Abnormal lung auscultation and percussion (ie, consolidation) • Infiltrate on chest radiograph
Pneumothorax	• Sudden sharp, pleuritic unilateral chest pain • Decreased breath sounds and hyperresonance of affected side • Chest radiograph: increased lucency and absence of pulmonary markings
Gastrointestinal	
Esophageal spasm	• Retrosternal pain, worsened by swallowing • History of dysphagia
Acute cholecystitis	• Right upper quadrant abdominal tenderness • Often accompanied by nausea • History of fatty food intolerance

ECG Abnormalities

ECG abnormalities, which reflect abnormal electrical currents during an ACS, are usually manifest in characteristic ways. In UA or NSTEMI, ST-segment depression and/or T-wave inversions may occur (Fig. 7-6). These abnormalities may be transient, occurring just for the duration of chest discomfort in UA, or they may persist in patients with NSTEMI. In contrast,

TABLE 7-6	Distinguishing Features of Acute Coronary Syndromes		
		Myocardial Infarction	
Feature	**Unstable Angina**	**NSTEMI**	**STEMI**
Typical symptoms	Crescendo, rest, or new-onset severe angina	Prolonged "crushing" chest pain, more severe and wider radiation than usual angina	
Serum biomarkers	No	Yes	Yes
Electrocardiogram initial findings	ST depression and/or T-wave inversion	ST depression and/or T-wave inversion	ST elevation (and Q waves later)

NSTEMI, non–ST-elevation myocardial infarction; STEMI, ST-elevation myocardial infarction.

as described in Chapter 4, STEMI presents with a temporal sequence of abnormalities: initial ST-segment elevation, followed over the course of several hours by inversion of the T wave and the appearance of pathologic Q waves (Fig. 7-7). Importantly, these characteristic patterns of ECG abnormalities in ACS can be minimized or prevented by early therapeutic interventions.

Historically, MIs had been classified as "Q-wave" or "non–Q-wave" infarctions before the advent of the terms "STEMI" and "NSTEMI," respectively. The older terminology, which is still occasionally encountered, reflected the fact that pathologically transmural infarctions typically produce pathologic Q waves (after an initial period of ST elevation), whereas subendocardial infarctions do not. However, it is now known that the development of Q waves does not reliably correlate with pathologic findings and that much overlap exists among the types of infarction. Moreover, the finding of new pathologic Q waves to classify ACSs now has little therapeutic relevance because Q waves, when they occur, take hours to develop and therefore are not helpful in making acute treatment decisions.

Unstable Angina/Non–ST-Elevation Myocardial Infarction

Figure 7-6. ECG abnormalities in unstable angina and non–ST-segment-elevation myocardial infarction.

Serum Biomarkers of Infarction

Necrosis of myocardial tissue causes disruption of the sarcolemma, so that intracellular macromolecules leak into the cardiac interstitium and ultimately into the bloodstream. Detection of such molecules in the serum, particularly cardiac-specific troponins, serves important diagnostic and prognostic roles. In patients with STEMI or NSTEMI, these markers rise above a threshold level in a defined temporal sequence.

Cardiac-Specific Troponins

Troponin (Tn) is a regulatory protein in muscle cells that controls interactions between myosin and actin (see Chapter 1). It consists of three subunits: TnC, TnI, and TnT. Although these subunits are found in both skeletal and cardiac muscles, the cardiac forms of troponin I (cTnI) and troponin T (cTnT) are structurally unique, and highly specific and sensitive assays for their detection in the serum are available. Abnormal circulating levels of these biomarkers serve as evidence of cardiomyocyte injury, are diagnostic of infarction in the appropriate

ST-Elevation Myocardial Infarction

| Normal | Acute | Hours | Days 1-2 | Days later | Weeks later |

- ST elevation

- ST elevation
- ↓R Wave
- Q wave begins

- T-wave inversion
- Q wave deeper

- ST normalizes
- T wave inverted

- ST & T normal
- Q wave persists

Figure 7-7. ECG evolution during ST-segment-elevation myocardial infarction.

clinical setting, and convey powerful prognostic information. Newer-generation "high-sensitivity" troponin assays are able to reliably detect the most minor serum elevations in cardiac troponin. Such enhanced precision allows these assays to be used to detect myocardial injury based on either absolute levels above the normal range or sequential increases still within the normal range, and thus offer improved early sensitivity, allowing the diagnosis of MI to be made within hours of presentation. However, as these assays become ever more sensitive, small serum elevations can also be detected in conditions other than MI, related to acute cardiac strain or inflammation (eg, in heart failure, myocarditis, hypertensive crises, or pulmonary embolism [due to right ventricular strain]). Therefore, while an elevated serum troponin level indicates myocardial injury, it is the clinician's role to determine if the cause is an ACS.

Creatine Kinase

The enzyme creatine kinase (CK) is found in the heart, skeletal muscle, brain, and other organs. Injury to any of these tissues may lead to elevation in serum concentrations of the enzyme. There are, however, three *isoenzymes* of CK that improve diagnostic specificity of its origin: CK-MM (found mainly in skeletal muscle), CK-BB (located predominantly in the brain), and **CK-MB** (localized mainly in the heart). Elevation of CK-MB is highly suggestive of myocardial injury. To facilitate the diagnosis of MI using this biomarker, it is common to calculate the ratio of CK-MB to total CK.. The ratio is usually >2.5% in the setting of myocardial injury and less than that when CK-MB elevation is from another source. The serum level of CK-MB starts to rise ~3-8 hours following infarction, peaks at ~24 hours, and returns to normal within 48-72 hours. As CK-MB is neither as sensitive nor as specific for detection of myocardial injury as cardiac troponin, the latter is the preferred diagnostic biomarker in clinical use.

Imaging

Sometimes, the early diagnosis of MI can remain uncertain even after careful evaluation of the patient's history, ECG, and serum biomarkers. In such a situation, an additional diagnostic study that may be useful in the acute setting is *echocardiography*, which often reveals new abnormalities of ventricular contraction in the region of ischemia or infarction.

TREATMENT OF ACUTE CORONARY SYNDROMES

Successful management of ACS requires rapid initiation of therapy to limit myocardial damage and minimize complications. Therapy must address the intracoronary thrombus that incited the syndrome and provide antiischemic measures to restore the balance between myocardial oxygen supply and demand. Although certain therapeutic aspects are common to all ACS, there is a critical difference in the approach to patients who present with ST-segment elevation (STEMI) compared with those without ST-segment elevation (UA and NSTEMI). Patients with STEMI typically have total occlusion of a coronary artery and require immediate reperfusion therapy (mechanical or pharmacologic), whereas patients without ST-segment elevation generally do not (see Fig. 7-8 and as discussed later in the chapter).

General in-hospital measures for any patient with an ACS include admitting the patient to an intensive or intermediate care setting where **continuous ECG monitoring** for arrhythmias is undertaken. The patient is initially maintained at bed rest to minimize myocardial oxygen demand, while supplemental **oxygen** is provided (by face mask or nasal cannula), if there is any degree of hypoxemia, to improve oxygen supply. Analgesics, such as **morphine**, may be administered to reduce chest pain and associated anxiety.

ACUTE TREATMENT OF UNSTABLE ANGINA AND NON–ST-ELEVATION MYOCARDIAL INFARCTION

The management of UA and NSTEMI is essentially the same and is therefore discussed as one entity, whereas the approach to STEMI is described later. The primary treatment of UA and

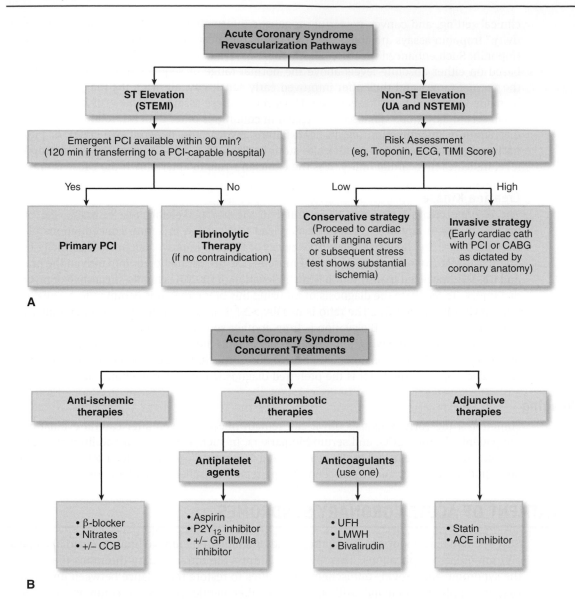

Figure 7-8. Initial management strategies in acute coronary syndromes (ACSs). A. Revascularization options. Primary percutaneous coronary intervention (PCI) is the preferred approach for STEMI patients if it is available rapidly. In UA/NSTEMI, early invasive assessment is advised in patients with high-risk features. **B.** Pharmacologic agents that are typically indicated in ACS. Platelet P2Y₁₂ inhibitors include clopidogrel, ticagrelor, and prasugrel. Note that when a glycoprotein (GP) IIb/IIIa receptor antagonist is used as an additional antiplatelet agent, it is typically initiated at the time of PCI. Bivalirudin is an anticoagulant option for patients with ACS undergoing PCI. ECG, electrocardiogram; CCB, calcium channel blocker; LMWH, low molecular weight heparin; UFH, unfractionated intravenous heparin; ACE, angiotensin-converting enzyme.

NSTEMI consists of *antiischemic* medications to restore the balance between myocardial oxygen supply and demand, and *antithrombotic* therapy to prevent further growth, and to facilitate resolution of, the underlying partially occlusive coronary thrombus.

Anti-ischemic Therapy

The same pharmacologic agents used to decrease myocardial oxygen demand in chronic stable angina are appropriate in UA and NSTEMI but are often administered more aggressively. **β-Blockers** decrease sympathetic drive to the myocardium, thus reducing oxygen demand,

and contribute to electrical stability. This group of drugs reduces the likelihood of progression from UA to MI and lowers mortality rates in patients who present with infarction. In the absence of contraindications (eg, marked bradycardia, bronchospasm, decompensated heart failure, or hypotension), an oral β-blocker is usually initiated in the first 24 hours to achieve a target heart rate of ~60 beats/min. Such therapy is usually continued indefinitely after hospitalization because of proven long-term mortality benefits following an MI.

Nitrates help bring about anginal relief through venodilation, which lowers myocardial oxygen demand by diminishing venous return to the heart (reducing preload and therefore lowering ventricular wall stress). Nitrates may also improve coronary flow and prevent vasospasm through coronary vasodilation. In UA or NSTEMI, nitroglycerin is often initially administered by the sublingual route, followed as needed by a continuous intravenous infusion. In addition to providing symptomatic relief of angina, intravenous nitroglycerin is useful as a vasodilator in patients with ACS accompanied by heart failure or severe hypertension.

Nondihydropyridine **calcium channel antagonists** (ie, verapamil and diltiazem) exert antiischemic effects by decreasing heart rate and contractility and through their vasodilatory properties (see Chapter 6). These agents do not confer mortality benefit to patients with ACS and are reserved for those in whom ischemia persists despite β-blocker and nitrate therapies or for those with contraindications to β-blocker use. They should *not* be prescribed to patients with LV systolic dysfunction, because clinical trials have shown adverse outcomes in that case.

Antithrombotic Therapy

The purpose of antithrombotic therapy, including antiplatelet and anticoagulant medications, is to prevent further propagation of the partially occlusive intracoronary thrombus while facilitating its dissolution by endogenous mechanisms.

Antiplatelet Drugs

The majority of patients with UA or NSTEMI should receive at least two forms of antiplatelet therapy, typically aspirin and an inhibitor of the platelet $P2Y_{12}$ ADP receptor.

Aspirin inhibits platelet synthesis of thromboxane A_2, a potent mediator of platelet activation (see Chapter 17), and is one of the most important interventions to reduce mortality in patients with all forms of ACS. It should be administered immediately on presentation and continued indefinitely in patients without contraindications to its use (eg, allergy or underlying bleeding disorder).

Aspirin inhibits only a single pathway of platelet activation. Another important agonist is ADP, which activates platelets in part by binding to the platelet $P2Y_{12}$ receptor (see Chapter 17). Antagonists of this receptor inhibit platelet activation and include oral clopidogrel, prasugrel, and ticagrelor. **Clopidogrel** is a thienopyridine derivative (described in Chapter 17) that further reduces cardiovascular death, recurrent MI, and stroke rates in patients with UA or NSTEMI who are treated with aspirin.

However, not all patients respond to clopidogrel with similar benefit as it is a prodrug that requires cytochrome P-450–mediated biotransformation to its active metabolite. Patients with reduced function polymorphisms of the *CYP2C19* gene produce lower concentrations of clopidogrel's activate metabolite, less platelet inhibition, and attenuated clinical benefits. Thus, newer $P2Y_{12}$ ADP receptor blockers have been developed that do not have this metabolic shortcoming, have more rapid onsets of action, and achieve greater degrees of platelet inhibition than clopidogrel. For example, **prasugrel** is also a thienopyridine derivative. Compared to clopidogrel, it reduces coronary event rates in patients with ACS who undergo percutaneous coronary intervention (PCI), but because it is more potent, it also increases the risk of bleeding complications.

Both clopidogrel and prasugrel are *irreversible* platelet inhibitors. **Ticagrelor** is a nonthienopyridine drug that is a *reversible* $P2Y_{12}$ ADP receptor blocker. Compared to clopidogrel, it has been shown to further decrease major cardiovascular events and mortality, without an increased risk of life-threatening bleeding episodes; minor bleeding is, however, more common than with clopidogrel. Thus, ticagrelor and prasugrel are preferred over clopidogrel in patients with ACS.

In some circumstances, even more powerful antiplatelet agents are utilized in ACSs. The **glycoprotein (GP) IIb/IIIa receptor antagonists** (which include the monoclonal antibody *abciximab* and the small molecules *eptifibatide* and *tirofiban*) are potent intravenous antiplatelet agents that block the final common pathway of platelet aggregation (see Chapter 17). These agents are effective in reducing adverse coronary events in patients undergoing PCI. In patients presenting with UA or NSTEMI, their benefit is manifest primarily in those at the highest risk of complications (eg, recurrent episodes of chest pain despite other antithrombotic therapies). When used, GP IIb/IIIa receptor antagonists are most commonly initiated in the cardiac catheterization laboratory at the time of PCI.

Anticoagulant Drugs

Intravenous **unfractionated heparin (UFH)** has long been standard anticoagulant therapy for UA and NSTEMI. It binds to antithrombin, which greatly increases the potency of that plasma protein in the inactivation of clot-forming thrombin. UFH additionally inhibits coagulation factor Xa, slowing thrombin formation and thereby further impeding clot development. In patients with UA or NSTEMI, UFH improves cardiovascular outcomes and reduces the likelihood of progression from UA to MI. It is administered as a weight-based bolus, followed by continuous intravenous infusion. Because of a high degree of pharmacodynamic variability, its anticoagulant effect must be monitored and its dose adjusted through serial measurements of the serum activated partial thromboplastin time (aPTT).

To overcome the pharmacologic shortcomings of UFH, **low molecular weight heparins (LMWHs)** were developed. Like UFH, LMWHs also interact with antithrombin but preferentially inhibit coagulation factor Xa. They provide a more predictable pharmacologic response than UFH. As a result, LMWHs are easier to use, prescribed as one or two daily subcutaneous injections based on the patient's weight. Unlike UFH, repeated monitoring of blood tests and dosage adjustments are not generally necessary. In clinical trials in patients with UA or NSTEMI, the LMWH *enoxaparin* (see Chapter 17) has demonstrated reduced death and ischemic event rates compared with UFH.

Bivalirudin is another type of anticoagulant that has been shown to be beneficial in UA and NSTEMI and is sometimes used in place of UFH or LMWH. It acts as an intravenous direct thrombin inhibitor (see Chapter 17), and it may may cause less bleeding than UFH.

With all of these choices, the decision of which anticoagulant to prescribe to an individual patient often depends on whether an initial conservative vs invasive approach is followed.

Conservative vs Early Invasive Management of UA and NSTEMI

Many patients with UA or NSTEMI stabilize following institution of the therapies described in the previous section, while others have recurrent ischemic events. There is currently no definitive way to predict which direction a patient will take or to quickly determine which individuals have such severe underlying CAD that coronary revascularization is warranted. These uncertainties have led to two therapeutic strategies in UA/NSTEMI: (1) an early invasive approach, in which urgent cardiac catheterization is performed and coronary revascularization undertaken as indicated, and (2) a conservative approach, in which the patient is managed with medications (as detailed in the previous section) and undergoes angiography only if ischemic episodes spontaneously recur or if the results of a subsequent stress test indicate substantial residual inducible ischemia. The conservative approach offers the advantage of avoiding costly and potentially risky invasive procedures. Conversely, an early invasive strategy allows rapid identification and definitive treatment (ie, revascularization) for those with critical coronary disease.

In general, an early invasive approach is recommended to patients with refractory angina, with complications such as shock or ventricular arrhythmias, or those with the most concerning clinical features. Risk assessment algorithms consider such features and help identify patients at high likelihood of a poor outcome. One commonly used tool is the **Thrombolysis in Myocardial Infarction (TIMI) risk score** that employs seven variables to predict a patient's risk level:

1. Age > 65 years old
2. ≥3 risk factors for coronary artery disease (as described in Chapter 5)
3. Known coronary stenosis of ≥50% by prior angiography
4. ST-segment deviations on the ECG at presentation
5. At least two anginal episodes in prior 24 hours
6. Use of aspirin in prior 7 days (ie, implying resistance to aspirin's effect)
7. Elevated serum troponin or CK-MB

Clinical studies have confirmed that a patient's TIMI risk score predicts the likelihood of death or subsequent ischemic events, such that an early invasive strategy is recommended in patients with higher scores (≥3). If an early invasive approach is adopted, the patient should undergo angiography within 72 hours, or within 24 hours for patients at especially high risk.

ACUTE TREATMENT OF ST-SEGMENT ELEVATION MYOCARDIAL INFARCTION

In contrast to UA and NSTEMI, the culprit artery in STEMI is typically *completely* occluded. Thus, to limit myocardial damage, the major focus of acute treatment is to achieve very rapid reperfusion of the jeopardized myocardium using either percutaneous coronary mechanical revascularization or fibrinolytic drugs. These approaches reduce the extent of myocardial necrosis and greatly improve survival. To be effective, they must be undertaken as soon as possible; the earlier the intervention occurs, the greater the amount of myocardium that can be salvaged. Decisions about therapy must be made within minutes of a patient's assessment, based on the history and electrocardiographic findings, often before serum markers of necrosis would be expected to rise.

In addition, as is the case in UA and NSTEMI, specific medications should be initiated promptly to prevent further thrombosis and to restore the balance between myocardial oxygen supply and demand. For example, antiplatelet therapy with **aspirin** decreases mortality rates and rates of reinfarction after STEMI. It should be administered immediately on presentation (by chewing a tablet to facilitate absorption) and continued orally daily thereafter. An **anticoagulant** (eg, intravenous UFH) is typically initiated to help maintain patency of the coronary vessel and is an important adjunct to PCI and fibrinolytic regimens. **β-Blockers** reduce myocardial oxygen demand and lower the risk of recurrent ischemia, arrhythmias, and reinfarction. In the absence of contraindications (eg, asthma, hypotension, or significant bradycardia), an oral β-blocker should be administered to achieve a heart rate of 50-60 beats/min. Intravenous β-blocker therapy should generally be avoided, as that route of administration has been associated with an increased risk of cardiogenic shock in STEMI. **Nitrate** therapy, usually intravenous nitroglycerin, is used to help control ischemic pain and also serves as a beneficial vasodilator in patients with heart failure or severe hypertension.

Primary Percutaneous Coronary Intervention

The preferred method of reperfusion therapy in patients with acute STEMI is immediate cardiac catheterization and PCI of the lesion responsible for the infarction. This approach, termed *primary PCI*, is a very effective method for reestablishing coronary perfusion and, in clinical trials performed at highly experienced medical centers, has achieved optimal flow in the infarct-related artery in more than 95% of patients. During the procedure, performed under fluoroscopy, a catheter is inserted into a peripheral artery and directed to the site of coronary occlusion. A balloon at the end of the catheter is then inflated, compressing the thrombus and atherosclerotic plaque, and a stent is usually inserted (see Chapter 6), thereby restoring and maintaining coronary blood flow. In order to salvage as much myocardium as possible, the goal is that the time from first medical contact to PCI be <90 minutes. At medical centers without PCI availability, the decision to transfer a patient to a PCI-capable hospital or to treat with fibrinolytic therapy (discussed in next section) must be made rapidly. A delay in reperfusion leads to worse outcomes for patients regardless of the mechanism chosen, and the longer the delay, the less benefit primary PCI has over fibrinolytic therapy. Generally, transfer to a PCI-capable hospital is recommended if the procedure can be performed within 120 minutes of first medical contact.

To reduce thrombotic complications, patients undergoing primary PCI receive a combination of medications. **Aspirin** and a **P2Y$_{12}$ receptor inhibitor** (eg, ticagrelor, prasugrel, or clopidogrel) are the antiplatelet agents typically administered prior to the procedure. A more potent **GP IIb/IIIa platelet inhibitor** is also sometimes used with PCI. Anticoagulation therapy consists of either **UFH** or **bivalirudin** as the primary choices.

After primary PCI, aspirin is continued indefinitely. For patients who receive coronary stents during PCI, a prolonged course of a P2Y$_{12}$ receptor inhibitor reduces the risk of ischemic complications and stent thrombosis.

Fibrinolytic Therapy

Primary PCI is the preferred reperfusion approach in acute STEMI, as it leads to greater survival with lower rates of reinfarction and bleeding when compared to fibrinolytic therapy. However, if PCI is not available or is likely to be delayed, fibrinolytic therapy is the reperfusion alternative. Fibrinolytic drugs accelerate lysis of the occlusive intracoronary thrombus in STEMI, thereby restoring blood flow and limiting myocardial damage. This section does *not* pertain to patients with UA or NSTEMI, as such individuals *do not* benefit from fibrinolytic therapy.

Currently used fibrinolytic agents include **recombinant tissue–type plasminogen activator (alteplase, tPA), reteplase (rPA)**, and **tenecteplase (TNK-tPA)**. Each drug functions by stimulating the natural fibrinolytic system, transforming the inactive precursor plasminogen into the active protease plasmin, which lyses fibrin clots. Although the intracoronary thrombus is the target, plasmin has poor substrate specificity and can degrade other proteins, including fibrin's precursor fibrinogen. As a result, bleeding is the most common complication of these drugs. Administration of fibrinolytic agents in the early hours of an acute STEMI restores blood flow in most (70%-80%) coronary occlusions and significantly reduces the extent of tissue damage. Improved artery patency translates into substantially increased survival rates and fewer postinfarction complications. The rapid initiation of fibrinolysis is crucial: patients who receive therapy within 2 hours of the onset of symptoms of STEMI have *half* the mortality rate of those who receive it after 6 hours.

To prevent immediate vessel reocclusion after successful thrombolysis, anticoagulants (UFH or LMWHs), and antiplatelet therapy, including aspirin and a platelet P2Y$_{12}$ inhibitor, are administered. For those initially treated with fibrinolytic therapy who do not demonstrate an adequate acute response, including expeditious resolution of symptoms and ST-segment elevations, transfer of the patient to a hospital capable of performing "rescue" PCI is recommended as soon as possible.

Because the major risk of thrombolysis is bleeding, contraindications to such therapy include situations in which *necessary* fibrin clots within the circulation would be jeopardized (eg, patients with active peptic ulcer disease or an underlying bleeding disorder, patients who have had a recent stroke, or patients who are recovering from recent surgery). Consequently, ~30% of patients may not be suitable candidates for thrombolysis.

Adjunctive Therapies

Angiotensin-converting enzyme (ACE) inhibitors limit adverse ventricular remodeling and reduce the incidence of heart failure, recurrent ischemic events, and mortality following an MI. Their benefit is additive to that of aspirin and β-blocker therapies, and they have shown favorable improvements especially in higher-risk patients—those with anterior wall infarctions or LV systolic dysfunction. In patients who are intolerant of ACE inhibitors, **angiotensin receptor blockers (ARBs)** can be substituted.

Cholesterol-lowering **statins** (HMG-CoA reductase inhibitors) reduce mortality rates of patients with coronary artery disease (see Chapter 5). Clinical trials of patients with ACS have demonstrated that it is safe to begin statin therapy early during hospitalization and that a high-intensity lipid-lowering regimen, designed to reduce low-density lipoprotein (LDL) cholesterol levels by >50% (ideally to <70 mg/dL), provides greater protection against subsequent cardiovascular events and death than less intense regimens. The benefits of statin therapy may extend beyond lipid lowering, because this group of drugs has attributes that can improve endothelial dysfunction, inhibit platelet aggregation, and impair thrombus formation. Additional LDL cholesterol lowering with the cholesterol absorption inhibitor *ezetimibe* and/or a *PCSK9 inhibitor* (both described in Chapter 17) after an ACS further reduces subsequent cardiovascular event rates.

As discussed later in the chapter, impaired ventricular contractility after MI can lead to heart failure. Patients with a LV ejection fraction of <40% and symptoms of heart failure after STEMI should be considered for therapy with an **aldosterone antagonist** (spironolactone or eplerenone) in addition to an ACE inhibitor and beta-blocker. Aldosterone augments sodium reabsorption from the distal nephron (contributing to fluid retention, an undesired effect in heart failure) and also promotes inflammation and myocardial fibrosis. Chronic administration of an aldosterone antagonist mitigates these effects and has been shown to decrease mortality following MI in patients with LV dysfunction.

COMPLICATIONS

In UA, potential complications include death, or progression to infarction over the ensuing days and weeks. Once infarction has transpired, especially STEMI, complications can result from the inflammatory, mechanical, and electrical abnormalities induced by regions of necrosing myocardium (Fig. 7-9). Early complications result from myocardial necrosis itself. Those that develop several days to weeks later reflect the inflammation and healing of necrotic tissue.

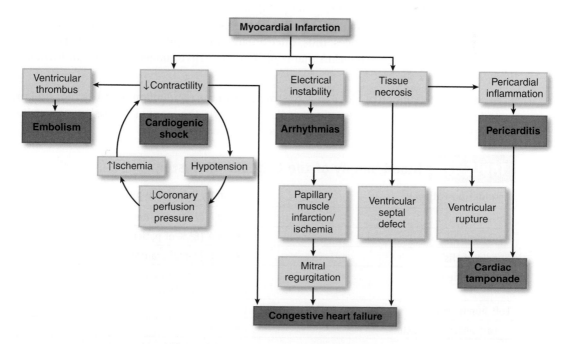

Figure 7-9. Complications of MI. Infarction may result in decreased contractility, electrical instability, and tissue necrosis, which can lead to the indicated sequelae.

TABLE 7-7   Arrhythmias in Acute Myocardial Infarction

Rhythm	Cause
Sinus bradycardia	• ↑Vagal tone • ↓SA nodal artery perfusion
Sinus tachycardia	• Pain and anxiety • Heart failure • Volume depletion • Chronotropic drugs (eg, dopamine)
APBs, atrial fibrillation	• Heart failure • Atrial ischemia
VPBs, VT, VF	• Ventricular ischemia • Heart failure
AV block (1°, 2°, 3°)	• IMI: ↑vagal tone and ↓AV nodal artery flow • AMI: extensive destruction of conduction tissue

AMI, anterior myocardial infarction; APBs, atrial premature beats; AV, atrioventricular; IMI, inferior myocardial infarction; SA, sinoatrial; VPBs, ventricular premature beats; VF, ventricular fibrillation; VT, ventricular tachycardia.

RECURRENT ISCHEMIA

Postinfarction angina has been reported in 20%-30% of patients following an MI. This rate has not been reduced by the use of thrombolytic therapy, but it is lower in those who have undergone acute percutaneous coronary revascularization. Indicative of inadequate residual coronary blood flow, it is a poor prognostic indicator and correlates with an increased risk for reinfarction. Such patients usually require urgent cardiac catheterization, often followed by revascularization by percutaneous techniques or coronary artery bypass surgery.

ARRHYTHMIAS

Arrhythmias occur frequently during acute MI and are a major source of mortality prior to hospital arrival. Fortunately, modern cardiac care units are highly attuned to the detection and treatment of rhythm disturbances; thus, once a patient is hospitalized, arrhythmia-associated deaths are uncommon. Mechanisms that contribute to arrhythmogenesis after MI include the following (Table 7-7):

1. Anatomic interruption of blood flow to structures of the conduction pathway (eg, sinoatrial node, atrioventricular node, and bundle branches); the normal perfusion of pertinent components of the conduction system is summarized in Table 7-8.

TABLE 7-8   Blood Supply of the Conduction System

Conduction Pathway	Primary Arterial Supply
SA node	• RCA (70% of patients)
AV node	• RCA (85% of patients)
Bundle of His	• LAD (septal branches)
Right bundle branch	• Proximal portion by LAD • Distal portion by RCA
Left bundle branch	
Left anterior fascicle	• LAD
Left posterior fascicle	• LAD and PDA

AV, atrioventricular; LAD, left anterior descending coronary artery; PDA, posterior descending artery; RCA, right coronary artery; SA, sinoatrial.

2. Accumulation of toxic metabolic products (eg, cellular acidosis) and abnormal transcellular ion concentrations owing to membrane leaks.

3. Autonomic stimulation (sympathetic and parasympathetic).

4. Administration of potentially arrhythmogenic drugs (eg, dopamine).

Ventricular Fibrillation

Ventricular fibrillation (rapid, disorganized electrical activity of the ventricles) is largely responsible for sudden cardiac death during the course of acute MI. Most fatal episodes occur before hospital arrival, which can be mitigated by increasing availability of automatic external defibrillators in public places. Episodes of ventricular fibrillation that occur during the first 48 hours of MI are often related to transient electrical instability, and the long-term prognosis of survivors of such events is not adversely affected. However, ventricular fibrillation occurring later than 48 hours after the acute MI usually reflects severe LV dysfunction and is associated with high subsequent mortality rates.

Ventricular ectopic beats, ventricular tachycardia, and ventricular fibrillation during an acute MI arise from either reentrant circuits or enhanced automaticity of ventricular cells (see Chapter 11). Ventricular ectopic beats are common and usually not treated unless they become consecutive, multifocal, or frequent. Cardiac care unit personnel are proficient at arrhythmia detection and institution of treatment should more malignant ventricular arrhythmias develop. Therapy for ventricular arrhythmias is described in Chapter 12.

Supraventricular Arrhythmias

Supraventricular arrhythmias are also common in acute MI. *Sinus bradycardia* results from either excessive vagal stimulation or sinoatrial nodal ischemia, usually in the setting of an inferior wall MI. *Sinus tachycardia* occurs frequently and may result from pain and anxiety, heart failure, drug administration (eg, dopamine), or intravascular volume depletion. Because sinus tachycardia increases myocardial oxygen demand and could exacerbate ischemia, identifying and treating its cause are important. *Atrial premature beats* and *atrial fibrillation* (see Chapter 12) may result from atrial ischemia or atrial distention secondary to LV failure.

Conduction Blocks

Conduction blocks (atrioventricular nodal block and bundle branch blocks) develop commonly in acute MI. They may result from ischemia or necrosis of conduction tracts, or in the case of atrioventricular blocks, they may develop transiently because of increased vagal tone. Vagal activity may be increased because of stimulation of afferent fibers by the inflamed myocardium or as a result of generalized autonomic activation in association with the discomfort of an acute MI.

MYOCARDIAL DYSFUNCTION

Heart Failure

Acute cardiac ischemia results in impaired ventricular contractility (systolic dysfunction) and increased myocardial stiffness (diastolic dysfunction), both of which may lead to symptoms of heart failure. In addition, ventricular remodeling, arrhythmias, and acute mechanical complications of MI (described later in the chapter) may culminate in heart failure. Signs and symptoms of such decompensation include dyspnea, pulmonary rales, and a third heart sound (S_3). Treatment consists of standard heart failure therapy, which typically includes diuretics for relief of volume overload, and ACE inhibitor and β-blocker therapies for long-term mortality benefit (see Chapter 9). As noted earlier, for patients with post-MI heart failure and an LV ejection fraction <40%, an aldosterone antagonist (spironolactone or eplerenone—described in Chapter 17) should be considered. However, when an aldosterone antagonist is prescribed concurrently with an ACE inhibitor, the serum potassium level should be carefully monitored to prevent hyperkalemia.

Cardiogenic Shock

Cardiogenic shock is a condition of severely decreased cardiac output and hypotension (systolic blood pressure < 90 mm Hg) with inadequate perfusion of peripheral tissues. It may develop when a large portion of LV mass has infarcted, or when certain severe mechanical complications of MI occur as described later in this chapter. Cardiogenic shock is self-perpetuating because (1) hypotension leads to decreased coronary perfusion, which exacerbates ischemic damage and (2) reduced stroke volume increases LV size and therefore augments myocardial oxygen demand (see Fig. 7-9). Cardiogenic shock occurs in ∼5%-7% of patients after MI, and the mortality rate is very high (30%-40%). Early cardiac catheterization and revascularization are critical to improving outcomes from cardiogenic shock.

Patients in cardiogenic shock generally require intravenous inotropic agents (eg, dobutamine) and/or vasopressors (eg, norepinephrine) to increase cardiac output and support arterial pressure. For patients with cardiogenic shock that is refractory to pharmacologic treatment, percutaneous **mechanical circulatory support (MCS)** devices provide therapeutic options. An **intra-aortic balloon pump (IABP)** is a type of MCS device consisting of an inflatable balloon chamber that is inserted (usually through the femoral artery) into the aorta and is set to rhythmically inflate during diastole to increase intra-aortic pressure, thus augmenting perfusion of the coronary arteries. During systole, the balloon deflates to create a "vacuum" that serves to reduce the afterload of the left ventricle, thus aiding the ejection of blood into the aorta, improving cardiac output and peripheral tissue perfusion. Historically, IABPs have been the preferred form of MCS device used to treat cardiogenic shock. However, contemporary randomized controlled trials have failed to demonstrate that this type of therapy improves cardiovascular outcomes and it is used now used in a more limited subset of patients. Newer mechanical approaches that provide more robust hemodynamic support include **percutaneous left ventricular assist devices (LVADs)** and **extracorporeal membrane oxygenation (ECMO)**, which are increasingly used for the treatment of cardiogenic shock. Although there are multiple types of these devices, each with a unique design and operation, all serve to "bypass" or assist the heart by transporting oxygenated blood to the aorta or its major branches using motor pumps.

Right Ventricular Infarction

Approximately one-third of patients with infarction of the LV inferior wall also develop necrosis of portions of the right ventricle. This is because the same coronary artery (usually the right coronary) perfuses both regions in most individuals. The resulting abnormal contraction and decreased compliance of the right ventricle lead to signs of right-sided heart failure, out of proportion to signs of left-sided failure. In addition, profound hypotension may result when right ventricular dysfunction impairs blood flow through the lungs, leading to the left ventricle becoming underfilled. In this case, intravenous volume infusion serves to correct hypotension, often guided by hemodynamic measurements via a transvenous pulmonary artery catheter (see Chapter 3).

Mechanical Complications

Mechanical complications following MI result from cardiac tissue ischemia and necrosis.

Papillary Muscle Rupture

Ischemic necrosis and rupture of an LV papillary muscle may be rapidly fatal because of acute severe mitral regurgitation, as the valve leaflets lose their anchoring attachments. *Partial* rupture, with more moderate regurgitation, is not immediately lethal but may result in symptoms of heart failure or pulmonary edema. Because it has a more precarious blood supply, the posteromedial LV papillary muscle is more susceptible to infarction than its anterolateral counterpart.

Ventricular Free Wall Rupture

An infrequent but deadly complication, rupture of the LV free wall through a tear in necrotic myocardium may occur within the first 2 weeks following MI. It is more common among women and patients with a history of hypertension. Hemorrhage into the pericardial space owing to LV free wall rupture results in rapid cardiac tamponade, in which blood fills the pericardial space and severely restricts ventricular filling (see Chapter 14). Survival is rare.

On occasion, a **pseudoaneurysm** results if rupture of the free wall is incomplete and held in check by thrombus formation that "plugs" the hole in the myocardium. This situation is the cardiac equivalent of a time bomb, because subsequent complete rupture into the pericardium and tamponade could follow. If detected (usually by imaging studies), surgical repair may prevent an otherwise disastrous outcome.

Ventricular Septal Rupture

This complication is analogous to LV free wall rupture, but the abnormal flow of blood is not directed across the LV wall into the pericardium. Rather, blood is shunted across the ventricular septum from the left ventricle to the right ventricle, usually precipitating congestive heart failure because of subsequent volume overload of the pulmonary capillaries. A loud systolic murmur at the left sternal border, representing transseptal flow, is common in this situation. Although each results in a systolic murmur, ventricular septal rupture can be differentiated from acute mitral regurgitation by the location of the murmur (see Fig. 2-11), by Doppler echocardiography, or by measuring the O_2 saturation of blood in the right-sided heart chambers through a transvenous catheter. If there is shunting of oxygenated blood from the left ventricle across the septal defect, the O_2 content in the right ventricle is abnormally higher than that in the right atrium.

True Ventricular Aneurysm

A late complication of MI, a true ventricular aneurysm, may come to attention weeks to months after an acute infarction. It develops as the ventricular wall is weakened, but not perforated, by the phagocytic clearance of necrotic tissue, and it results in a localized outward bulge (dyskinesis) when the residual viable heart muscle contracts. Unlike the pseudoaneurysm described earlier, a true aneurysm does not involve communication between the LV cavity and the pericardium, so that rupture and tamponade do not develop. Instead, potential complications of LV aneurysm include (1) thrombus formation within this region of stagnant blood flow, serving as a source of emboli to peripheral organs; (2) ventricular arrhythmias associated with the stretched myofibers; and (3) heart failure resulting from reduced forward cardiac output, because some of the LV stroke volume is "wasted" by filling the aneurysmal segment during systole.

Clues to the presence of an LV aneurysm include persistent ST-segment elevations on the ECG weeks after an acute ST-segment elevation MI and a bulge at the LV border on chest radiography. The abnormality can be confirmed by echocardiography or other imaging modalities.

Pericarditis

Acute pericarditis may occur in the early (in-hospital) post-MI period as inflammation extends from the myocardium to the adjacent pericardium. Sharp pain, fever, and a pericardial friction rub are typically present in this situation and help distinguish pericarditis from the discomfort of recurrent myocardial ischemia (see Chapter 14). The symptoms usually respond promptly to aspirin therapy. Anticoagulants are relatively contraindicated in MI complicated by pericarditis to avoid hemorrhage from the inflamed pericardial lining. The frequency of MI-associated pericarditis has declined since the introduction of acute reperfusion strategies, because those approaches limit the extent of myocardial damage and inflammation.

Dressler Syndrome

Dressler syndrome is now a rare form of pericarditis that can occur weeks following an MI. The cause is unclear, but an immune process directed against damaged myocardial tissue is suspected to play a role. The syndrome is heralded by fever, malaise, and sharp, pleuritic chest pain typically accompanied by leukocytosis; an elevated erythrocyte sedimentation rate; and a pericardial effusion. Similar to other forms of acute pericarditis, Dressler syndrome generally responds to aspirin or other nonsteroidal anti-inflammatory therapies.

Thromboembolism

Stasis of blood flow in regions of impaired LV contraction after an MI may result in intracavity thrombus formation, especially when the infarction involves the LV apex or when a true aneurysm has formed. Subsequent thromboemboli can result in infarction of peripheral organs (eg, a cerebrovascular event [stroke] caused by embolism to the brain).

RISK STRATIFICATION AND MANAGEMENT FOLLOWING MYOCARDIAL INFARCTION

The most important predictor of post-MI outcome is the extent of LV dysfunction. Other features that portend adverse outcomes include early recurrence of ischemic symptoms, a large volume of residual myocardium still at risk because of severe underlying coronary disease, and high-grade ventricular arrhythmias.

To identify patients at high risk for complications who may benefit from cardiac catheterization and revascularization, exercise treadmill testing is often performed (unless the patient has already undergone catheterization and corrective percutaneous revascularization for the presenting coronary syndrome). Patients with significantly abnormal results, or those who demonstrate an early spontaneous recurrence of angina, are customarily referred for cardiac catheterization to define their coronary anatomy.

Standard postdischarge therapy for the long-term includes aspirin, a β-blocker, and a high-intensity HMG-CoA reductase inhibitor (statin). A $P2Y_{12}$ platelet inhibitor is continued for 12 months or longer. ACE inhibitors are prescribed to patients who have LV contractile dysfunction; an aldosterone antagonist should be considered in those with LV contractile dysfunction and heart failure symptoms. Rigorous attention to underlying cardiac risk factors, such as smoking, hypertension, and diabetes, is mandatory, and a formal exercise rehabilitation program speeds convalescence.

Patients who have an LV ejection fraction of ≤30% after MI are at high risk of sudden cardiac death and are candidates for prophylactic placement of an implantable cardioverter-defibrillator. Current guidelines recommend postponing such implantation for at least 40 days post-MI (or for at least 3 months post-MI when a patient undergoes coronary revascularization) because clinical trials have not shown a survival benefit at earlier stages.

Summary

- Acute coronary syndromes (ACSs) include **unstable angina** (UA), **non–ST-segment elevation myocardial infarction** (NSTEMI), and **ST-segment elevation myocardial infarction** (STEMI).

- Most ACS episodes are precipitated by **intracoronary thrombus formation** at the site of atherosclerotic plaque disruption.

- Distinctions among types of ACS are based on the severity of ischemia and whether myocardial necrosis results: STEMI is associated with an occlusive thrombus and severe ischemia with necrosis, whereas ACSs without ST-segment elevation (NSTEMI and UA) usually result from partially occlusive thrombi with less severe ischemia. Compared with UA, the insult in NSTEMI is of sufficient magnitude to cause some myocardial necrosis.

- ACSs result in biochemical and mechanical changes that **impair systolic contraction**, **decrease myocardial compliance**, and **predispose to arrhythmias**; infarction initiates an inflammatory response that clears necrotic tissue and leads to scar formation.

- Diagnosis of the specific type of ACS relies on the **patient's history, ECG abnormalities**, and the presence of specific **biomarkers** in the serum (eg, cardiac troponin T or troponin I).

- Acute treatment of UA and NSTEMI includes **anti-ischemic therapy** to restore the balance between myocardial oxygen supply and demand (eg, β-blockers, nitrates), **antithrombotic therapy** to facilitate resolution of the intracoronary thrombus (eg, aspirin, a $P2Y_{12}$ ADP receptor antagonist, and an **anticoagulant** [eg, intravenous or low molecular weight heparin]), and high-intensity **statin** therapy.

- **Early coronary angiography**, with subsequent coronary revascularization, is beneficial for UA or NSTEMI patients with high-risk features.

- **Acute treatment of STEMI includes rapid coronary reperfusion**, ideally with a percutaneous catheter-based intervention if available, or else fibrinolytic therapy.

- Other important therapies for STEMI include **antiplatelet therapy** (aspirin, $P2Y_{12}$ receptor antagonist), an **anticoagulant**, a **β-blocker**, sometimes nitrate therapy, and a **statin**; an **ACE inhibitor** is also frequently appropriate.

- Potential complications of infarction include arrhythmias (eg, **ventricular tachycardia** and **fibrillation,** and **supraventricular tachycardias**) and conduction blocks (**atrioventricular blocks** and **bundle branch blocks**).

- **Heart failure** or **cardiogenic shock** may develop because of ventricular dysfunction or mechanical complications (eg, acute mitral regurgitation or ventricular septal defect).

- **Right ventricular infarction** results in signs of right heart failure out of proportion to left heart failure, often with intravascular volume sensitivity and hypotension.

- Standard pharmacologic therapy following discharge from the hospital after an ACS includes measures to reduce the risks of thrombosis (**aspirin and a $P2Y_{12}$ receptor antagonist**), recurrent ischemia (a **β-blocker**), progressive atherosclerosis (high-intensity **statin**), and adverse ventricular remodeling (an **ACE inhibitor**, especially if left ventricular [LV] dysfunction is present).

- Adding an **aldosterone antagonist** should be considered for patients with LV systolic dysfunction and heart failure.

- Systemic anticoagulation is indicated if an **intraventricular thrombus** is present.

Review Questions

1. Which of the following histologic changes can be detected within 3 hours of transmural myocardial infarction (MI)?

   a. Coagulation necrosis
   b. Fibrosis
   c. Polymorphonuclear (PMN) cell infiltration
   d. Wavy myofibers

2. A 54-year-old woman presents to the emergency department with persistent substernal chest pain, nausea, and diaphoresis. Her ECG reveals 2-mm ST-segment depressions in the anterior chest leads, and the troponin level is abnormally elevated. Which of the following medications should NOT be administered to this patient?

   a. Nitroglycerin
   b. A fibrinolytic agent (eg, tissue plasminogen activator)
   c. A $P2Y_{12}$ receptor antagonist (eg, clopidogrel)
   d. An anticoagulant (eg, unfractionated heparin)

3. A 68-year-old man presents with 12 hours of continuous substernal chest pain. His heart rate is 110 beats/min and blood pressure is 80/50 mm Hg. Physical exam reveals a regular rhythm with no murmurs, clear lungs, and elevated jugular venous pressure (12 cm). The ECG identifies 3-mm ST-segment elevations in the inferior leads (II, III, and aVF). What is the most likely explanation for the patient's low blood pressure?

   a. Severe left ventricular dysfunction
   b. Right ventricular infarction
   c. Papillary muscle rupture
   d. Ventricular septal rupture

Answers to Review Questions

1. **Choice d is correct.** One of the earliest histologic changes of myocardial infarction (1-3 hours) is the appearance of wavy myofibers, which is visualized as intercellular edema separating myocardial cells that are tugged about by the surrounding, functional myocardium. An acute inflammatory response with PMN infiltration (4-12 hours) and coagulation necrosis (18-24 hours) are subsequent early histologic changes. Late pathologic changes include yellow softening (due to necrotic tissue resorption by macrophages) and fibrosis.

2. **Choice b is correct.** This patient presents with a non-ST-segment elevation myocardial infarction (NSTEMI). The initial management strategy for patients with NSTEMI includes anti-ischemic therapies (including a β-blocker and nitrate), antiplatelet therapies (including aspirin and a $P2Y_{12}$ receptor antagonist), an anticoagulant, and adjunctive therapies (including a statin and ACE inhibitor). High-risk patients with NSTEMI should undergo early cardiac catheterization and revascularization of the culprit coronary artery. Unlike patients with ST-segment elevation MI, those with NSTEMI do not benefit from fibrinolytic therapy.

3. **Choice b is correct.** This patient presents with an inferior wall ST-segment elevation myocardial infarction (STEMI) and has signs of right-sided heart failure (ie, elevated jugular venous pressure), without signs of left-sided heart failure (ie, lungs are clear). These findings are suggestive of infarction of the right ventricle (which is adjacent to, and shares blood supply with the LV inferior wall) that can lead to profound hypotension as impaired RV function leads to underfilling of the left ventricle. Papillary muscle rupture and ventricular septal rupture are potential mechanical complications of MI that can also lead to hypotension, but both would be expected to cause a systolic murmur.

Acknowledgments

Contributors to previous editions of this chapter were Jayme Wilder, MD; June-Wha Rhee, MD; Haley Naik, MD; Anurag Gupta, MD; J. G. Fletcher, MD; William Carlson, MD; and Patrick T. O'Gara, MD.

Additional Reading

Amsterdam EA, Wenger NK, Brindis RG, et al. 2014 AHA/ACC Guideline for the management of patients with non–ST-elevation acute coronary syndromes: a report of the American College of Cardiology/American Heart Association Task Force on Practice Guidelines. *Circulation*. 2014;130:e344-e426.

Anderson JL, Morrow DA. Acute myocardial infarction. *N Engl J Med*. 2017;376:2053-2064.

Gallone G, Baldetti L, Pagnesi M, et al. Medical therapy for long-term prevention of atherothrombosis following an acute coronary syndrome. *J Am Coll Cardiol*. 2018;72:2886-2903.

Ibanez B, James S, Agewall S, et al. 2017 ESC Guidelines for the management of acute myocardial infarction in patients presenting with ST-segment elevation: the Task Force for the management of acute myocardial infarction in patients presenting with ST-segment elevation of the European Society of Cardiology (ESC). *Eur Heart J*. 2018;39:119-177.

Mehta SR, Wood DA, Storey RF, et al. Complete revascularization with multivessel PCI for myocardial infraction. *N Engl J Med*. 2019;381:1411-1421.

Neumann JT, Twerenbold R, Ojeda F, et al. Application of high-sensitivity troponin in suspected myocardial infarction. *N Engl J Med*. 2019;380:2529-2540.

O'Gara PT, Kushner FG, Ascheim DD, et al. 2013 ACCF/AHA Guideline for the management of ST-elevation myocardial infarction: Executive summary: a report of the American College of Cardiology Foundation/American Heart Association Task Force on Practice Guidelines. *Circulation*. 2013;127:529-555.

Sandoval Y, Jaffe AS. Type 2 myocardial infarction. *J Am Coll Cardiol*. 2019;73:1846-1860.

Schüpke S, Neumann FJ, Menichelli M, et al. Ticagrelor or prasugrel in patients with acute coronary syndromes. *N Engl J Med*. 2019;381:1524-1534.

Valvular Heart Disease

8

Diana M. Lopez | Patrick T. O'Gara | Leonard S. Lilly

This chapter describes the pathophysiologic abnormalities in patients with common valvular heart diseases. Each condition is discussed separately because unifying principles do not govern the behavior of all stenotic or regurgitant valves. Effective patient management requires accurate identification of the valve lesion, a determination of its severity, and a clear understanding of the pathophysiologic consequences and natural history of the condition.

The evaluation of a patient with suspected valvular disease begins at the bedside with a careful history and physical examination from which the trained clinician can usually identify the type of abnormality present. Definitive diagnosis is most often achieved with transthoracic echocardiography (TTE), which allows for staging of disease severity. In selected patients, additional investigation with transesophageal echocardiography (TEE), exercise testing, or cardiac catheterization may be necessary to fully define the significance of the condition and guide therapy.

Management of patients with heart valve disease often involves serial clinical and imaging assessments. Pharmacologic therapy is sometimes prescribed for symptomatic improvement, but recognition of timely indications for invasive valve repair or replacement is essential, as will be described for each valve lesion.

MITRAL VALVE DISEASE

MITRAL STENOSIS

Etiology

Mitral stenosis (MS) refers to a narrowed mitral valve orifice, and by far, the most common cause is prior rheumatic fever (Box 8-1). Approximately 50%-70% of patients with symptomatic MS provide a history of acute rheumatic fever occurring, on average, 20 years before presentation. Other rare etiologies of MS include calcification of the mitral annulus that extends onto the leaflets, infective endocarditis (IE) with large vegetations that obstruct the valve orifice, and rare congenital stenosis of the valve.

Box 8-1 **Rheumatic Fever**

Acute rheumatic fever (ARF) is an inflammatory condition that primarily affects the heart, skin, and connective tissues. Its incidence has waned greatly in the past century in industrialized societies, where it is now rare, but it remains a major burden in developing countries. ARF arises as a complication of pharyngitis caused by group A beta-hemolytic streptococci and mainly afflicts children and young adults. During prior epidemics, ~3% of patients with acute streptococcal pharyngitis developed ARF 2-3 weeks after the initial throat infection. Common presenting symptoms are chills, fever, fatigue, and migratory arthritis. The cardinal clinical manifestations that establish the diagnosis are known as **Jones criteria** (see Table below).

Involvement of the heart is thought to result from autoimmune cross-reactivity between bacterial and cardiac antigens. Pathologically, carditis (cardiac inflammation) afflicts all layers of the heart (pericardium, myocardium, and endocardium). Histopathologic examination may demonstrate **Aschoff bodies**, areas of focal fibrinoid necrosis surrounded by inflammatory cells (see Figure below) that later resolve to form fibrous scar tissue. During the acute episode, carditis may cause tachycardia, impaired ventricular contractility, a pericardial friction rub, and transient heart murmurs that reflect turbulent flow across inflamed valve leaflets. Doppler echocardiography helps establish the presence of cardiac involvement. Treatment of the acute episode includes high-dose aspirin to reduce inflammation and penicillin to eliminate residual streptococcal infection.

The most important sequela of ARF is chronic rheumatic heart disease (RHD) characterized by permanent deformity and impairment of one or more cardiac valves. Symptoms of valvular dysfunction, however, do not manifest until 10-30 years after ARF has subsided. This latency period may be shorter with more aggressive disease sometimes observed in developing countries. RHD affects the mitral valve in almost all cases, the aortic valve in 20%-30%, and rarely the tricuspid valve as well. Stenosis and/or regurgitation of each valve can result.

Management of RHD includes prophylaxis against recurrent streptococcal infection and treatment of the chronic valve lesions. Recurrences of ARF can incite further cardiac damage, so individuals with ARF should receive preventive low-dose penicillin prophylaxis at least until early adulthood, by which time exposure and susceptibility to streptococcal infections have diminished.

Histopathology of an Aschoff body in acute rheumatic carditis. Mononuclear inflammatory cells surround a center of focal necrosis. (Courtesy of Dr. Frederick J. Schoen, Brigham and Women's Hospital, Boston.)

Criteria for Diagnosis of Rheumatic Fever[a]

Major criteria
Carditis (inflammation of all three heart layers)
Migratory arthritis (mainly large joints)[b]
Sydenham chorea (involuntary movements)
Erythema marginatum (skin rash with advancing edge and clearing center)
Subcutaneous nodules

Minor criteria
Arthralgias
Fever
Elevated acute-phase reactants (ESR, CRP)
Prolonged PR interval on electrocardiogram

Evidence of group A streptococcal infection
Antistreptolysin O antibodies
Positive throat culture or rapid antigen test

[a]Diagnosis requires evidence of streptococcal infection and either two major criteria or one major plus two minor criteria.
[b]In moderate- to high-risk populations, arthritis of a single joint is a sufficient criterion.
ESR, erythrocyte sedimentation rate; CRP, C-reactive protein.

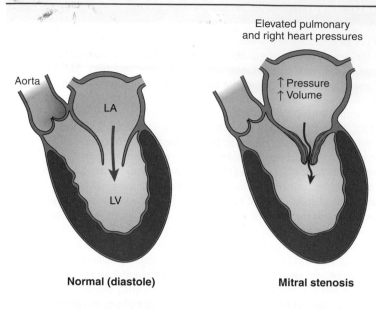

Normal (diastole)   Mitral stenosis

Figure 8-1. Pathophysiology of mitral stenosis. In the normal heart, blood flows freely from the left atrium (LA) into the left ventricle (LV) during diastole (*blue arrow*). In mitral stenosis, there is obstruction to LA emptying (*red arrow*). Thus, the LA pressure increases, which in turn elevates pulmonary and right heart pressures.

Pathology

RHD causes valvular inflammation that ultimately results in fibrous thickening and calcification of the valves, fusion of the commissures (the borders where the leaflets meet), and thickening and shortening of the chordae tendineae.

Pathophysiology

vIn early diastole in the normal heart, the mitral valve opens and blood flows freely from the left atrium (LA) into the left ventricle (LV), such that there is a negligible pressure difference between the two chambers. In MS, however, there is obstruction to blood flow across the valve such that emptying of the LA is impeded and there is an abnormal pressure gradient between the LA and LV (Figs. 8-1 and 8-2). As a result, the left atrial pressure increases.

Figure 8-2. Hemodynamic profile of mitral stenosis. The left atrial (LA) pressure (*red curve*) is elevated, and there is a pressure gradient (*shaded area*) between the LA and left ventricle (LV) during diastole. Compare with schematic of normal tracing (see Fig. 2-1). Abnormal heart sounds are present: there is a diastolic opening snap (OS) that corresponds to the opening of the mitral valve, followed by a decrescendo murmur. There is an accentuation of the murmur just before S_1 owing to the increased pressure gradient when the LA contracts in patients in sinus rhythm (presystolic accentuation).

Hemodynamic changes become apparent when the cross-sectional area of the valve, normally 4-6 cm^2, is reduced to <2 cm^2.

The high left atrial pressure in MS is transmitted retrograde to the pulmonary circulation, resulting in increased pulmonary venous and capillary pressures (see Fig. 8-1). This elevation of hydrostatic pressure in the pulmonary vasculature may cause transudation of plasma into the lung interstitium and alveoli. The patient may therefore experience dyspnea and other symptoms of heart failure (as described in Chapter 9). In severe cases, significant elevation of pulmonary venous pressure leads to the opening of collateral channels between the pulmonary and bronchial veins. Subsequently, an engorged bronchial vein may rupture into a bronchus, resulting in hemoptysis (coughing up blood).

The elevation of left atrial pressure in MS can result in two distinct forms of pulmonary hypertension: passive and reactive. Most patients with MS exhibit *passive* pulmonary hypertension, related to the backward transmission of the elevated LA pressure into the pulmonary vasculature as described in the previous paragraph. This actually represents an "obligatory" increase in pulmonary artery pressure that preserves forward flow in the setting of increased left atrial and pulmonary venous pressures. Additionally, ~40% of patients with MS demonstrate *reactive* pulmonary hypertension with medial hypertrophy and intimal fibrosis of the pulmonary arterioles. Reactive pulmonary hypertension initially serves a "beneficial" role because the increased arteriolar resistance impedes blood flow into the engorged pulmonary capillary bed and thus reduces capillary hydrostatic pressure (thereby "protecting" the pulmonary capillaries from even higher pressures). However, this benefit is at the cost of decreased blood flow through the pulmonary vasculature and elevation of the right-sided heart pressures, as the right ventricle pumps against the increased resistance. Chronic elevation of right ventricular pressure leads to hypertrophy and dilatation of that chamber and ultimately to right-sided heart failure.

Chronic pressure overload of the LA in MS leads to left atrial enlargement. Left atrial dilatation stretches the atrial conduction fibers and may disrupt the integrity of the cardiac conduction system, resulting in *atrial fibrillation* (a rapid irregular heart rhythm; see Chapter 12). Atrial fibrillation contributes to a decline in cardiac output in MS because the increased heart rate shortens diastole. This reduces the time available for blood to flow across the obstructed mitral valve to fill the LV and, at the same time, further augments the elevated left atrial pressure. In addition, with atrial fibrillation, there is a loss of the late diastolic atrial contraction that normally contributes to LV filling.

The relative stagnation of blood flow in the dilated LA in MS, especially when combined with the development of atrial fibrillation, predisposes to intra-atrial thrombus formation. Thromboemboli to the brain and other organs may follow, leading to devastating complications such as cerebrovascular occlusion (stroke). Thus, MS patients who develop atrial fibrillation require chronic anticoagulation therapy.

The consequences of MS primarily affect the LA and the pulmonary vasculature, as described above. Left ventricular pressures are usually normal, but impaired filling of the chamber through the stenotic valve may reduce LV stroke volume and cardiac output.

Clinical Manifestations and Evaluation
Presentation
The natural history of MS is variable. Survival exceeds 80% in asymptomatic or minimally symptomatic patients at 10 years. However, the 10-year survival of untreated patients after onset of symptoms is only 50%-60%. Longevity is much more limited for patients with advanced symptoms and is dismal for those who develop significant pulmonary hypertension, with a mean survival of <3 years.

The clinical presentation of MS depends largely on the degree of reduction of the valve area. The more severe the stenosis, the greater the symptoms related to elevation of left atrial and pulmonary venous pressures. The earliest manifestations are those of dyspnea and reduced exercise capacity. In mild MS, dyspnea may be absent at rest; however, it develops on exertion as LA pressure rises with the exercise-induced increase in blood flow through the heart and faster heart rate (ie, decreased diastolic filling time). Other conditions and activities that augment heart rate and cardiac blood flow and precipitate or exacerbate symptoms of MS include fever, anemia, hyperthyroidism, pregnancy, rapid arrhythmias such as atrial fibrillation, emotional stress, and sexual intercourse.

With more severe MS (ie, a smaller valve area), dyspnea occurs even at rest. Increasing fatigue and more severe signs of pulmonary congestion, such as orthopnea and paroxysmal nocturnal dyspnea (described in Chapter 9), occur. With advanced MS and pulmonary hypertension, signs of right-sided heart failure ensue, including jugular venous distention, hepatomegaly, ascites, and peripheral edema. Compression of the recurrent laryngeal nerve by an enlarged pulmonary artery or LA may cause hoarseness (known as *Ortner syndrome*).

Less often, the diagnosis of MS is heralded by one of its complications: atrial fibrillation, thromboembolism, endocarditis, or hemoptysis, as described in the earlier section on pathophysiology.

Examination

On examination, there are several typical findings of MS. Palpation of the chest may reveal a right ventricular "heave" next to the sternum in patients with increased right ventricular pressure. Auscultation discloses a loud S_1 (the first heart sound, corresponding to mitral valve closure) in the early stages of the disease. The increased S_1 results from the high pressure gradient between the atrium and ventricle, which keeps the mobile portions of the mitral valve leaflets widely separated throughout diastole; at the onset of systole, ventricular contraction abruptly slams the leaflets together from a relatively wide position, causing the closure sound to be more prominent. In late stages of the disease, the intensity of S_1 may normalize or become reduced as the valve leaflets progressively thicken, calcify, and become less mobile.

A main feature of auscultation in MS is a high-pitched "opening snap" (OS) that follows S_2. The OS is thought to result from the sudden tensing of the chordae tendineae and stenotic leaflets on opening of the abnormal valve. The interval between S_2 and the OS relates inversely to the severity of MS. That is, the more severe the MS, the higher the LA pressure and the earlier the valve is forced open in diastole. The OS is followed by a low-frequency decrescendo murmur (termed a *diastolic rumble*) caused by turbulent flow across the stenotic valve during diastole (see Fig. 8-2). The duration, but not the intensity, of the diastolic murmur relates to the severity of MS. That is, the more severe the stenosis, the longer it takes for the LA to empty and for the gradient between the LA and LV to dissipate. Near the end of diastole, contraction of the LA in patients in sinus rhythm causes the pressure gradient between the LA and LV to rise again (see Fig. 8-2); therefore, the murmur briefly becomes louder at that time (termed *presystolic accentuation*). This final accentuation of the murmur does not occur if atrial fibrillation has developed because there is no effective atrial contraction in that situation.

Diagnostic Studies

The *electrocardiogram* in MS routinely shows left atrial enlargement and, if pulmonary hypertension has developed, right ventricular hypertrophy. Atrial fibrillation may be present. The *chest radiograph* reveals left atrial enlargement, pulmonary vascular redistribution, interstitial edema, and Kerley B lines resulting from edema within the pulmonary septae (see Chapter 3). With the development of pulmonary hypertension, right ventricular enlargement and prominence of the pulmonary arteries appear.

Echocardiography is of major diagnostic value in MS. Structural findings include thickened mitral leaflets with abnormal fusion of their commissures and restricted separation during diastole. The degree of left atrial enlargement can be quantified, and if present, intra-atrial thrombus may be visualized. The mitral valve area can be measured directly on cross-sectional views or calculated from Doppler velocity measurements. Patients can be stratified into stages of disease severity based partly on the mitral valve area. A normal mitral valve orifice measures between 4 and 6 cm². Current guidelines define clinically important "severe" MS as a valve area ≤1.5 cm², a state that is typically accompanied by LA enlargement and elevated pulmonary artery systolic pressure. A valve area ≤1.0 cm² is termed "very severe" MS. If the findings determined by echocardiography seem milder than the patient's history and examination suggest, an *exercise test* with accompanying Doppler assessment or *cardiac catheterization* may be warranted to further define hemodynamic measurements.

Treatment

Salt intake restriction and diuretic therapy may improve symptoms due to vascular congestion. Heart rate slowing agents, such as β-blockers or nondihydropyridine calcium channel blockers (eg, diltiazem or verapamil, see Chapter 17), increase diastolic LV filling time and therefore ease symptoms that occur during exercise. These drugs, or digoxin, are similarly useful to slow the ventricular rate in patients with accompanying rapid atrial fibrillation. Anticoagulant therapy to prevent thromboembolism is recommended for MS patients with atrial fibrillation, an identified atrial thrombus, or prior embolic events.

Percutaneous or surgical valve interventions are the only treatments that alter the natural history of MS and are indicated in patients with severe, symptomatic MS. *Percutaneous balloon mitral valvuloplasty* is the treatment of choice in appropriately selected patients (those without advanced anatomic deformity of the valve, mitral regurgitation [MR], or left atrial thrombus). During this procedure, a balloon catheter is advanced from the femoral vein into the right atrium, across the atrial septum (by intentionally puncturing the septum), and through the narrowed mitral valve orifice. The balloon is then rapidly inflated, thereby "cracking" open the fused commissures. The short- and long-term results of this procedure are typically excellent and compare favorably with those of surgical treatment in anatomically appropriate patients. In young adults with the most suitable anatomy for the procedure, the event-free survival rate approaches 80%-90% over 3-7 years of follow-up. Approximately 5% of patients undergoing balloon mitral valvuloplasty are left with a residual atrial septal defect due to the transseptal puncture. Less frequent complications include cerebral emboli at the time of valvuloplasty, cardiac perforation by the catheter, or the unintentional creation of substantial MR.

Open mitral valve commissurotomy (an operation in which the stenotic commissures are separated under direct visualization) may be undertaken in patients for whom percutaneous balloon valvuloplasty is not feasible or successful. It is effective in relieving obstruction, and restenosis occurs in fewer than 20% of patients over 10-20 years of follow-up. Perioperative mortality rates are low (2%). *Mitral valve replacement* is considered in patients who are not appropriate candidates for balloon valvuloplasty or open commissurotomy.

Mitral Regurgitation

Etiology

The mitral valve apparatus is a complex structure composed of an annulus, two leaflets, chordae tendineae, and papillary muscles, supported by the adjacent myocardium to which the annulus and papillary muscles are attached (Fig. 8-3). Disruption to the structural integrity of any of these components or their coordinated action can result in abnormal closure of the valve during systole, with ensuing MR. MR is categorized as *primary* if it is due to a structural defect of one or more of the valve components or *secondary* if the valve is structurally normal, but regurgitation instead results from left ventricular enlargement. In the latter case, MR

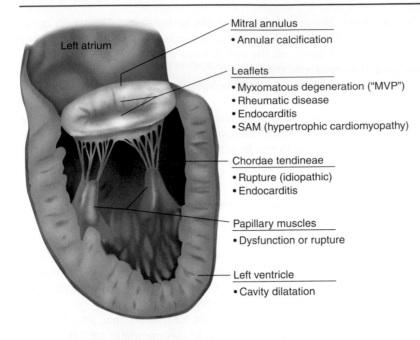

Mitral annulus
• Annular calcification

Left atrium

Leaflets
• Myxomatous degeneration ("MVP")
• Rheumatic disease
• Endocarditis
• SAM (hypertrophic cardiomyopathy)

Chordae tendineae
• Rupture (idiopathic)
• Endocarditis

Papillary muscles
• Dysfunction or rupture

Left ventricle
• Cavity dilatation

Figure 8-3. The mitral valve apparatus and associated common etiologies of mitral regurgitation. MVP, mitral valve prolapse; SAM, systolic anterior motion.

arises from abnormal coaptation and closure of the mitral leaflets owing to dilatation of the mitral annulus by the enlarged LV, and/or spatial separation of the papillary muscles, which places traction of the chordae and attached leaflets. Furthermore, depending on the nature of the valvular insult, MR can present as an "acute" or "chronic" condition, with different pathophysiologic consequences.

Most cases of *acute MR* are primary in nature and result from sudden damage to components of the valve apparatus. For example, rupture of an infarcted papillary muscle can occur within days of an acute ST-segment elevation MI, often resulting in severe MR (see Chapter 7). Acute MR due to sudden rupture of chordae tendineae can result from endocarditis, blunt trauma to the chest, or from degeneration of the chordae owing to connective tissue disorders such as Marfan syndrome.

Chronic MR has multiple primary causes, including myxomatous degeneration of the valve, in which "floppy" leaflets allow regurgitation to occur by bowing excessively into the LA during systole (termed "mitral valve prolapse" [MVP] and described in the next section). Other causes of chronic primary MR include rheumatic deformity of the valve, congenital valve defects, and extensive calcification of the mitral annulus, which prevents normal movement of the valve leaflets, thus interfering with valve closure.

Secondary (also termed "functional") chronic MR results from LV enlargement and/or dysfunction as described above, as may occur with prior myocardial infarction, chronic ischemic heart disease, or dilated cardiomyopathy (see Chapter 10).

Pathophysiology

In MR, a portion of the left ventricular stroke volume is abnormally ejected backward into the low-pressure LA during systole (Fig. 8-4). As a result, the forward cardiac output (into the aorta) is less than the LV's total output (forward flow plus backward leak). Therefore, the direct consequences of MR include (1) an elevation of left atrial volume and pressure, (2) a reduction of forward cardiac output, and (3) a volume-related stress on the LV because the regurgitant volume returns to the LV in diastole along with the normal pulmonary venous return. To meet normal circulatory needs and to eject the additional volume, LV stroke volume

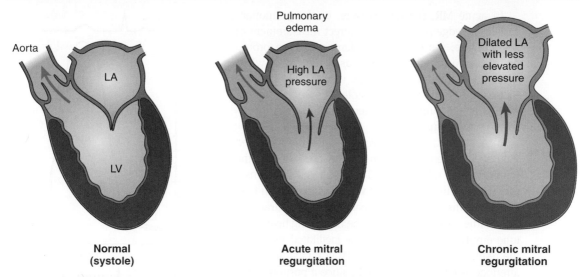

Figure 8-4. Pathophysiology of mitral regurgitation. In the normal heart, left ventricular (LV) contraction during systole forces blood exclusively through the aortic valve into the aorta (*green arrows*); the closed mitral valve prevents regurgitation into the left atrium (LA). In mitral regurgitation (MR), a portion of LV output is forced backward into the LA (*red arrows*), so that forward cardiac output into the aorta is reduced. In *acute* MR, the LA is of normal size and is relatively noncompliant, such that the LA pressure rises significantly and pulmonary edema may result. In *chronic* MR, the LA has enlarged and is more compliant, so that the LA pressure is less elevated and pulmonary congestive symptoms are less common. However, LV enlargement and eccentric hypertrophy result from the chronically elevated volume load.

must rise. This increase is accomplished by the Frank-Starling mechanism (see Chapter 9), whereby the elevated LV diastolic volume augments myofiber stretch and stroke volume. The hemodynamic consequences of MR vary depending on the degree of regurgitation and how long it has been present.

The severity of MR and the ratio of forward cardiac output to backward flow are dictated by five factors: (1) the size of the mitral orifice during regurgitation, (2) the systolic pressure gradient between the LV and LA, (3) the systemic vascular resistance opposing forward LV blood flow, (4) left atrial compliance, and (5) the duration of regurgitation with each systolic contraction.

The *regurgitant fraction* in MR is defined as follows:

$$\frac{\text{Volume of MR}}{\text{Total LV stroke volume}}$$

This ratio rises whenever the resistance to aortic outflow is increased (ie, blood follows the path of least resistance). For example, high systemic blood pressure or the presence of aortic stenosis (AS) will increase the regurgitant fraction. The extent to which left atrial pressure rises in response to the regurgitant volume is determined by the left atrial compliance. Compliance is a measure of the chamber's pressure-volume relationship, reflecting the ease or difficulty with which the chamber can be filled (see Table 9-1).

In *acute MR*, left atrial compliance undergoes little immediate change. Because the LA is a relatively stiff chamber, its pressure increases substantially when it is suddenly exposed to a regurgitant volume load (see Fig. 8-4). This elevated pressure is transmitted backward to the pulmonary circulation and can result in rapid pulmonary edema, a medical emergency.

In acute MR, the LA pressure, or the pulmonary capillary wedge pressure (an indirect measurement of LA pressure; see Chapter 3), demonstrates a prominent v wave (often referred to as a "cv" wave when it merges with the preceding c wave), reflecting the increased LA filling during systole (Fig. 8-5). Additionally, as in MS, pulmonary artery and right heart pressures passively rise.

In acute MR, the LV accommodates the increased volume load returning from the LA according to the Frank-Starling relationship. The result is a compensatory increase in the LV stroke volume and ejection fraction, such that at the end of each systolic contraction, LV volume remains normal in the nonfailing heart. Systolic emptying of the ventricle is facilitated in MR by the reduced total impedance to LV contraction (ie, the afterload is lower than normal), since a portion of the LV output is directed into the relatively low-impedance LA, rather than into the higher-pressure aorta.

In contrast to the acute situation, the more gradual development of *chronic MR* permits the LA to undergo compensatory changes that lessen the effects of regurgitation on the pulmonary circulation (see Fig. 8-4). In particular, the LA dilates and its compliance increases such that the chamber is able to accommodate a larger volume without a substantial increase in pressure. Left atrial dilatation is therefore adaptive in that it limits significant increases in pulmonary vascular pressures. However, this adaptation occurs at the cost of reduced forward cardiac output, because the compliant LA becomes a preferred low-pressure "sink" for left ventricular ejection, compared with the aorta. Consequently, as progressively larger fractions of blood regurgitate into the LA, symptoms of chronic MR include those of low forward cardiac output (eg, weakness and fatigue). In addition, chronic left atrial dilatation predisposes to the development of atrial fibrillation.

To reiterate, major pathophysiologic differences between acute and chronic MR relate to a great extent to left atrial size and compliance:

Acute MR: Normal LA size and compliance → High LA pressure → High pulmonary venous pressure → Pulmonary congestion and edema

Chronic MR: Increased LA size and compliance → Relatively normal LA and pulmonary venous pressures, but decreased forward cardiac output

In chronic MR, the LV also undergoes gradual compensatory dilatation in response to the volume load through eccentric hypertrophy (see Chapter 9). Compared with acute MR, the resulting increased ventricular compliance accommodates the augmented filling volume with relatively normal diastolic pressures. Forward output in chronic MR is preserved to near-normal levels for an extended period by maintaining a higher stroke volume via the Frank-Starling mechanism. Over years, however, chronic volume overload results in deterioration of systolic ventricular function, a decline in forward output, and symptoms of heart failure.

Figure 8-5. Hemodynamic profile of mitral regurgitation (MR). A large systolic v wave is noted in the left atrial (LA) pressure tracing. A holosystolic murmur is present in chronic MR (as shown here), beginning at the first heart sound (S_1) and continuing through the second heart sound (S_2). In acute severe MR, the systolic murmur may have a decrescendo quality, reflecting rapid equilibration of LV and LA pressures owing to the relatively low LA compliance. ECG, electrocardiogram; LV, left ventricle.

Clinical Manifestations and Evaluation

Presentation

As described in the pathophysiology section, patients with acute MR usually present with symptoms of pulmonary edema (see Chapter 9). The symptoms of chronic MR are predominantly due to low cardiac output, especially during exertion, and include fatigue and weakness. Patients with severe MR or those who develop LV contractile dysfunction often complain of dyspnea, orthopnea, and/or paroxysmal nocturnal dyspnea. In chronic severe MR, symptoms of right heart failure (eg, increased abdominal girth, peripheral edema) may develop as well.

Examination

The physical examination of a patient with *chronic* MR typically reveals an apical holosystolic (also termed pansystolic) murmur that often radiates to the axilla. The holosystolic nature of the murmur reflects the continued pressure gradient between LV and LA throughout systole (see Fig. 8-5). This description, accurate for rheumatic MR, has several exceptions. For example, in patients with isolated posterior mitral leaflet prolapse, the regurgitant jet is directed anteriorly. In this setting, the murmur may instead radiate to the base of the heart and could be confused with the murmur of AS in that location. Fortunately, the distinction between the systolic murmur of MR and that of AS can be made by simple bedside maneuvers. If the patient is instructed to clench his/her fists and forearms, systemic vascular resistance will increase and the murmur of MR will intensify, whereas the murmur of AS will not. Even more helpful in this distinction is the effect of varying cardiac cycle length (the time between consecutive heart beats) on the intensity of the systolic murmur. In a patient with atrial fibrillation or with frequent premature beats, the LV fills to a degree that directly depends on the preceding cycle length (ie, a longer cycle length permits greater left ventricular filling). The systolic murmur of AS becomes louder in the beat after a long cycle length because even small pressure gradients are amplified as more blood is ejected across the reduced aortic orifice. In MR, however, the intensity of the murmur does not vary significantly because the change in the LV-LA pressure gradient is minimally affected by alterations in the cycle length.

In addition to the systolic murmur, a common finding in chronic MR is the presence of an S_3, which reflects increased volume returning to the LV in early diastole (see Chapter 2). Additionally, in chronic MR, the cardiac apical impulse is often laterally displaced toward the axilla because of LV enlargement.

In patients with severe *acute* MR, the character of the systolic murmur is often different, occurring in early to mid systole with a decrescendo quality. The length and quality of the murmur are dictated by the systolic pressure gradient between the LV and the relatively noncompliant LA. That is, as the LA pressure rises in systole in acute MR, the LV and LA pressures quickly equalize, thus truncating the murmur. Patients with acute MR often display signs of pulmonary congestion.

Diagnostic Studies

The *chest radiograph* may display pulmonary edema in acute MR but in chronic asymptomatic MR more likely demonstrates left ventricular and atrial enlargement, without pulmonary congestion. Calcification of the mitral annulus may be seen if that is the cause of the MR. In chronic MR, the *electrocardiogram* typically demonstrates left atrial enlargement and signs of left ventricular hypertrophy. *Echocardiography* can often identify the structural cause of MR and assess its severity. *Cardiac catheterization* is used to identify accompanying coronary artery disease, and left ventriculography is sometimes performed to confirm MR severity. The characteristic hemodynamic finding is a large systolic *v* wave in the pulmonary capillary wedge pressure tracing (reflective of LA pressure—see Chapter 3). The *v* wave becomes less conspicuous, however, with progressive LA dilatation and greater compliance over time.

Natural History and Treatment

Acute severe MR is a surgical emergency with a poor prognosis, even with appropriate treatment, with a 30-day mortality rate of 20%-25%. The natural history of chronic MR is related to its underlying cause. For example, in rheumatic valve disease, the course is one of very slow progression with a 15-year survival rate of 70%. On the other hand, abrupt worsening of chronic MR of any cause may occur with superimposed complications, such as rupture of chordae tendineae or endocarditis, and can result in an immediate life-threatening situation.

The treatment of acute MR almost always requires corrective surgery. Pharmacologic therapy is useful only to temporarily stabilize patients. For example, intravenous nitroprusside is a potent vasodilator that decreases arterial resistance, thereby augmenting forward flow and diminishing the regurgitant volume. In this way, cardiac output and pulmonary congestion may improve, at least transiently. Surgical intervention consists of either mitral valve repair (reconstruction of the native valve) or replacement, depending on the underlying cause and valve anatomy.

Management of chronic MR depends on the etiology. In chronic *primary* MR, the continuous left ventricular volume overload can slowly impair left ventricular contractile function, ultimately, resulting in heart failure. Medical treatment with vasodilators is less useful than in acute MR and has not been shown to delay the need for valve surgery in chronic MR. Surgical intervention should be undertaken in symptomatic patients or at the earliest sign of LV contractile dysfunction on imaging studies (eg, a fall in EF to <60% by echocardiography) even before symptoms develop. Per current guidelines, surgical intervention is also reasonable in patients with chronic asymptomatic severe primary MR with (1) the development of atrial fibrillation or pulmonary hypertension; or (2) patients with normal EF but a progressive increase in end-systolic LV size or decline in EF towards 60% on serial imaging studies; or (3) for patients in whom the likelihood of successful valve repair (without replacement) is >95% at highly skilled centers.

Surgical options for chronic primary MR include mitral valve repair or replacement. *Mitral valve repair* is the preferred operative technique when feasible and involves the reconstruction of parts of the valve responsible for the regurgitation. For example, a perforated leaflet may be patched with transplanted autologous pericardium, or ruptured chordae may be reattached to a papillary muscle. Mitral repair preserves native valve tissue and eliminates many of the problems associated with artificial valves described later in the chapter. In patients who undergo repair, the postoperative survival rate appears to be better than the natural history of MR and has provided impetus toward earlier surgical intervention. Operative mortality rates for unselected patients with MR are <2% for mitral valve repair and 5%-7% for mitral valve replacement. These rates are higher if concurrent coronary artery bypass grafting is performed.

In patients with chronic, severe, symptomatic primary MR who are at prohibitive operative risk, a recently developed technique of transcatheter mitral valve repair (TMVR) can be considered. In this procedure, a catheter is advanced percutaneously from the femoral vein into the right side of the heart, then into the LA via a puncture through the interatrial septum (similar to mitral balloon valvuloplasty), and advanced into the LV. A mechanical clip is then deployed, which grasps and tethers the anterior and posterior mitral leaflets together and is left in place, reducing the size of the regurgitant orifice. The procedure has been shown to be safe and effective in prospective observational studies of high surgical risk patients, with improvement in the severity of MR and functional status. However, in a randomized trial of percutaneous repair vs valve surgery for patients with severe primary MR, surgery proved more effective and remains the intervention of choice in patients who are acceptable candidates for an operation.

Because chronic, *secondary* MR is often a result of left ventricular dysfunction (ie, not a structural valve abnormality), pharmacologic rather than surgical intervention is the mainstay of treatment, using standard heart failure medications, including diuretics, drugs that interfere with the renin-angiotensin system, beta-blockers, and aldosterone antagonists (see Chapter 9). Invasive valve intervention is considered only when a patient with chronic, severe secondary MR has persistent symptoms despite optimal medical therapy and underlying causes of LV dysfunction have been addressed (eg, coronary artery revascularization in patients with ischemic disease). Recent trial data showed that a specific TMVR approach (using a transcatheter mitral clip to lessen regurgitation) reduced hospitalizations for heart failure and mortality in patients with symptomatic secondary moderate-to-severe MR, and is now approved for that purpose. There are limited data on the safety and efficacy of isolated mitral valve surgery for secondary MR, which is therefore not routinely performed.

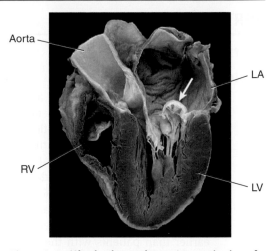

Figure 8-6. Mitral valve prolapse. Long-axis view of the left ventricle (LV) demonstrates a myxomatous, elongated appearance of the mitral valve with prolapse of the posterior leaflet (*arrow*) into the left atrium (LA). RV, right ventricle. (From Schoen FJ, Mitchell RN. The heart. In: Kumar V, Abbas A, Aster JC, eds. *Robbins and Cotran Pathologic Basis of Disease*. 9th ed. Philadelphia, PA: Elsevier Saunders; 2015.)

MITRAL VALVE PROLAPSE

MVP is characterized by abnormal billowing of a portion of one or both mitral leaflets into the LA during ventricular systole and is frequently accompanied by MR (Fig. 8-6). MVP may be inherited as a primary autosomal dominant disorder with variable penetrance, or it may accompany certain connective tissue diseases, such as Marfan syndrome or Ehlers-Danlos syndrome. Pathologically, the valve leaflets, particularly the posterior leaflet, are enlarged, and the normal dense collagen and elastin matrix of the valvular fibrosa is fragmented and replaced with loose myxomatous connective tissue. Additionally, in more severe lesions, elongated or ruptured chordae, annular enlargement, or thickened leaflets may be present. By echocardiographic criteria, MVP is found in about 2% of the population and is more common in women.

MVP is often asymptomatic, but affected individuals may describe chest pain or palpitations because of associated arrhythmias. Most often it is identified on routine physical examination by the presence of a midsystolic click and late systolic murmur heard best at the cardiac apex. The midsystolic click is thought to correspond to the sudden tensing of the involved mitral leaflet or chordae tendineae as the leaflet is forced back toward the LA; the murmur corresponds to regurgitant flow through the incompetent valve. The click and murmur are characteristically altered during dynamic auscultation at the bedside: maneuvers that increase the volume of the LV (eg, sudden squatting, which increases venous return) place traction of the chordae tendineae, limiting and delaying the occurrence of prolapse in systole, and cause the click and murmur to occur later (ie, further from S_1). Conversely, if the volume of blood in the LV is decreased (eg, by standing, which decreases venous return), prolapse occurs earlier, and the click and murmur move closer to S_1.

Confirmation of the diagnosis is obtained by *echocardiography*, which demonstrates posterior displacement of a portion of one or both mitral leaflets into the LA during systole. The *electrocardiogram* and *chest radiograph* are usually normal unless chronic MR has resulted in left atrial and left ventricular enlargement.

The clinical course of MVP is most often benign. Treatment consists of reassurance about the usually good prognosis and monitoring for the development of progressive MR. Occasionally, rupture of myxomatous chordae in this condition can cause sudden, severe regurgitation and pulmonary edema. Other potential complications include endocarditis, peripheral emboli owing to microthrombus formation on the redundant valve tissue, and atrial or ventricular arrhythmias.

AORTIC VALVE DISEASE

AORTIC STENOSIS

Etiology

Among adult patients, there are three major causes of AS: (1) degenerative calcification of a previously normal trileaflet aortic valve, (2) calcification of a congenitally bicuspid aortic valve, and (3) rheumatic aortic valve disease. Degenerative disease of a trileaflet valve shares many pathologic features with atherosclerosis, as described below. Bicuspid aortic valves are present in 1%-2% of the population (with men affected more commonly than women), and such patients typically develop signs of severe valve disease about a decade earlier than patients with the trileaflet, degenerative type of AS. Rheumatic aortic valve disease is now uncommon in developed countries. It is nearly always accompanied by rheumatic involvement of the mitral valve.

Figure 8-7. Pathophysiology of aortic stenosis (AS). The impediment to left ventricular (LV) outflow in AS results in elevated LV pressures and secondary concentric ventricular hypertrophy.

Pathology

The pathologic appearance in AS is dependent on its etiology. Degenerative, calcific AS results from a dynamic process of endothelial dysfunction, lipid accumulation, inflammation, and alteration of signaling pathways that appear similar to atherogenesis. Over time, valvular myofibroblasts differentiate into osteoblasts and deposit calcium hydroxyapatite crystals, resulting in leaflet thickening and stiffening. This process is likely exacerbated by abnormal shear forces, as occurs with congenitally deformed (bicuspid) valves, and could explain the earlier presentation of such patients. As with atherosclerosis, risk factors for calcific, degenerative AS include dyslipidemia, smoking, and hypertension (see Chapter 5).

In rheumatic AS, endocardial inflammation leads to organization and fibrosis of the valve and ultimately to fusion of the commissures and formation of calcified masses within the aortic cusps.

Figure 8-8. Hemodynamic profile of aortic stenosis. A systolic pressure gradient (*shaded area*) is present between the left ventricle (LV) and aorta. The second heart sound (S_2) is diminished in intensity, and there is a crescendo-decrescendo systolic murmur that does not extend beyond S_2. ECG, electrocardiogram.

Pathophysiology

In AS, blood flow across the aortic valve is impeded during systole (Fig. 8-7). Progressive reduction of the aortic valve area requires elevation of left ventricular systolic pressure to overcome the impedance to flow to drive blood into the aorta (Fig. 8-8).

Since the obstruction in AS develops gradually, the LV is able to compensate by undergoing concentric hypertrophy in response to the increased pressure load. Initially, such hypertrophy serves an important role in reducing LV wall stress (remember from Chapter 6 that wall stress = $(P \times r) \div 2h$, in which h represents wall thickness). Over time, however, it also reduces the compliance of the ventricle. The resulting elevation of diastolic LV pressure causes the LA to hypertrophy, which facilitates filling of the "stiffened" LV. Whereas left atrial contraction contributes only a small portion of the left ventricular stroke volume in normal individuals, it may provide more than 25% of the stroke volume to the stiffened LV in AS patients. Thus, left atrial hypertrophy is beneficial, and the loss of effective atrial contraction (eg, development of atrial fibrillation) can cause marked clinical deterioration.

Three major manifestations occur in patients with advanced AS: (1) angina, (2) exertional syncope, and (3) heart failure, all of which can be explained on the basis of the underlying pathophysiology. Each manifestation, in order, heralds an increasingly ominous prognosis (Table 8-1).

AS may result in *angina* because it creates a substantial imbalance between myocardial oxygen supply and demand. Myocardial oxygen *demand* is increased in two ways. First, the muscle mass of the hypertrophied LV is increased, requiring greater-than-normal perfusion. Second, wall stress is increased because of the elevated systolic ventricular pressure. In addition, AS reduces myocardial oxygen *supply* because the elevated left ventricular diastolic pressure reduces the coronary perfusion pressure gradient between the aorta and the myocardium.

AS may cause *syncope* during exertion. Although left ventricular hypertrophy allows the chamber to generate a high pressure and maintain a normal cardiac output at rest, the ventricle cannot significantly increase its cardiac output during exercise because of the fixed stenotic aortic orifice. In addition, exercise leads to vasodilatation of the peripheral muscle beds. Thus, the combination of peripheral vasodilatation and the inability to augment cardiac output contributes to decreased cerebral perfusion pressure and, potentially, loss of consciousness on exertion.

Finally, AS can result in symptoms of *heart failure*. Early in the course of AS, an abnormally increased left atrial pressure occurs primarily at the end of diastole, when the LA contracts into the thickened noncompliant LV. As a result, the mean left atrial pressure and pulmonary venous pressure are not greatly affected early in the disease. However, with progression of stenosis, the LV may develop contractile dysfunction because of the insurmountably high afterload, leading to increased left ventricular diastolic volume and pressure. The accompanying marked elevation of LA and pulmonary venous pressures incites pulmonary alveolar congestion and symptoms of heart failure.

A normal aortic valve has a cross-sectional area of 3-4 cm^2 and a mean systolic pressure gradient between the LV and aorta of <5 mm Hg. As the valve area decreases in AS, the pressure gradient rises. When the valve area declines to <1.0 cm^2, or the mean pressure gradient increases to >40 mm Hg, a patient is considered to have severe AS, and symptoms typically appear.

Clinical Manifestations and Evaluation

Presentation

Angina, syncope, and/or heart failure may appear after many asymptomatic years of slowly progressive valve stenosis. Once these symptoms develop, they confer a significantly decreased survival if invasive correction of AS is not undertaken (see Table 8-1).

TABLE 8-1	Median Survival Time in Symptomatic Severe Aortic Stenosis (Without Procedural Intervention)	
Clinical Symptoms	**Median Survival**	
Angina	5 y	
Syncope	3 y	
Heart failure	2 y	

Derived from Ross J Jr, Braunwald E. Aortic stenosis. *Circulation.* 1968;38(suppl v):61.

Examination

Physical examination often permits accurate detection and estimation of the severity of AS. The key features of advanced AS include (1) a coarse late-peaking systolic ejection murmur and (2) a weakened (*parvus*) and delayed (*tardus*) upstroke of the carotid artery owing to the obstructed LV outflow. Other common findings on cardiac examination include the presence of an S_4 (because of atrial contraction into the "stiff" LV—see Chapter 2) and reduced intensity, or complete absence, of the aortic component of the second heart sound (see Fig. 8-8).

Diagnostic Studies

On the *electrocardiogram*, left ventricular hypertrophy is common in advanced AS. *Echocardiography* is a more sensitive technique to assess LV wall thickness and displays the abnormal anatomy and reduced excursion of the stenotic valve leaflets. The transvalvular pressure gradient and aortic valve area can be readily calculated by Doppler echocardiography (see Chapter 3). *Cardiac catheterization* is sometimes used to confirm the severity of AS and also to define the coronary anatomy, because concurrent coronary artery bypass surgery may be appropriate at the time of aortic valve replacement (AVR) in patients with coexisting coronary disease.

Natural History and Treatment

Mild, asymptomatic AS has a slow rate of progression such that over a 20-year period, only 20% of patients will progress to severe or symptomatic disease. There is no current effective medical therapy for slowing the rate of progression of AS. Since the natural history of severe, symptomatic, uncorrected AS is very poor (see Table 8-1), effective treatment requires replacement of the valve.

AVR is indicated when a patient with severe AS develops symptoms, or when there is evidence of progressive LV dysfunction in the absence of symptoms. The left ventricular ejection fraction almost always increases after valve replacement, even in patients with impaired preoperative left ventricular function. The effect of surgical AVR on the natural history of AS is dramatic, as the 10-year survival rate rises to ~60%.

Unlike its successful role in MS, *percutaneous balloon valvuloplasty* has been disappointing as a sole treatment of adults with calcific AS. Although balloon dilatation of the aortic valve orifice can fracture calcified masses leading to a slight reduction in valve obstruction, up to 50% of patients develop restenosis within 6 months. Valvuloplasty is occasionally used as a temporizing measure in patients too ill to proceed directly to valve replacement and can also be an effective treatment in young patients with noncalcified bicuspid AS.

In distinction, *transcatheter aortic valve replacement* (*TAVR*) has emerged as a successful minimally invasive treatment option, instead of open surgical AVR, for many patients with severe symptomatic AS. This technique involves percutaneous insertion of a specially designed bioprosthetic valve that is maneuvered into the narrowed orifice of the stenotic native valve, whereupon expansion of the prosthetic valve fixes the device in place, producing a larger aortic valve opening. The procedure is much less invasive than surgical AVR, with generally rapid recovery. TAVR has been validated in randomized prospective trials, and for inoperable patients, TAVR outcomes are superior to standard medical therapy. In high and intermediate surgical risk patients, TAVR is as effective as surgical AVR with similar survival and stroke rates. And recently published randomized studies involving low surgical risk patients demonstrated similar or superior mortality and stroke outcomes with TAVR compared to surgical AVR. TAVR outcomes are best when transfemoral artery access is possible for catheter insertion. Notable potential complications of the procedure include vascular complications of catheter insertion, conduction system trauma with heart block requiring pacemaker implantation, and aortic regurgitation (AR) around the prosthesis.

The decision of whether to perform surgical AVR vs TAVR for an individual patient with severe symptomatic AS should involve an experienced heart team of invasive cardiologists and cardiac surgeons. For most patients who are at high or intermediate surgical risk, TAVR is the preferred option, especially if femoral artery access is feasible. For low surgical risk patients who are at least 65 years old, TAVR is generally preferred over surgical AVR if there is acceptable femoral artery access, and aortic root anatomy is conducive for the procedure. Patients for whom surgical AVR may be preferred include those with other indications for open chest surgery (eg, coronary artery bypass or required repair of other heart valves or the aorta), those for whom femoral artery catheter access is not feasible, those with anatomic limitations of the aortic root or coronary ostia that would preclude transcatheter valve placement, and younger individuals, for whom surgical placement of a mechanical valve prosthesis offers a long-term durable solution (long-term durability of transcatheter bioprosthetic valves is not yet known, and mechanical valves cannot be placed via the transcatheter route).

Of note, patients with AS due to a bicuspid aortic valve were excluded from many of the major TAVR clinical trials. A recent analysis found that the mortality rate of TAVR for bicuspid valves is no different than for patients with trileaflet valves, but the stroke rate and procedural complications requiring conversion to an open-heart operation were greater in this population. Thus, patients with AS resulting from a known bicuspid valve need to be considered for TAVR on an individual basis by the structural heart team.

Aortic Regurgitation

Etiology

AR, also termed *aortic insufficiency*, may result either from abnormalities of the aortic valve leaflets or from dilatation of the aortic root. Primary *valvular* causes include (1) bicuspid aortic valve (in some patients AR predominates over AS), (2) endocarditis (due to perforation or erosion of a leaflet), and (3) rheumatic valve disease (due to thickening and shortening of the aortic valve cusps). Primary *aortic root* disease results in AR when the aortic annulus dilates sufficiently to cause separation of the leaflets, preventing normal coaptation in diastole. Examples include age-related degenerative dilation of the aortic root, aortic aneurysms, and aortic dissection, which are described in Chapter 15.

Pathophysiology

In AR, abnormal regurgitation of blood occurs from the aorta into the LV during diastole. Therefore, with each contraction, the LV must pump that regurgitant volume plus the normal quantity of blood entering from the LA. Hemodynamic compensation relies on the Frank-Starling mechanism to augment stroke volume. Factors influencing the severity of AR are analogous to those of MR: (1) the size of the regurgitant aortic orifice, (2) the pressure gradient across the aortic valve during diastole, and (3) the duration of diastole.

As in MR, the hemodynamic abnormalities and symptoms differ in acute and chronic AR (Fig. 8-9). In *acute AR*, the LV is of normal size and relatively noncompliant. Thus, the volume load of regurgitation causes the LV diastolic pressure to rise substantially. The sudden high diastolic LV pressure is transmitted to the LA and pulmonary circulation, often producing dyspnea and pulmonary edema. Thus, acute severe AR is usually a surgical emergency, requiring immediate valve replacement.

In *chronic AR*, the LV undergoes compensatory adaptation in response to the long-standing regurgitation. AR subjects the LV primarily to volume overload but also to an excessive pressure load; therefore, the ventricle compensates through chronic dilatation (eccentric hypertrophy, with replication of sarcomeres in series—see Chapter 9) and, to a lesser degree, increased thickness. Over time, the dilatation increases the compliance of the LV and allows it to accom-

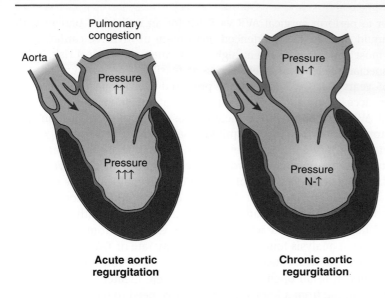

Figure 8-9. Pathophysiology of acute and chronic aortic regurgitation (AR). Abnormal regurgitation of blood from the aorta into the left ventricle (LV) is shown in each schematic drawing (*red arrows*). In acute AR, the LV is of normal size and relatively low compliance, such that its diastolic pressure rises significantly; this pressure increase is reflected back to the left atrium (LA) and pulmonary vasculature, resulting in pulmonary congestion or edema. In chronic AR, adaptive LV and LA enlargement have occurred, such that a greater volume of regurgitation can be accommodated with less of an increase in diastolic LV pressure, so that pulmonary congestion is less likely. N, normal.

modate a larger regurgitant volume with less of an increase in diastolic pressure, reducing the pressure transmitted into the LA and pulmonary circulation. However, by accommodating the large regurgitant volume, the aortic (and therefore systemic arterial) diastolic pressure drops substantially. The combination of a high LV stroke volume (causing increased systolic arterial pressure) with a reduced aortic diastolic pressure produces a widened *pulse pressure* (the difference between arterial systolic and diastolic pressures), a hallmark of chronic AR (Fig. 8-10). As a result of the decreased aortic diastolic pressure, the coronary artery perfusion pressure falls, potentially reducing myocardial oxygen supply. This, coupled with the increase in LV size (which causes increased wall stress and myocardial oxygen demand), can produce angina, even in the absence of atherosclerotic coronary disease.

Compensatory left ventricular dilatation and hypertrophy are generally adequate to meet the demands of chronic AR for many years, during which affected patients are asymptomatic. Gradually, however, progressive remodeling of the LV occurs, resulting in systolic dysfunction. This causes decreased forward cardiac output as well as an increase in left atrial and pulmonary vascular pressures. At that point, the patient develops symptoms of heart failure.

Clinical Manifestations and Assessment

Presentation

Common symptoms of chronic AR include dyspnea on exertion, fatigue, decreased exercise tolerance, and the uncomfortable sensation of a forceful heartbeat associated with the high pulse pressure.

Examination

Physical examination may show bounding pulses and other stigmata of the widened pulse pressure (Table 8-2), in addition to a hyperdynamic LV impulse and a blowing murmur of AR in early diastole along the left sternal

Figure 8-10. Hemodynamic profile of aortic regurgitation. During diastole, the aortic pressure falls rapidly (*arrow*), and left ventricular (LV) pressure rises as blood regurgitates from the aorta into the LV. A diastolic decrescendo murmur, beginning at the second heart sound (S_2), corresponds with the abnormal regurgitant flow. ECG, electrocardiogram.

TABLE 8-2	**Examples of Physical Findings Associated with Widened Pulse Pressure in Chronic Aortic Regurgitation**	
Name	**Description**
Bisferiens pulse	Double systolic impulse in carotid or brachial artery
Corrigan pulse	"Water hammer" pulses with marked distention and collapse
Hill sign	Popliteal systolic pressure more than 60 mm Hg greater than brachial systolic pressure
Quincke sign	Capillary pulsations visible at the lip or proximal nail beds

border (see Fig. 8-10). It is best heard with the patient leaning forward, after exhaling. In addition, a low-frequency middiastolic rumbling sound may be auscultated at the cardiac apex in some patients with severe AR. Known as the *Austin Flint murmur*, it is thought to reflect turbulence of blood flow through the *mitral* valve during diastole owing to downward displacement of the mitral anterior leaflet by the regurgitant stream of AR. It can be distinguished from the murmur of MS by the absence of an OS or presystolic accentuation.

Diagnostic Studies

In chronic AR, the *chest radiograph* shows an enlarged left ventricular silhouette. This is usually absent in acute AR, in which pulmonary vascular congestion is the more likely finding. *Doppler echocardiography* can identify and quantify the degree of AR and often can identify its cause. If echocardiographic imaging is suboptimal, *cardiac magnetic resonance imaging* can be obtained for quantification of the degree of AR and assessment of LV volumes and function.

Treatment

Data from natural history studies indicate that clinical progression of patients with asymptomatic chronic AR and normal LV contractile function is very slow. Therefore, asymptomatic patients are monitored with periodic examinations and assessment of LV function, usually by serial echocardiography. Patients with asymptomatic severe AR may benefit from afterload reducing vasodilators (eg, a calcium channel blocker or an angiotensin-converting enzyme inhibitor) for treatment of accompanying hypertension. However, such agents do not prolong the compensated stage of chronic AR.

Symptomatic patients, or asymptomatic patients with severe AR and impaired LV systolic function (ie, LV ejection fraction <0.50), should be offered surgical AVR to prevent progressive deterioration. Studies of such patients show that without surgery, death usually occurs within 4 years after the development of angina or 2 years after the onset of heart failure symptoms. AVR is also reasonable for asymptomatic patients with normal LV systolic function who have developed severe LV enlargement (defined as LV end-systolic diameter >50 mm) due to the regurgitation.

TRICUSPID VALVE DISEASE

TRICUSPID STENOSIS

Tricuspid stenosis (TS) is rare and is usually a long-term consequence of rheumatic fever. The OS and diastolic murmur of TS are similar to those of MS, but the murmur is heard closer to the sternum, and it intensifies on inspiration because of increased right heart blood flow. In TS, the neck veins are distended and may show a large *a* wave as a result of right atrial contraction against the stenotic tricuspid valve orifice when sinus rhythm is present (see Chapter 2).

Patients may develop abdominal distention and hepatomegaly owing to passive venous congestion. Percutaneous balloon dilatation or surgical correction (valvuloplasty or valve replacement) is usually required.

TRICUSPID REGURGITATION

Tricuspid regurgitation (TR) is usually *functional* rather than structural in nature; that is, it most commonly results from right ventricular enlargement (eg, owing to pressure or volume overload) rather than from primary valve disease. Among patients with rheumatic MS, 20% also have significant TR (of whom 80% have functional TR because of pulmonary hypertension with right ventricular enlargement, and 20% have structural TR resulting from rheumatic involvement of the tricuspid valve). A rare cause of TR is *carcinoid syndrome*, in which a type of gastrointestinal neuroendocrine tumor releases serotonin metabolites into the bloodstream. These metabolites are thought to be responsible for the formation of endocardial plaques in the right side of the heart. Involvement of the tricuspid valve immobilizes the leaflets, often resulting in substantial TR and, less often, TS.

The most common physical signs of TR are prominent *v* waves in the jugular veins (see Chapter 2) and a pulsatile liver because of regurgitation of right ventricular blood into the systemic veins. The systolic murmur of TR is heard at the lower left sternal border. It is often soft but becomes louder on inspiration. Doppler echocardiography readily detects TR and can quantify it. The treatment of functional TR is directed at the conditions responsible for the elevated right ventricular size or pressure and diuretic therapy; surgical repair of the valve is indicated in severe cases.

PULMONIC VALVE DISEASE

PULMONIC STENOSIS

Pulmonic stenosis (PS) is rare, and its cause is almost always congenital deformity of the valve (see Chapter 16). Carcinoid syndrome, described in the previous section, is another rare etiology, in which encasement and immobilization of the valve leaflets can occur. The systolic crescendo-decrescendo murmur of PS is usually loudest at the second or third left intercostal space close to the sternum. It may radiate to the neck or left shoulder and is often preceded by an ejection click (see Chapter 2).

PS is considered to be severe if the peak systolic pressure gradient across the valve is >64 mm Hg, moderate if the gradient is 36-64 mm Hg, and mild if the gradient is <36 mm Hg. Only patients with moderate-to-severe gradients are symptomatic. In such cases, transcatheter balloon valvuloplasty is usually effective therapy.

PULMONIC REGURGITATION

Pulmonic regurgitation most commonly develops in the setting of pulmonary hypertension and results from dilatation of the valve ring by the enlarged pulmonary artery. Auscultation reveals a high-pitched decrescendo murmur along the left sternal border that is often indistinguishable from AR (the two conditions are easily differentiated by Doppler echocardiography). Treatment focuses on addressing the underlying cause of pulmonary hypertension.

SURGICAL PROSTHETIC VALVES

The patient who undergoes valve replacement surgery often benefits dramatically from hemodynamic and symptomatic improvement but also acquires a new set of potential

Figure 8-11. Examples of prosthetic heart valves. A. SJM™ Masters Series mechanical heart valve. (SJM is a trademark of Abbott or its related companies. Reproduced with permission of Abbott, © 2020. All rights reserved.) **B.** A bioprosthetic aortic valve with leaflets in the closed position. (Reproduced with permission of Medtronic, Inc.)

complications related to the valve prosthesis itself. Since all available valve substitutes have certain limitations, valve replacement surgery is not a true "cure."

Currently available valve substitutes include mechanical and bioprosthetic (derived from animal or human tissue) devices (Fig. 8-11). One example of a mechanical valve is the St. Jude prosthesis, a hinged bileaflet valve consisting of two pyrolytic carbon discs that open opposite one another. Mechanical valves are very durable, but present foreign thrombogenic surfaces to the circulating blood and require lifelong anticoagulation to prevent thromboembolism.

In contrast, bioprosthetic valves display a very low rate of thromboembolism and do not require long-term anticoagulation therapy. The most commonly used bioprostheses are made from glutaraldehyde-fixed porcine (pig) valves secured in a support frame. In addition, bovine (cow) pericardium and human homograft (aortic valves harvested and cryopreserved from cadavers) prostheses are used. For patients who undergo AVR because of endocarditis, human homograft replacements are especially useful because they have low rates of subsequent reinfection.

Bioprosthetic valves have limited durability compared with mechanical valves, and structural failure occurs in up to 50% by 15 years after implantation. The principal causes of failure are leaflet tears and calcification. Failure rates vary greatly depending on the position of the valve. For example, bioprosthetic valves in the mitral position deteriorate more rapidly than those in the aortic position. This is likely because the mitral valve is exposed to higher closing forces, resulting in greater leaflet stress than that experienced by aortic prostheses. Of note, select patients with symptomatic deterioration of a bioprosthetic valve who are at high risk of reoperation can be effectively treated by inserting a new transcatheter valve into the failing valve (termed a "valve-in-valve" procedure).

Common to all types of valve replacement is the risk of infective endocarditis (discussed in the next section), which occurs with an incidence of 1%-2% per patient per year. If endocarditis occurs in the first 60 days after valve surgery, the mortality rate is exceedingly high (50%-80%). If endocarditis occurs later, mortality rates range from 20% to 50%. Reoperation is usually required when endocarditis involves a mechanical prosthesis because an adjacent abscess is frequently present. Some cases of bioprosthetic valve endocarditis may respond to antibiotic therapy alone.

Given their respective advantages and disadvantages, the mortality and complication rates of mechanical and bioprosthetic valves are similar for the first 10 years after replacement. In 20-year follow-up studies of randomized, controlled trials, mechanical valves have been shown to be superior to bioprosthetic valves for event-free survival, except for bleeding complications related to anticoagulation therapy. Therefore, the decision about which type of prosthesis to use in a patient often centers on (1) the patient's expected lifespan in comparison to the functional longevity of the valve, (2) risk-vs-benefit considerations of chronic anticoagulation therapy, and (3) patient and surgeon preferences. Mechanical valves are often recommended for younger patients and for those who will be tolerant of, and compliant with, anticoagulant therapy. Bioprosthetic valves are generally suitable choices for patients ~70 years of age or older and for patients with contraindications to chronic anticoagulation.

INFECTIVE ENDOCARDITIS

Infection of the endocardial surface of the heart, including the cardiac valves, can lead to extensive tissue damage and is often fatal. IE carries an overall 6-month mortality rate of 20%-25%, even with appropriate therapy, and a 100% mortality rate if it is not recognized and treated correctly.

There are three clinically useful ways to classify IE: (1) by clinical course, (2) by host substrate, and (3) by the specific infecting microorganism. In the first classification scheme, IE is termed **acute bacterial endocarditis (ABE)** when the syndrome presents as a rapidly progressive fulminant infection, and a highly virulent and invasive organism such as *Staphylococcus aureus* is causal. Because of the aggressiveness of the responsible microorganism, ABE may occur on previously healthy heart valves. When IE presents with a more insidious clinical course, it is termed **subacute bacterial endocarditis (SBE)** and less virulent organisms, such as viridans streptococci, are typically involved. SBE most frequently occurs in individuals with prior underlying valvular damage.

The second means of classification of IE is according to the host substrate: (1) native valve endocarditis, (2) prosthetic valve endocarditis, or (3) endocarditis in the setting of intravenous drug abuse. Native valve endocarditis accounts for the majority of these. Different microorganisms and clinical courses are associated with each of these categories. For example, the skin contaminant *Staphylococcus epidermidis* is a common cause of prosthetic valve endocarditis, but that is rarely the case when endocarditis occurs on a native heart valve. Intravenous drug users have a propensity for *S. aureus* endocarditis of the tricuspid valve (the mitral and aortic valves may also become infected in such patients).

The third classification of IE is according to the specific infecting microorganism (eg, *S. aureus* endocarditis). As described below, the most common responsible organisms are gram-positive cocci. Certain bacterial strains that cause endocarditis are associated with particular anatomic sources. For example, viridans group streptococci usually originate from oropharyngeal tissue. Endocarditis due to *Streptococcus gallolyticus* (formerly termed *S. bovis*) commonly arises from the gastrointestinal tract and should prompt investigation for colonic polyps or colorectal carcinoma.

PATHOGENESIS

The pathogenesis of native valve endocarditis requires several conditions: (1) endocardial surface injury, (2) platelet-fibrin-thrombus formation at the site of injury, (3) bacterial entry into the circulation, and (4) bacterial adherence to the injured endocardial surface. The first two conditions provide an environment favorable to infection, whereas the latter two permit implantation of the organism on the endocardial surface. The most common cause of endothelial injury is turbulent blood flow resulting from preexisting cardiac or intravascular abnormalities, including acquired valvular heart lesions (eg, MR or AS), congenital heart diseases, and hypertrophic cardiomyopathy (see Chapter 10).

Once an endocardial surface is injured, platelets adhere to the exposed subendocardial connective tissue and initiate the formation of a sterile thrombus (termed a *vegetation*) through fibrin deposition. This process is referred to as *nonbacterial thrombotic endocarditis* (NBTE). NBTE makes the endocardium more hospitable to microbes in two ways. First, the platelet-fibrin deposits provide a surface for adherence by bacteria. Second, the fibrin covers adherent organisms and protects them from host defenses by inhibiting chemotaxis and migration of phagocytes.

When NBTE is present, the delivery of microorganisms in the bloodstream to the injured surface can lead to IE. Three factors determine the ability of an organism to induce IE: (1) access to the bloodstream, (2) survival of the organism in the circulation, and (3) adherence of the bacteria to the endocardium. Bacteria can be introduced into the bloodstream whenever a mucosal or skin surface harboring an organism is traumatized, such as from the mouth during dental procedures, or from the skin during illicit intravenous drug use. However, while transient bacteremia is a relatively common event, only microorganisms suited for survival in the circulation and able to adhere to the platelet-fibrin mesh overlying the endocardial defect will cause IE. For example, gram-positive organisms account for the majority of cases of endocarditis largely because of their resistance to destruction in the circulation by complement and their tendency to adhere to endothelial and platelet surface proteins. Table 8-3 lists the most common infectious causes of endocarditis compiled from hospitals in multiple international locations; staphylococci (especially *S. aureus*) and streptococci are the most frequent. In recent decades, antibiotic resistant strains such as methicillin-resistant *S. aureus* and vancomycin-resistant enterococci have become increasingly common and are associated with increased mortality rates from IE.

Once organisms adhere to the injured surface, they may be protected from phagocytic activity by overlying fibrin. The organisms are then free to multiply, which enlarges the infected vegetation. The latter provides a source for continuous bacteremia and can lead to several complications, including (1) mechanical cardiac injury, (2) thrombotic or septic emboli, and

TABLE 8-3 Microbiology of Infective Endocarditis (*n* = 2781)	
Organism	**Incidence (%)**
Staphylococci	
S. aureus	31
Coagulase negative	11
Streptococci	
Viridans	17
Enterococci	10
S. bovis	6
Other streptococci	6
Other organisms (eg, gram-negative bacteria, fungi)	8
Culture negative or polymicrobial	11

Derived from Murdoch DR, Corey GR, Hoen B, et al. Clinical presentation, etiology, and outcome of infective endocarditis in the 21st century: the International Collaboration on Endocarditis-Prospective Cohort Study. *Arch Intern Med*. 2009;169:463.

(3) immune injury mediated by antigen-antibody deposition. For example, local extension of the infection within the heart can result in progressive valvular damage, abscess formation, or erosion into the cardiac conduction system. Portions of a vegetation may embolize, often to the central nervous system, kidneys, or spleen, and incite infection or infarction of the target organs. Additionally, immune complex deposition can result in glomerulonephritis, arthritis, or vasculitis.

CLINICAL MANIFESTATIONS

A patient with *acute* IE is likely to report an explosive and rapidly progressive illness with high fever and shaking chills. In contrast, *subacute* IE presents less dramatically with low-grade fever often accompanied by nonspecific constitutional symptoms such as fatigue, anorexia, weakness, myalgia, and night sweats. These symptoms are not specific for IE and could easily be mistaken for influenza or an upper respiratory tract infection. Thus, the diagnosis of subacute IE requires a high index of suspicion. A history of a valve lesion or other condition known to predispose to endocarditis is helpful. A thorough history should also inquire about injection drug use, prior valvular disease, recent dental procedures, and other potential sources of bacteremia.

Cardiac examination may reveal a murmur representing underlying valvular pathology that predisposed the patient to IE or a new murmur of valvular insufficiency owing to IE-induced damage. The development of right-sided valve lesions (eg, TR), although rare in normal hosts, is particularly common in endocarditis associated with intravenous drug abuse. During the course of endocarditis, severe valvular destruction may result in signs of heart failure, which is the leading cause of death in patients with IE.

Other physical findings that may appear in IE are those associated with septic embolism or immune complex deposition. Central nervous system emboli occur in up to 40% of patients, often resulting in new neurologic findings on physical examination. Injury to the kidneys, of embolic or immunologic origin, may manifest as flank pain, hematuria, or renal failure. Lung infarction (septic pulmonary embolism) or infection (pneumonia) is particularly common in endocarditis that involves right-sided valves.

Embolic infarction and seeding of the vasa vasorum of arteries can cause localized aneurysm formation (termed a *mycotic aneurysm*) that weakens the vessel wall and may rupture. Mycotic aneurysms may be found in the aorta, viscera, or peripheral organs and are particularly dangerous in cerebral vessels, because rupture there can result in fatal intracranial hemorrhage.

Skin findings resulting from septic embolism or immune complex vasculitis are often collectively referred to as *peripheral stigmata* of endocarditis. For example, petechiae may appear as tiny, circular, red-brown discolorations on mucosal surfaces or skin. *Splinter hemorrhages*, the result of subungual microemboli, are small, longitudinal hemorrhages found beneath finger nails. Other peripheral stigmata of IE, which are now rarely encountered, include painless, flat, irregular discolorations found on the palms and soles called *Janeway lesions*; tender, pea-sized, erythematous nodules found primarily in the pulp space of the fingers and toes termed *Osler nodes*; and emboli to the retina that produce *Roth spots*, microinfarctions that appear as white dots surrounded by hemorrhage.

The systemic inflammatory response produced by the infection is responsible for fever and splenomegaly, as well as for a number of laboratory findings, including an elevated white blood cell count with a leftward shift (increase in proportion of neutrophils and immature granulocytes), an elevated erythrocyte sedimentation rate and C-reactive protein level, and in ∼50% of cases, an elevated serum rheumatoid factor.

The *electrocardiogram* may help identify extension of the infection into the cardiac conduction system, manifested by various degrees of heart block or new arrhythmias. *Echocardiography* is used to visualize vegetations, valvular dysfunction, and associated abscess formation.

Echocardiographic assessment can consist of transthoracic echocardiography (TTE) or transesophageal echocardiography (TEE), as described in Chapter 3. TTE is useful in detecting large vegetations and has the advantage of being noninvasive and easy to obtain. However, while the *specificity* of TTE for vegetations is high, the *sensitivity* for finding small vegetations is <65%. TEE, on the other hand, is much more sensitive (>90%) for the detection of vegetations and myocardial abscess formation and can be particularly useful for the evaluation of infection involving prosthetic valves.

Central to the diagnosis and appropriate treatment of endocarditis is the identification of the responsible microorganism by blood culture. Once positive culture results are obtained, treatment can be tailored to the causative organism according to its antibiotic sensitivities. A specific etiologic agent is identified ~90% of the time. However, blood cultures may return negative if antibiotics have already been administered or if the organism has unusual growth requirements.

Even after a careful history, examination, and evaluation of laboratory data, the diagnosis of IE can be elusive. Therefore, attempts have been made to standardize the diagnosis, resulting in the widely used Duke criteria (Table 8-4). By this standard, the diagnosis of endocarditis rests on the presence of either two major criteria, one major and three minor criteria,

TABLE 8-4	Modified Duke Criteria for Diagnosis of Infective Endocarditis (IE)[a]
Major Criteria	**Minor Criteria**

I. Positive blood culture, defined as either A or B
  A. Typical microorganism for IE from two separate blood cultures:
    1. *Streptococcus viridans*, *S. bovis*, HACEK group
    2. *Staphylococcus aureus* or enterococci, in the absence of a primary focus
  B. Microorganisms consistent with IE from persistently positive blood cultures:
    1. Blood cultures drawn >12 h apart
    2. All of three, or most of four, separate cultures drawn at least 1 h apart
    3. Single positive blood culture for *Coxiella burnetii* or antiphase I IgG antibody titer >1:800
II. Evidence of endocardial involvement, defined as A or B:
  A. Echocardiogram positive for endocarditis:
    1. Oscillating intracardiac mass
    2. Myocardial abscess
    3. New partial detachment of prosthetic valve
  B. New valvular regurgitation
	Predisposing cardiac condition or intravenous drug use
	Fever (≥38.0°C)
	Vascular phenomena (septic arterial or pulmonary emboli, mycotic aneurysm, intracranial hemorrhage, conjunctival hemorrhage, Janeway lesions)
	Immunologic phenomena (glomerulonephritis, Osler nodes, Roth spots, rheumatoid factor)
	Positive blood cultures not meeting major criteria or serologic evidence of infection with organism consistent with IE

[a]Clinical diagnosis of definite endocarditis requires two major criteria, one major plus three minor criteria, or five minor criteria. Possible endocarditis requires one major plus one minor criteria or three minor criteria.
HACEK, *Haemophilus* spp., *Actinobacillus actinomycetemcomitans*, *Cardiobacterium hominis*, *Eikenella* spp., and *Kingella kingae*.
Derived from Li JS, Sexton DJ, Mick N, et al. Proposed modifications to the Duke criteria for the diagnosis of infective endocarditis. *Clin Infect Dis*. 2000;30:633-638.

or five minor criteria. Positive blood cultures and endocardial involvement detected by echo-cardiography provide the strongest evidence for IE and are considered major criteria. Minor criteria relate to clinical risk factors and findings on physical examination.

TREATMENT

Treatment of endocarditis entails 4-6 weeks of high-dose intravenous antibiotic therapy. Although empiric broad-spectrum antibiotics may be used initially (after blood cultures are obtained) for patients who are severely ill or hemodynamically unstable, specific, directed therapy is appropriate once the causative microorganism has been identified. Current studies are assessing the role of substituting oral antibiotics after a shortened course of intravenous therapy for patients with stable endocarditis. Surgical intervention, usually with valve replacement, is indicated for patients with persistent bacteremia or fever despite appropriate antibiotic therapy, for those with severe valvular dysfunction leading to heart failure, and for individuals who develop myocardial abscesses or recurrent endocarditis-related thromboemboli.

PREVENTION

An additional essential concept is *prevention* of endocarditis by administering antibiotics to certain susceptible individuals before invasive procedures that are likely to result in bacteremia. The American Heart Association recommends such antibiotic prophylaxis for the cardiac conditions that place them at the highest risk for developing an adverse outcome from IE, as delineated in Table 8-5, when such individuals are subjected to procedures listed in the table.

TABLE 8-5   Antibiotic Prophylaxis for Infective Endocarditis

Cardiac conditions for which antibiotic prophylaxis is reasonable[a]
1. Presence of a prosthetic heart valve or prior valve repair with prosthetic material
2. Prior history of endocarditis
3. Certain congenital heart diseases (CHD):
   - Unrepaired cyanotic CHD (described in Chapter 16)
   - Completely repaired congenital heart defects with prosthetic material, during the first 6 mo after the procedure (ie, prior to protective endothelialization)
   - Repaired CHD with residual defects adjacent to the site of prosthetic material (which inhibits endothelialization)
4. Cardiac transplant recipients who develop cardiac valve abnormalities

Procedures that warrant antibiotic therapy for conditions listed above
1. Dental procedures that involve manipulation of gingival tissue, manipulation of periapical region of the teeth, or perforation of the oral mucosa
2. Upper respiratory tract procedures, *only if* involves incision or biopsy of mucosa (eg, tonsillectomy, bronchoscopy with biopsy)
3. Genitourinary or gastrointestinal procedures, *only if* infections of those systems are present
4. Procedures on *infected* skin or musculoskeletal tissue

[a]The conditions on this list have the highest risk of adverse outcomes from endocarditis.
Derived from Wilson W, Taubert KA, Gewitz M, et al. Prevention of infective endocarditis: guidelines from the American Heart Association: a guideline from the American Heart Association Rheumatic Fever, Endocarditis, and Kawasaki Disease Committee, Council on Cardiovascular Disease in the Young, and the Council on Clinical Cardiology, Council on Cardiovascular Surgery and Anesthesia, and the Quality of Care and Outcomes Research Interdisciplinary Working Group. *Circulation.* 2007;116:1736-1754.

Summary

- Effective management of valvular heart disease requires identification of the valve abnormality, a determination of its severity, and an understanding of the pathophysiologic consequences and natural history of the condition (Table 8-6).

- Diagnosis of valvular disease is assisted by transthoracic echocardiography (TTE) and/or transesophageal echocardiography (TEE); in selected patients, additional imaging may be necessary.

- Management of patients with stenotic or regurgitant valves involves serial clinical and echocardiographic assessments; pharmacologic therapy is sometimes prescribed for symptomatic improvement, but recognition of timely indications for valve repair or replacement is essential.

- **Mitral stenosis** usually results from prior rheumatic fever; left atrial (LA) enlargement and atrial fibrillation are common.

- **Mitral regurgitation** (MR) arises from disruption of the structural integrity of any of the components of the mitral valve apparatus or their coordinated action; with chronic MR, LA enlargement and left ventricular (LV) volume overload are typical.

- In **mitral valve prolapse**, the valve leaflets are elongated, and the normal dense collagen and elastin matrix of the valvular fibrosa is fragmented and replaced with loose myxomatous connective tissue; one or both leaflets bow into the LA during systole resulting in lack of coaptation and mitral regurgitation.

- **Aortic stenosis** has three primary causes: (1) degenerative calcification of a previously normal trileaflet aortic valve, (2) calcification of a congenitally bicuspid aortic valve, and (3) rheumatic valve disease; the primary hemodynamic consequence is LV pressure overload with compensatory LV hypertrophy; cardinal symptoms are chest discomfort, exertional dyspnea, and exertional light-headedness.

- **Aortic regurgitation** may result either from abnormalities of the aortic valve leaflets or from dilatation of the aortic root; the primary hemodynamic perturbation is LV volume overload.

- **Tricuspid stenosis** is rare and is usually a delayed consequence of rheumatic fever.

- **Tricuspid regurgitation** is typically functional (due to RV enlargement) rather than structural in nature.

- **Pulmonic stenosis** is rare, and its cause is almost always congenital deformity of the valve.

- **Pulmonic regurgitation** most commonly develops in the setting of severe pulmonary hypertension and results from dilatation of the valve ring by an enlarged pulmonary artery.

- The pathogenesis of **endocarditis** requires endocardial surface injury, platelet-fibrin-thrombus formation at the site of injury, bacterial entry into the circulation, and bacterial adherence to the injured endocardial surface.

TABLE 8-6 Summary of Major Valvular Conditions

Valve Lesion	Causes	Symptoms	Physical Findings	Murmur Diagram
Mitral stenosis (MS)	Sequelae of rheumatic fever	Symptoms of left-sided (and later right-sided) heart failure[a]	• Loud S₁ (in early MS) • Opening snap • Diastolic rumble (loudest in left lateral decubitus position)	
Mitral regurgitation (MR)	*Acute:* • Endocarditis • Ruptured chordae • Papillary muscle rupture *Chronic:* • Rheumatic • Mitral prolapse • Calcified annulus • LV dilatation • Adverse remodeling after MI	*Acute:* • Pulmonary edema *Chronic:* • Symptoms of left-sided heart failure[a] and low cardiac output (eg, fatigue)	• Holosystolic murmur at apex (may be decrescendo in *acute* MR) • Murmur accentuated by hand grip	
Aortic stenosis (AS)	• Degenerative calcific • Congenital • Rheumatic	• Chest pain • Syncope • Dyspnea on exertion	• Carotids: delayed upstroke and decreased volume • Palpation: suprasternal thrill *Auscultation:* • Soft A₂ • Systolic ejection–type murmur (loudest at upper right sternal border)	
Aortic regurgitation (AR)	• Congenital (eg, bicuspid valve) • Endocarditis • Rheumatic • Aortic root dilatation	• Dyspnea on exertion • Chest pain (sometimes)	• Wide pulse pressure • Bounding pulses • Early diastolic decrescendo murmur (heard best at end expiration, with patient leaning forward)	

[a]Symptoms of left-sided heart failure include exertional dyspnea, orthopnea, and paroxysmal nocturnal dyspnea; symptoms of right-sided heart failure include peripheral edema, abdominal bloating, and right upper quadrant tenderness (hepatic enlargement).

A₂, aortic component of second heart sound; LV, left ventricular; S₁, first heart sound; S₂, second heart sound.

Review Questions

1. Which of the following valvular conditions presents primarily a pressure load to the left ventricle?

   a. Mitral stenosis
   b. Chronic mitral regurgitation
   c. Aortic stenosis
   d. Chronic aortic regurgitation

2. Which of the following statements regarding right-sided cardiac valvular disease is true?

   a. Most cases of pulmonic stenosis are acquired later in life.
   b. Endocarditis associated with intravenous drug use most commonly affects the tricuspid valve.
   c. Tricuspid regurgitation more commonly arises from a primary valvular abnormality than as a result of right ventricular pressure or volume overload.
   d. Pulmonic regurgitation is most often due to rheumatic deformity of the valve.

3. For which of the following patients would it be appropriate to prescribe antibiotic prophylaxis for the prevention of bacterial endocarditis?

   a. A 35-year-old woman with a mechanical mitral valve scheduled for a routine dental cleaning
   b. A 47-year-old man with history of endocarditis undergoing a cervical lymph node biopsy
   c. A 58-year-old man with an aortic bioprosthetic aortic valve undergoing cystoscopy for evaluation of hematuria
   d. A 40-year-old woman with mitral valve prolapse and severe mitral regurgitation about to undergo root canal dental surgery

4. (Advanced question) A 71-year-old man with known aortic stenosis has developed progressive shortness of breath with exertion. Transthoracic echocardiography shows the following: LV ejection fraction = 35% (normal LV ejection fraction is ≥55%, as described in Chapter 9), mean pressure gradient across the aortic valve = 26 mm Hg, and calculated aortic valve area = 0.7 cm² (normal is >3.0 cm²). Should this patient be referred for aortic valve replacement?

   a. Yes—The aortic valve area (AVA) is <1.0 cm², consistent with severe aortic stenosis.
   b. No—Although the AVA is <1.0 cm², the low mean pressure gradient across the valve indicates that severe aortic stenosis is not present.
   c. Yes—Severe aortic stenosis is the cause of the reduced LV ejection fraction, which is an indication for aortic valve replacement.
   d. Additional testing is needed to determine if this patient truly has severe aortic stenosis.

Answers to Review Questions

1. **Choice c is correct.** Obstruction to left ventricular outflow in aortic stenosis presents a pressure load to the left ventricle, which compensates through concentric hypertrophy. Mitral and aortic regurgitation each present primarily a *volume* load to the LV, ultimately resulting in chamber dilatation out of proportion to increased wall thickness (eccentric

hypertrophy). Mitral stenosis impairs filling of the LV and presents neither a pressure nor volume load on the chamber.

2. **Choice b is correct.** Endocarditis resulting from intravenous drug abuse most commonly affects the tricuspid valve; mitral and aortic involvement occurs less frequently. Most cases of pulmonic stenosis are congenital in nature and are present at birth. Tricuspid regurgitation is most often functional, due to RV volume or pressure overload, rather than a result of a primary structural valve disorder. Significant pulmonic regurgitation typically develops as a result of pulmonary hypertension.

3. **Choice a is correct.** This patient in choice "a" has a mechanical valve prosthesis that places her at risk of endocarditis from transient bacteremia that can occur during dental cleaning, thus antibiotic prophylaxis is appropriate. Lymph node biopsy and genitourinary procedures in the absence of a urinary tract infection do not generally result in bacteremia so that antibiotic prophylaxis for endocarditis prevention is not recommended in those scenarios. Mitral valve prolapse and mitral regurgitation are not indications for antibiotic prophylaxis per current guidelines.

4. **Choice d is correct.** This patient has a markedly reduced calculated aortic valve area suggestive of severe aortic stenosis, but the mean transvalvular gradient (<40 mm Hg) does not confirm that diagnosis. Of note, in the setting of this patient's poor contractile function (EF < 40%), the left ventricular stroke volume may be too low to generate the high pressure gradient typically present in true severe aortic stenosis (a condition termed "low-flow low-gradient aortic stenosis"). In this scenario, it is important to determine if the low ejection fraction is a result of truly severe AS or if there is an underlying heart muscle disorder (a form of cardiomyopathy, as described in Chapter 9) causing the low EF and shortness of breath and, in turn, resulting in underestimation of the transvalvular gradient and calculated aortic valve area. Additional testing is needed to differentiate these two possibilities.

This patient therefore underwent dobutamine stress echocardiography (described in Chapter 3), during which the infusion of the ionotrope dobutamine augmented contractility and thus LV stroke volume. During the infusion, the LV ejection fraction rose, the transvalvular mean gradient increased to >40 mm Hg, while the calculated AVA remained <1.0 cm^2, confirming the diagnosis of truly severe aortic stenosis, and he was referred for aortic valve replacement. Had an underlying cardiomyopathy been the cause of the low EF and pressure gradient, dobutamine infusion would have augmented the EF, and the calculated AVA would have increased >1.0 cm^2 as a result of more forceful contraction, showing that the valve was not truly severely stenotic.

Acknowledgments

Contributors to previous editions of this chapter were Elizabeth Ryznar, MD; Christopher A. Miller, MD; Mia M. Edwards, MD; Patrick Yachimski, MD; Stephen K. Frankel, MD; Edward Chan, MD; Elia Duh, MD; Brian Stidham, MD; and John A. Bittl, MD.

Additional Reading

Habib G, Lancellotti P, Antunes MJ, et al. 2015 ESC Guidelines for the management of infective endocarditis. *Eur Heart J.* 2015;36:3075-3128.

Iversen K, Ihlemann N, Gill SU, et al. Partial oral versus intravenous antibiotic treatment of endocarditis. *N Engl J Med.* 2019;380:415-424.

Mack MJ, Leon MB, Thourani VH, et al. Transcatheter aortic-valve replacement with a balloon-expandable valve in low risk patients. *N Engl J Med.* 2019;380:1695-1705.

Nishimura RA, Otto CM, Bonow RO, et al. 2017 AHA/ACC Focused Update of the 2014 AHA/ACC Guideline for the management of patients with valvular heart disease. *J Am Coll Cardiol.* 2017;70:252-289.

Rudasill SE, Sanaiha Y, Mardock AL, et al. Clinical outcomes of infective endocarditis in injection drug users. *J Am Coll Cardiol.* 2019;73(5):559.

Watkins DA, Beaton AZ, Carapetis JR, et al. Rheumatic heart disease worldwide. *J Am Coll Cardiol.* 2018;72:1397-1416.

Wilson W, Taubert KA, Gewitz M, et al. Prevention of infective endocarditis: guidelines from the American Heart Association. *Circulation.* 2007;116:1736-1754.

Heart Failure

Lauren A. Eberly | Eldrin F. Lewis | Leonard S. Lilly

The heart normally accepts blood at low filling pressures during diastole and then propels it forward at higher pressures in systole. Heart failure is present when the heart is unable to pump blood forward at a sufficient rate to meet the metabolic demands of the body or is able to do so only if cardiac filling pressures are abnormally high. Although conditions outside the heart may cause this definition to be met through inadequate tissue perfusion (eg, severe hemorrhage) or increased metabolic demands (eg, hyperthyroidism), in this chapter, only cardiac causes of heart failure are considered.

Heart failure results in a clinical syndrome of fatigue, shortness of breath, and often volume overload. It may be the final and most severe manifestation of nearly every form of cardiac disease, including coronary atherosclerosis, myocardial infarction, valvular diseases, hypertension, congenital heart disease, and the cardiomyopathies. The current prevalence of heart failure in the United States is 6.2 million, and the number of patients with this condition is increasing, not only because the population is aging but also because of interventions that prolong survival after damaging cardiac insults such as myocardial infarction. As a result, heart failure accounts for more than 16 million outpatient visits annually and is one of the most common diagnoses of hospitalized patients aged 65 years and older.

Heart failure most commonly results from conditions of impaired left ventricular function. Thus, this chapter begins by reviewing the physiology of normal myocardial contraction and relaxation.

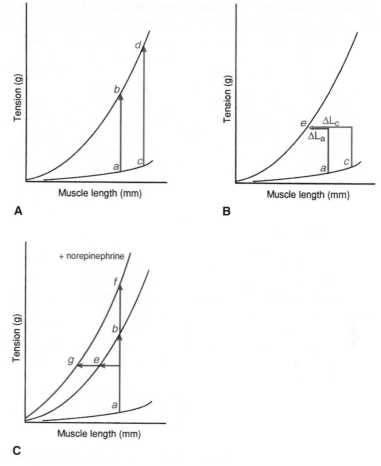

Figure 9-1. Physiology of normal cardiac muscle segments. A. Passive (*lower curve*) and total (*upper curve*) length-tension relations for isolated cat papillary muscle. Lines *ab* and *cd* represent the force developed during isometric contractions. Initial passive muscle length *c* is longer (ie, has been stretched more) than length *a* and therefore has a greater passive tension. When the muscle segments are stimulated to contract, the muscle with the longer initial length generates greater total tension (point *d* vs point *b*). **B.** If the muscle fiber preparation is allowed to shorten against a fixed load, the length at the end of the contraction is dependent on the load but not the initial fiber length; stimulation at point *a* or *c* results in the same final fiber length (*e*). Thus, the muscle that starts at length *c* shortens a greater distance (ΔL_c) than the muscle at length *a* (ΔL_a). **C.** The uppermost curve is the length-tension relation in the presence of the positive inotropic agent norepinephrine. For any given initial length, an isometric contraction in the presence of norepinephrine generates greater force (point *f*) than one in the absence of norepinephrine (point *b*). When contracting against a fixed load, the presence of norepinephrine causes greater muscle fiber shortening and a smaller final muscle length (point *g*) compared with contraction in the absence of the inotropic agent (point *e*). (Adapted from Downing SE, Sonnenblick EH. Cardiac muscle mechanics and ventricular performance: force and time parameters. *Am J Physiol.* 1964;207:705-715.)

PHYSIOLOGY

Experimental studies of isolated cardiac muscle segments have revealed several important principles that can be applied to the intact heart. As a muscle segment is stretched apart, the relation between its length and the tension it passively develops is curvilinear, reflecting its intrinsic elastic properties (Fig. 9-1A, lower curve). If the muscle is first passively stretched and then stimulated to contract while its ends are held at fixed positions (termed an *isometric* contraction), the total tension (the sum of active plus passive tension) generated by the fibers is proportional to the length of the muscle at the time of stimulation (see Fig. 9-1A, upper curve). That is, stretching the muscle before stimulation optimizes the overlap and interaction of myosin and actin filaments, increasing the number of cross bridges and the force of contraction. Stretching cardiac muscle fibers also increases the sensitivity of the myofilaments to calcium, augmenting force development.

This relationship between the initial fiber length and force development is of great importance in the intact heart: within a physiologic range, the larger the ventricular volume during diastole, the more the fibers are stretched before stimulation and the greater the force of the next contraction. This is the basis of the **Frank-Starling relationship**, the observation that ventricular output increases in relation to the **preload** (the stretch on the myocardial fibers before contraction).

A second observation from isolated muscle experiments arises when the fibers are not tethered at a fixed length but are allowed to shorten during stimulation against a fixed load (termed the **afterload**). In this situation (termed an *isotonic* contraction), the final length of the muscle at the end of contraction is determined by the magnitude of the load but is *independent* of the length of the muscle before stimulation (see Fig. 9-1B). That is, (1) the tension generated by the fiber is equal to the fixed load; (2) the greater the load opposing contraction, the less the muscle fiber can shorten; (3) if the fiber is stretched to a longer length before stimulation but the afterload is kept constant, the muscle will shorten a greater distance to attain the same final length at the end of contraction; and (4) the maximum tension that can be produced during isotonic contraction (ie, using a load sufficiently great such that the muscle is just unable to shorten) is the same as the force produced by an isometric contraction at that initial fiber length.

This concept of afterload is also relevant to the intact heart: the pressure generated by the ventricle and the size of the chamber at the end of each contraction depend on the load against which the ventricle contracts but are independent of the stretch on the myocardial fibers before contraction.

A third key experimental observation relates to myocardial **contractility**, which accounts for changes in the force of contraction independent of the initial fiber length and afterload. Contractility reflects chemical and hormonal influences on cardiac contraction, such as exposure to catecholamines. When contractility is enhanced pharmacologically (eg, by a norepinephrine infusion), the relation between initial fiber length and force developed during contraction is shifted upward (see Fig. 9-1C) such that a greater total tension develops with isometric contraction at any given preload. Similarly, when contractility is augmented and the cardiac muscle is allowed to shorten against a fixed afterload, the fiber contracts to a greater extent and achieves a shorter final fiber length compared with the baseline state. At the molecular level, enhanced contractility is likely related to an increased cycling rate of actin-myosin cross-bridge formation.

DETERMINANTS OF CONTRACTILE FUNCTION IN THE INTACT HEART

In a healthy person, cardiac output (CO) is matched to the body's total metabolic need. CO is equal to the product of stroke volume (SV, the volume of blood ejected with each contraction) and the heart rate (HR):

$$CO = SV \times HR$$

The three major determinants of SV are preload, afterload, and myocardial contractility, as shown in Figure 9-2.

Preload

The concept of preload (Table 9-1) in the intact heart was described by physiologists Frank and Starling a century ago. In experimental preparations, they showed that within physiologic limits, the more a normal ventricle is distended (ie, filled with blood) during diastole, the greater the volume that is ejected during the next systolic contraction. This relationship is illustrated graphically by the Frank-Starling curve, also known as the ventricular function curve (Fig. 9-3). The graph relates a measurement of cardiac performance (such as CO or SV) on the vertical axis as a function of preload on the horizontal axis. As described earlier,

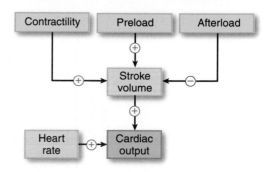

Figure 9-2. Key mediators of cardiac output. Determinants of the stroke volume include contractility, preload, and afterload. Cardiac output = heart rate × stroke volume.

the preload can be thought of as the amount of myocardial stretch at the end of diastole, just before contraction. Measurements that correlate with myocardial stretch, and that are often used to indicate the preload on the horizontal axis, are the ventricular end-diastolic volume (EDV) or end-diastolic pressure (EDP). Conditions that decrease intravascular volume, and thereby reduce ventricular preload (eg, dehydration or severe hemorrhage), result in a smaller EDV and hence a reduced SV during contraction. Conversely, an increased volume within the left ventricle (LV) during diastole (eg, a large intravenous fluid infusion) results in a greater-than-normal SV.

TABLE 9-1	Terms Related to Cardiac Performance
Term	**Definition**
Preload	The ventricular wall tension at the end of diastole. In clinical terms, it is the stretch on the ventricular fibers just before contraction, often approximated by the end-diastolic volume or end-diastolic pressure
Afterload	The ventricular wall tension during contraction; the force that must be overcome for the ventricle to eject its contents
Contractility (inotropic state)	Property of heart muscle that accounts for changes in the strength of contraction, independent of the preload and afterload. Reflects chemical or hormonal influences on the force of contraction
Stroke volume (SV)	Volume of blood ejected from the ventricle with each systolic contraction SV = end-diastolic volume − end-systolic volume
Ejection fraction (EF)	The fraction of end-diastolic volume ejected from the ventricle during each systolic contraction (normal range = 55%-75%) EF = stroke volume ÷ end-diastolic volume
Cardiac output (CO)	Volume of blood ejected from the ventricle per minute CO = SV × heart rate
Compliance	Intrinsic property of a chamber that describes its pressure-volume relationship during filling. Reflects the ease or difficulty with which the chamber can be filled. Compliance = Δvolume ÷ Δpressure

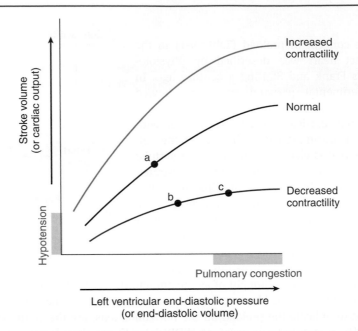

Figure 9-3. Left ventricular (LV) performance (Frank-Starling) curves relate preload, measured as LV end-diastolic volume (EDV) or pressure (EDP), to cardiac performance, measured as ventricular stroke volume or cardiac output. On the curve of a normal heart (*middle line*), cardiac performance continuously increases as a function of preload. States of increased contractility (eg, norepinephrine infusion) are characterized by an augmented stroke volume at any level of preload (*upper line*). Conversely, decreased LV contractility (associated with a major form of heart failure) is characterized by a curve that is shifted downward (*lower line*). Point *a* is an example of a normal person at rest. Point *b* represents the same person after developing systolic dysfunction and heart failure (eg, after a large myocardial infarction): stroke volume has fallen, and the decreased LV emptying results in elevation of the EDV. Because point *b* is on the ascending portion of the curve, the elevated EDV serves a compensatory role because it results in an increase in subsequent stroke volume, albeit less than if operating on the normal curve. Further augmentation of LV filling (eg, increased circulating volume) in the heart failure patient is represented by point *c*, which resides on the relatively flat part of the curve: stroke volume is only slightly augmented, but the significantly increased EDP results in pulmonary congestion.

Afterload

Afterload (see Table 9-1) in the intact heart reflects the force that the ventricle must overcome to empty its contents. It is more accurately defined as the ventricular wall stress that develops during systolic ejection. Wall stress (σ), like pressure, is expressed as force per unit area and, for the LV, may be estimated from Laplace relationship:

$$\sigma = \frac{P \times r}{2h}$$

where P is ventricular pressure, r is ventricular chamber radius, and h is ventricular wall thickness. Thus, ventricular wall stress rises in response to a higher pressure load (eg, hypertension) or an increased chamber size (eg, a dilated LV). Conversely, as would be expected from the Laplace relationship, an increase in wall thickness (h) serves a compensatory role in *reducing* wall stress, because the force is distributed over a greater mass per unit surface area of ventricular muscle.

Contractility (Also Termed "Inotropic State")

In the intact heart, as in the isolated muscle preparation example, contractility accounts for changes in myocardial force for a given set of preload and afterload conditions, resulting from chemical and hormonal influences. By relating a measure of ventricular performance (SV or CO) to preload (left ventricular EDP or EDV), each Frank-Starling curve is a reflection of the heart's current inotropic state (see Fig. 9-3). The effect on SV by an alteration in preload is reflected by a change in position along a particular Frank-Starling curve. Conversely, a change in contractility shifts the entire curve in an upward or downward direction. Thus, when contractility is enhanced pharmacologically (eg, by an infusion of norepinephrine), the ventricular performance curve is displaced upward such that at any given preload, the SV is increased. Conversely, when a drug that reduces contractility is administered, or the ventricle's contractile function is impaired (as in certain types of heart failure), the curve shifts in a downward direction, leading to reductions in SV and CO at any given preload.

PRESSURE-VOLUME LOOPS

Another useful graphic display to illustrate the determinants of cardiac function is the ventricular pressure-volume loop, which relates changes in ventricular volume to corresponding changes in pressure throughout the cardiac cycle (Fig. 9-4). In the LV, filling of the chamber begins after the mitral valve (MV) opens in early diastole (point *a*). The curve between points *a* and *b* represents diastolic filling. As the volume increases during diastole, it is associated

Figure 9-4. Example of a normal left ventricular (LV) pressure-volume loop. At point *a*, the MV opens and filling of the LV commences. During passive diastolic filling of the LV (line *ab*), its volume increases with a gradual rise in pressure. When ventricular contraction commences and its pressure exceeds that of the left atrium, the MV closes (point *b*) and isovolumetric contraction of the LV ensues (the aortic valve is not yet open, and no blood leaves the chamber), as shown by line *bc*. When LV pressure rises to that in the aorta, the aortic valve (AV) opens (point *c*), and ejection begins. The volume within the LV declines during ejection (line *cd*), but LV pressure continues to rise until ventricular relaxation commences, and then it begins to lessen. At point *d*, the LV pressure during relaxation falls below that in the aorta, and the AV closes, leading to isovolumetric relaxation (line *da*). As LV pressure declines further to below that in the left atrium, the MV reopens (point *a*). Point *b* represents the end-diastolic volume (EDV) and pressure, and point *d* is the end-systolic volume (ESV) and pressure. Stroke volume is calculated as the difference between the EDV and ESV.

with a small rise in pressure, in accordance with the passive length-tension properties or **compliance** (see Table 9-1) of the myocardium, analogous to the lower curve in Figure 9-1A for an isolated muscle preparation.

Next, the onset of left ventricular systolic contraction causes the ventricular pressure to rise. When the pressure in the LV exceeds that of the left atrium (point *b*), the MV is forced to close. As the pressure continues to increase, the ventricular volume does not immediately change, because the aortic valve has not yet opened and blood is neither entering nor leaving the chamber; therefore, this phase is called **isovolumetric contraction**. When the rise in ventricular pressure reaches the aortic diastolic pressure, the aortic valve is forced to open (point *c*), and ejection of blood into the aorta commences. During ejection, the volume within the ventricle decreases, but its pressure continues to rise until ventricular relaxation begins. The pressure against which the ventricle ejects (a component of afterload) is represented by the curve *cd*. Ejection ends during the relaxation phase, when the ventricular pressure falls below that of the aorta and the aortic valve closes (point *d*).

As the ventricle continues to relax, its pressure declines while its volume remains constant because the MV has not yet opened (this phase is known as **isovolumetric relaxation**). When the ventricular pressure falls below that of the left atrium, the MV opens again (point *a*), and the cycle repeats.

Note that point *b* represents the pressure and volume at the end of diastole, whereas point *d* represents the pressure and volume at the end of systole. The difference between the EDV and end-systolic volume (ESV) represents the quantity of blood ejected during contraction (ie, the stroke volume).

Changes in any of the determinants of cardiac function are reflected by alterations in the pressure-volume loop. By analyzing the effects of a change in an individual parameter (preload, afterload, or contractility) on the pressure-volume relationship, the resulting modifications in ventricular pressure and SV can be predicted (Fig. 9-5).

Alterations in Preload

If afterload and contractility are held constant but preload is caused to increase (eg, by administration of intravenous fluid), left ventricular EDV rises. This increase in preload augments the SV via the Frank-Starling mechanism such that the ESV achieved is the same as it was before increasing the preload (see Fig. 9-5A). This means that the normal LV is able to adjust its SV and effectively empty its contents to match its diastolic filling volume, as long as contractility and afterload are kept constant.

Although EDV and EDP are often used interchangeably as markers of preload, the relationship between filling volume and pressure (ie, ventricular compliance; see Table 9-1) largely governs the extent of ventricular filling. If ventricular compliance is reduced (eg, in severe LV hypertrophy), the slope of the diastolic filling curve (segment *ab* in Fig. 9-4) becomes steeper. A "stiff" or poorly compliant ventricle reduces the ability of the chamber to fill during diastole, resulting in a lower-than-normal ventricular EDV. In this circumstance, the SV will be reduced while the ESV remains unchanged.

Alterations in Afterload

If preload and contractility are held constant and afterload is augmented (eg, in high-impedance states such as hypertension or aortic stenosis), the pressure generated by the LV during ejection increases. In this situation, more ventricular work is expended in overcoming the resistance to ejection, and therefore less fiber shortening takes place. As shown in Figure 9-5B, an increase in afterload results in a higher ventricular systolic pressure and a greater-than-normal LV ESV. Thus, in the setting of increased afterload, the ventricular stroke volume (EDV-ESV) is reduced.

Figure 9-5. The effect of varying preload, afterload, and contractility on the pressure-volume loop.
A. When arterial pressure (afterload) and contractility are held constant, sequential increases (lines *1*, *2*, and *3*) in preload (measured in this case as end-diastolic volume [EDV]) are associated with loops that have progressively higher stroke volumes but a constant end-systolic volume (ESV). **B.** When the preload (EDV) and contractility are held constant, sequential increases (points *1*, *2*, and *3*) in arterial pressure (afterload) are associated with loops that have progressively lower stroke volumes and higher end-systolic volumes. There is a nearly linear relationship between the afterload and ESV, termed the end-systolic pressure-volume relation (ESPVR). **C.** A positive inotropic intervention shifts the end-systolic pressure-volume relation upward and leftward from ESPVR-1 to ESPVR-2, resulting in loop 2, which has a larger stroke volume and a smaller end-systolic volume than the original loop 1.

The dependence of the ESV on afterload is approximately linear: the greater the afterload, the higher the ESV. This relationship is depicted in Figure 9-5 as the **end-systolic pressure-volume relation (ESPVR)** and is analogous to the total tension curve in the isolated muscle experiments described earlier.

Alterations in Contractility

The slope of the ESPVR line on the pressure-volume loop graph is a function of cardiac contractility. In conditions of increased contractility, the ESPVR slope becomes steeper; that is, it shifts upward and toward the left. Hence, at any given preload or afterload, the ventricle empties more completely (the SV increases) and results in a smaller-than-normal ESV (see Fig. 9-5C). Conversely, in situations of reduced contractility, the ESPVR line shifts downward, consistent with a decline in SV and a higher ESV. Thus, the ESV is *dependent* on the afterload against which the ventricle contracts and the inotropic state but is *independent* of the EDV prior to contraction.

The important physiologic concepts in this section are summarized as follows:

1. Ventricular SV is a function of preload, afterload, and contractility. SV rises when there is an increase in preload, a decrease in afterload, or augmented contractility.
2. Ventricular EDV (or EDP) is used as a representation of preload. The EDV is influenced by the chamber's compliance.
3. Ventricular ESV depends on the afterload and contractility but not on the preload.

PATHOPHYSIOLOGY

Chronic heart failure may result from a wide variety of cardiovascular insults. The etiologies can be grouped into those that (1) impair ventricular contractility, (2) increase afterload, or (3) impair ventricular relaxation and filling (Fig. 9-6). Heart failure that results from an

Figure 9-6. Conditions that cause left-sided heart failure through impairment of ventricular systolic or diastolic function. [a]Note that in chronic stable stages, the conditions in this box (aortic stenosis, hypertension) may instead result in heart failure with *preserved* EF, due to compensatory ventricular hypertrophy and increased diastolic stiffness (diastolic dysfunction).

abnormality of ventricular emptying (due to impaired contractility or greatly excessive after-load) is termed *systolic dysfunction*, whereas heart failure caused by abnormalities of diastolic relaxation or ventricular filling is termed *diastolic dysfunction*. However, there is much over-lap, and many patients demonstrate both systolic and diastolic abnormalities. As a result, it is common to categorize heart failure patients into two general categories based on the left ven-tricular ejection fraction (LVEF), a measure of cardiac performance (see Table 9-1): (1) **heart failure with reduced ejection fraction (EF)** (ie, primarily systolic dysfunction) and (2) **heart failure with preserved EF** (ie, primarily diastolic dysfunction). In the United States, approxi-mately one-half of patients with heart failure fall into each of these categories.

Heart Failure With Reduced EF (HFrEF)

In states of systolic dysfunction, the affected ventricle has a diminished capacity to eject blood because of impaired myocardial contractility or pressure overload (ie, excessive after-load). Loss of contractility may result from destruction of myocytes, abnormal myocyte func-tion, or fibrosis. Pressure overload impairs ventricular ejection by significantly increasing resistance to flow.

Figure 9-7A depicts the effects of systolic dysfunction due to impaired contractility on the pressure-volume loop. The ESPVR is shifted downward such that systolic emptying ceases at a higher-than-normal ESV. As a result, the SV falls. When normal pulmonary venous return is added to the increased ESV that has remained in the ventricle because of incomplete empty-ing, the diastolic chamber volume increases, resulting in a higher-than-normal EDV and pres-sure. While that increase in preload induces a compensatory rise in SV (via the Frank-Starling mechanism), impaired contractility and the reduced EF cause the ESV to remain elevated.

During diastole, the persistently elevated LV pressure is transmitted to the left atrium (through the open MV) and to the pulmonary veins and capillaries. An elevated pulmonary

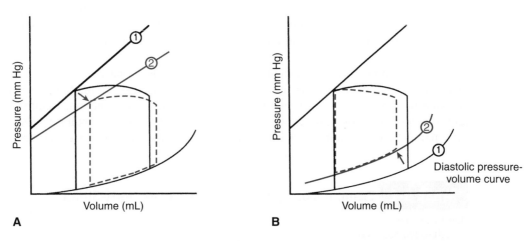

Figure 9-7. The pressure-volume loop in systolic and diastolic dysfunction. A. The normal pressure-volume loop (*solid line*) is compared with one demonstrating systolic dysfunction (*dashed line*). In systolic dysfunction caused by decreased cardiac contractility, the end-systolic pressure-volume relation is shifted downward and rightward (from line *1* to line *2*). As a result, the end-systolic volume (ESV) is increased (*arrow*). As normal venous return is added to that greater-than-normal ESV, there is an obligatory increase in the end-diastolic volume (EDV) and pressure (preload), which serves a compensatory function by partially elevating stroke volume toward normal via the Frank-Starling mechanism. **B.** The pressure-volume loop of diastolic dysfunction results from increased stiffness of the ventricle (*dashed line*). The passive diastolic pressure-volume curve is shifted upward (from line *1* to line *2*) such that at any diastolic volume, the ventricular pressure is higher than normal. The result is a decreased EDV (*arrow*) because of reduced filling of the stiffened ventricle at a higher-than-normal end-diastolic pressure.

capillary hydrostatic pressure, when sufficiently high (usually >20 mm Hg), results in the transudation of fluid into the pulmonary interstitium and symptoms of pulmonary congestion.

HEART FAILURE WITH PRESERVED EF (HFpEF)

Patients who exhibit heart failure with preserved EF frequently demonstrate abnormalities of ventricular diastolic function: impaired early diastolic relaxation (an active, energy-dependent process), increased stiffness of the ventricular wall (a passive property), or both. Acute myocardial ischemia is an example of a condition that *transiently* inhibits energy delivery and diastolic relaxation. Conversely, left ventricular hypertrophy, fibrosis, or restrictive cardiomyopathy (see Chapter 10) causes the LV walls to become *chronically* stiffened. Certain pericardial diseases (cardiac tamponade and pericardial constriction, as described in Chapter 14) present an external force that limits ventricular filling and represent potentially reversible forms of diastolic dysfunction. The effect of impaired diastolic function is reflected in the pressure-volume loop (see Fig. 9-7B): in diastole, filling of the ventricle occurs at higher-than-normal pressures because the lower part of the loop is shifted upward as a result of reduced chamber compliance. Patients with diastolic dysfunction often manifest signs of vascular congestion because the elevated diastolic pressure is transmitted retrograde to the pulmonary and systemic veins.

RIGHT-SIDED HEART FAILURE

Whereas the physiologic principles described above may be applied to both right-sided and left-sided heart failure, there are distinct differences in function between the two ventricles. Compared with the LV, the right ventricle (RV) is a thin-walled, highly compliant chamber that accepts its blood volume at low pressures and ejects against a low pulmonary vascular resistance. As a result of its high compliance, the RV has little difficulty accepting a wide range of filling volumes without marked changes in filling pressure. Conversely, the RV is quite susceptible to failure in situations that present a sudden increase in afterload, such as acute pulmonary embolism.

The most common cause of right-sided heart failure is actually the presence of left-sided heart failure (Table 9-2). In this situation, excessive afterload confronts the RV because of the elevated pulmonary vascular pressures that result from LV dysfunction. *Isolated* right heart failure is less common and usually reflects increased RV afterload owing to diseases of the lung parenchyma or pulmonary vasculature. Right-sided heart disease that results from a

TABLE 9-2   Examples of Conditions That Cause Right-Sided Heart Failure

Cardiac causes
    Left-sided heart failure
    Pulmonic valve stenosis
    Right ventricular infarction

Pulmonary parenchymal diseases
    Chronic obstructive pulmonary disease
    Interstitial lung disease (eg, sarcoidosis)
    Chronic lung infection or bronchiectasis

Pulmonary vascular diseases
    Pulmonary embolism
    Pulmonary arteriolar hypertension

primary pulmonary process is known as cor pulmonale, which may lead to symptoms of right heart failure.

When the RV fails, the elevated diastolic pressure is transmitted retrograde to the right atrium with subsequent congestion of the systemic veins, accompanied by signs of right-sided heart failure as described below. Indirectly, isolated right heart failure may also influence left heart function: the decreased right ventricular output reduces blood return to the LV (ie, diminished preload), causing left ventricular SV to decline.

COMPENSATORY MECHANISMS

Several natural compensatory mechanisms are called into action in patients with heart failure that buffer the fall in CO and help preserve sufficient blood pressure (BP) to perfuse vital organs. These compensations include (1) the Frank-Starling mechanism, (2) neurohormonal alterations, and (3) the development of ventricular hypertrophy and remodeling (Fig. 9-8).

FRANK-STARLING MECHANISM

As shown in Figure 9-3, heart failure caused by impaired left ventricular contractile function causes a downward shift of the ventricular performance curve. Consequently, at a given preload, SV is decreased compared with normal. The reduced SV results in incomplete chamber emptying so that the volume of blood that accumulates in the ventricle during diastole is higher than normal (see Fig. 9-3, point *b*). This increased stretch on the myofibers, acting via the Frank-Starling mechanism, induces a greater SV on subsequent contraction, which helps to empty the enlarged LV and preserve forward CO (see Fig. 9-8).

This beneficial compensatory mechanism has its limits, however. In the case of severe heart failure with marked depression of contractility, the curve may be nearly flat at higher diastolic volumes, reducing the augmentation of CO achieved by the increased chamber filling. Concurrently in such a circumstance, marked elevation of the EDV and pressure (which is transmitted retrograde to the left atrium, pulmonary veins, and capillaries) may result in pulmonary congestion and edema (see Fig. 9-3, point *c*).

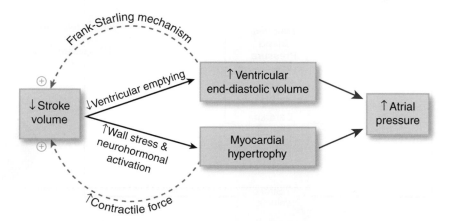

Figure 9-8. Compensatory mechanisms in heart failure. Both the Frank-Starling mechanism (which is invoked by the rise in ventricular end-diastolic volume) and increased contractile force (due to myocardial hypertrophy from augmented wall stress and neurohormonal activation) serve to maintain forward stroke volume (*dashed green arrows*). However, the chronic rise in end-diastolic volume and myocardial hypertrophy passively augment atrial pressure (*red arrows*), which may in turn contribute to symptoms of heart failure (eg, pulmonary congestion in the case of left-sided heart failure).

NEUROHORMONAL ALTERATIONS

Several important neurohormonal compensatory mechanisms are activated in heart failure in response to the decreased CO (Fig. 9-9). Three of the most important involve (1) the adrenergic nervous system, (2) the renin-angiotensin-aldosterone system, and (3) increased production of antidiuretic hormone (ADH). In part, these mechanisms serve to increase systemic vascular resistance, which helps to maintain arterial perfusion to vital organs, even in the setting of a reduced CO. That is, because BP is equal to the product of CO and total peripheral resistance (TPR),

$$BP = CO \times TPR$$

a rise in TPR induced by these compensatory mechanisms can nearly balance the fall in CO and, in the early stages of heart failure, maintain fairly normal BP. In addition, neurohormonal activation results in salt and water retention, which in turn increases intravascular volume and left ventricular preload, maximizing SV via the Frank-Starling mechanism.

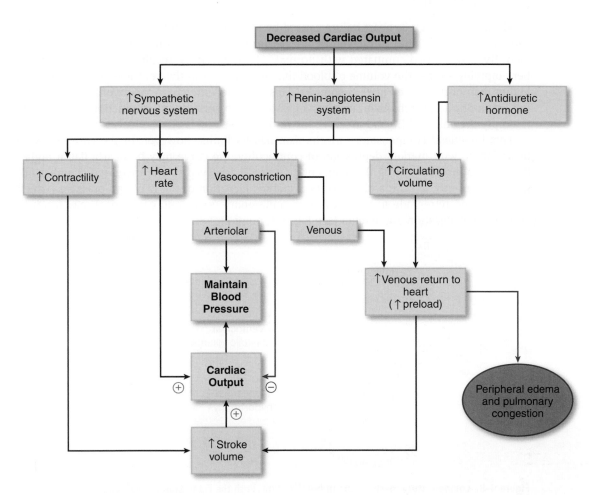

Figure 9-9. Compensatory neurohormonal stimulation develops in response to the reduced forward cardiac output and blood pressure of heart failure. Increased activity of the sympathetic nervous system, renin-angiotensin-aldosterone system, and antidiuretic hormone serves to support the cardiac output and blood pressure (*boxes*). However, adverse consequences of these activations (*red lines*) include an increase in afterload from excessive vasoconstriction (which may impede cardiac output) and excess fluid retention, which contribute to peripheral edema and pulmonary congestion.

Although the acute effects of neurohormonal stimulation are compensatory and beneficial, chronic activation of these mechanisms often ultimately proves deleterious to the failing heart and contributes to a progressive downhill course, as described later.

Adrenergic Nervous System

The fall in CO in heart failure is sensed by baroreceptors in the carotid sinus and aortic arch. These receptors decrease their rate of firing in proportion to the fall in BP, and the signal is transmitted by the 9th and 10th cranial nerves to the cardiovascular control center in the medulla. As a consequence, sympathetic outflow to the heart and peripheral circulation is enhanced, and parasympathetic tone is diminished. There are three immediate consequences (see Fig. 9-9): (1) an increase in HR, (2) augmentation of ventricular contractility, and (3) vasoconstriction caused by stimulation of α-receptors on the systemic veins and arteries.

The increased HR and ventricular contractility directly augment CO (see Fig. 9-2). Vasoconstriction of the venous and arterial circulations is also initially beneficial. *Venous* constriction augments blood return to the heart, which increases preload and raises SV through the Frank-Starling mechanism, as long as the ventricle is operating on the ascending portion of its ventricular performance curve. *Arteriolar* constriction increases the peripheral vascular resistance and therefore helps maintain blood pressure (BP = CO × TPR). The regional distribution of α-receptors is such that during sympathetic stimulation, blood flow is redistributed to vital organs (eg, heart and brain) at the expense of the skin, splanchnic viscera, and kidneys.

Renin-Angiotensin-Aldosterone System

This system is also activated early in patients with heart failure (see Fig. 9-9), mediated by increased renin release. The main stimuli for renin secretion from the juxtaglomerular cells of the kidney in heart failure patients include (1) decreased renal artery perfusion pressure secondary to low CO, (2) decreased salt delivery to the macula densa of the kidney owing to alterations in intrarenal hemodynamics, and (3) direct stimulation of juxtaglomerular β-receptors by the activated adrenergic nervous system.

Renin is an enzyme that acts on circulating angiotensinogen to form angiotensin I, which is then rapidly cleaved by endothelial cell–bound angiotensin-converting enzyme (ACE) to form angiotensin II (AII), a potent vasoconstrictor (see Chapter 13). Increased AII constricts arterioles and raises TPR, thereby serving to maintain systemic BP. In addition, AII acts to increase intravascular volume by two mechanisms: (1) at the hypothalamus, it stimulates thirst and therefore water intake, and (2) at the adrenal cortex, it increases aldosterone secretion. The latter hormone promotes sodium reabsorption from the distal convoluted tubule of the kidney into the circulation (see Chapter 17), serving to augment intravascular volume. The elevation of intravascular volume increases left ventricular preload and thereby raises CO via the Frank-Starling mechanism in patients on the ascending portion of the ventricular performance curve (see Fig. 9-3).

Antidiuretic Hormone

Secretion of this hormone (also termed *vasopressin*) by the posterior pituitary is increased in many patients with heart failure, presumably mediated through arterial baroreceptors, and by increased levels of AII. ADH contributes to increased intravascular volume because it promotes water retention in the distal nephron. The increased intravascular volume serves to augment left ventricular preload and CO.

Although each of these neurohormonal alterations in heart failure is *initially* beneficial, continued activation ultimately proves harmful. For example, the increased circulating volume and augmented venous return to the heart may eventually *worsen* engorgement of the lung vasculature, exacerbating congestive pulmonary symptoms. Furthermore, the elevated arteriolar resistance increases the load against which the failing LV contracts and may therefore ultimately *impair* SV and reduce CO (see Fig. 9-9). In addition, the increased HR augments metabolic demand and can therefore further reduce the performance of the failing heart. Continuous sympathetic activation results in down-regulation of cardiac β-adrenergic receptors and up-regulation of inhibitory G proteins, contributing to a decrease in the myocardium's sensitivity to circulating catecholamines and a *reduced* inotropic response.

Chronically elevated levels of AII and aldosterone have additional detrimental effects. They provoke the production of cytokines (small proteins that mediate cell-cell communication and immune responses), activate macrophages, and stimulate fibroblasts, resulting in fibrosis and adverse remodeling of the failing heart.

Because the undesired consequences of chronic neurohormonal activation eventually outweigh the benefits, much of today's pharmacologic therapy of heart failure is designed to moderate these "compensatory" mechanisms, as examined later in the chapter.

Natriuretic Peptides

In contrast to the ultimately adverse consequences of the neurohormonal alterations described in the previous section, the natriuretic peptides are natural "beneficial" hormones secreted in heart failure in response to increased intracardiac pressures. The best studied of these are atrial natriuretic peptide (ANP) and B-type natriuretic peptide (BNP). ANP is stored in atrial cells and is released in response to atrial distention. BNP is not detected in healthy hearts with normal loading conditions but is produced when ventricular myocardium is subjected to hemodynamic stress (eg, in heart failure or during myocardial infarction). The prohormone proBNP generates both BNP and another compound that is inert: N-terminal proBNP (NT-proBNP). Clinical studies have shown a close relationship between serum BNP or NT-proBNP levels and the severity of heart failure.

Actions of the natriuretic peptides are mediated by specific natriuretic receptors and are largely opposite to those of the other hormone systems activated in heart failure. They result in excretion of sodium and water, vasodilatation, inhibition of renin secretion, and antagonism of the effects of AII on aldosterone and vasopressin levels. Although these effects are beneficial to patients with heart failure, they are usually not sufficient to fully counteract the vasoconstriction and volume-retaining effects of the other activated hormonal systems.

Other Peptides

Among other peptides that are generated in heart failure is **endothelin 1**, a potent vasoconstrictor, derived from endothelial cells lining the vasculature (see Chapter 6). In patients with heart failure, the plasma concentration of endothelin 1 correlates with disease severity and adverse outcomes. Drugs designed to inhibit endothelin receptors (and therefore blunt adverse vasoconstriction) improve LV function, but long-term clinical benefits have not been demonstrated in heart failure patients.

VENTRICULAR HYPERTROPHY AND REMODELING

Ventricular hypertrophy and remodeling are important compensatory processes that develop over time in response to hemodynamic burdens. Wall stress (as defined earlier) is often increased in developing heart failure because of either LV dilatation (increased chamber radius) or the need to generate high systolic pressures to overcome excessive afterload (eg, in aortic stenosis or hypertension). A sustained increase in wall stress (along with neurohormonal and cytokine alterations) stimulates the development of myocardial hypertrophy and deposition of extracellular matrix. This increased mass of muscle fibers serves as a compensatory mechanism that helps to maintain contractile force and *counteracts* the elevated ventricular wall stress (recall that wall thickness is in the denominator of the Laplace wall stress formula). However, because of the increased stiffness of the hypertrophied wall, these benefits come at the expense of higher-than-normal diastolic ventricular pressures, which are transmitted to the left atrium and pulmonary vasculature (see Fig. 9-8).

The pattern of compensatory hypertrophy and remodeling that develops depends on whether the ventricle is subjected to chronic volume or pressure overload. Chronic chamber dilatation owing to *volume* overload (eg, chronic mitral or aortic regurgitation) results in the synthesis of new sarcomeres in series with the old, causing the myocytes to elongate. The radius of the ventricular chamber therefore enlarges, doing so in proportion to the increase in wall thickness, and is termed **eccentric hypertrophy**. Chronic *pressure* overload (eg, caused by hypertension or aortic stenosis) results in the synthesis of new sarcomeres in *parallel* with the old (ie, the myocytes thicken), termed **concentric hypertrophy**. In this situation, the wall thickness increases without proportional chamber dilatation, and wall stress may therefore be reduced substantially.

Such hypertrophy and remodeling help to reduce wall stress and maintain contractile force, but ultimately, ventricular function may decline further, allowing the chamber to dilate out of proportion to wall thickness. When this occurs, the excessive hemodynamic burden on the contractile units produces a downward spiral of deterioration with progressive heart failure symptomatology.

MYOCYTE LOSS AND CELLULAR DYSFUNCTION

Impairment of ventricular function in heart failure may result from the actual loss of myocytes and/or impaired function of living myocytes. The loss of myocytes may result from cellular *necrosis* (eg, from myocardial infarction or exposure to cardiotoxic drugs such as doxorubicin) or *apoptosis* (programmed cell death). In apoptosis, genetic instructions activate intracellular pathways that cause the cell to fragment and undergo phagocytosis by other cells, without an inflammatory response. Implicated triggers of apoptosis in heart failure include elevated catecholamines, AII, inflammatory cytokines, and mechanical strain on the myocytes owing to the augmented wall stress.

Even viable myocardium in heart failure is abnormal at the ultrastructural and molecular levels. Mechanical wall stress, neurohormonal activation, and inflammatory cytokines, such as tumor necrosis factor (TNF), are believed to alter the genetic expression of contractile proteins, ion channels, catalytic enzymes, surface receptors, and secondary messengers in the myocyte. Experimental evidence has demonstrated such changes at the subcellular level that affect intracellular calcium handling by the sarcoplasmic reticulum, decrease the responsiveness of the myofilaments to calcium, impair excitation-contraction coupling, and alter cellular energy production. Cellular mechanisms currently considered the most important contributors to dysfunction in heart failure include (1) a reduced cellular ability to maintain calcium homeostasis and/or (2) changes in the production, availability, and utilization of high-energy phosphates. However, the exact subcellular alterations that result in heart failure have not been fully unraveled, and this is an active area of cardiovascular research.

PRECIPITATING FACTORS

Many patients with heart failure remain asymptomatic for extended periods either because the impairment is mild or because cardiac dysfunction is balanced by the compensatory mechanisms described earlier. Often, clinical manifestations are precipitated by circumstances that increase the cardiac workload and tip the balanced state into one of decompensation.

Common precipitating factors are listed in Table 9-3. For example, conditions of increased metabolic demand such as fever or infection may not be matched by a sufficient increase in output by the failing heart so that symptoms of cardiac insufficiency are precipitated.

TABLE 9-3	Factors That May Precipitate Symptoms in Patients With Chronic Compensated Heart Failure

Increased metabolic demands
  Fever
  Infection
  Anemia
  Tachycardia
  Hyperthyroidism
  Pregnancy

Increased circulating volume (increased preload)
  Excessive sodium content in diet
  Excessive fluid administration
  Renal failure

Conditions that increase afterload
  Uncontrolled hypertension
  Pulmonary embolism (increased right ventricular afterload)

Conditions that impair contractility
  Negative inotropic medications
  Myocardial ischemia or infarction
  Excessive ethanol ingestion

Failure to take prescribed heart failure medications

Excessively slow heart rate

Tachyarrhythmias precipitate heart failure by decreasing diastolic ventricular filling time and by increasing myocardial oxygen demand. Excessively low HRs directly cause a drop in CO (remember, cardiac output = stroke volume × heart rate). An increase in salt ingestion, renal dysfunction, or failure to take prescribed diuretic medications may increase the circulating volume, thus promoting systemic and pulmonary congestion. Uncontrolled hypertension depresses systolic function because of excessive afterload. A large pulmonary embolism results in both hypoxemia (and therefore decreased myocardial oxygen supply) and augmented right ventricular afterload. Ischemic insults (ie, myocardial ischemia or infarction), ethanol ingestion, or negative inotropic medications (eg, large doses of β-blockers) can all depress myocardial contractility and precipitate symptoms in the otherwise compensated heart failure patient.

CLINICAL MANIFESTATIONS

The clinical manifestations of heart failure result from impaired forward CO and/or elevated venous pressures and relate to the ventricle that has failed (Table 9-4). A patient may present with the chronic progressive symptoms of heart failure described here or, in certain cases, with sudden decompensation of left-sided heart function (eg, acute pulmonary edema, as described later in the chapter).

Symptoms

The most prominent manifestation of chronic left ventricular failure is *dyspnea* (breathlessness) on exertion. Controversy regarding the cause of this symptom has centered on whether it results primarily from pulmonary venous congestion or from decreased forward CO. A pulmonary venous pressure that exceeds ~20 mm Hg leads to transudation of fluid into the pulmonary interstitium and congestion of the lung parenchyma. The resulting reduced

TABLE 9-4	Common Symptoms and Physical Findings in Heart Failure
Symptoms	**Physical Findings**
Left sided	
Dyspnea	Diaphoresis (sweating)
Orthopnea	Tachycardia, tachypnea
Paroxysmal nocturnal dyspnea	Pulmonary crackles (rales)
Fatigue	Loud P_2
	S_3 gallop (in systolic dysfunction)
	S_4 gallop (in diastolic dysfunction)
Right sided	
Peripheral edema	Jugular venous distention
Right upper quadrant discomfort	Hepatomegaly
(because of hepatic enlargement)	Peripheral edema

pulmonary compliance increases the work of breathing to move the same volume of air. Moreover, the excess fluid in the interstitium compresses the walls of the bronchioles and alveoli, increasing the resistance to airflow and requiring greater effort of respiration. In addition, juxtacapillary receptors (J receptors) are stimulated and mediate rapid shallow breathing. The heart failure patient can also suffer from dyspnea even in the absence of pulmonary congestion, because reduced blood flow to overworked respiratory muscles and accumulation of lactic acid may also contribute to that sensation. Heart failure may initially cause dyspnea only on exertion, but more severe dysfunction results in symptoms at rest as well.

Other manifestations of low forward output in heart failure may include *dulled mental status* because of reduced cerebral perfusion and *impaired urine output* during the day because of decreased renal blood flow. The latter often gives way to increased urinary frequency at night (*nocturia*) when, while supine, blood flow is redistributed to the kidney, promoting renal perfusion and diuresis. Reduced skeletal muscle perfusion may result in *fatigue* and *weakness*.

Other congestive manifestations of heart failure include *orthopnea, paroxysmal nocturnal dyspnea (PND)*, and *nocturnal cough*. Orthopnea is the sensation of labored breathing while lying flat and is relieved by sitting upright. It results from the redistribution of intravascular blood from the gravity-dependent portions of the body (abdomen and lower extremities) toward the lungs after lying down. The degree of orthopnea is generally assessed by the number of pillows on which the patient sleeps to avoid breathlessness. Sometimes, orthopnea is so significant that the patient may try to sleep upright in a chair.

PND is severe breathlessness that awakens the patient from sleep 2 to 3 hours after retiring to bed. This frightening symptom results from the gradual reabsorption into the circulation of lower extremity interstitial edema after lying down, with subsequent expansion of intravascular volume and increased venous return to the heart and lungs. A nocturnal cough is another symptom of pulmonary congestion and is produced by a mechanism similar to orthopnea. Hemoptysis (coughing up blood) may result from rupture of engorged bronchial veins.

In right-sided heart failure, the elevated systemic venous pressures can result in *abdominal discomfort* because the liver becomes engorged and its capsule stretched. Similarly, anorexia (decreased appetite) and nausea may result from edema within the gastrointestinal tract. *Peripheral edema*, especially in the ankles and feet, also reflects increased hydrostatic venous pressures. Because of the effects of gravity, it tends to worsen while the patient is upright during the day and is often improved by morning after lying supine at night. Even before peripheral edema develops, the patient may note an unexpected *weight gain* resulting from the accumulation of interstitial fluid.

The symptoms of heart failure are commonly graded according to the New York Heart Association (NYHA) classification (Table 9-5), and patients may shift from one class to another, in

TABLE 9-5	New York Heart Association Classification of Chronic Heart Failure
Class	**Definition**
I	No limitation of physical activity
II	Slight limitation of activity. Dyspnea and fatigue with moderate exertion (eg, walking upstairs quickly)
III	Marked limitation of activity. Dyspnea with minimal exertion (eg, slowly walking upstairs)
IV	Severe limitation of activity. Symptoms are present even at rest

either direction, over time. Another system classifies patients according to their stage in the temporal course of heart failure (Table 9-6). In this system, progression is in only one direction, from Stage A to Stage D, reflecting the typical sequence of heart failure manifestations in clinical practice.

PHYSICAL SIGNS

The physical signs of heart failure depend on the severity and chronicity of the condition and can be divided into those associated with left or right heart dysfunction (see Table 9-4). Patients with only mild impairment may appear well. However, a patient with severe chronic heart failure may demonstrate *cachexia* (a frail, wasted appearance) owing in part to poor appetite and to the metabolic demands of the increased effort in breathing. In decompensated left-sided heart failure, the patient may appear *dusky* (decreased CO) and *diaphoretic* (sweating because of increased sympathetic nervous activity), and the extremities are cool because of peripheral arterial vasoconstriction. *Tachypnea* (rapid breathing) is common. The pattern of Cheyne-Stokes respiration may also be present in advanced heart failure, characterized by periods of hyperventilation separated by intervals of apnea (absent breathing). This pattern is related to the prolonged circulation time between the lungs and respiratory center of the brain in heart failure that interferes with the normal feedback mechanism of systemic oxygenation. *Sinus tachycardia* (resulting from increased sympathetic nervous system activity) is also common. Pulsus alternans (alternating strong and weak contractions detected in the peripheral pulse) may be present as a sign of advanced ventricular dysfunction.

TABLE 9-6	Stages of Chronic Heart Failure
Stage	**Description**
A	The patient is at risk of developing heart failure but has not yet developed structural cardiac dysfunction (eg, patient with coronary artery disease, hypertension, or family history of cardiomyopathy)
B	The patient with structural heart disease associated with heart failure but has not yet developed symptoms
C	The patient with current or prior symptoms of heart failure associated with structural heart disease
D	The patient with structural heart disease and *refractory* heart failure symptoms despite maximal medical therapy who requires advanced interventions (eg, cardiac transplantation)

Derived from Yancy C, Jessup M, Bozkurt B, et al. 2013 ACCF/AHA Guideline for the Management of Heart Failure: Executive Summary A Report of the American College of Cardiology Foundation/American heart Association Task Force on Practice Guidelines. *Circulation*. 2013;128:1810-1852.

In left-sided heart failure, the auscultatory finding of *pulmonary crackles* (also termed "rales") is created by the "popping open" of small airways during inspiration that had been closed off by edema fluid. This finding is initially apparent at the lung bases, where hydrostatic forces are greatest; however, more severe pulmonary congestion is associated with additional crackles higher in the lung fields. Compression of conduction airways by pulmonary congestion may produce coarse rhonchi and wheezing; the latter finding in heart failure is termed *cardiac asthma*.

Depending on the cause of heart failure, palpation of the heart may show that the left ventricular impulse is not focal but diffuse (in dilated cardiomyopathy), sustained (in pressure overload states such as aortic stenosis or hypertension), or lifting in quality (in volume overload states such as mitral regurgitation). Because elevated left heart filling pressures result in increased pulmonary vascular pressures, the pulmonic component of the second heart sound is often louder than normal. An *early diastolic sound* (S_3) is frequently heard in adults with systolic heart failure and is caused by abnormal filling of the dilated chamber (see Chapter 2). A *late diastolic sound* (S_4) results from forceful atrial contraction into a stiffened ventricle and is common in states of decreased LV compliance (diastolic dysfunction). The murmur of *mitral regurgitation* is sometimes auscultated in left-sided heart failure if LV dilatation has stretched the valve annulus and spread the papillary muscles apart from one another, thus preventing proper closure of the mitral leaflets in systole.

In right-sided heart failure, different physical findings may be present. Cardiac examination may reveal a palpable parasternal *right ventricular heave*, representing RV enlargement, or a *right-sided S_3 or S_4 gallop*. The murmur of *tricuspid regurgitation* may be auscultated and is due to right ventricular enlargement, analogous to mitral regurgitation that develops in patients with LV dilatation. The elevated systemic venous pressure produced by right heart failure is manifested by *distention of the jugular veins* as well as *hepatic enlargement* with abdominal right upper quadrant tenderness. *Edema* accumulates in the dependent portions of the body, beginning in the ankles and feet of ambulatory patients and in the presacral regions of those who are bedridden.

Pleural effusions may develop in either left- or right-sided heart failure, because the pleural veins drain into both the systemic and pulmonary venous beds. The presence of pleural effusions is suggested on physical examination by dullness to percussion over the posterior lung bases.

DIAGNOSTIC STUDIES

A normal mean left atrial (LA) pressure is ≤10 mm Hg (see Fig. 3-13). If the LA pressure exceeds ~15 mm Hg, the chest radiograph shows *upper-zone vascular redistribution*, such that the vessels supplying the upper lobes of the lung are larger than those supplying the lower lobes (see Fig. 3-5). This is explained as follows: when a patient is in the upright position, blood flow is normally greater to the lung bases than to the apices because of the effect of gravity. Redistribution of flow occurs with the development of interstitial and perivascular edema, because such edema is most prominent at the lung bases (where the hydrostatic pressure is the highest), such that the blood vessels in the bases are compressed, whereas flow into the upper lung zones is less affected.

When the LA pressure surpasses ~20 mm Hg, interstitial edema is usually manifested on the chest radiograph as indistinctness of the vessels and the presence of *Kerley B lines* (short linear markings at the periphery of the lower lung fields indicating interlobular edema—see Fig. 3-5C). If the LA pressure exceeds 25 to 30 mm Hg, alveolar pulmonary edema may develop, with opacification of the air spaces. The relationship between LA pressure and chest radiograph findings is modified in patients with *chronic* heart failure because of enhanced lymphatic drainage, such that higher pressures can be accommodated with fewer radiologic signs.

Depending on the cause of heart failure, the chest radiograph may show *cardiomegaly*, defined as a cardiothoracic ratio >0.5 on the posteroanterior image. A high right atrial pressure also causes enlargement of the azygos vein silhouette. Pleural effusions may be present.

Assays for BNP and NT-proBNP, described earlier in the chapter, correlate well with the degree of LV dysfunction and prognosis. Furthermore, an elevated serum level of BNP or NT-proBNP can help distinguish heart failure from other causes of dyspnea, such as pulmonary parenchymal diseases.

The cause of heart failure is often evident from the history, such as a patient who has sustained a large myocardial infarction, or by physical examination, as in a patient with a murmur of valvular heart disease. When the cause is not clear from clinical evaluation, the first step is to determine whether systolic ventricular function is normal or depressed (see Fig. 9-6). Of the several noninvasive tests that can help make this determination, echocardiography is especially useful and readily available.

PROGNOSIS

The prognosis of heart failure is dismal in the absence of a correctable underlying cause. The 5-year mortality rate following the diagnosis ranges between 45% and 60%, with men having worse outcomes than women. Patients with severe symptoms (ie, NYHA class III or IV) fare the least well, having a 1-year survival rate of only 40%. The greatest mortality is due to refractory heart failure, but many patients die suddenly, presumably because of associated ventricular arrhythmias. Heart failure patients with preserved EF have similar rates of hospitalization, in-hospital complications, and mortality as those with reduced EF.

Ventricular dysfunction usually begins with an inciting insult but is a progressive process, contributed to by the maladaptive activation of neurohormones, cytokines, and continuous ventricular remodeling. Thus, it should not be surprising that measures of neurohormonal and cytokine stimulation predict survival in heart failure patients. For example, adverse prognosis correlates with the serum norepinephrine level (marker of sympathetic nervous system activity), serum sodium (reduced level reflects activation of renin-angiotensin-aldosterone system and alterations in intrarenal hemodynamics), endothelin 1, BNP, and TNF levels.

Despite the generally bleak prognosis, a heart failure patient's outlook can be substantially improved by specific interventions, as discussed in the following sections.

TREATMENT OF HEART FAILURE WITH REDUCED EJECTION FRACTION

There are five main goals of therapy in patients with chronic HFrEF:

1. *Identification and correction of the underlying condition causing heart failure.* In some patients, this may require surgical repair or replacement of dysfunctional cardiac valves, coronary artery revascularization, aggressive treatment of hypertension, or cessation of alcohol consumption.
2. *Elimination of the acute precipitating cause of symptoms* in a patient with heart failure who was previously in a compensated state. This may include treating acute infections or arrhythmias, removing sources of excessive salt intake, or eliminating drugs that can aggravate symptomatology (eg, certain calcium channel blockers, which have a negative inotropic effect, or nonsteroidal anti-inflammatory drugs, which can contribute to volume retention).
3. Management of heart failure symptoms and improvement in quality of life:
   a. *Treatment of pulmonary and systemic vascular congestion.* This is most readily accomplished by dietary sodium restriction and diuretic medications.
   b. *Measures to increase forward cardiac output* and perfusion of vital organs through the use of vasodilators and positive inotropic drugs.

4. *Modulation of the neurohormonal response* to prevent adverse ventricular remodeling in order to slow the progression of LV dysfunction.

5. *Prolongation of long-term survival.* There is strong evidence from clinical trials that longevity is enhanced by specific therapies, as described below.

DIURETICS

The mechanisms of action of diuretic drugs are summarized in Chapter 17. By promoting the elimination of sodium and water through the kidney, diuretics reduce intravascular volume and thus venous return to the heart. As a result, the preload of the LV is decreased, and its diastolic pressure falls out of the range that promotes pulmonary congestion (Fig. 9-10, point *b*). The intent is to reduce the EDP (and therefore hydrostatic forces contributing to pulmonary congestion) without a significant fall in SV. The judicious use of diuretics does not significantly reduce SV and CO in this setting, because the failing ventricle is operating on the "flat" portion of a depressed Frank-Starling curve. However, overly vigorous diuresis *can* lower LV filling pressures into the steep portion of the ventricular performance curve, resulting in an undesired fall in CO (see Fig. 9-10, point *b'*). Thus, diuretics should be used only if there is evidence of pulmonary congestion (rales) or peripheral interstitial fluid accumulation (eg, edema).

Agents that act primarily at the renal loop of Henle (eg, furosemide, torsemide, and bumetanide) are the most potent diuretics in heart failure. Thiazide diuretics (eg,

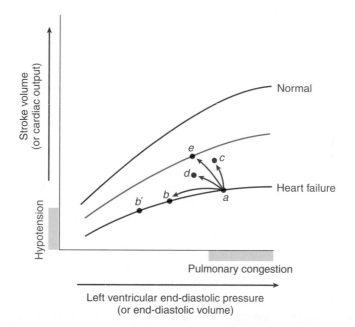

Figure 9-10. The effect of treatment on the left ventricular (LV) Frank-Starling curve in patients who have heart failure with reduced EF. Point *a* represents the failing heart on a curve that is shifted downward compared with normal. The stroke volume is reduced (with blood pressure bordering on hypotension), and the LV end-diastolic pressure (LVEDP) is increased, resulting in symptoms of pulmonary congestion. Therapy with a diuretic or pure venous vasodilator (point *b* on the same Frank-Starling curve) reduces LV pressure without much change in stroke volume (SV). However, excessive diuresis or venous vasodilatation may result in an undesired fall in SV with hypotension (point *b'*). Inotropic drug therapy (point *c*) and arteriolar (or "balanced") vasodilator therapy (point *d*) augment SV, and because of improved LV emptying during contraction, the LVEDP lessens. Point *e* represents the potential added benefit of combining an inotrope and vasodilator together. The *middle curve* shows one example of how the Frank-Starling relationship shifts upward during inotropic/vasodilator therapy but does not achieve the level of a normal ventricle.

hydrochlorothiazide and metolazone) are also useful but are less effective in the setting of decreased renal perfusion, which is often present in this condition.

The potential adverse effects of diuretics are described in Chapter 17. The most important in heart failure patients include overly vigorous diuresis resulting in a fall in CO and electrolyte disturbances (particularly hypokalemia and hypomagnesemia), which may promote arrhythmias. In patients with acute heart failure exacerbations, diuretics should be administered intravenously (either by bolus injections or continuous infusion) because venous congestion can limit the absorption of oral diuretics from the gut.

VASODILATORS

One of the most important cardiac advances in the late twentieth century was the introduction of vasodilator therapy for the treatment of heart failure, particularly ACE inhibitors and similar agents. As indicated earlier, neurohormonal compensatory mechanisms in heart failure often lead to excessive vasoconstriction, volume retention, and ventricular remodeling, with progressive deterioration of cardiac function. Vasodilator drugs help to reverse these adverse consequences. Moreover, multiple studies have shown that certain vasodilator regimens significantly extend survival in patients with heart failure. The pharmacology of these drugs is described in Chapter 17.

Venous vasodilators (eg, nitrates) increase venous capacitance and thereby decrease venous return to the heart and left ventricular preload. Consequently, LV diastolic pressures fall, and the pulmonary capillary hydrostatic pressure declines, similar to the hemodynamic effects of diuretic therapy. As a result, pulmonary congestion improves, and as long as the heart failure patient is on the relatively "flat" part of the depressed Frank-Starling curve (see Fig. 9-10), the CO does not fall despite the reduction in ventricular filling pressure. However, venous vasodilatation in a patient who is operating on the steeper part of the curve may result in an undesired fall in SV, CO, and BP.

Pure *arteriolar vasodilators* (eg, hydralazine) reduce systemic vascular resistance and therefore LV afterload, which in turn permits increased ventricular muscle fiber shortening during systole (see Fig. 9-5B). This results in an augmented SV and is represented on the Frank-Starling diagram as a shift in an upward direction (see Fig. 9-10, point *d*). Although an arterial vasodilator might be expected to reduce BP—an undesired effect in patients with heart failure who may already be hypotensive—this generally does not happen. As resistance is reduced by arteriolar vasodilatation, a concurrent *rise* in CO usually occurs, such that BP remains constant or decreases only mildly.

Some groups of drugs result in vasodilatation of *both* the venous and arteriolar circuits ("balanced" vasodilators). Of these, the most important are agents that inhibit the renin-angiotensin-aldosterone system. **Angiotensin-converting enzyme inhibitors** (ACE inhibitors, described in Chapters 13 and 17) interrupt the production of AII, thereby modulating the vasoconstriction incited by that hormone in heart failure patients. In addition, because aldosterone levels fall in response to ACE inhibitor therapy, sodium elimination is facilitated, resulting in reduced intravascular volume and improvement of systemic and pulmonary vascular congestion. ACE inhibitors also augment circulating levels of bradykinin (see Chapter 17), which is thought to contribute to beneficial vasodilatation in heart failure. As a result of these effects, ACE inhibitors limit maladaptive ventricular remodeling in patients with chronic heart failure and following acute myocardial infarction (see Chapter 7).

Supporting the beneficial hemodynamic and neurohormonal blocking effects of ACE inhibitors, many large clinical trials have shown that these drugs improve heart failure symptoms, reduce the need for hospitalization, and most importantly, extend survival in patients with HFrEF. Thus, ACE inhibitors are standard first-line chronic therapy for patients with LV systolic dysfunction.

The renin-angiotensin-aldosterone system can also be therapeutically inhibited by **angiotensin II receptor blockers (ARBs)**, as described in Chapters 13 and 17. Since AII can be formed by pathways other than ACE, ARBs provide a more complete inhibition of the system than ACE inhibitors, through blockade of the actual AII receptor (see Fig. 17-6). Conversely, ARBs do not cause the potentially beneficial rise in serum bradykinin. The net result is that the hemodynamic effects and mortality benefit of ARBs in heart failure are similar to those of ACE inhibitors. Thus, they are prescribed to heart failure patients mainly when ACE inhibitors are not tolerated (eg, because of bradykinin-mediated side effects such as cough).

A newer derivative of ARB therapy in heart failure is an **angiotensin receptor-neprilysin inhibitor (ARNI)**, which combines the ARB valsartan with sacubitril, an inhibitor of the enzyme neprilysin. Neprilysin is a membrane-bound enzyme that degrades endogenous vasoactive peptides, including natriuretic peptides and bradykinin. By blocking the action of neprilysin, sacubitril causes the concentration of these vasoactive substances to increase, beneficially enhancing vasodilation and sodium excretion in heart failure patients. In a study of patients with chronic symptomatic HF with reduced EF, the ARNI sacubitril-valsartan reduced mortality compared to patients treated with an ACE inhibitor. Therefore, this medication is now often recommended as a replacement for ACE inhibitor or ARB therapy in patients with chronic symptomatic HFrEF.

Chronic therapy using the combination of the venous dilator **isosorbide dinitrate** plus the arteriolar dilator **hydralazine** has also been shown to improve survival in patients with moderate symptoms of heart failure. However, when the ACE inhibitor enalapril was compared with the hydralazine-isosorbide dinitrate (H-ISDN) combination, the ACE inhibitor was shown to produce the greater improvement in survival. Thus, H-ISDN is generally substituted when a patient cannot tolerate ACE inhibitor or ARB therapy (eg, because of renal insufficiency or hyperkalemia). Of note, the African American Heart Failure trial demonstrated that the *addition* of H-ISDN to standard heart failure therapy (including a diuretic, β-blocker, and ACE inhibitor or ARB) in black patients with heart failure further improved functional status and survival.

Nesiritide (human recombinant BNP) is an intravenous vasodilator drug available for hospitalized patients with decompensated heart failure. It causes rapid and potent vasodilatation, reduces elevated intracardiac pressures, and augments forward CO. However, it is an expensive drug that does not improve outcomes and may worsen renal function, so is rarely used.

POSITIVE INOTROPIC DRUGS

Inotropic drugs include β-adrenergic agonists, phosphodiesterase type 3 inhibitors (see Chapter 17), and digitalis glycosides. By increasing the availability of intracellular calcium, each of these drug groups enhances the force of ventricular contraction and therefore shifts the Frank-Starling curve in an upward direction (see Fig. 9-10). As a result, SV and CO are augmented at any given ventricular EDV. Thus, these agents may be useful in treating patients with systolic dysfunction, but typically not those with heart failure with preserved EF.

β-**Adrenergic agonists** (eg, dobutamine and dopamine) are administered intravenously for temporary hemodynamic support in acutely ill, hospitalized patients. Their long-term use is limited by the lack of an oral form of administration and by the development of drug tolerance. The latter refers to the progressive decline in effectiveness during continued administration of the drug, possibly owing to down-regulation of myocardial adrenergic receptors. Likewise, the role of **phosphodiesterase 3 inhibitors** (eg, milrinone) is limited to the brief intravenous treatment of congestive heart failure in acutely ill patients. Despite the initial promise of effective *oral* phosphodiesterase 3 inhibitors for chronic therapy, studies thus far actually demonstrate *reduced* survival among patients receiving this form of treatment.

One of the oldest forms of inotropic therapy is **digitalis** (see Chapter 17), which can be administered intravenously or orally. Digitalis preparations enhance contractility, reduce cardiac enlargement, improve symptoms, and augment CO in patients with systolic heart failure.

Digitalis also increases the sensitivity of the baroreceptors so that the compensatory sympathetic drive in heart failure is blunted, a desired effect that reduces left ventricular afterload. By slowing AV nodal conduction and thereby reducing the rate of ventricular contractions, digitalis has an added benefit in patients with congestive heart failure who have concurrent atrial fibrillation. Although digitalis can improve symptomatology and reduce hospitalizations in heart failure patients, it has not been shown to improve long-term survival. Thus, its use is limited to a small number of patients who remain symptomatic despite other standard therapies or to help slow the ventricular rate if atrial fibrillation is also present. Digitalis is *not* useful in the treatment of heart failure with preserved EF because it does not improve ventricular relaxation properties.

β-Blockers

Historically, β-blockers were thought to be contraindicated in patients with systolic dysfunction because their negative inotropic effect would be expected to worsen symptomatology. However, clinical trials have actually shown that long-term β-blocker therapy has important *benefits* in patients with stable chronic HFrEF, including augmented CO, reduced hemodynamic deterioration, the need for fewer hospitalizations, and improved survival. The explanation for these desired effects remains conjectural but may relate to the drug effects on reducing HR and blunting chronic sympathetic activation or to their anti-ischemic properties.

The three β-blockers that have been shown to be beneficial in randomized clinical trials of heart failure include **carvedilol** (a nonselective β-blocker with weak α-blocking properties—see Chapter 17) and the β_1-selective agents **metoprolol succinate** and **bisoprolol**. These drugs are well tolerated in stable patients (ie, those without recent deterioration of heart failure symptoms or active volume overload). Nonetheless, β-blockers should always be used cautiously in heart failure to prevent acute deterioration related to their negative inotropic effect. Regimens should be started at low dosage and augmented gradually.

Aldosterone Antagonist Therapy

There is evidence that chronic excess of aldosterone in heart failure contributes to cardiac fibrosis and adverse ventricular remodeling. Antagonists of this hormone (which have been used historically as mild diuretics—see Chapter 17) have shown clinical benefit in heart failure patients. For example, in a trial of patients with advanced heart failure (ie, NYHA class III to IV) who were already taking an ACE inhibitor and diuretics, the aldosterone receptor antagonist **spironolactone** substantially reduced mortality rates and improved heart failure symptoms. **Eplerenone**, a more specific aldosterone receptor inhibitor, has been shown to improve survival of patients with congestive heart failure after acute myocardial infarction (see Chapter 7) as well as patients with more mild forms of chronic heart failure (ie, NYHA class II to III). Although aldosterone antagonists have been well tolerated in carefully controlled studies, the serum potassium level must be monitored to prevent hyperkalemia, especially if there is renal impairment or concomitant ACE inhibitor therapy.

In summary, standard therapy of chronic HFrEF should include several drugs, the cornerstones of which are an ACE inhibitor and a β-blocker (see Fig. 9-11). An accepted sequence of therapy is to start with an ACE inhibitor as well as a diuretic if pulmonary or systemic congestive symptoms are present. If the patient is unable to tolerate the ACE inhibitor, then an ARB (or hydralazine plus isosorbide dinitrate) may be substituted. ARNI therapy should be considered in place of the ACE inhibitor or ARB for patients with persistent chronic heart failure symptoms. For patients without recent clinical deterioration in symptoms, a β-blocker should also be prescribed. Those with persistent symptomatic heart failure may benefit further with the addition of an aldosterone antagonist. For refractory symptoms, digoxin is used on rare occasion for its hemodynamic benefit.

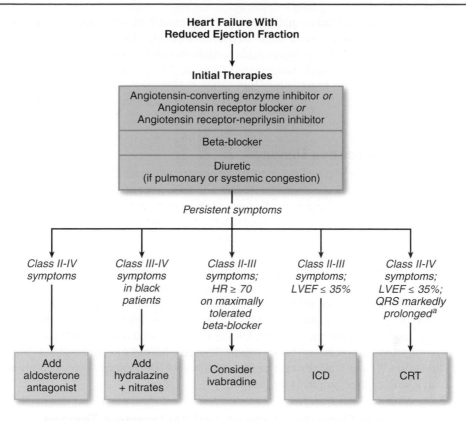

Figure 9-11. General approach to treatment of heart failure with reduced ejection fraction (HFrEF). The foundation of therapy should include an angiotensin-converting enzyme inhibitor (or angiotensin receptor blocker, or angiotensin receptor-neprilysin inhibitor), β-blocker, and a diuretic if volume overload is present. For persistent symptoms, one or more additional therapies are appropriate as indicated. The listed heart failure severity classes are described in Table 9-5. Patients who remain severely symptomatic despite these measures may be candidates for implanted mechanical ventricular assist devices or cardiac transplantation. CRT, cardiac resynchronization therapy; ICD, implantable cardioverter defibrillator. [a]Especially for QRS duration ≥150 msec with left bundle branch block morphology.

ADDITIONAL THERAPIES

Ivabradine

Ivabradine is an inhibitor of the sinoatrial node I_f pacemaker current (I_f is described in Chapter 1). It slows the HR, without affecting ventricular contractile function, and has been demonstrated to reduce hospitalizations for heart failure, but does not lower mortality. Its role is as a second-line agent for patients with HFrEF with LVEF <35%, who are in sinus rhythm with a persistent rate heart >70 bpm, despite beta-blocker therapy.

Arrhythmia Management

Atrial and ventricular arrhythmias frequently accompany chronic heart failure. For example, atrial fibrillation is very common in this setting, and conversion back to sinus rhythm (see Chapter 11) can substantially improve CO. Ventricular arrhythmias are also frequent in heart failure and may lead to sudden death. Amiodarone is the antiarrhythmic drug that is most effective at suppressing arrhythmias and least likely to provoke other dangerous rhythm disorders in heart failure patients. However, studies of amiodarone for the treatment of asymptomatic ventricular arrhythmias in heart failure have not shown a consistent survival benefit.

In addition, heart failure patients with symptomatic or sustained ventricular arrhythmias, or those with inducible ventricular tachycardia during electrophysiologic testing, benefit more from the insertion of an *implantable cardioverter-defibrillator (ICD*; see Chapter 11). Based on the results of large-scale randomized trials, ICD implantation is indicated for many patients with symptomatic heart failure and LVEF ≤ 35%, regardless of the presence of ventricular arrhythmias, because this approach reduces the likelihood of sudden cardiac death in this population.

Cardiac Resynchronization Therapy

Intraventricular conduction abnormalities with widened QRS complexes (especially left bundle branch block) are common in patients with advanced heart failure. Such abnormalities can actually contribute to cardiac symptoms because of the resultant uncoordinated pattern of right and left ventricular contraction. Advanced pacemakers have been developed that stimulate both ventricles simultaneously, thus resynchronizing the contractile effort. This technique of biventricular pacing, also termed *cardiac resynchronization therapy (CRT)*, has been shown to augment left ventricular systolic function, improve exercise capacity, and reduce the frequency of heart failure exacerbations and mortality. Thus, CRT is appropriate for selected patients with advanced systolic dysfunction (LVEF ≤ 35%), a prolonged QRS duration (especially patients with QRS ≥ 150 msec with left bundle branch block morphology, and also some patients with QRS ≥ 120 msec who require multiple hospitalizations) and continued symptoms of heart failure despite pharmacologic therapies. Since patients who receive CRT are typically also candidates for an ICD, modern devices combine both functions in a single, small implantable unit.

Cardiac Mechanical Circulatory Support and Replacement Therapy

A patient with severe LV dysfunction whose condition remains refractory to maximal medical management may be a candidate for *cardiac transplantation*. However, only ~4000 transplants are performed worldwide each year because of a shortage of donor hearts, many fewer than the number of patients with refractory heart failure symptoms. For certain patients who are too ill to wait for a heart donor, or who are not eligible for a transplant, alternative mechanical therapies are in selected use. *Ventricular assist devices (VADs)* and implantable *total artificial hearts* can be used to support cardiac pump function in such patients. Recent technological advances in continuous-flow left-sided VADs have resulted in 2-year survival rates of ~80%, compared to <10% survival rates in similar groups of advanced heart failure patients treated with medical therapy alone.

TREATMENT OF HEART FAILURE WITH PRESERVED EJECTION FRACTION

The goals of therapy in heart failure with preserved EF include (1) the relief of pulmonary and systemic congestion and (2) addressing correctable causes of the impaired diastolic function (eg, hypertension, coronary artery disease). Diuretics reduce pulmonary congestion and peripheral edema but must be used cautiously to avoid under filling of the LV. A stiffened LV relies on higher-than-normal pressures to achieve adequate diastolic filling (see Fig. 9-7B), and excessive diuresis could reduce filling and therefore impair SV and CO (see Fig. 9-10, point *b′*).

Unlike patients with impaired systolic function, β-blockers, ACE inhibitors, and ARBs have no demonstrated mortality benefit in patients with heart failure with preserved EF. The aldosterone antagonist spironolactone has been shown to reduce the frequency of hospitalizations for heart failure in this population, but did not improve the survival rate in a large clinical trial. Since contractile function is preserved, inotropic drugs have no therapeutic role in this syndrome.

ACUTE HEART FAILURE

In contrast to the findings of chronic heart failure described to this point, patients with acute heart failure are those who present with urgent and often life-threatening symptomatology. Acute heart failure may develop in a previously asymptomatic patient (eg, resulting from an acute coronary syndrome [Chapter 7], severe hypertension [Chapter 13], or acute valvular regurgitation [Chapter 8]), or it may complicate chronic compensated heart failure following a precipitating trigger (see Table 9-3). Management of acute heart failure typically requires hospitalization and prompt interventions.

↑LV filling Pressures
(Pulmonary and/or Systemic Congestion)

		No	Yes
Reduced Cardiac Output and Vasoconstriction	No	Profile A "Warm and Dry"	Profile B "Warm and Wet"
	Yes	Profile L "Cold and Dry"	Profile C "Cold and Wet"

Figure 9-12. Hemodynamic profiles in acute heart failure. (Derived from Nohria A, Tsang SW, Fang JC, et al. Clinical assessment identifies hemodynamic profiles that predict outcomes in patients admitted with heart failure. *J Am Coll Cardiol.* 2003;41:1797-1804.)

The classification of patients with acute heart failure, and the approach to therapy, can be tailored based on the presence or absence of two major findings at the bedside: (1) volume overload (ie, "wet" vs "dry") as a reflection of elevated LV filling pressures and (2) signs of decreased CO with reduced tissue perfusion ("cold" vs "warm" extremities). Examples of a "wet" profile, indicative of volume overload, include pulmonary crackles, jugular venous distension, and edema of the lower extremities. Figure 9-12 shows how patients with acute heart failure can be divided into four profiles based on observations of these parameters.

Profile A indicates normal hemodynamics. Cardiopulmonary symptoms in such patients would be due to factors other than heart failure, such as parenchymal lung disease or transient myocardial ischemia. Profiles B and C are typical of patients with acute pulmonary edema (described below). Those with Profile B have "wet" lungs but preserved ("warm") tissue perfusion. Profile C is more serious; in addition to congestive findings, impaired forward CO results in marked systemic vasoconstriction (eg, activation of the sympathetic nervous system) and therefore "cold" extremities. Patients with Profile C have a prognosis worse than those with Profile B, who in turn have poorer outcomes than those with Profile A.

Patients with Profile L do not represent an extension of this continuum. Rather, they display "cold" extremities due to low output (hence the label "L") but no signs of vascular congestion. This profile may arise in patients who are actually volume deplete or those with very limited cardiac reserve in the absence of volume overload (eg, a patient with a dilated LV and mitral regurgitation who becomes short of breath with activity because of the inability to generate adequate forward CO). These profiles of acute heart failure should not be confused with the classification of chronic heart failure (stages A through D) presented in Table 9-6.

The goals of therapy in acute heart failure are to (1) normalize ventricular filling pressures and (2) restore adequate tissue perfusion. Identification of the patient's profile type guides therapeutic interventions. For example, a patient with Profile B would require diuretic and/or vasodilator therapy for pulmonary edema (described in the next section), and those with Profile C may additionally require intravenous inotropic medications to strengthen CO. Patients with Profile L may require volume expansion. The presence of profile A would prompt a search for contributions to the patient's symptoms other than heart failure.

Acute Pulmonary Edema

A common manifestation of acute left-sided heart failure (eg, typical of Profiles B and C) is cardiogenic pulmonary edema, in which elevated capillary hydrostatic pressure causes rapid accumulation of fluid within the interstitium and alveolar spaces of the lung. In the presence of normal plasma oncotic pressure, pulmonary edema develops when the pulmonary capillary wedge pressure, which reflects LV diastolic pressure, exceeds ~25 mm Hg.

This condition is frequently accompanied by hypoxemia because of shunting of pulmonary blood flow through regions of hypoventilated alveoli. Like other manifestations of acute heart failure, pulmonary edema may appear suddenly in a previously asymptomatic person (eg, in the setting of an acute myocardial infarction) or in a patient with chronic compensated congestive heart failure following a precipitating event (see Table 9-3). Pulmonary edema is a horrifying experience for the patient, resulting in severe dyspnea and anxiety while struggling to breathe.

On examination, the patient is tachycardic and may demonstrate cold, clammy skin owing to peripheral vasoconstriction in response to increased sympathetic outflow (ie, profile C). Tachypnea and coughing of "frothy" sputum represent transudation of fluid into the alveoli. Crackles are auscultated initially at the bases and later throughout the lung fields, sometimes accompanied by wheezing because of edema within the conductance airways.

Pulmonary edema is a life-threatening emergency that requires immediate improvement of systemic oxygenation and elimination of the underlying cause. The patient should be seated upright to permit pooling of blood within the systemic veins of the lower body, thereby reducing venous return to the heart. Supplemental oxygen is provided by a face mask. Morphine sulfate is administered intravenously to reduce anxiety and also acts as a venous dilator to facilitate pooling of blood peripherally. A rapidly acting diuretic, such as intravenous furosemide, is administered to further reduce LV preload and pulmonary capillary hydrostatic pressure. Other means of reducing preload include administration of nitrates (often intravenously). Intravenous inotropic drugs (eg, dopamine) may increase forward CO and are used primarily in patients with profile C. During resolution of the pulmonary congestion and hypoxemia, attention should be directed at identifying and treating the underlying precipitating cause.

An easy-to-remember mnemonic for the principal components of management of pulmonary edema is the alphabetic sequence LMNOP:

Lasix (trade name for furosemide)
Morphine
Nitrates
Oxygen
Position (sit upright)

Summary

- **Ventricular stroke volume** (SV) is a function of preload, afterload, and contractility; SV rises when there is an increase in preload, a decrease in afterload, or augmented contractility.
- **Cardiac output** = heart rate × stroke volume.
- Ventricular **end-diastolic volume** (or end-diastolic pressure) represents preload and is influenced by the chamber's compliance.

- Ventricular **end-systolic volume** depends on afterload and contractility but not on preload.

- **Heart failure** is a clinical syndrome in which CO fails to meet the metabolic demands of the body or meets those demands only if cardiac filling pressures are abnormally high.

- Chronic heart failure may be classified into two categories: (1) **heart failure with reduced EF** (HFrEF) owing to impaired left ventricular systolic function and (2) **heart failure with preserved EF** (HFpEF), generally a result of diastolic dysfunction.

- **Compensatory mechanisms** in heart failure that initially maintain circulatory function include (1) preload augmentation with increased SV via the Frank-Starling mechanism, (2) activation of neurohormonal systems, and (3) ventricular hypertrophy; however, these compensations eventually become maladaptive, contributing to adverse ventricular remodeling and progressive deterioration of ventricular function.

- Symptoms of heart failure may be exacerbated by **precipitating factors** that increase metabolic demand (eg, tachycardia), increase circulating volume, augment afterload, or decrease contractility.

- **Treatment** of heart failure includes addressing the underlying cause of the condition, eliminating precipitating factors, and modulating detrimental neurohormonal activations.

- Standard therapy of symptomatic heart failure with *reduced* EF includes an **ACE inhibitor**, **β-blocker**, and sometimes an **aldosterone antagonist**. For patients who *do not* tolerate an ACE inhibitor, an **AII receptor blocker** (ARB) or the combination of **hydralazine plus nitrates** can be prescribed instead. For those who *do* tolerate an ACE inhibitor or ARB, substitution with an **angiotensin receptor-neprilysin inhibitor** (ARNI; eg, valsartan-sacubitril) should be considered to further improve cardiovascular outcomes.

- **Diuretics** should be used to treat volume overload, and **inotropic drugs** are typically reserved for acute "rescue" management of low CO states.

- For patients with heart failure with reduced EF who meet specific criteria, an **implantable cardioverter-defibrillator** and/or **cardiac resynchronization therapy** (biventricular pacing) may be indicated.

- For refractory end-stage heart failure, **cardiac transplantation** and/or **mechanical circulatory support** should be considered in selected patients.

- **Therapy for heart failure with *preserved* EF** relies primarily on diuretics to relieve pulmonary congestion, but such therapy must be administered cautiously to avoid excess reduction of preload and hypotension.

- **Acute heart failure** can be profiled by, and treatment decisions based on, the presence or absence of (1) elevated left heart filling pressures (wet vs dry) and (2) reduced systemic tissue perfusion with elevated systemic vascular resistance (ie, cold vs warm).

Review Questions

1. Regarding the pressure volume loop in Part A of the figure, answer the following questions:

A   **B**

  A. What is the stroke volume?
  B. What is the ejection fraction?
  C. In Part B of the figure, which of the following would explain the shift from the original pressure-volume loop (drawn in blue) to the pressure-volume loop drawn in green?
    a. Severe uncontrolled hypertension
    b. Large myocardial infarction
    c. Intravenous fluid administration
    d. Intravenous infusion of dobutamine

2. A 72-year-old woman presents with dyspnea on exertion, labored breathing while lying in bed, and severe breathlessness that awakes her from sleep at about 2 AM each night. Which of the following would be more suggestive of heart failure with preserved ejection fraction (HFpEF) than heart failure with reduced ejection fraction (HFrEF)?

  a. Presence of a third heart sound (S_3) on physical examination
  b. Increased left ventricular end-diastolic volume on echocardiography
  c. Normal left ventricular end-systolic volume on echocardiography
  d. Mortality reduction with angiotensin-converting enzyme (ACE) inhibitor therapy

3. A 64-year-old man presents with shortness of breath, orthopnea, and lower extremity swelling in recent months. Examination is notable for jugular venous distention, bibasilar crackles, an S_3 heart sound, and symmetric pitting edema from the knees to the ankles bilaterally. Echocardiography is performed and demonstrates a left ventricular ejection fraction of 30%. Which of the following medications would improve survival when administered chronically?

  a. Metoprolol succinate
  b. Furosemide
  c. Digoxin
  d. Dopamine

Answers to Review Questions

1. **A. The stroke volume is 90 mL.** Stroke volume (SV) = end-diastolic volume (EDV) − end-systolic volume (ESV). In a pressure-volume loop, the right vertical line represents end-diastolic volume and the right vertical line represents end-systolic volume (see Fig. 9-4). In this case, EDV is 135 mL and ESV is 45 mL, such that SV = 135 − 45 = 90 mL.

   B. The ejection fraction is 67%. The ejection fraction = SV/EDV = 90 mL/135 mL = 67%.

   C. Choice d is correct. The green loop demonstrates an increase in contractility (in this cause due to the positive inotrope dobutamine) compared to the baseline blue loop. Increased contractility produces a larger SV and results in a smaller end systolic volume (see Fig. 9-5C). A large myocardial infarction would decrease contractility, having the opposite effect (smaller SV, larger end-systolic volume). Severe uncontrolled hypertension would cause an increase in afterload, which would be associated with a loop with lower SV and higher end-systolic volume (see Fig. 9-5B). Intravenous fluid administration would increase preload, leading to higher EDV and SV but unchanged end-systolic volume (see Fig. 9-5A).

2. **Choice c is correct.** HFpEF is characterized by impaired diastolic relaxation and/or increased ventricular stiffness leading to higher diastolic ventricular pressure at any diastolic volume. In HFpEF there is normal, or reduced, ventricular EDV, normal ejection fraction, and normal ventricular end-systolic volume (see Fig. 9-7B). A fourth heart sound (S_4) is common in this condition, reflecting atrial contraction into the stiffened ventricle. An S_3 is more suggestive of HFrEF.

   ACE inhibitors reduce mortality in patients with HFrEF, but this benefit does not extend to patients with HFpEF.

3. **Choice a is correct.** This patient has HFrEF and presents with volume overload as demonstrated by jugular venous distension, pulmonary congestion (crackles), and systemic interstitial fluid accumulation (lower extremity edema). While diuretic therapy is indicated to decrease preload and for symptomatic relief, it does not provide a mortality benefit. Pharmacologic agents that improve symptoms and mortality in HFrEF include ACE inhibitors (as well as ARBs and the angiotensin receptor-neprilysin inhibitor valsartan-sacubitril), certain β-blockers, and aldosterone antagonists (eg, spironolactone). Although digoxin decreases the frequency of heart failure hospitalizations, it does not improve long-term survival. Inotropic agents such as dopamine are administered for temporary hemodynamic support in acutely ill, hospitalized patients, but do not improve long-term survival.

Acknowledgments

Contributors to previous editions of this chapter were David Miranda, MD; Gregory D. Lewis, MD; Neal Anjan Chatterjee; Ravi V. Shah, MD; George S. M. Dyer, MD; Stephen K. Frankel, MD; Arthur Coday Jr., MD; Vikram Janakiraman, MD; and Michael A. Fifer, MD.

Additional Reading

Braunwald E. Heart failure. *JACC Heart Fail.* 2013;1:1-20.

Ellison DH, Felker GM. Diuretic treatment in heart failure. *N Engl J Med.* 2017;377:1964-1975.

Redfield MM. Heart failure with preserved ejection fraction. *N Engl J Med.* 2016;375:1868-1877.

Rossignol P, Hernandez AF, Solomon SD, et al. Heart failure drug treatment. *Lancet.* 2019;393:1034-1044.

Shah KS, Xu H, Matsouaka RA, et al. Heart failure with preserved, borderline, and reduced ejection fraction: 5-year outcomes. *J Am Coll Cardiol*. 2017;70:2476-2486.

Tromp J, Westinbrink BD, Ouwerkerk W, et al. Identifying pathophysiological mechanisms in heart failure with reduced versus preserved ejection fraction. *J Am Coll Cardiol*. 2018;72:1081-1090.

Velazquez EJ, Morrow DA, DeVore AD, et al. Angiotensin-neprilysin inhibition in acute decompensated heart failure. *N Engl J Med*. 2019;380:539-548.

Yancy CW, Jessup M, Bozkurt B, et al. 2017 ACC/AHA/HFSA focused update of the 2013 ACCF/AHA guideline for the management of heart failure: a report of the American College of Cardiology/American Heart Association Task Force on Clinical Practice Guidelines and the Heart Failure Society of America. *Circulation*. 2017;136:e137-e161.

10

The Cardiomyopathies

Lauren A. Eberly | **Neal K. Lakdawala** |
Leonard S. Lilly

Cardiomyopathies are a diverse set of heart muscle disorders that affect myocardial systolic and/or diastolic function. These conditions may result in inappropriate ventricular dilatation, hypertrophy, and/or stiffness, and progressive heart failure and cardiovascular death are potential end manifestations. Cardiomyopathies can involve the heart alone or may be a component of a systemic syndrome.

Cardiomyopathies traditionally have been classified into three main types based on the anatomic appearance and abnormal physiology of the left ventricle (LV) (Fig. 10-1). **Dilated** cardiomyopathy (DCM) is characterized by ventricular chamber enlargement with impaired *systolic* contractile function; **hypertrophic** cardiomyopathy (HCM), by an abnormally thickened ventricular wall with abnormal *diastolic* relaxation but usually intact systolic function; and **restrictive** cardiomyopathy, by an abnormally stiffened myocardium (because of fibrosis or an infiltrative process) leading to impaired *diastolic* relaxation, but systolic contractile function is typically normal or near normal.

While this phenotype-based classification describes general features of cardiomyopathies, it does not specify their genetic underpinnings, other organ involvement, or risk stratification. A newer classification scheme, the MOGE(S) system, seeks to delineate morphology (M), organ involvement (O), genetic inheritance pattern (G), etiologic annotation (E), and the functional status (S) of the disease. However, this chapter is organized by the traditional phenotype-based classification, as it is still the system predominantly utilized in clinical settings.

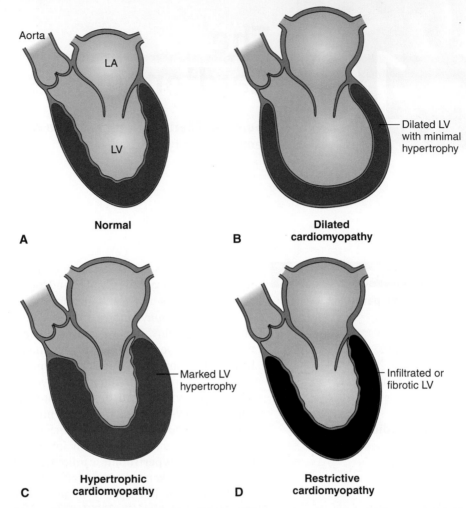

Figure 10-1. Anatomic appearance of the cardiomyopathies (CMPs). A. Normal heart demonstrating the left ventricle (LV) and left atrium (LA). **B.** Dilated CMP is characterized by ventricular enlargement with only mildly increased thickness. **C.** Hypertrophic CMP demonstrates marked ventricular hypertrophy, either asymmetrically or symmetrically (as drawn here). **D.** Restrictive CMP is caused by infiltration or fibrosis of the ventricles, usually without chamber enlargement. LA enlargement is common to all three types of CMP.

DILATED CARDIOMYOPATHY

ETIOLOGY

Myocyte damage and cardiac enlargement in DCM result from a wide spectrum of etiologies (Table 10-1). Although many cases are classified as idiopathic (ie, the cause is undetermined), examples of defined conditions that can result in DCM include specific genetic mutations, viral myocarditis, excessive alcohol ingestion, the peripartum state, and exposure to cardiotoxic antineoplastic agents.

Genetic abnormalities are the most common identifiable causes of DCM. Several familial forms have been identified and are responsible for ~40% of what was once classified as idiopathic disease. Autosomal dominant inheritance is predominant, but autosomal recessive, X-linked, and mitochondrial patterns of inheritance also occur. Culprit mutations lead to abnormalities of contractile force generation, force transmission, energy production, and

TABLE 10-1	Etiologies of Dilated Cardiomyopathies

Genetic
Familial cardiomyopathies (eg, mutations in cytoskeletal, sarcomeric, nuclear membrane genes)
Muscular/myotonic dystrophies (eg, mutations in sarcolemmal membrane genes)

Inflammatory myocarditis
Infective (especially viral)
Noninfective
   Granulomatous inflammatory disease
      Sarcoidosis
      Giant cell myocarditis
   Connective tissue diseases
   Immune checkpoint inhibitor cancer therapy

Toxic
Chronic alcohol ingestion
Cocaine
Chemotherapeutic agents (eg, anthracyclines, trastuzumab)

Metabolic
Hypothyroidism
Chronic hypocalcemia or hypophosphatemia
Hemochromatosis

Miscellaneous
Peripartum cardiomyopathy

myocyte viability. Many responsible mutations have been identified in genes that code for cardiac cytoskeletal, myofibrillar, and nuclear membrane proteins (Table 10-2), with the most frequent being truncating mutations in the large sarcomeric gene titin (*TTN*), accounting for 20%-25% of all DCM patients.

Other causes of DCM include forms of inflammatory myocarditis. For example, acute **viral myocarditis** generally afflicts young, previously healthy people. Implicated viruses include coxsackievirus group B, parvovirus B19, and adenovirus, among many others. Viral myocarditis is usually a self-limited illness with full recovery, but some patients progress to a postviral form of DCM. It is hypothesized that myocardial destruction and fibrosis result from immune-mediated injury triggered by viral constituents. Transvenous ventricular biopsy during acute viral myocarditis may demonstrate active inflammation, but specific viral genomic sequences have been demonstrated in only a minority of patients.

Noninfective causes of myocardial inflammation include sarcoidosis and giant cell myocarditis. **Sarcoidosis** is a multisystem inflammatory disease. Evidence suggests that it is caused by an immunologic response to an unclear trigger and is characterized by noncaseating granulomas on histopathology. Cardiac involvement occurs in ~25% of patients with systemic sarcoidosis, potentially resulting in conduction abnormalities, ventricular arrhythmias, and heart failure. **Giant cell myocarditis**, a rare and rapidly progressive disease, is caused by T-cell–mediated inflammation and destruction of myocytes. Heart failure, arrhythmias, and conduction disturbances are common. Myocarditis also manifests occasionally in patients with **connective tissue diseases** (eg, systemic lupus erythematosus) and after administration of **immune checkpoint inhibitors** (recently developed antineoplastic therapies that inhibit negative immune regulation).

DCM arises in some people who consume **alcohol** excessively and chronically. Although the pathogenesis is unknown, ethanol is thought to impair cellular function by impacting mitochondrial oxidative function, myofilament protein synthesis, cytosolic calcium levels,

TABLE 10-2	Examples of Familial Forms of Dilated and Hypertrophic Cardiomyopathies	
Protein	**Mutations Identified in DCM**	**Mutations Identified in HCM**
Cytoskeletal/sarcolemmal membrane proteins		
Desmin	√	
Dystrophin	√	
Sarcomeric proteins		
β-Myosin heavy chain	√	√
Myosin-binding protein C		√
Cardiac troponin T	√	√
Cardiac troponin I	√	√
Titin	√	
α-Tropomyosin	√	√
Essential myosin light chain		√
Nuclear membrane protein		
Lamin A/C	√	

and myocyte apoptosis. While its clinical presentation and histologic features are similar to those of other dilated cardiomyopathies, alcoholic cardiomyopathy is important to identify because it is potentially reversible; cessation of ethanol consumption can lead to dramatic recovery of ventricular function.

Cocaine use can also lead to cardiomyopathy, the mechanism of which is not fully understood. Contributing factors include increased myocardial demand and oxidative stress through sympathomimetic effects, decreased coronary flow, and increased platelet aggregation potentially leading to coronary thrombus formation.

Other toxin-mediated causes of DCM include some types of cancer **chemotherapy**, including a dose-dependent toxicity of anthracyclines (eg, doxorubicin). Metabolic causes of DCM, which are often reversible, include hypothyroidism, chronic hypocalcemia or hypophosphatemia, and hemochromatosis, a condition of iron overload that can include toxic iron deposition in the myocardium.

Peripartum cardiomyopathy is a form of DCM that presents with heart failure symptoms between the last trimester of pregnancy and up to 6 months postpartum. Risk factors include older maternal age, African ancestry, and having multiple pregnancies. A unifying etiology of this condition has not been identified, but ~15% of patients have truncating mutations in the *TTN* gene, suggesting a possible genetic predisposition. Ventricular function returns to normal in ~50% of affected women over the months following pregnancy, but recurrences of DCM with subsequent pregnancies may occur.

Stress cardiomyopathy (also termed *apical ballooning syndrome* or *takotsubo cardiomyopathy*) is a form of temporary DCM. This condition is characterized by acute and transient left ventricular dysfunction that typically arises after a severe emotional or physically stressful event and occurs primarily in older women. Typically, the dysfunction is regional, most commonly affecting the entire LV apical region, in distinction to vigorous contraction of the unaffected portions of the ventricle. The presentation may mimic that of an acute myocardial infarction, but the regional wall motion abnormality does not follow a normal coronary anatomic distribution, and in most cases LV dysfunction resolves completely within days to weeks. During the acute phase, some patients may develop heart failure, arrhythmias, hypotension, and even cardiac arrest. The exact pathogenesis of stress cardiomyopathy remains unknown, but suspected factors include an excessive sympathetic response leading to coronary vasoconstriction and microvascular dysfunction.

PATHOLOGY

Although enlargement of all four cardiac chambers is common in DCM (Fig. 10-2), LV dysfunction and enlargement are most often primary. Microscopically, findings are non-specific with evidence of myocyte degeneration with irregular hypertrophy and atrophy of myofibers. Interstitial and perivascular fibrosis is often extensive.

Figure 10-2. Transverse sections of a normal heart (right) and a heart from a patient with dilated cardiomyopathy (DCM). In the DCM specimen, there is biventricular dilatation without a proportional increase in wall thickness. LV, left ventricle; RV, right ventricle. (Modified from Emmanouilides GC, ed. *Moss and Adams' Heart Disease in Infants, Children, and Adolescents*. 5th ed. Baltimore, MD: Lippincott Williams & Wilkins; 1995:86.)

PATHOPHYSIOLOGY

The hallmark of DCM is left ventricular dilatation with decreased contractile function (Fig. 10-3), but with disease progression, the right ventricle (RV) may also be involved.

As ventricular stroke volume and cardiac output decline because of impaired myocyte contractility, compensatory actions are triggered, including (1) the Frank-Starling mechanism, in which the elevated ventricular diastolic volume increases the stretch of the myofibers, thereby increasing the subsequent stroke volume, and (2) neurohormonal activation, initially mediated by the sympathetic nervous system (see Chapter 9). The latter contributes to an increased heart rate and contractility, which help to buffer the fall in cardiac output. These compensations may render the patient asymptomatic during the early stages of ventricular dysfunction. However, as progressive myocyte degeneration and volume overload ensue, clinical symptoms of heart failure develop.

With a persistent reduction of cardiac output, the decline in renal blood flow prompts the kidneys to increase secretion of renin. This activation of the renin-angiotensin-aldosterone axis increases peripheral vascular resistance (mediated through angiotensin II) and

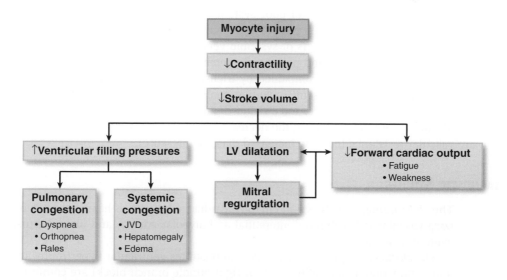

Figure 10-3. Pathophysiology of dilated cardiomyopathy. The reduced ventricular stroke volume results in decreased forward cardiac output and increased ventricular filling pressures. The listed clinical manifestations follow. LV, left ventricle; JVD, jugular venous distention.

intravascular volume (because of increased aldosterone). As described in Chapter 9, these effects are also initially helpful in buffering the fall in cardiac output.

Ultimately, however, the "compensatory" effects of neurohormonal activation prove detrimental. Arteriolar vasoconstriction and increased systemic resistance render it more difficult for the LV to eject blood in the forward direction, and the rise in intravascular volume further burdens the ventricles, resulting in pulmonary and systemic congestion. In addition, chronically elevated levels of angiotensin II and aldosterone directly contribute to pathologic myocardial remodeling and fibrosis.

As the cardiomyopathic process causes the ventricles to enlarge over time, the mitral and tricuspid valves may fail to coapt properly in systole, and valvular regurgitation ensues. Such regurgitation has three detrimental consequences: (1) excessive volume and pressure loads are placed on the atria, causing them to dilate, often leading to atrial fibrillation; (2) regurgitation of blood into the left atrium further decreases forward stroke volume into the aorta and systemic circulation; and (3) when the regurgitant volume returns to the LV during each diastole, an even greater volume load is presented to the dilated LV.

CLINICAL FINDINGS

The clinical manifestations of DCM are primarily those of heart failure. Pulmonary congestion results in dyspnea, orthopnea, and paroxysmal nocturnal dyspnea, whereas chronic systemic venous congestion causes ascites and peripheral edema. Because these symptoms may develop insidiously, the patient may complain only of recent weight gain (because of interstitial edema) and shortness of breath on exertion. Less common are symptoms of low forward cardiac output and reduced tissue perfusion, including fatigue and light-headedness.

PHYSICAL EXAMINATION

Signs of pulmonary and/or systemic venous congestion are often present. Pulmonary venous congestion results in auscultatory crackles (rales), and dullness to percussion at the lung bases may be present because of pleural effusions. Cardiac examination shows an enlarged heart with leftward displacement of the apical impulse. On auscultation, a third heart sound (S3) is common as a sign of poor systolic function and volume overload. The murmur of mitral regurgitation is often present as a result of left ventricular dilatation. If right ventricular failure has developed, signs of systemic venous congestion include jugular vein distention, hepatomegaly, ascites, and peripheral edema. Right ventricular enlargement and contractile dysfunction are often accompanied by tricuspid valve regurgitation. Signs of decreased cardiac output may be present, including cool extremities (owing to peripheral vasoconstriction), low arterial pressure, and a reduced pulse pressure (the difference between systolic and diastolic pressure), reflecting the decreased cardiac output combined with elevated systemic vascular resistance (causing increased diastolic pressure).

DIAGNOSTIC STUDIES

The *chest radiograph* shows an enlarged cardiac silhouette. If heart failure is present, pulmonary vascular redistribution, interstitial and alveolar edema, and pleural effusions are often evident (see Fig. 3-5).

The *electrocardiogram* (ECG) often demonstrates ventricular hypertrophy and interventricular conduction abnormalities (left or right bundle branch block) are common. With disease progression, the QRS voltage may lessen due to attrition of cardiomyocytes. Patchy fibrosis of the myocardium contributes to arrhythmias, most importantly atrial fibrillation and ventricular tachycardia.

Echocardiography in DCM typically demonstrates enlargement of the affected ventricle(s) with little concentric hypertrophy and reduced systolic function. Left atrial enlargement and functional mitral regurgitation (due to LV enlargement) are common.

Cardiac catheterization or CT angiography is often performed to determine whether coronary artery disease is contributing to the impaired ventricular function. This is most useful diagnostically in patients who have symptoms of angina or evidence of prior myocardial infarction on the ECG. Hemodynamic measurements typically show elevated right- and left-sided diastolic pressures and diminished cardiac output. In select cases, transvenous biopsy of the RV may be performed in the cardiac catheterization laboratory to clarify the etiology of the cardiomyopathy.

Cardiac magnetic resonance imaging (MRI) is helpful in the evaluation of DCM, particularly to distinguish between contributors such as ischemic damage, myocardial inflammation, and iron overload (hemochromatosis). *Positron emission tomography* (PET) is useful in the diagnosis of cardiac sarcoidosis (see Chapter 3).

TREATMENT

The goal of therapy in DCM is to promote reverse remodeling of dilated ventricles, enhance myocardial function, relieve symptoms, prevent complications, and improve long-term survival. Thus, in addition to treating any identified underlying cause of DCM, therapeutic considerations include those described in the following sections.

Medical Treatment of Heart Failure Symptoms

Approaches for the relief of vascular congestion are the same as standard therapies for heart failure (see Chapter 9). Initial therapy typically includes salt restriction and *diuretics* if volume overload is present. After decongestion is achieved, appropriate treatment includes vasodilator therapy with an *angiotensin-converting enzyme (ACE) inhibitor, angiotensin II receptor blocker (ARB), or angiotensin receptor-neprilysin inhibitor (ARNI)*, as well as a *β-blocker* in hemodynamically stable patients. For patients with persistent symptoms, the addition of an *aldosterone antagonist* should be considered. These measures have been shown to improve symptoms and reduce mortality in patients with heart failure secondary to DCM.

Prevention and Treatment of Arrhythmias

Atrial and ventricular arrhythmias are common in advanced DCM. It is important to maintain serum electrolytes (notably, potassium and magnesium) within their normal ranges, especially during diuretic therapy, to avoid provoking serious arrhythmias. Studies have shown that available antiarrhythmic drugs do not prevent death from ventricular arrhythmias in DCM. In fact, when used in patients with poor LV function, many antiarrhythmic drugs have dangerous *proarrhythmic* effects. *Amiodarone* is the antiarrhythmic drug studied most extensively in patients with DCM. Whereas there is no convincing evidence that it reduces mortality in DCM, it is the safest of the antiarrhythmics for suppressing atrial fibrillation and ventricular tachycardia in this population. In contrast to antiarrhythmic drugs, the placement of an *implantable cardioverter-defibrillator* (ICD) does reduce arrhythmic deaths in patients with DCM. Patients with prior sustained ventricular tachycardia or cardiac arrest have a class I indication for ICD therapy. Based on large-scale randomized trials, an ICD is also recommended for patients with chronic symptomatic DCM and at least moderately reduced systolic function (eg, LV ejection fraction ≤35%), regardless of whether ventricular arrhythmias have been detected.

Many patients with DCM have conduction abnormalities (eg, left bundle-branch block) that contribute to dyssynchronous ventricular contraction and reduced cardiac output. Electronic pacemakers capable of stimulating both ventricles simultaneously have been devised to better coordinate systolic contraction as an adjunct to medical therapy (termed *cardiac resynchronization therapy*, as described in Chapter 9). Demonstrated benefits of this approach include improved quality of life and exercise tolerance, fewer hospitalizations for heart failure, and reduced mortality, particularly in those with pretreatment left bundle branch block and a markedly prolonged QRS duration (≥150 ms).

Prevention of Thromboembolic Events

Patients with DCM are at increased risk of thromboembolic complications for reasons that include (1) blood stasis in the ventricles resulting from poor systolic function, (2) stasis in the atria due to chamber enlargement or atrial fibrillation, and (3) systemic venous stasis because of poor circulatory flow. Peripheral venous or right ventricular thrombi may lead to pulmonary emboli, whereas thromboemboli of left ventricular origin may lodge in a systemic artery, resulting in cerebral, myocardial, or renal infarctions. In DCM with heart failure, systemic anticoagulation should be considered for patients with a history of venous or systemic thromboembolism, atrial fibrillation, or those with left ventricular thrombi identified by cardiac imaging.

Cardiac Transplantation

In suitable patients with refractory heart failure, cardiac transplantation offers a substantially better 5-year prognosis than do the standard therapies for DCM described above. The 1- and 11-year survival rates after transplantation are ~90% and ~50%, respectively. However, the scarcity of donor hearts greatly limits the availability of this approach. Thus, other mechanical options have been developed and continue to undergo refinements. Implanted left ventricular assist devices are used for hemodynamic support in patients awaiting cardiac transplantation or as longer-term "destination" therapy in some patients with predominant left heart failure.

HYPERTROPHIC CARDIOMYOPATHY

With an estimated prevalence of 1 out of every 500 adults, HCM is characterized by left ventricular hypertrophy that is not caused by chronic pressure overload (ie, *not* the result of hypertension or aortic stenosis [AS]). In this condition, systolic LV contraction is typically normal or vigorous, but the affected muscle is thickened and stiff, resulting in impaired ventricular relaxation and elevated LV filling pressure. While HCM is the most common cause of sudden death in young patients, the prognosis tends to be more benign when HCM is diagnosed in older individuals.

ETIOLOGY

HCM most often arises from autosomal dominant mutations in genes that code for components of the sarcomere. The most frequently mutated genes encode β-myosin heavy chain (β-MHC) and myosin-binding protein C, with other sarcomeric genes implicated less often (examples of which are listed in Table 10-2). Mutations that cause HCM lead to *augmented* systolic function, diminished relaxation, and increased energy utilization. These fundamental changes in contractile function precede overt hypertrophic remodeling and fibrosis.

PATHOLOGY

Although hypertrophy in HCM may involve any portion of the ventricles, *asymmetric hypertrophy* of the ventricular septum (Fig. 10-4) is most common. Less often, ventricular hypertrophy is concentric or is localized to the apex or midregion of the LV.

Unlike ventricular hypertrophy resulting from hypertension in which the myocytes enlarge uniformly and remain orderly, the histology of HCM is unusual. The myocardial fibers are in a pattern of extensive disarray (Fig. 10-5). Short, wide, hypertrophied fibers are oriented in chaotic directions and are surrounded by numerous cardiac fibroblasts and extracellular matrix. Such myocyte disarray and fibrosis play a role in the abnormal diastolic stiffness and arrhythmogenesis that are common in this disorder.

Figure 10-4. Postmortem heart specimen from a patient with hypertrophic cardiomyopathy. Marked left ventricular hypertrophy is present, especially of the interventricular septum (IVS).

PATHOPHYSIOLOGY

The predominant feature of HCM is ventricular hypertrophy that reduces the compliance and diastolic relaxation properties of the LV (Fig. 10-6). Patients who have asymmetric hypertrophy of the proximal interventricular septum may display additional findings related to transient obstruction of left ventricular outflow during systole. It is useful to consider the pathophysiology of HCM based on whether such systolic outflow tract obstruction is present.

A   **B**   **C**

Figure 10-5. Light microscopy of hypertrophic myocardium. A. Normal myocardium. **B.** Hypertrophied myocytes in a patient with valvular heart disease. **C.** Myocyte disarray with fibrosis in a patient with hypertrophic cardiomyopathy.

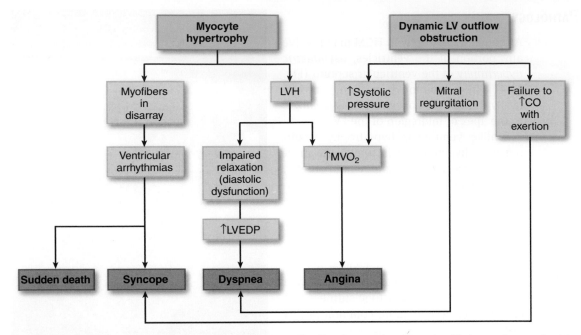

Figure 10-6. Pathophysiology of hypertrophic cardiomyopathy. The disarrayed and hypertrophied myocytes may lead to ventricular arrhythmias (which can cause syncope or sudden death) and impaired diastolic left ventricular (LV) relaxation (which causes elevated LV filling pressures and dyspnea). If dynamic LV outflow obstruction is present, mitral regurgitation often accompanies it (which contributes to dyspnea), and the impaired ability to raise cardiac output with exertion can lead to exertional syncope. The thickened LV wall and increased systolic pressure associated with outflow tract obstruction each contribute to increased myocardial oxygen consumption (MVO_2) and can precipitate angina. CO, cardiac output; LVEDP, LV end-diastolic pressure; LVH, LV hypertrophy.

HCM Without Outflow Tract Obstruction

Although systolic contraction of the LV is usually vigorous in HCM, reduced ventricular compliance alters the normal pressure-volume relationship, causing the passive diastolic filling curve to shift upward (see Fig. 9-7B). The associated rise in diastolic LV pressure is transmitted backward, leading to elevated left atrial, pulmonary venous, and pulmonary capillary pressures. Dyspnea, especially during exertion, is thus a common symptom in this disorder.

HCM With Outflow Obstruction

Approximately 60% of patients with HCM manifest systolic outflow tract obstruction at rest or with provocation. The mechanism of systolic obstruction involves abnormal motion of the anterior mitral valve leaflet toward the LV outflow tract where the thickened septum protrudes (Fig. 10-7). The process is explained as follows: (1) during ventricular contraction, ejection of blood toward the aortic valve is more rapid than usual, because it must flow through an outflow tract that is narrowed by the thickened septum; (2) this rapid flow creates Venturi forces that abnormally draw the anterior mitral leaflet toward the septum during contraction; and (3) the anterior mitral leaflet approaches and abuts the hypertrophied septum, causing transient obstruction of blood flow into the aorta. Although generally less, the pressure gradient generated across the LV outflow tract can exceed 100 mm Hg.

In patients with outflow obstruction, elevated left atrial and pulmonary capillary wedge pressures result from both the decreased ventricular compliance and the outflow obstruction during contraction. The high ventricular systolic pressure increases wall stress and myocardial oxygen consumption, which can result in angina (see Fig. 10-6). In addition, because obstruction is caused by abnormal motion of the anterior mitral leaflet toward the septum

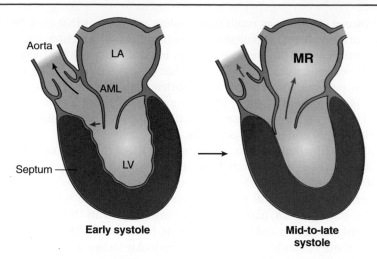

Figure 10-7. Pathophysiology of left ventricular (LV) outflow obstruction and mitral regurgitation (MR) in hypertrophic cardiomyopathy. Left panel. The LV outflow tract is abnormally narrowed between the hypertrophied interventricular septum and the anterior leaflet of the mitral valve (AML). Rapid ejection velocity through the narrowed tract in early systole draws the AML toward the septum (*short red arrow*). LA, left atrium. **Right panel.** As the mitral valve anterior leaflet abnormally moves toward and contacts the septum, outflow into the aorta is transiently obstructed (*short blue arrow*). Because the mitral leaflets do not coapt normally in systole, MR also results (*long red arrow*).

(and therefore *away* from the posterior mitral leaflet), the mitral valve may not close properly during systole, and mitral regurgitation may result. Such regurgitation further elevates left atrial and pulmonary venous pressures and may worsen symptoms of dyspnea, as well as contribute to the development of atrial fibrillation.

The systolic pressure gradient observed in obstructive HCM is dynamic in that its magnitude varies during contraction and depends, at any given time, on the distance between the anterior leaflet of the mitral valve and the hypertrophied septum. Situations that *decrease* LV cavity size (eg, reduced venous return owing to intravascular volume depletion) bring the mitral leaflet and septum into closer proximity and *promote* obstruction. Conversely, conditions that *enlarge* the LV (eg, augmented intravascular volume) increase the distance between the anterior mitral leaflet and septum and *reduce* the obstruction. Positive inotropic drugs (which augment the force of contraction; see Chapter 17) also force the mitral leaflet and septum into closer proximity and contribute to obstruction, whereas negative inotropic drugs (eg, β-blockers) have the opposite effect.

CLINICAL FINDINGS

The symptoms of HCM vary widely from none to marked physical limitations (see Fig. 10-6). The average age of presentation is the mid-20s.

The most frequent symptom is *dyspnea* owing to elevated diastolic LV (and pulmonary capillary) pressure. This symptom is further exacerbated by the high systolic LV pressure and mitral regurgitation found in patients with outflow tract obstruction.

Angina may be described by patients with HCM, even in the absence of obstructive coronary artery disease. Myocardial ischemia may be contributed to by (1) the high oxygen demand of the increased muscle mass and (2) the narrowed small branches of the coronary arteries within the hypertrophied ventricular wall. If outflow tract obstruction is present, the high systolic ventricular pressure increases myocardial oxygen demand because of the increased wall stress and contributes further to ischemia.

Syncope in HCM may result from cardiac arrhythmias that arise because of the structurally abnormal myofibers. In patients with outflow tract obstruction, syncope may also be induced by exertion, when the pressure gradient is made worse by the increased force of contraction, thereby causing a transient fall in cardiac output. Orthostatic light-headedness is also common in patients with outflow tract obstruction. This occurs because venous return to the heart is reduced on standing by the gravitational pooling of blood in the lower extremities. The LV thus decreases in size and outflow tract obstruction intensifies, transiently reducing cardiac output and cerebral perfusion.

When arrhythmias occur, symptoms of HCM may be exacerbated. For example, *atrial fibrillation* is not well tolerated because the loss of normal atrial contraction further impairs diastolic filling and can therefore worsen symptoms of pulmonary congestion. Of greatest concern, the first clinical manifestation of HCM may be *ventricular fibrillation*, resulting in *sudden cardiac death*, particularly in young adults with HCM during strenuous physical exertion. Risk factors for sudden death among patients with HCM include a history of syncope, a family history of sudden death, prior ventricular tachycardia, and extreme hypertrophy of the LV wall (>30 mm in thickness).

PHYSICAL EXAMINATION

A patient with a mild form of HCM may have a normal cardiac examination. Otherwise, a common finding is a fourth heart sound (S4), generated by left atrial contraction into the stiffened LV (see Chapter 2). The forceful atrial contraction may also result in a palpable presystolic impulse over the cardiac apex (a "double apical impulse").

Other findings are typical in patients with systolic outflow obstruction. The carotid pulse rises briskly in early systole but then quickly declines as obstruction to cardiac outflow appears. The characteristic systolic murmur of LV outflow obstruction is rough and crescendo-decrescendo in shape, is heard best at the left lower sternal border (in proximity to the turbulent flow through the narrowed outflow tract), and, unlike AS, does not typically radiate to the carotid arteries. In addition, as the stethoscope is moved toward the apex, the holosystolic blowing murmur of accompanying mitral regurgitation may be auscultated. Although the LV outflow obstruction murmur may be soft at rest, bedside maneuvers that alter preload and afterload can dramatically increase its intensity and help differentiate this murmur from other conditions, such as AS (Table 10-3).

A commonly used technique in this regard is the *Valsalva maneuver*, produced by asking the patient to "bear down" (forceful exhalation against a closed glottis). The Valsalva maneuver increases intrathoracic pressure, which decreases venous return to the heart and transiently reduces LV size. This action brings the hypertrophied septum and anterior leaflet of the mitral valve into closer proximity, creating greater obstruction to forward flow. Thus, during Valsalva, the murmur of HCM increases in intensity. In contrast, the murmur of AS decreases in intensity during Valsalva because of the reduced flow across the stenotic valve.

Conversely, a change from standing to a *squatting position* suddenly augments venous return to the heart (which increases preload) while simultaneously increasing the systemic

TABLE 10-3	Effect of Maneuvers on Murmurs of AS and HCM		
	Valsalva	**Squatting**	**Standing**
HCM murmur	↑	↓	↑
AS murmur	↓	↑	↓

HCM, hypertrophic cardiomyopathy; AS, aortic stenosis.

vascular resistance. The increased preload raises the stroke volume and therefore causes the murmur of AS to become louder. In contrast, the transient increase in LV size during squatting reduces the LV outflow tract obstruction in HCM and softens the intensity of that murmur. Sudden *standing* from a squatting position has the opposite effect on each of these murmurs (see Table 10-3).

DIAGNOSTIC STUDIES

The *ECG* typically shows left ventricular hypertrophy and often T-wave inversions in the precordial leads. Deep, narrow Q waves may appear in the lateral leads, the reciprocal of prominent septal forces. In some patients, diffuse T-wave inversions are present, which can predate clinical, echocardiographic, or other electrocardiographic manifestations of HCM. Atrial fibrillation is present in up to 25% of older HCM patients. Episodes of nonsustained ventricular tachycardia, when present, may be detected by ambulatory electrocardiographic monitoring.

Echocardiography is crucial in the evaluation of HCM. The degree of LV hypertrophy can be measured and regions of asymmetrical wall thickness identified. When present, left ventricular outflow obstruction is detected, including abnormal anterior motion of the mitral valve as it is drawn toward the hypertrophied septum during systole and partial closure of the aortic valve in midsystole as flow across it is transiently obstructed. Doppler recordings during echocardiography accurately measure the outflow pressure gradient and quantify any associated mitral regurgitation.

Cardiac catheterization is reserved for occasional patients in whom LV outflow tract obstruction cannot be distinguished from valvular aortic stenosis by echocardiography or more commonly if percutaneous septal ablation (described in "Treatment" section) is planned. The major feature in patients with obstruction is the finding of a pressure gradient within the outflow portion of the LV, either at rest or during maneuvers that transiently reduce LV size and promote outflow tract obstruction. Myocardial biopsy in HCM is neither diagnostic nor of prognostic value and is generally not advised unless it is required to differentiate HCM from other suspected disorders (eg, amyloidosis).

Finally, genetic testing can be helpful in establishing, or excluding, the diagnosis of HCM in family members of an affected patient when a specific mutation in that family has been identified.

TREATMENT

β-Blockers are standard therapy for HCM because they (1) reduce myocardial oxygen demand by slowing the heart rate and the force of contraction (and therefore diminish angina and dyspnea), (2) lessen any LV outflow gradient during exercise by reducing the force of contraction (allowing the chamber size to increase, thus separating the anterior leaflet of the mitral valve from the ventricular septum), and (3) increase passive diastolic ventricular filling time owing to the decreased heart rate. Despite their antiarrhythmic effect, β-blockers do not prevent sudden arrhythmic death in this condition, nor have they been shown to slow disease progression.

L-type *calcium channel antagonists* (ie, verapamil and diltiazem) may have beneficial effects on ventricular relaxation and filling and are sometimes useful in improving exercise capacity in patients who fail to respond to β-blockers. Patients who develop pulmonary congestion may benefit from mild diuretic therapy, but these drugs must be administered cautiously to avoid volume depletion; reduced intravascular volume decreases LV size and could exacerbate outflow tract obstruction. Vasodilators (including nitrates) similarly reduce LV size and should be avoided.

Atrial fibrillation is poorly tolerated in HCM and should be controlled aggressively, initially with *antiarrhythmic drugs*. Effective and useful antiarrhythmics for atrial fibrillation in HCM include amiodarone and disopyramide (a class IA antiarrhythmic drug that also possesses negative inotropic properties that may help reduce LV outflow tract obstruction; see Chapter 17). Digitalis should be avoided in HCM because its positive inotropic effect increases the force of contraction and can worsen LV outflow tract obstruction.

Sudden cardiac death in HCM is an occasional occurrence and almost always results from ventricular tachycardia or fibrillation. As there is a propensity for sudden death in HCM to occur during physical exertion, strenuous exercise and competitive sports should generally be avoided. Since medical therapy has not been shown to prevent sudden death in HCM, patients judged to be at high risk for sudden death (see risk factors in "Clinical Findings") are referred for placement of an ICD.

Surgical therapy (*septal myectomy*) is considered for patients whose symptoms do not respond adequately to pharmacologic therapy. This procedure involves excision of portions of the hypertrophied septal muscle mass and usually improves outflow tract obstruction, symptoms, and exercise capacity. While myectomy is the "gold-standard" approach to treatment of refractory symptoms in this condition, a less invasive alternative in select patients is *percutaneous septal ablation*. This procedure is performed in the cardiac catheterization laboratory during which dehydrated ethanol is injected directly into the first major septal coronary artery (a branch of the left anterior descending artery), causing a small, controlled myocardial infarction. The desired and often achieved result is reduction of septal thickness and improvement in outflow tract obstruction.

Finally, genetic counseling should be provided to all patients with HCM. Because it is an autosomal dominant disease, children of affected persons have a 50% chance of inheriting the abnormal gene. First-degree relatives of patients with HCM should be screened by physical examination, electrocardiography, echocardiography, and sometimes genetic testing. Even asymptomatic HCM patients are at risk of complications, including sudden death.

Prognosis

Clinical expression of HCM varies from asymptomatic patients with normal longevity to early death from cardiac arrest, heart failure, or stroke. The prognosis in the general population is better than that reported in early studies of patients at referral centers, and the current risk of sudden death in adults with HCM is <1% per year. Approximately 5% of patients will develop adverse LV remodeling and develop a progressive decline in *systolic* function ("end-stage" HCM). In general, the clinical course is worse for HCM patients with a sarcomere mutation and for those diagnosed early in life.

RESTRICTIVE CARDIOMYOPATHY

Restrictive cardiomyopathies (RCM) are characterized by abnormally rigid (but not necessarily thickened) ventricles with impaired diastolic filling. Systolic function is usually normal, or near normal. Causes of restrictive cardiomyopathy include *infiltration* of an abnormal substance between myocytes (eg, amyloid fibrils), *storage* of an abnormal substance within myocytes (eg, iron overload in hemochromatosis), *myocardial fibrosis* (eg, after radiation therapy), and *endomyocardial disorders* (Table 10-4). Some causes of RCM (eg, sarcoidosis and hemochromatosis) can also present as dilated cardiomyopathies. *Primary* (idiopathic) RCM is a very rare condition that can be familial (eg, resulting from mutations in the *DES* gene, which encodes the intermediate filament desmin).

The most common recognized cause of restrictive cardiomyopathy in nontropical countries is **amyloidosis.** In this systemic disease, insoluble misfolded amyloid fibrils deposit within

TABLE 10-4 Examples of Restrictive Cardiomyopathy

Infiltrative
Amyloidosis
Sarcoidosis (more commonly causes dilated cardiomyopathy [DCM])

Storage diseases
Hemochromatosis (iron overload—is also a cause of DCM)
Inherited metabolic diseases

Fibrotic
Radiation therapy
Scleroderma

Endomyocardial disease
Tropical endomyocardial fibrosis
Hypereosinophilic syndrome

Idiopathic (may be familial)

tissues, including the heart, causing organ dysfunction. Amyloid deposition is diagnosed histologically from biopsy of the myocardium or other tissues, with the type of amyloid protein defined by immunohistochemistry.

Amyloid fibrils can arise from several different proteins that distinguish the categories of disease. *Primary amyloidosis* is caused by deposition of immunoglobulin light-chain AL fragments, such as those secreted by a plasma cell tumor (usually multiple myeloma) with infiltration of the heart, peripheral nerves, liver, kidneys, and vascular endothelium. In contrast, in *transthyretin-related (TTR) amyloidosis*, amyloid fibrils form from transthyretin, a transport protein produced by the liver, with infiltration typically restricted to the heart and peripheral nerves. There are two types of TTR-related amyloidosis. *Hereditary TTR amyloidosis* is an autosomal dominant condition in which amyloid fibrils form from point mutations in the *TTR* gene that encodes transthyretin. *Wild-type TTR amyloidosis* is a disease predominantly of older men, in which amyloid is generated from nonmutated transthyretin. In each form of amyloidosis, cardiac involvement is marked by deposition of extracellular amyloid between myocardial fibers in the ventricles and atria, in the walls of coronary arteries, and in the valvular endocardium.

Restrictive cardiomyopathy develops in cardiac amyloidosis due to infiltrating amyloid protein. Diastolic dysfunction is the prominent cardiac abnormality; systolic dysfunction may develop later in the course of the disease. Orthostatic hypotension may be present, contributed to by amyloid deposition in the autonomic nervous system and peripheral blood vessels.

PATHOPHYSIOLOGY

Reduced compliance of the ventricles in restrictive cardiomyopathy, whether due to infiltration or fibrosis, results in an upward shift of the passive ventricular filling curve (see Fig. 9-7B), leading to abnormally high diastolic pressures. This has two major consequences: (1) elevated systemic and pulmonary venous pressures, with signs of right- and left-sided vascular congestion, and (2) reduced ventricular cavity size with decreased filling, stroke volume, and cardiac output.

CLINICAL FINDINGS

It follows from the underlying pathophysiology that signs of left- and right-sided heart failure are common (Fig. 10-8). Decreased cardiac output is manifested by fatigue and decreased exercise tolerance. Systemic congestion (often more prominent than pulmonary congestion

Figure 10-8. Pathophysiology of restrictive cardiomyopathy. The rigid myocardium results in elevated ventricular diastolic pressures and decreased ventricular filling. The resultant symptoms can be predicted from these abnormalities. CO, cardiac output.

in this condition) leads to jugular venous distention, peripheral edema, and ascites with a large, tender liver. Arrhythmias, including atrial fibrillation, are common. RCM etiologies that involve the cardiac conduction system (eg, sarcoidosis) can cause conduction blocks (described in Chapter 12).

PHYSICAL EXAMINATION

Signs of congestive heart failure are often present, including pulmonary rales, distended neck veins, ascites, and peripheral edema. Similar to constrictive pericarditis (see Chapter 14), jugular venous distention may paradoxically worsen with inspiration (the *Kussmaul sign*) because the stiffened RV cannot accommodate the increased venous return.

DIAGNOSTIC STUDIES

The *chest radiograph* usually shows a normal-sized heart with signs of pulmonary congestion. The *ECG* displays nonspecific ST- and T-wave abnormalities; conduction disturbances such as atrioventricular block or a bundle branch block may be present. The ECG voltage in cardiac amyloidosis is often strikingly reduced, owing to infiltration of the myocardium by amyloid fibrils, while in distinction *echocardiography* shows an often thickened myocardium. The diminished QRS amplitude is a feature that helps distinguish increased echocardiographic LV wall thickness in amyloidosis from HCM (which causes *augmented* QRS amplitude on the ECG). *Technetium pyrophosphate nuclear imaging* is both sensitive and specific for the presence of TTR forms of amyloidosis.

The RCM share nearly identical symptoms, physical signs, and hemodynamic profiles with constrictive pericarditis, as described in Chapter 14. The most useful diagnostic tools to differentiate these two conditions are transvenous endomyocardial biopsy, computed tomography (CT), and MRI. For example, in RCM, transvenous endomyocardial biopsy may demonstrate the cause of the condition (eg, the presence of amyloid fibrils in amyloidosis or iron deposits in patients with hemochromatosis). *CT* or *MRI* scans accurately identify the thickened pericardium present in most patients with constrictive pericarditis, a finding that is not present in states causing restrictive cardiomyopathy.

TREATMENT

Restrictive cardiomyopathy typically has a poor prognosis, except when treatment can target an underlying cause. Symptomatic therapy for all etiologies includes salt restriction and cautious use of diuretics to improve symptoms of systemic and pulmonary congestion. Unlike the dilated cardiomyopathies, vasodilators (including inhibitors of the renin-angiotensin system) are not beneficial. Maintenance of sinus rhythm (eg, converting atrial fibrillation to sinus rhythm) is important to maximize diastolic filling and forward cardiac output. Patients with RCM and atrial fibrillation are at high risk for atrial thrombus formation and thromboembolism and should be treated with an anticoagulant. Some RCM are prone to intraventricular thrombus formation, thus warranting chronic oral anticoagulant therapy. In the case of primary (AL) amyloidosis, antineoplastic therapy (eg, bortezomib, cyclophosphamide, and dexamethasone) prolongs survival. For TTR-related amyloidosis, recent clinical trials have demonstrated that medications that bind and stabilize TTR (eg, tafamidis) reduce mortality.

OTHER FORMS OF CARDIOMYOPATHY

Not all forms of cardiac muscle disease fit into the traditional categories of cardiomyopathy described in this chapter. Examples include (1) left ventricular noncompaction (LVNC) and (2) arrhythmogenic right ventricular cardiomyopathy (ARVC).

LEFT VENTRICULAR NONCOMPACTION

LVNC is a rare condition that has been recognized with greater frequency in recent years due to higher resolution of cardiac imaging techniques. It is manifested by a thickened myocardium with very prominent trabeculae and deep recesses that extend from the LV cavity into the intertrabecular spaces. The abnormal regions of the myocardium contract poorly, often demonstrate characteristics of impaired diastolic relaxation, and predispose to rhythm disturbances and thrombus formation. Patients may present in childhood or adulthood with symptoms of heart failure (due to systolic and/or diastolic dysfunction), ventricular arrhythmias, or thromboembolism. A number of mutations in sarcomeric and other genes have been associated with this condition. Management is aimed at treating symptoms and complications as there is no corrective therapy for LVNC itself. Depending on the manifestations, approaches include standard treatment of heart failure (Chapter 9), ICD implantation for management of life-threatening ventricular arrhythmias, chronic anticoagulation for those with atrial fibrillation or significant contractile dysfunction to prevent thromboembolism, and cardiac transplantation for advanced, refractory heart failure.

ARRHYTHMOGENIC RIGHT VENTRICULAR CARDIOMYOPATHY

ARVC is another genetic form of cardiomyopathy. It is characterized by replacement of right ventricular (and occasionally left ventricular) myocardium with adipose and fibrous tissue, resulting in rhythm disturbances and contractile dysfunction. Ventricular arrhythmias originating from the abnormal ventricle are common and may result in palpitations and syncope. Symptoms often begin in the teen years, and ARVC is a potential cause of sudden death among young athletes.

Both autosomal dominant and recessive inheritance forms of ARVC have been identified. The majority of mutations occur in genes that encode components of desmosomes, cell membrane structures responsible for cell-to-cell adhesion, leading to fibrosis and aberrant signaling with proliferation of adipose tissue in the myocardium. ARVC diagnostic criteria rely on family history, ECG abnormalities (see Chapter 12, Box 12-1), the presence of arrhythmias emanating from the RV, morphologic abnormalities detected by imaging studies (especially echocardiography and cardiac MRI), and genetic testing. Management of ARVC typically includes ICD implantation because the disease is progressive and life-threatening ventricular tachycardia is common.

Summary

- Cardiomyopathies are a group of disorders that impair normal myocardial function and may result in inappropriate ventricular dilatation, hypertrophy, or stiffness (Table 10-5); heart failure and cardiovascular death are potential complications.
- **Dilated cardiomyopathies** are characterized by progressive ventricular chamber enlargement with impaired *systolic* contractile function, often leading to symptomatic heart failure, ventricular arrhythmias, and/or embolic complications.
- **Hypertrophic cardiomyopathy** is characterized by an abnormally thickened ventricular wall with abnormal *diastolic* relaxation but usually intact systolic function; dynamic LV outflow tract obstruction during systole may be present, and the most common symptoms are dyspnea and exertional angina.
- Ventricular arrhythmias in HCM may lead to **sudden cardiac death**.
- **Restrictive cardiomyopathies** are characterized by an abnormally stiffened myocardium (because of fibrosis or an infiltrative process) leading to impaired *diastolic* relaxation, but systolic contractile function is typically normal or near normal; symptoms of heart failure are typical.

TABLE 10-5   Summary of the Cardiomyopathies

	Dilated Cardiomyopathy	Hypertrophic Cardiomyopathy	Restrictive Cardiomyopathy
Ventricular morphology	Dilated LV with little concentric hypertrophy	Marked hypertrophy, often asymmetric	Fibrotic or infiltrated myocardium
Etiology examples	Genetic, inflammatory, toxic, metabolic, peripartum	Genetic	Amyloidosis, genetic
Symptoms	Fatigue, weakness, dyspnea, orthopnea, PND	Dyspnea, angina, syncope	Dyspnea, fatigue
Physical exam	Pulmonary crackles, S3; if RV failure present: JVD, hepatomegaly, peripheral edema	S4; if outflow obstruction present: systolic murmur loudest at the left sternal border, accompanied by mitral regurgitation	Predominantly signs of RV failure: JVD, hepatomegaly, peripheral edema
Pathophysiology	Impaired systolic contraction	Impaired diastolic relaxation; LV systolic function vigorous, often with dynamic obstruction	"Stiff" LV with impaired diastolic relaxation but usually normal systolic function
Cardiac size on chest radiograph	Enlarged	Normal or enlarged	Usually normal
Echocardiogram	Dilated, poorly contractile LV	LV hypertrophy, often more pronounced at the septum; systolic anterior movement of MV with mitral regurgitation	Usually normal systolic contraction; the myocardium may have enhanced echogenicity in infiltrative disorders

LV, left ventricle; PND, paroxysmal nocturnal dyspnea; RV, right ventricle; JVD, jugular venous distention; MV, mitral valve.

Review Questions

1. A 76-year old woman with multiple myeloma (bone marrow cancer of plasma cells) presents with dyspnea and lower extremity edema. Her ECG demonstrates low-voltage QRS complexes in each lead. Echocardiography shows markedly increased ventricular thickness, enlargement of both atria, and a normal left ventricular ejection fraction. What is the most likely diagnosis?

   a. Hypertrophic cardiomyopathy
   b. Arrhythmogenic right ventricular cardiomyopathy
   c. Dilated cardiomyopathy
   d. Cardiac amyloidosis causing restrictive cardiomyopathy

2. A 40-year-old man presents with progressive exertional dyspnea. Cardiac examination is notable for an S4 and a harsh systolic crescendo-decrescendo murmur along the left sternal border while supine, which increases in intensity after standing. Which of the following statements is correct?

   a. A dilated cardiomyopathy is likely present.
   b. He has advanced valvular aortic stenosis.
   c. Echocardiography would likely demonstrate asymmetric septal hypertrophy.
   d. β-Blocker therapy should be avoided.

3. Which of the following is *not* a recognized cause of dilated cardiomyopathy?

   a. Excess ethanol consumption
   b. Mitral stenosis
   c. Anthracycline chemotherapy
   d. Viral myocarditis

Answers to Review Questions

1. **Choice d is correct.** Cardiac amyloidosis is a cause of restrictive cardiomyopathy and heart failure symptoms, and primary AL-type amyloidosis is associated with plasma cell dyscrasias such as multiple myeloma. There is typically increased ventricular wall thickness, but often paradoxically low QRS voltage on the ECG owing to the infiltrating amyloid protein. Hypertrophic cardiomyopathy also causes increased ventricular thickness, but the ECG would demonstrate *increased* QRS voltage, representing LV hypertrophy.

2. **Choice c is correct.** This patient likely has hypertrophic cardiomyopathy (HCM) with LV outflow tract obstruction related to asymmetric septal hypertrophy. In this condition, the harsh systolic murmur increases in intensity upon standing or during a Valsalva maneuver (see Table 10-3) because reduced LV size during these maneuvers further narrows the outflow tract. In aortic stenosis, the murmur *softens* with maneuvers that decrease LV filling. An S4 is common in HCM, generated by left atrial contraction into the stiffened, hypertrophied LV. β-Blockers are standard therapy for HCM.

3. **Choice b is correct.** Each of these conditions, except mitral stenosis, can result in dilated cardiomyopathy with reduced LV contractile function (see Table 10-1).

Acknowledgments

Contributors to previous editions of this chapter were P. Connor Johnson, MD; Christopher T. Lee, MD; Marc N. Wein, MD; Yi-Bin Chen, MD; David Grayzel, MD; Kay Fang, MD; and G. William Dec, MD.

Additional Reading

Arbustini E, Narula J, Tavazzi J, et al. The MOGE(S) classification of cardiomyopathy for clinicians. *J Am Coll Cardiol.* 2014;64:304-318.

Birnie DH, Nery PB, Ha AC, et al. Cardiac Sarcoidosis. *J Am Coll Cardiol.* 2016;68:411-421.

Bonaca MP, Olenchock BA, Salem JE, et al. Myocarditis in the setting of cancer therapeutics. *Circulation.* 2019;140:80-91.

Hanna M, Huded C, Rodriguez ER, et al. Progress in diagnosing and managing cardiac amyloidosis. *Cleve Clin J Med.* 2019;86: 29-46.

Maron BJ. Clinical course and management of hypertrophic cardiomyopathy. *N Engl J Med.* 2018;379:655-668.

Maron BJ, Maron MS, Maron BA, et al. Moving beyond the sarcomere to explain heterogeneity in hypertrophic cardiomyopathy. *J Am Coll Cardiol.* 2019;73:1978-1986.

Maurer MS, Schwartz JH, Gundapaneni B, et al. Tafamidis treatment for patients with transthyretin amyloid cardiomyopathy. *N Engl J Med.* 2018;379:1007-1016.

Ruberg FL, Grogan M, Hanna M, et al. Transthyretin amyloid cardiomyopathy: JACC state-of-the-art review. *J Am Coll Cardiol.* 2019;73:2872-2891.

11

Mechanisms of Cardiac Arrhythmias

Victor Nauffal | Leonard S. Lilly

Normal cardiac function relies on the flow of electric impulses through the heart in an exquisitely coordinated fashion. Abnormalities of the electric rhythm are known as *arrhythmias* (also termed *dysrhythmias*) and are among the most common clinical problems encountered. The presentations of arrhythmias range from common benign palpitations to severe symptoms of low cardiac output and death. Therefore, a thorough understanding of these disorders is important to the daily practice of medicine.

Abnormally slow heart rhythms are termed *bradycardias* (or *bradyarrhythmias*). Fast rhythms are known as tachycardias (or *tachyarrhythmias*). Tachycardias are further characterized as *supraventricular* when they involve the atrium or atrioventricular (AV) node and designated *ventricular* when they originate from the His-Purkinje system or ventricles. This chapter extends the description of basic cardiac electrophysiology presented in Chapter 1 and explains the mechanisms by which arrhythmias develop, followed by a general approach to their management. Chapter 12 describes specific rhythm disorders, including how to recognize and treat them.

Disorders of heart rhythm result from alterations of **impulse formation**, **impulse conduction**, or both. The chapter first addresses how abnormalities of impulse formation and conduction occur and under what circumstances they cause arrhythmias. Figure 11-1 provides an organizational schema for this presentation.

While studying the concepts in this chapter, it is important to recall that cardiac tissue is composed of cells that are electrically coupled and operate as a syncytium. As myocytes depolarize and ionic currents result in individual action potentials, the electrical activity rapidly propagates from one cell to the next with minimal resistance, spreading through a large mass of tissue. As a result, the leading edge of a depolarization may be located several centimeters ahead of its trailing edge, and this property plays an important role in the genesis of certain arrhythmias, as will be described.

NORMAL IMPULSE FORMATION

As described in Chapter 1, electric impulse formation in the heart arises from the intrinsic automaticity of specialized cardiac cells. **Automaticity** refers to a cell's ability to spontaneously depolarize to a threshold voltage to generate an action potential. Although atrial and ventricular myocytes do not have this property under normal conditions, the cells of the specialized conducting system do possess natural automaticity and are therefore termed **pacemaker cells**. The specialized conducting system includes the sinoatrial (SA) node, the AV node, the bundle of His, the bundle branches, and Purkinje fibers. In pathologic situations, myocardial cells outside the conducting system may also acquire automaticity.

Ionic Basis of Automaticity

Cells with natural automaticity do not have a static resting voltage. Rather, they inherently display gradual depolarization during phase 4 of the action potential (Fig. 11-2). If this spontaneous depolarization reaches the threshold value, an action potential upstroke is generated. An important ionic current largely responsible for phase 4 spontaneous depolarization is known as the **pacemaker current (I_f)**. The channels that carry this current are activated by hyperpolarization (increasingly negative voltages) and mainly conduct sodium ions. I_f channels begin to open when the membrane voltage becomes more negative than approximately -50 mV and are *different* entities than the fast sodium channels responsible for rapid phase 0 depolarization in ventricular and atrial myocytes. The inward flow of Na^+ through these slow channels, driven by its concentration gradient and the negative intracellular potential, depolarizes the membrane toward threshold.

In the pacemaker cells of the SA node, three other ionic currents also contribute to phase 4 gradual depolarization: (1) a slowly increasing inward calcium current, carried mostly by L-type Ca^{++} channels that become activated at voltages reached near the end of phase 4; (2) a progressively declining outward potassium current; and (3) an additional inward sodium

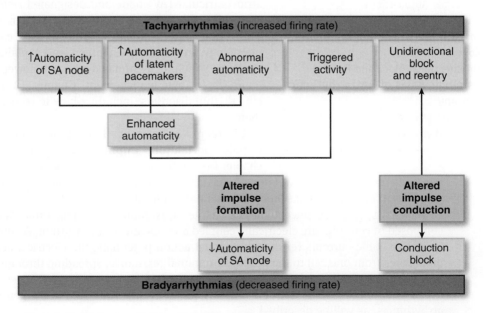

Figure 11-1. Arrhythmias result from alterations in impulse formation and/or impulse conduction. Tachyarrhythmias result from enhanced automaticity, triggered activity, or unidirectional block with reentry. Bradyarrhythmias result from decreased automaticity or conduction block. SA, sinoatrial.

Figure 11-2. The action potential (AP) of a pacemaker cell (eg, the sinus node). The spontaneous phase 4 depolarization results primarily from the I_f (pacemaker) inward current, which drives the cell to threshold (approximately −40 mV). The upstroke of the AP is caused by the slow inward current of Ca^{++} ions. Reduction of the Ca^{++} current (owing to inactivation of calcium channels) and K$^+$ efflux through voltage-gated potassium channels is responsible for repolarization. MDP, maximum negative diastolic potential; TP, threshold potential.

current mediated by activation of the electrogenic sodium-calcium exchanger by calcium release from the sarcoplasmic reticulum.

When the membrane potential of a pacemaker cell reaches the threshold condition, the upstroke of the action potential is generated. In contrast to the phase 0 upstroke of cells in the Purkinje system, that of cells in the sinus and AV nodes is much slower (see Fig. 11-2). The reason for the difference is that the membrane potential determines the proportion of fast sodium channels that are in a resting state capable of depolarization, compared with an inactivated state. The number of available (or resting-state) fast sodium channels decreases as the resting (diastolic) membrane potential becomes less negative. Because sinus and AV nodal cells have less negative maximum diastolic membrane voltages (−50 to −60 mV) than do Purkinje cells (−90 mV), the large majority of fast sodium channels is inactivated in these pacemaker cells. Thus, the action potential upstroke relies to a great extent on a smaller *calcium* current (through the relatively slower opening of L-type Ca^{++} channels) and has a less rapid rate of rise than do cells of the Purkinje system or ventricular myocardium. The repolarization phase of pacemaker cells results from both the inactivation of the open calcium channels and the opening of voltage-gated potassium channels that permit efflux of potassium from the cells (see Fig. 11-2).

NATIVE AND LATENT PACEMAKERS

The distinct populations of automatic cells in the specialized conduction pathway have different intrinsic rates of firing. These rates are determined by three variables that influence how fast the membrane potential reaches the threshold condition: (1) the rate (ie, the slope) of phase 4 spontaneous depolarization, (2) the maximum negative diastolic potential, and (3) the threshold potential. A more negative maximum diastolic potential, or a less negative threshold potential, slows the rate of impulse initiation because it takes longer to reach the threshold value (Fig. 11-3). Conversely, the greater the I_f, the steeper the slope of phase 4 and the faster the cell depolarizes. The size of I_f depends on the number and opening kinetics of the individual pacemaker channels through which this current flows.

Since all healthy myocardial cells are electrically connected by gap junctions, an action potential generated in one part of the myocardium will ultimately spread to all other regions. When an impulse arrives at a cell that is not yet close to threshold, the current from the depolarized cell will bring the adjacent cell's membrane potential to the threshold level so that it will fire (regardless of how close its intrinsic I_f has brought it to threshold). Thus, the pacemaker cells with the fastest rate of depolarization set the heart rate. In the normal heart, the dominant pacemaker is the *SA node*, which at rest initiates impulses at a rate of 60-100 bpm. Because the sinus node rate is faster than that of the other tissues that possess automaticity, its repeated discharges prevent spontaneous firing of other potential pacemaker sites.

Figure 11-3. Determinants of cell firing rates. A. Alterations in the pacemaker current (I_f) and in the magnitude of the maximum diastolic potential (MDP) alter the cell firing rate. (*a*) The normal action potential (AP) of a pacemaker cell. (*b*) Reduced I_f renders the slope of phase 4 less steep; thus, the time required to reach threshold potential (TP) is increased. (*c*) The MDP is more negative; therefore, the time required to reach TP is increased. **B.** Alterations in TP change the firing rate of the cell. Compared with the normal TP (*a*), the TP in *b* is less negative; thus, the duration of time to achieve threshold is increased, and the firing rate decreases.

The SA node is known as the **native pacemaker** because it normally sets the heart rate. Other cells within the specialized conduction system harbor the potential to act as pacemakers if necessary and are therefore called **latent pacemakers** (or **ectopic pacemakers**). In contrast to the SA node, the AV node and the bundle of His have intrinsic firing rates of 50-60 bpm, and cells of the Purkinje system have rates of ~30-40 bpm. These latent sites may initiate impulses and take over the pacemaker function if the SA node slows or fails to fire or if conduction abnormalities block the normal wave of depolarization from reaching them.

OVERDRIVE SUPPRESSION

Not only does the cell population with the fastest intrinsic rhythm preempt all other automatic cells from spontaneously firing, but it also directly *suppresses* their automaticity. This phenomenon is called overdrive suppression. Cells maintain their transsarcolemmal ion distributions because of the continuously active Na^+K^+-ATPase that extrudes three Na^+ ions from the cell in exchange for two K^+ ions transported in (Fig. 11-4). Because its net transport effect is one positive charge in the outward direction, Na^+K^+-ATPase creates a *hyperpolarizing* current (ie, it tends to make the inside of the cell *more negative*). As the cell potential becomes increasingly negative, additional time is required for spontaneous phase 4 depolarization to reach the threshold voltage (see Fig. 11-3A), and therefore, the rate of spontaneous firing is decreased. Although the hyperpolarizing current moves the membrane voltage away from threshold, pacemaker cells firing at their own intrinsic rate have an I_f current sufficiently large to overcome this hyperpolarizing influence (see Fig. 11-4).

The hyperpolarizing current increases when a cell is caused to fire more frequently than its intrinsic pacemaker rate. The more often the cell is depolarized, the greater the quantity of Na^+ ions that enter the cell per unit time. As a result of the increased intracellular Na^+ content, Na^+K^+-ATPase becomes more active, thereby tending to restore the normal transmembrane Na^+ gradient. This increased pump activity provides a larger hyperpolarizing current, opposing the depolarizing current I_f, and further decreases the rate of spontaneous depolarization. Thus, overdrive suppression decreases a cell's automaticity when that cell is driven to depolarize faster than its intrinsic discharge rate.

ELECTROTONIC INTERACTIONS

In addition to overdrive suppression, *anatomic connections* between pacemaker and nonpacemaker cells are important in determining how adjacent cells suppress latent pacemaker foci. Myocardial cells in the ventricle and Purkinje system repolarize to a resting potential of approximately −90 mV, whereas pacemaker cells in the sinus and AV nodes repolarize to a maximum diastolic potential of about −60 mV. When these two cell types are adjacent to one another, they are *electrically cou-*

Figure 11-4. Competition between the depolarizing pacemaker current (If) and Na+K+-ATPase, which produces a hyperpolarizing current. Na+K+-ATPase transports three Na+ ions outside the cell in exchange for two K+ ions transported inward. This hyperpolarizing current acts to suppress automaticity by antagonizing I_f and contributes to overdrive suppression in cells that are stimulated more rapidly than their intrinsic firing rate.

pled through low-resistance gap junctions concentrated in their intercalated discs. This coupling results in a compromise of electric potentials owing to electrotonic current flow between the cells, causing relative *hyperpolarization* of the pacemaker cell and relative *depolarization* of the nonpacemaker cell (Fig. 11-5). Hyperpolarization moves the diastolic potential further

Figure 11-5. Electrotonic interaction between pacemaker (eg, AV nodal) and nonpacemaker (myocardial) cells. A. Pacemaker cells that are not coupled to myocardial cells have a maximum diastolic potential (MDP) of approximately −60 mV, whereas myocardial cells have a resting potential (RP) of approximately −90 mV. **B.** When pacemaker cells and myocytes are neighbors, they may be connected electrically by gap junctions at their intercalated discs (eg, at the AV node). In this situation, electric current flows between the pacemaker cell and the myocardial cell, tending to hyperpolarize the former and depolarize the latter, driving their membrane potentials closer to one another. The hyperpolarizing current renders the MDP more negative, causing it to take longer for spontaneous depolarization to reach the threshold value, thereby suppressing automaticity. If a disease state impairs coupling between cells, the influence of surrounding myocytes on the pacemaker cell is reduced, allowing I_f to depolarize to threshold more readily and enhancing automaticity. TP, threshold potential.

from threshold and thus slows the heart rate (as shown in Fig. 11-3A). Electrotonic effects may be particularly important in suppressing automaticity in the AV node (via connections between atrial myocytes and AV nodal cells) and in the distal Purkinje fibers (which are coupled to ventricular myocardial cells). In contrast, cells in the center of the SA node are less tightly coupled to atrial myocytes; thus, their automaticity is less subject to electrotonic interactions.

Decoupling of normally suppressed cells, such as those in the AV node (eg, by ischemic damage), may reduce the inhibitory electrotonic influence and *enhance* automaticity, producing ectopic rhythms by the latent pacemaker tissue.

ALTERED IMPULSE FORMATION

Arrhythmias may arise from altered impulse formation at the SA node or from other sites, including the specialized conduction pathways or regions of cardiac muscle. The main abnormalities of impulse initiation that lead to arrhythmias are (1) **altered automaticity** (of the sinus node or latent pacemakers within the specialized conduction pathway), (2) **abnormal automaticity** in atrial or ventricular myocytes, and (3) **triggered activity**.

ALTERATIONS IN SINUS NODE AUTOMATICITY

The rate of impulse initiation by the sinus node, as well as by the latent pacemakers of the specialized conducting system, is regulated primarily by neurohumoral factors.

Increased Sinus Node Automaticity

The most important modulator of normal sinus node automaticity is the autonomic nervous system. Sympathetic stimulation, acting through β_1-adrenergic receptors, increases the open probability of the pacemaker channels (Fig. 11-6), through which I_f can flow. The increase in I_f leads to a steeper slope of phase 4 depolarization, causing the SA node to reach threshold and fire earlier than normal and the heart rate to increase.

In addition, sympathetic stimulation shifts the action potential threshold to more negative voltages by increasing the probability that voltage-sensitive Ca^{++} channels are capable of opening (recall that calcium carries the current of phase 0 depolarization in pacemaker cells). Therefore, phase 4 depolarization reaches the threshold potential earlier. Sympathetic activity thus increases sinus node automaticity both by increasing the rate of pacemaker depolarization via I_f and by causing the action potential threshold to become more negative. Examples of this normal physiologic effect occur during physical exercise or emotional stress, when sympathetic stimulation appropriately increases the heart rate.

Figure 11-6. Effect of sympathetic and parasympathetic (cholinergic) stimulation on pacemaker current channels. The channels through which the pacemaker current (I_f) flows are voltage gated, opening at more negative membrane potentials. At any given voltage, there exists a probability between 0 and 1 that a specific channel will be open. Compared with normal baseline behavior (*curve A*), sympathetic stimulation (*curve B*) or treatment with anticholinergic drugs shifts this probability to a higher value for any given level of membrane voltage, thus increasing the number of open channels and the rate at which the cell will fire. *Curve C* shows that parasympathetic cholinergic stimulation (or treatment with a β-blocker, which antagonizes sympathetic stimulation) has the opposite effect, decreasing the probability of a channel being open and therefore inhibiting depolarization.

Decreased Sinus Node Automaticity

Normal decreases in SA node automaticity are mediated by reduced sympathetic stimulation and by increased activity of the parasympathetic nervous system. Whereas activation of the sympathetic nervous system has a major role in increasing the heart rate during times of stress, the parasympathetic nervous system is the major controller of the heart rate at rest.

Cholinergic (ie, parasympathetic) stimulation via the vagus nerve acts at the SA node to reduce the probability of pacemaker channels being open (see Fig. 11-6). Thus, I_f and the slope of phase 4 depolarization are reduced, and the intrinsic firing rate of the cell is slowed. In addition, the probability of the Ca^{++} channels being open is decreased, such that the action potential threshold increases to a less negative potential. Furthermore, cholinergic stimulation increases the probability of acetylcholine-sensitive K^+ channels being open at rest. Positively charged K^+ ions exit through these "inward rectifier" channels, which differ from the K^+ channels that are active in phase 3 repolarization (see Chapter 1), producing an outward current that drives the diastolic potential more negative. The overall effect of reduced I_f, a more negative maximum diastolic potential, and a less negative threshold level is a slowing of the intrinsic firing rate and therefore a reduced heart rate.

It follows that the use of pharmacologic agents that modify these effects of the autonomic nervous system will also affect the firing rate of the SA node. For example, β-receptor blocking drugs ("β-blockers") antagonize the β-adrenergic sympathetic effect; therefore, they *decrease* the rate of phase 4 depolarization of the SA node and slow the heart rate. Conversely, atropine, an anticholinergic (antimuscarinic) drug, has the opposite effect: by blocking parasympathetic activity, the rate of phase 4 depolarization *increases* and the heart rate accelerates.

ESCAPE RHYTHMS

If the sinus node becomes suppressed and fires much less frequently than normal, the site of impulse formation may shift to a latent pacemaker within the specialized conduction pathway. An impulse initiated by a latent pacemaker because the SA node rate has slowed is called an **escape beat**. Persistent impairment of the SA node will allow a continued series of escape beats, termed an **escape rhythm**. Escape rhythms are protective in that they prevent the heart rate from becoming pathologically slow when SA node firing is impaired.

As discussed in the previous section, suppression of sinus node activity may occur because of increased parasympathetic tone. Different regions of the heart have varied sensitivities to parasympathetic (vagal) stimulation. The SA node and the AV node are most sensitive to such an influence, followed by atrial tissue. The ventricular conducting system is the least sensitive. Therefore, moderate parasympathetic stimulation slows the sinus rate and allows the pacemaker to shift to the AV node. However, very strong parasympathetic stimulation suppresses excitability at both the SA node and AV node and may therefore result in the emergence of a ventricular escape pacemaker.

ENHANCED AUTOMATICITY OF LATENT PACEMAKERS

Another means by which a latent pacemaker can assume control of impulse formation is if it develops an intrinsic rate of depolarization *faster* than that of the sinus node. Termed an **ectopic beat**, such an impulse is *premature* relative to the normal rhythm, whereas an escape beat is *late* and terminates a pause caused by a slowed sinus rhythm. A sequence of similar ectopic beats is called an **ectopic rhythm**.

Ectopic beats may arise in several circumstances. For example, high catecholamine concentrations can enhance the automaticity of latent pacemakers, and if the resulting rate of depolarization exceeds that of the sinus node, then an ectopic rhythm will develop. Ectopic beats are also commonly induced by hypoxemia, ischemia, electrolyte disturbances, and certain drug toxicities (such as digitalis, as described in Chapter 17).

ABNORMAL AUTOMATICITY

Cardiac tissue injury may lead to pathologic changes in impulse formation, whereby myocardial cells *outside* the specialized conduction system acquire automaticity and spontaneously depolarize. Although such activity may appear similar to impulses originating from latent pacemakers within the specialized conduction pathways, these ectopic beats arise from cells that do not usually possess automaticity. If the rate of depolarization of such cells exceeds that of the sinus node, they transiently take over the pacemaker function and become the source of an abnormal ectopic rhythm.

Because these myocardial cells have few or no activated pacemaker channels, they do not normally carry I_f. How injury allows such cells to spontaneously depolarize has not been fully elucidated. However, when cardiac tissue becomes injured, its cellular membranes become "leaky." As such, they are unable to maintain the concentration gradients of ions, and the resting potential becomes less negative (ie, the cell partially depolarizes). When a cell's membrane potential is reduced to a value less negative than -60 mV, gradual phase 4 depolarization can be demonstrated even among nonpacemaker cells. This spontaneous depolarization probably results from a very slowly inactivating calcium current, a decrease in the outward potassium current that normally acts to repolarize the cell, and less effect of the inward rectifier K^+ current that normally holds cells at a more negative potential range.

TRIGGERED ACTIVITY

Under certain conditions, an action potential can "trigger" abnormal depolarizations that result in extra heart beats or tachyarrhythmias. This process may occur when the first action potential leads to oscillations of the membrane voltage known as *afterdepolarizations*. Unlike the *spontaneous* activity seen when enhanced automaticity occurs, this type of automaticity is *stimulated* by a preceding action potential. As illustrated in Figures 11-7 and 11-8, there are two types of afterdepolarizations depending on their timing after the inciting action potential: *early* afterdepolarizations occur during the repolarization phase of the inciting beat, whereas *delayed* afterdepolarizations occur shortly after repolarization has been completed. In either case, abnormal action potentials are triggered if the afterdepolarization reaches a threshold voltage.

Early afterdepolarizations are changes of the membrane potential in the positive direction that interrupt normal repolarization (see Fig. 11-7). They can occur either during the plateau of the action potential (phase 2) or during rapid repolarization (phase 3). Early afterdepolarizations are more likely to develop in conditions that prolong the action potential duration

Figure 11-7. Triggered activity. An early afterdepolarization (*arrow*) occurs before the action potential (AP) has fully repolarized. Repetitive afterdepolarizations (*dashed curve*) may produce a rapid sequence of triggered action potentials and hence a tachyarrhythmia.

Figure 11-8. Triggered activity. A delayed afterdepolarization (*arrow*) arises after the cell has fully repolarized. If the delayed afterdepolarization reaches the threshold voltage, a propagated action potential (AP) is triggered (*dashed curve*).

(and therefore the electrocardiographic QT interval), as may occur during therapy with certain drugs (see Chapter 17) and in the inherited long QT syndromes (see Chapter 12).

The ionic current responsible for an early afterdepolarization depends on the membrane voltage at which the triggered event occurs. If the early afterdepolarization occurs during phase 2 of the action potential, when most of the Na^+ channels are still in an inactivated state, the upstroke of the triggered beat relies mostly on an inward Ca^{++} current. If, however, the afterdepolarization occurs during phase 3 (when the membrane voltage is more negative), there is partial recovery of the inactivated Na^+ channels, which then contribute more to the current underlying the triggered beat.

An early afterdepolarization-triggered action potential can be self-perpetuating and lead to a series of depolarizations and therefore a tachyarrhythmia (see Fig. 11-7). Early afterdepolarizations appear to be the initiating mechanism of the polymorphic ventricular tachycardia known as torsades de pointes, which is described in Chapter 12.

Delayed afterdepolarizations may appear shortly after repolarization is complete (see Fig. 11-8). They most commonly develop in states of *high intracellular calcium*, as may be present with digitalis intoxication (see Chapter 17), or during marked catecholamine stimulation. It is thought that intracellular Ca^{++} accumulation causes the activation of chloride currents, or of the Na^+-Ca^{++} exchanger, that results in brief inward currents that generate the delayed afterdepolarization.

As with early afterdepolarizations, if the amplitude of the delayed afterdepolarization reaches a threshold voltage, an action potential will be generated. Such action potentials can be self-perpetuating and lead to tachyarrhythmias. Some idiopathic ventricular tachycardias that occur in otherwise structurally normal hearts are likely due to this mechanism, as are atrial and ventricular tachycardias associated with digitalis toxicity (see Chapter 17).

ALTERED IMPULSE CONDUCTION

Alterations in impulse conduction also lead to arrhythmias. Conduction blocks generally slow the heart rate (bradyarrhythmias); however, under certain circumstances, the process of reentry (described later) can ensue and produce abnormal fast rhythms (tachyarrhythmias).

CONDUCTION BLOCK

A propagating impulse is blocked when it encounters a region of the heart that is electrically unexcitable. Conduction block can be either transient or permanent and may be unidirectional (ie, conduction proceeds when the involved region is stimulated from one direction but not when stimulated from the opposite direction) or bidirectional (conduction is blocked in both directions). Various conditions may cause conduction block, including ischemia, fibrosis, inflammation, and certain drugs. When conduction block occurs because a propagating impulse encounters cardiac cells that are still refractory from a previous depolarization, the block is said to be *functional*. A propagating impulse that arrives a short time later, when the tissue is no longer refractory, may be conducted appropriately. For example, antiarrhythmic drugs that prolong the action potential duration (described in Chapter 17) tend to produce functional conduction blocks. Conversely, when conduction block is caused by a barrier imposed by fibrosis or scarring that replaces myocytes, the block is said to be *fixed*.

Conduction block within the specialized conducting system of the AV node or the His-Purkinje system prevents normal propagation of the cardiac impulse from the sinus node to more distal sites. This atrioventricular block (AV block) removes the normal overdrive suppression that keeps latent pacemakers in the His-Purkinje system in check. Thus, conduction block usually results in emergence of escape beats or escape rhythms, as the more distal sites assume the pacemaker function.

AV block is common, and certain types of AV block necessitate implantation of an artificial pacemaker, as discussed in Chapter 12.

UNIDIRECTIONAL BLOCK AND REENTRY

A common mechanism by which altered impulse conduction leads to tachyarrhythmias is termed **reentry**. During such a rhythm, an electric impulse circulates repeatedly around a reentry path, recurrently depolarizing a region of cardiac tissue.

During normal cardiac conduction, each electric impulse that originates in the SA node travels in an orderly, sequential fashion through the rest of the heart, ultimately depolarizing all the myocardial fibers. The refractory period of each cell prevents immediate reexcitation from adjacent depolarized cells so that the impulse stops when all of the heart muscle has been excited. However, conduction blocks that prevent rapid depolarization of parts of the myocardium can create an environment conducive to continued impulse propagation and reentry, as illustrated in Figure 11-9.

The figure depicts electric activity as it flows through a branch point anywhere within the conduction pathways. Panel A shows propagation of a normal action potential. At point *x*, the impulse branches into two pathways (α and β) and travels down each into the more distal conduction tissue. In the normal heart, the α and β pathways have similar conduction velocities and refractory periods such that portions of the wave fronts that pass through them may collide in the distal conduction tissue and extinguish each other, as shown by the red line.

Panel B shows what happens if conduction is blocked in one limb of the pathways. In this example, the action potential is obstructed when it encounters the β pathway from above and therefore propagates only down the α tract into the distal tissue. As the impulse continues to spread, it encounters the distal end of the β pathway (at point *y*). If the tissue in the distal β tract is also unable to conduct, the impulse simply continues to propagate into the deeper tissues, and reentry does not occur. However, if the impulse at point *y* is able to propagate retrogradely (backward) into pathway β, one of the necessary conditions for reentry is met.

When an action potential can conduct in a retrograde direction in a conduction pathway, whereas it had been prevented from doing so in the forward direction, **unidirectional block** is said to be present. Unidirectional block tends to occur in regions where the refractory periods of adjacent cells are heterogeneous, such that some cells recover before others. In addition, unidirectional block may occur in states of cellular dysfunction and in regions where fibrosis has altered the myocardial structure.

As shown in panel C of Figure 11-9, if the impulse is able to propagate retrogradely up the β pathway, it will again arrive at point *x*. At that time, if the α pathway has not yet repolarized from the previous action potential that had occurred moments earlier, that limb is refractory to repeat stimulation, and the returning impulse simply stops there.

However, panel D illustrates what happens if the velocity of retrograde conduction in the diseased β path is not normal but *slower than normal*. In that case, sufficient time may elapse

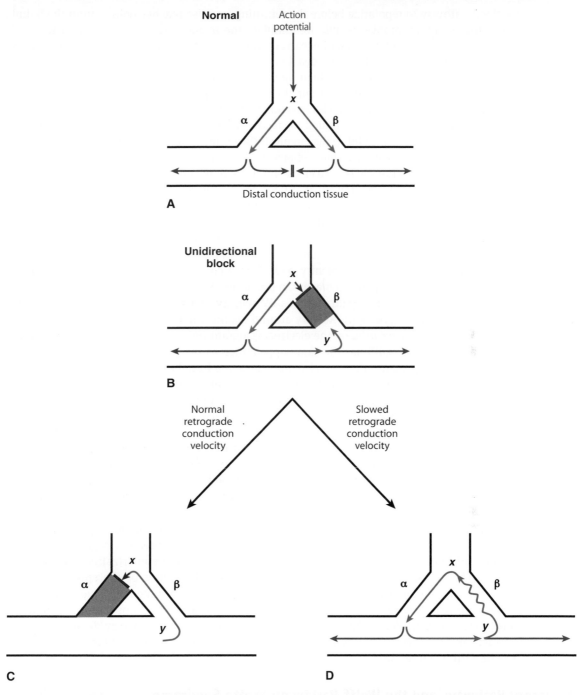

Figure 11-9. Mechanism of reentry. A. Normal conduction. When an action potential (AP) reaches a branch in the conduction pathway (point *x*), the impulse travels down both fibers (α and β) to excite distal conduction tissue. **B.** Unidirectional block. Forward passage of the impulse is blocked in the β pathway but proceeds normally down the α pathway. When the impulse reaches point *y*, if retrograde conduction of the β pathway is intact, the AP can enter β from below and conduct in a retrograde fashion. **C.** When point *x* is reached again, if the α pathway has not had sufficient time to repolarize, then the impulse stops. **D.** However, if conduction through the retrograde pathway is sufficiently slow (*jagged line*), it reaches point *x* after the α pathway has recovered. In that circumstance, the impulse is able to excite the α pathway again, and a reentrant loop is formed.

for the α pathway to repolarize before the returning impulse reaches point x from the β limb. Then, the invading impulse is able to stimulate the α pathway once again, and the cycle repeats itself. This circular stimulation can continue indefinitely, and each pass of the impulse through the loop excites cells of the distal conduction tissue, which propagates to the rest of the myocardium, at an abnormally high rate, resulting in a tachyarrhythmia.

For the mechanism of reentry to occur, the propagating impulse must continuously encounter excitable tissue. Thus, the time it takes for the impulse to travel around the reentrant loop must be greater than the time required for recovery (the refractory period) of the tissue, and this must be true for each point in the circuit. If the conduction time is shorter than the recovery time, the impulse will encounter refractory tissue and stop. Because normal conduction velocity in ventricular muscle is ~ 50 cm/s and the average effective refractory period is about 0.2 seconds, a reentry path circuit would need to be at least 10 cm long for reentry to occur in a normal ventricle. However, with *slower* conduction velocities, a shorter reentry circuit is possible. Most clinical cases of reentry occur within small regions of tissue because the conduction velocity within the reentrant loop is, in fact, abnormally slow.

In summary, the two critical conditions for reentry are (1) unidirectional block and (2) slowed conduction through the reentry path. These conditions commonly occur in regions where fibrosis has developed, such as infarction scars. In some cases, reentry occurs over an anatomically fixed circuit or path, such as AV reentry using an accessory pathway (as discussed in the following section). Reentry around distinct anatomic pathways usually appears as a *monomorphic tachycardia* on the electrocardiogram (ECG); that is, in the case of ventricular tachycardia, each QRS has the same appearance as the preceding and subsequent QRS complexes. This is because the reentry path is the same from beat to beat, producing a stable, regular tachycardia. This is the most common mechanism of ventricular tachycardia associated with areas of ventricular scar, as may result from a prior myocardial infarction.

Other types of reentry do not require a stable, fixed path. For example, one form can occur in electrically heterogeneous myocardium, in which waves of reentrant excitation spiral through the tissue, continually changing direction. These so-called spiral waves can be initiated when a wave front of depolarization encounters a broad region of functional block, which could be refractory from a preceding wave front, be poorly excitable tissue due to myocardial ischemia, or be under the influence of certain antiarrhythmic medications. Forward propagation of the wave front is asymmetrically blocked by this region, as the remainder of the front proceeds around the block. As the region repolarizes and becomes excitable again, parts of the wave front then spread retrogradely through it and continue in a spiral path following in the wake of the depolarization that had just passed. Unlike an anatomically fixed reentrant tract, the center of the spiral wave can move through the myocardium and even split into two or more reentry waves. In the ventricles, the resulting tachycardia has a continually changing QRS appearance, producing *polymorphic ventricular tachycardia*. If such activation is rapid and very disorganized, no distinct QRS complexes will be discernable, and the rhythm is *ventricular fibrillation* (as described in Chapter 12).

Accessory Pathways and the Wolff-Parkinson-White Syndrome

The mechanism of reentry is dramatically illustrated by the **Wolff-Parkinson-White (WPW) syndrome**. In the normal heart, an impulse generated by the SA node propagates through atrial tissue to the AV node, where expected slower conduction causes a short delay before continuing on to the ventricles. However, ~ 1 in 1500 people has the WPW syndrome and is born with an additional connection between an atrium and ventricle. Termed an accessory pathway (or bypass tract), this connection allows conduction between the atria and ventricles to bypass the AV node. The most common type of accessory pathway consists of microscopic

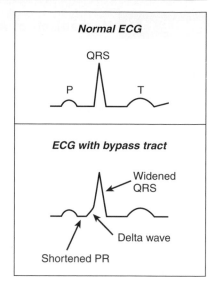

Figure 11-10. Accessory pathway (also termed a bypass tract). Example of an atrioventricular bypass tract (bundle of Kent), shown schematically, which can conduct impulses from the atrium directly to the ventricles, bypassing the AV node. The ECG demonstrates a shortened PR interval and a "delta wave" caused by early excitation of the ventricles via the accessory pathway. ECG, electrocardiogram; SA, sinoatrial.

fibers (known as a *bundle of Kent*) that span the AV groove somewhere along the mitral or tricuspid annuli, as shown in Figure 11-10.

Because accessory pathway tissue conducts impulses faster than the AV node, stimulation of the ventricles during sinus rhythm begins earlier than normal, and the PR interval of the ECG is therefore *shortened* (usually <0.12 seconds or <3 small boxes). In this situation, the ventricles are said to be "preexcited." However, the accessory pathway connects to ventricular myocardium rather than to the Purkinje system, such that the subsequent spread of the impulse through the ventricles from that site is slower than usual. In addition, because normal conduction over the AV node proceeds concurrently, ventricular depolarization represents a combination of the electric impulse traveling via the accessory tract *and* that conducted through the normal Purkinje system. As a result, the QRS complex in patients with WPW is wider than normal and demonstrates an abnormally slurred initial upstroke, known as a *delta wave* (Fig. 11-10).

During sinus rhythm, simultaneous conduction through the accessory pathway and AV node results in this interesting ECG appearance but causes no symptoms. The presence of the abnormal pathway, however, creates an ideal condition for reentry because the refractory period of the pathway is usually different from that of the AV node. An appropriately timed abnormal impulse (eg, a premature beat) may encounter block in the accessory pathway but conduct through the AV node or vice versa. If the propagating impulse then finds that the initially blocked pathway has recovered (unidirectional block), it can conduct in a retrograde direction up to the atrium and then down the other pathway back to the ventricles. Thus, a large anatomic loop is established, with the accessory pathway serving as one limb and the normal conduction pathway through the AV node as the other. The clinical characteristics of the WPW syndrome, including the types of reentrant tachycardia associated with it, are described in Chapter 12.

The mechanisms of altered impulse formation and conduction form the basis of all common arrhythmias, both abnormally slow rhythms (bradyarrhythmias) and abnormally fast ones (tachyarrhythmias). Table 11-1 lists the underlying mechanisms and examples of their commonly associated rhythm disturbances.

TABLE 11-1   Mechanisms of Arrhythmia Development

Abnormality	Mechanism	Examples
Bradyarrhythmias		
Altered impulse formation		
• Decreased automaticity	Decreased phase 4 depolarization (eg, parasympathetic stimulation)	Sinus bradycardia
Altered impulse conduction		
• Conduction blocks	Ischemic, anatomic, or drug-induced impaired conduction	First-, second-, and third-degree AV blocks
Tachyarrhythmias		
Altered impulse formation		
• Enhanced automaticity		
Sinus node	Increased phase 4 depolarization (eg, sympathetic stimulation)	Sinus tachycardia
AV node		AV junctional tachycardia
Ectopic focus	Acquires phase 4 depolarization	Ectopic atrial tachycardia and some forms of VT
• Triggered activity		
Early afterdepolarization	Prolonged action potential duration	Torsades de pointes
Delayed afterdepolarization	Intracellular calcium overload (eg, digitalis toxicity)	APBs, VPBs, digitalis-induced arrhythmias, "idiopathic" VT
Altered impulse conduction		
• Reentry	Unidirectional block plus slowed conduction	
Anatomical		Atrial flutter, AV nodal reentrant tachycardia, VT related to ventricular scar
Functional		Atrial fibrillation, polymorphic VT, ventricular fibrillation

AV, atrioventricular; APB, atrial premature beat; VPB, ventricular premature beat; VT, ventricular tachycardia.

PHYSIOLOGIC BASIS OF ANTIARRHYTHMIC THERAPY

Appropriate treatment of a rhythm disorder depends on its severity and its likely mechanism. When an arrhythmia produces severe hypotension or cardiac arrest, it must be immediately terminated to restore effective cardiac function. Therapy for termination may include electrical cardioversion (an electric "shock") for tachycardias, cardiac pacing for bradycardias, or administration of medications.

Additional therapy to prevent recurrences is guided by the etiology of the rhythm disturbance. Correctable factors that contribute to abnormal impulse formation and conduction (such as ischemia or electrolyte abnormalities) should be corrected. If there is a risk of recurrent arrhythmia, medications that alter automaticity, conduction, and/or refractoriness may be administered, or catheter or surgical ablation of conduction pathways is undertaken to physically disrupt the region responsible for the arrhythmia. Other advanced options include implantation of a permanent pacemaker for serious bradyarrhythmias or an implantable cardioverter-defibrillator (ICD) to automatically terminate malignant tachyarrhythmias should they recur. The following sections summarize the common therapeutic modalities, and Chapter 12 describes how they are used to address specific rhythm disorders.

BRADYARRHYTHMIAS

Not all slow heart rhythms require specific treatment. For those that do, pharmacologic therapy can increase the heart rate acutely, but the effect is transient. Electronic pacemakers are used when more sustained therapy is needed.

Pharmacologic Therapy

Pharmacologic therapy of bradyarrhythmias modifies the autonomic input to the heart in one of two ways:

1. *Anticholinergic drugs* (ie, antimuscarinic agents such as atropine). Vagal stimulation reduces the rate of sinus node depolarization (which slows the heart rate) and decreases conduction through the AV node, through the release of acetylcholine onto muscarinic receptors. Anticholinergic drugs competitively bind to muscarinic receptors and thereby reduce the vagal effect. This results in an increased heart rate and enhanced AV nodal conduction.

2. β_1-*Receptor agonists* (eg, isoproterenol). Mimicking the effect of endogenous catecholamines, these drugs increase heart rate and speed AV nodal conduction.

Atropine and isoproterenol are administered intravenously. Although these drugs are useful in managing certain slow heart rhythms emergently, it is not practical to continue them over the long term to treat persistent bradyarrhythmias.

Electronic Pacemakers

Electronic pacemakers apply repeated electric stimulation to the heart to initiate depolarizations at a desired rate, thereby assuming control of the rhythm. Pacemakers may be installed on a temporary or a permanent basis. Temporary units are used to stabilize patients who are awaiting implantation of a permanent pacemaker or to treat transient bradyarrhythmias, such as those caused by reversible drug toxicities.

There are two types of **temporary pacemakers**. *External* transcutaneous pacemakers deliver electric pulses to the patient's chest through large adhesive electrodes placed on the skin. The advantage of this technique is that it can be applied rapidly. Unfortunately, because the current used must be sufficient to initiate a cardiac depolarization, it stimulates thoracic nerves and skeletal muscle, which can be quite uncomfortable. Therefore, this form of pacing is usually used only on an emergency basis until another means of treating the arrhythmia can be implemented.

The other option for temporary pacing is a *transvenous* unit. In this case, an electrode-tipped catheter is inserted percutaneously into the venous system, passed into the heart, and connected to an external power source (termed a pulse generator). Electric pulses are applied directly to the heart through the electrode catheter, which is typically placed in the right ventricle or right atrium. This type of pacing is not painful and can be effective for days. There is, however, a risk of infection and/or thrombosis associated with the catheter.

Permanent pacemakers are more sophisticated than the temporary variety. Various configurations can sense and capture the electric activity of the atria and/or ventricles. With the most common types of permanent pacemakers, one or more wires (known as leads) with pacing electrodes are passed through an axillary or subclavian vein into the right ventricle and right atrium or through the coronary sinus into a cardiac vein (to stimulate the left ventricle). The pulse generator, similar in size to two silver dollars stacked on top of one another, is connected to the leads and then implanted under the skin, typically in the infraclavicular region. The pacemaker battery typically lasts about 10 years.

Modern permanent pacemakers sense cardiac activity and pace only when needed. They incorporate complex functions to track the patient's normal heart rate and can stimulate beats automatically in response to activity. They can also record useful data, such as whether fast rates have been sensed (which might indicate a tachyarrhythmia), the amount of pacing that has been required, and other parameters of pacemaker function. An external radiofrequency programming device is used to "interrogate" the pacemaker to obtain the recorded information and to adjust the pacing functions.

Although the most common indications for permanent pacemakers are bradyarrhythmias, pacemakers that incorporate a left ventricular pacing lead are also used to improve cardiac performance in some patients with heart failure (*cardiac resynchronization therapy*—see Chapter 9).

TACHYARRHYTHMIAS

The treatment of tachyarrhythmias is directed at the (1) protection of the patient from the consequences of the arrhythmia and (2) the specific mechanism responsible for the abnormal rhythm. Pharmacologic agents and cardioversion/defibrillation are commonly used approaches, but innovative electronic devices and transvenous catheter-based techniques to intentionally damage (ablate) arrhythmia-causing tissue have revolutionized treatment of these disorders.

Pharmacologic Therapy

Pharmacologic management of tachyarrhythmias is directed against the underlying mechanism (abnormal automaticity, reentrant circuits, or triggered activity). Many antiarrhythmic drugs are available, and the choice of which to use relies on the cause of the specific arrhythmia. From consideration of the arrhythmia mechanisms presented in this chapter, the following strategies emerge:

Desired Drug Effects to Eliminate Rhythms Caused by Increased Automaticity:

1. Reduce the slope of phase 4 spontaneous depolarization of the automatic cells.
2. Make the diastolic potential more negative (hyperpolarize).
3. Make the threshold potential less negative.

Desired Antiarrhythmic Effects to Interrupt Reentrant Circuits:

1. Inhibit conduction in the reentry circuit to the point that conduction fails, thus stopping the reentry impulse.
2. Increase the refractory period within the reentrant circuit so that a propagating impulse finds tissue within the loop unexcitable and the impulse stops.
3. Suppress premature beats that can initiate reentry.

Desired Drug Effects to Eliminate Triggered Activity:

1. Shorten the action potential duration (to prevent early afterdepolarizations).
2. Correct conditions of calcium overload (to prevent delayed afterdepolarizations).

Drugs used to achieve these goals modulate the action potential through interactions with ion channels, surface receptors, and transport pumps. Many drugs have multiple effects and may disrupt arrhythmias through more than one mechanism. The commonly used antiarrhythmic drugs and their actions are described in Chapter 17.

It is important to recognize that although these drugs suppress arrhythmias, they also have the potential to *aggravate* or provoke certain rhythm disturbances. This undesired consequence is referred to as **proarrhythmia** and is a major limitation of contemporary antiarrhythmic drug therapy. For example, antiarrhythmic agents that act therapeutically to prolong the action potential duration can, as an undesired effect, provoke early afterdepolarizations, the mechanism underlying the polymorphic ventricular tachycardia torsades de pointes (see Chapter 12). In addition, most agents used to treat tachyarrhythmias have the potential to aggravate bradyarrhythmias, and all antiarrhythmics have potentially toxic noncardiac side effects. These shortcomings have led to an increased reliance on nonpharmacologic treatment options, as described in the following sections.

Vagotonic Maneuvers

Many tachycardias involve transmission of impulses through the AV node, a structure that is sensitive to vagal modulation. Vagal tone can be transiently increased by a number of bedside maneuvers, and performing these may slow conduction, which terminates some reentrant tachyarrhythmias. For example, **carotid sinus massage** is performed by rubbing firmly for a few seconds over the carotid sinus, located at the bifurcation of the internal and external carotid arteries on either side of the neck. This maneuver stimulates the baroreceptor reflex (see Chapter 13), which elicits the desired increase in vagal tone and withdrawal of sympathetic tone. This maneuver should be performed on only one carotid sinus at a time (to prevent interference with brain perfusion) and is best avoided in patients with known advanced atherosclerosis involving the carotid arteries. Alternatively, the **Valsalva maneuver** can be performed to increase vagal tone by asking the patient to inhale and then to forcefully exhale against a closed glottis for ~10 seconds. Even more effective is the **modified Valsalva maneuver**, in which the Valsalva maneuver is undertaken in the semirecumbent position, immediately followed by shifting the patient to a supine position and lifting both of the patient's legs ("passive leg raising") for 45 seconds.

Electric Cardioversion and Defibrillation

Cardioversion and defibrillation involve the application of an electric shock to terminate a tachycardia. A shock with sufficient energy depolarizes the bulk of excitable myocardial tissue, interrupts reentrant circuits, establishes electric homogeneity, and allows the sinus node (the site of fastest spontaneous discharge) to regain pacemaker control. Tachyarrhythmias that are caused by reentry can usually be terminated by this procedure, whereas arrhythmias due to abnormal automaticity may simply persist.

External cardioversion is used to terminate supraventricular tachycardias or organized ventricular tachycardias. It is performed by briefly sedating the patient and then placing two large electrode paddles (or adhesive electrodes) against the chest on either side of the heart. The electric discharge is electronically *synchronized* to occur at the time of a QRS complex (ie, when ventricular depolarization occurs). This prevents the possibility of discharge during the T wave, when a shock could induce reentry (and lead to ventricular fibrillation) because regions of myocardium are in different phases of depolarization and recovery.

External defibrillation is performed to terminate ventricular fibrillation and polymorphic ventricular tachycardia (described in Chapter 12), employing the same equipment as that used for cardioversion. However, because there is no dominant organized QRS complex on which to synchronize the electric discharge, it is delivered using the "asynchronous" mode of the device.

Implantable Cardioverter-Defibrillators

ICDs automatically terminate dangerous ventricular arrhythmias using *internal* cardioversion-defibrillation or by way of a special type of artificial pacing. These devices are implanted, in a manner similar to that of permanent pacemakers, in patients at high risk of sudden cardiac death from ventricular arrhythmias. The device continuously monitors cardiac activity, and if the heart rate exceeds a certain programmable threshold for a specified time, the ICD delivers an appropriate intervention, such as an electric shock. Internal cardioversion or defibrillation requires substantially less energy than does external defibrillation but is still painful if the patient is conscious.

The majority of monomorphic ventricular tachycardias can be terminated by an ICD with a rapid burst of electric impulses, termed *antitachycardia pacing (ATP)*, rather than a shock. The goal is to artificially pace the heart at a rate faster than the tachycardia to prematurely depolarize a portion of a reentrant circuit, thereby rendering it refractory to further immediate stimulation. Consequently, when a reentrant impulse returns to the zone that has already been depolarized by the device, it encounters unexcitable tissue, it cannot propagate further, and the circuit is broken. An advantage of the ATP technique is that, unlike internal cardioversion, it is painless. However, ATP is not effective for terminating ventricular fibrillation, a situation in which the device is programmed to deliver an electric shock instead.

Catheter Ablation

If an arrhythmia originates from a distinct anatomical reentry circuit or an automatic focus, electrophysiologic mapping techniques can be used to localize the region of myocardium or conduction tissue responsible for the disturbance. It is then often possible to ablate the site via a catheter that applies radiofrequency current to heat and destroy the tissue. Such procedures have revolutionized the management of patients with many types of tachycardias, because they often offer a permanent therapeutic solution that spares patients from prolonged antiarrhythmic drug therapy. Additionally, for patients with ICDs and recurrent ventricular tachycardias causing defibrillator shocks, ablation is often effective in reducing the frequency of episodes.

Summary

- Arrhythmias result from disorders of **impulse formation**, **impulse conduction**, or both.
- **Bradyarrhythmias** (abnormally slow heart rhythms) develop because of decreased impulse formation (eg, sinus bradycardia) or decreased impulse conduction (eg, AV nodal conduction blocks).
- **Tachyarrhythmias** (abnormally fast rhythms) result from increased automaticity (of the SA node, latent pacemakers, or abnormal myocardial sites), triggered activity, or reentry.
- The two critical conditions for **reentry** are (1) unidirectional block and (2) slowed conduction through the reentry path; these conditions commonly occur in regions where fibrosis has developed, such as infarction scars.
- Bradyarrhythmias are usually treated acutely with drugs that accelerate the rate of sinus node discharge and enhance AV nodal conduction (eg, atropine, isoproterenol) or with temporary electronic pacemakers.
- **Permanent electronic pacemakers** are implanted when more sustained therapy for bradyarrhythmias is needed.
- Pharmacologic therapy for tachyarrhythmias is directed at the mechanism responsible for the rhythm disturbance.
- For refractory tachyarrhythmias, or in emergency situations, **electrical cardioversion or defibrillation** is utilized.
- Catheter-based **ablation techniques** are useful for long-term control of certain tachyarrhythmias.
- **ICDs** are lifesaving devices implanted in patients at high risk of arrhythmic sudden cardiac death.
- For patients with ICDs and recurrent ventricular tachycardias causing defibrillator shocks, ablation techniques are often effective in reducing the frequency of episodes.

Chapter 12 describes the diagnosis and management of the most common arrhythmias. Chapter 17 describes commonly used antiarrhythmic drugs.

Review Questions

1. Which of the following conditions are typically necessary for the development of a reentrant tachycardia?

   a. Bidirectional block
   b. Unidirectional block with slowed retrograde pathway conduction
   c. Fast retrograde pathway conduction
   d. Delayed afterdepolarizations

2. A 64-year-old woman with breast cancer was admitted to the hospital for chemotherapy. As part of her treatment, she received intravenous ondansetron, a medication for the prevention of nausea and vomiting. She was subsequently observed to have brief episodes of polymorphic ventricular tachycardia (torsades de pointes) on the cardiac monitor. When in sinus rhythm, the corrected QT interval was noted to be prolonged. Ondansetron was discontinued, the QT interval normalized, and no further arrhythmias were observed. What was the likely electrophysiologic basis of her tachyarrhythmia?

   a. Enhanced automaticity
   b. Delayed afterdepolarizations
   c. Early afterdepolarizations
   d. Reentry

3. A 54-year-old man with hypertension, diabetes mellitus, and prior myocardial infarction presents to the emergency department with episodic light-headedness. While undergoing examination, he suddenly loses consciousness. The blood pressure is 75/40 mm Hg. The electrocardiogram shows an organized form of ventricular tachycardia at a constant rate of 175 beats/min. Which of the following should be performed immediately?

   a. Carotid sinus massage
   b. Administer intravenous antiarrhythmic drug therapy
   c. Administer a β-blocker
   d. Synchronized electrical cardioversion

Answers to Review Questions

1. **Choice b is correct.** Unidirectional block and slow retrograde pathway conduction are the typical requirements for reentrant tachyarrhythmias (see Fig. 11-9). Slow retrograde conduction allows the initially depolarized limb of the pathway sufficient time to regain excitability in order to complete the reentrant circuit.

2. **Choice c is correct.** Prolongation of the QT interval from any cause can generate early afterdepolarizations, which may lead to torsades de pointes ("twisting of the points"), a form of polymorphic ventricular tachycardia (see Figs. 11-7 and 12-21), a potentially serious dysrhythmia. QT prolongation indicates a lengthened action potential duration that can be congenital (see Chapter 12) or result from electrolyte disturbances (hypokalemia, hypomagnesemia), persistent bradycardia, or certain drugs. Ondansetron is one of many medications that can prolong the action potential duration and the QT interval. It does so, at least in part, by blocking a repolarizing potassium channel current (I_{Kr}, described in Table 1-1).

3. Choice d is correct. Hemodynamically unstable patients with organized forms of ventricular tachyarrhythmia should undergo immediate synchronized electrical cardioversion. A synchronized discharge is electronically timed to occur at the time of a QRS complex, in order to avoid firing on the T wave, which could cause worsening of the dysrhythmia. In contrast, ventricular fibrillation or hemodynamically unstable polymorphic ventricular tachycardia should be treated with immediate defibrillation (otherwise termed *asynchronous* electrical cardioversion). Carotid sinus massage (a method to augment vagal tone), intravenous antiarrhythmic drug therapy, and β-blockers are not appropriate initial approaches for hemodynamically unstable arrhythmias.

Acknowledgments

Contributors to previous editions of this chapter were Mogan J. Prust, MD; Ranliang Hu, MD; Hillary K. Rolls, MD; Jennifer E. Ho, MD; Mark S. Sabatine, MD; Wendy Armstrong, MD; Nicholas Boulis, MD; Elliott M. Antman, MD; Leonard I. Ganz, MD; Gary R. Strichartz, PhD; and William G. Stevenson, MD.

Additional Reading

Appelboam A, Reuben A, Mann C, et al. Postural modification to the standard Valsalva manoeuvre for emergency treatment of supraventricular tachycardias (REVERT): a randomised controlled trial. *Lancet.* 2015;386:1747-1753.

DeSimone CV, Naksuk N, Asirvatham SJ. Supraventricular arrhythmias: clinical framework and common scenarios for the internist. *Mayo Clin Proc.* 2018;93:1825-1841.

Kusumoto FM, Schoenfeld MH, Barrett C, et al. 2018 ACC/AHA/HRS guideline on the evaluation and management of patients with bradycardia and cardiac conduction delay: a report of the American College of Cardiology/American Heart Association Task Force on Clinical Practice Guidelines and the Heart Rhythm Society. *Circulation.* 2019;140:e382-e482.

Qu Z, Weiss JN. Mechanisms of ventricular arrhythmias: from molecular fluctuations to electrical turbulence. *Annu Rev Physiol.* 2015;77:29-55.

Shivkumar K. Catheter ablation of ventricular arrhythmias. *N Engl J Med.* 2019;380:1555-1564.

Upadhyay GA, Alenghat FJ. Catheter ablation for atrial fibrillation in 2019. *JAMA.* 2019;322:686-687.

12
Clinical Aspects of Cardiac Arrhythmias

Victor Nauffal | Leonard S. Lilly

Chapter Outline

Bradyarrhythmias
Sinoatrial Node
Escape Rhythms
Atrioventricular Conduction System
Tachyarrhythmias
Supraventricular Arrhythmias
Ventricular Arrhythmias

Chapter 11 presented the mechanisms by which abnormal heart rhythms develop. This chapter describes how to recognize and treat specific arrhythmias. Table 12-1 categorizes the common rhythm disorders considered in this chapter.

There are five basic questions to consider when confronted with a patient with an abnormal heart rhythm, as detailed in the sections that follow:

1. Identification: What is the arrhythmia?
2. Pathogenesis: What is the underlying mechanism?
3. Precipitating factors: What conditions provoke it?
4. Clinical presentation: What symptoms and signs accompany the arrhythmia?
5. Treatment: What to do about it?

BRADYARRHYTHMIAS

In normal sinus rhythm, the heart rate ranges from 60 to 100 bpm, as described in Chapter 4. Bradyarrhythmias are rhythms in which the heart rate is <60 bpm. They arise from disorders of impulse formation or impaired impulse conduction, as described in Chapter 11.

SINOATRIAL NODE

Sinus Bradycardia

Sinus bradycardia (Fig. 12-1) is the slowing of the normal heart rhythm, as a result of decreased firing of the sinoatrial (SA) node, to a rate <60 bpm. Sinus bradycardia at rest or during sleep is normal and a benign finding in many people. Conversely, pathologic sinus bradycardia can result from either intrinsic SA node disease or extrinsic factors that affect the node. Depressed intrinsic automaticity can be caused by aging or any disease process that affects the atrium, including ischemic heart disease or cardiomyopathy. Extrinsic factors that suppress SA nodal activity include medications (eg, β-blockers and certain calcium channel blockers) and metabolic causes (eg, hypothyroidism).

Trained athletes often have elevated vagal tone, which results in physiologic and usually asymptomatic resting sinus bradycardia. Transient periods of high vagal tone can also occur in individuals as a reflex response to pain or fear, resulting in inappropriate sinus bradycardia.

Mild sinus bradycardia is usually asymptomatic and does not require treatment. However, a pronounced reduction of the heart rate can produce a fall in cardiac output with fatigue, light-headedness, confusion, or syncope. In such cases, any extrinsic provocative factors should be corrected, and specific therapy, as described in the next section, may be needed.

TABLE 12-1	Common Arrhythmias	
Location	**Bradyarrhythmias**	**Tachyarrhythmias**
SA node	Sinus bradycardia Sick sinus syndrome	Sinus tachycardia
Atria		Atrial premature beats Atrial flutter Atrial fibrillation Paroxysmal supraventricular tachycardias Focal atrial tachycardia Multifocal atrial tachycardia
AV node	Conduction blocks Junctional escape rhythm	Paroxysmal reentrant tachycardias (AV or AV nodal)
Ventricles	Ventricular escape rhythm	Ventricular premature beats Ventricular tachycardia Torsades de pointes Ventricular fibrillation

AV, atrioventricular; SA, sinoatrial.

Sick Sinus Syndrome

Intrinsic SA node dysfunction that causes periods of inappropriate bradycardia is known as sick sinus syndrome (SSS). This condition often produces symptoms of dizziness, confusion, or syncope. Patients with this syndrome (or any cause of symptomatic sinus bradycardia) can be treated acutely with intravenous anticholinergic drugs (eg, atropine) or β-adrenergic agonists (eg, isoproterenol), which transiently accelerate the heart rate. If the problem is chronic and not corrected by the removal of aggravating factors, placement of a permanent pacemaker is required.

SSS is common in elderly patients, who are also susceptible to supraventricular tachycardias (SVTs), most commonly atrial fibrillation (AF). This combination of slow and fast dysrhythmias is known as the **bradycardia-tachycardia syndrome** (Fig. 12-2) and is thought to result from atrial fibrosis that impairs function of the SA node and predisposes to AF and atrial flutter. During the tachyarrhythmia, overdrive suppression of the SA node occurs (as described in Chapter 11), and when the tachycardia terminates, a period of profound sinus bradycardia may ensue. Treatment generally requires the combination of antiarrhythmic drug therapy to suppress the tachyarrhythmias plus a permanent pacemaker to prevent bradycardia.

ESCAPE RHYTHMS

Cells in the atrioventricular (AV) node and His-Purkinje system are capable of automaticity but typically have slower firing rates than do those in the sinus node and are therefore suppressed during normal sinus rhythm. However, if SA node activity becomes impaired or if

Figure 12-1. Sinus bradycardia. The P wave and QRS complexes are normal, but the rate is <60 bpm.

Figure 12-2. Bradycardia-tachycardia syndrome. A brief irregular tachycardia is followed by slow sinus node discharge.

there is conduction block of the impulse from the SA node, escape rhythms can emerge from the more distal latent pacemakers (Fig. 12-3).

Junctional escape beats arise from the AV node or proximal bundle of His. They are characterized by a normal, narrow QRS complex and, when they occur in sequence (termed a **junctional escape rhythm**), appear at a rate of 40-60 bpm. The QRS complexes are not preceded by normal P waves because the impulse originates below the atria. However, *retrograde* P waves may be observed as an impulse propagates from the more distal pacemaker backward to the atrium. Retrograde P waves typically *follow* the QRS complex and are abnormally *inverted* (negative deflection on the electrocardiogram [ECG]) in limb leads II, III, and aVF, indicating activation of the atria starting from the AV node and proceeding superiorly.

Ventricular escape rhythms are characterized by even slower rates (30-40 bpm) and abnormally *widened* QRS complexes. The complexes are wide because the ventricles are not depolarized by the normal rapid simultaneous conduction over the right and left bundle branches but rather from a more distal point in the conduction system. The morphology that the QRS shows depends on the site of origin of the escape rhythm. For example, an escape rhythm originating from the left bundle branch will cause a right bundle-branch block QRS pattern, because the impulse depolarizes the left ventricle first and then spreads more slowly through the right ventricle (RV). Conversely, an escape rhythm originating in the right bundle branch causes the QRS to appear with a left bundle-branch block configuration. Escape rhythms that originate more distally, in the ventricular myocardium itself, are characterized by even wider QRS complexes because such impulses are conducted outside the rapidly propagating Purkinje fibers.

Figure 12-3. Escape rhythms. No P waves are evident. **A.** Junctional escape rhythm with normal-width QRS complexes. **B.** Wide QRS complexes typical of a ventricular escape rhythm.

Figure 12-4. First-degree AV block. The PR interval is prolonged.

Junctional and ventricular escape rhythms are protective backup mechanisms that maintain a heartbeat and cardiac output when the sinus node or normal AV conduction fails. The clinical findings and treatment of bradycardia associated with escape rhythms are identical to those of SSS described earlier.

ATRIOVENTRICULAR CONDUCTION SYSTEM

The AV conduction system includes the AV node, the bundle of His, and the left and right bundle branches. Impaired conduction between the atria and ventricles can result in three degrees (types) of AV conduction block.

First-Degree AV Block

First-degree AV block, shown in Figure 12-4, indicates prolongation of the normal delay between atrial and ventricular depolarization, such that the PR interval is lengthened (>0.2 seconds, which is >5 small boxes on the ECG). In this situation, the 1:1 relationship between P waves and QRS complexes is preserved. The impairment of conduction is usually within the AV node itself and can be caused by a transient reversible influence or a structural defect. *Reversible* causes include heightened vagal tone, transient AV nodal ischemia, and drugs that depress conduction through the AV node, including β-blockers, certain calcium channel antagonists, digitalis, and other antiarrhythmic medications. *Structural* causes of first-degree AV block include myocardial infarction and chronic degenerative diseases of the conduction system, which may occur with aging.

First-degree AV block is typically a benign, asymptomatic condition that does not require treatment. However, it can indicate disease in the AV node associated with susceptibility to higher degrees of AV block if drugs are administered that further impair AV conduction or if the conduction disease progresses.

Second-Degree AV Block

Second-degree AV block is characterized by *intermittent failure* of AV conduction, resulting in some P waves that are not followed by a QRS complex. There are two forms of second-degree AV block. In **type I** block (also termed **Wenckebach** block), shown in Figure 12-5, the degree of AV

Figure 12-5. Second-degree AV block: type I (Wenckebach). The P-wave rate is constant, but the PR interval progressively lengthens until a QRS is completely blocked (after the fourth P wave).

Figure 12-6. Second-degree AV block: type II. A QRS complex is blocked (after the fourth P wave) without gradual lengthening of the preceding PR intervals. While the QRS width in this example is normal, it is often widened in patients with type II block.

delay gradually increases with each beat until an impulse is completely blocked, such that there is no QRS after the P wave for a single beat. Therefore, the ECG shows a progressive increase in the PR interval from one beat to the next until a single QRS complex is absent, after which the PR interval shortens to its initial length, and the cycle starts again. Type I block almost always results from impaired conduction in the AV node (rather than more distally in the conduction system). It is usually benign and may be seen in children, trained athletes, and people with high vagal tone, particularly during sleep. It may also occur during an acute myocardial infarction because of increased vagal tone or ischemia of the AV node, but the block is usually temporary. Treatment of type I block is typically not necessary, but in symptomatic cases, administration of intravenous atropine or isoproterenol usually improves AV conduction transiently. Occasionally, placement of a permanent pacemaker is required for symptomatic block that does not resolve spontaneously or persists despite the correction of aggravating factors.

In contrast, **type II** second-degree AV block is a more serious condition. It is characterized by the sudden intermittent loss of AV conduction, *without* preceding gradual lengthening of the PR interval (Fig. 12-6). The block may persist for two or more beats (ie, two sequential P waves not followed by QRS complexes), in which case it is known as **high-grade** AV block (Fig. 12-7). Type II block is usually caused by conduction block distal to the AV node (in the bundle of His or more distally in the Purkinje system), and the QRS pattern often is widened. This type of block may arise from extensive myocardial infarction involving the septum or from chronic degeneration of the His-Purkinje system. It usually indicates severe disease and may progress to complete heart block without warning; therefore, a pacemaker is usually warranted, even in asymptomatic patients.

Third-Degree AV Block

Third-degree AV block, also termed **complete** heart block (Fig. 12-8), is present when there is *complete* failure of conduction between the atria and ventricles. In adults, the most common causes are acute myocardial infarction and chronic degeneration of the conduction pathways with advanced age. Third-degree AV block electrically disconnects the atria and ventricles; there is no relationship between the P waves and QRS complexes because the atria depolarize

Figure 12-7. High-grade AV block. Sequential QRS complexes are blocked (after the second and third P waves).

Figure 12-8. Third-degree AV block. The P wave and QRS rhythms are independent of one another. The QRS complexes are widened as they originate within the distal ventricular conduction system, not at the bundle of His. The second and fourth P waves are superimposed on normal T waves.

in response to SA node activity, while a more distal escape rhythm drives the ventricles independently. Thus, the P waves "march out" at a rate that is not related to the intervals at which QRS complexes appear. Depending on the site of the escape rhythm, the QRS complexes may be of normal width and occur at 40-60 bpm (originating from the AV node) or may be widened and occur at slower rates (originating from the His-Purkinje system). As a result of the slow rate, patients frequently experience light-headedness or syncope. Permanent pacemaker implantation is almost always necessary.

The term **AV dissociation** is a general description that refers to any situation in which the atria and ventricles beat independently, without any direct relationship between P waves and QRS complexes. Third-degree AV block is one example of AV dissociation.

TACHYARRHYTHMIAS

When the heart rate is >100 bpm for three beats or more, a tachyarrhythmia is present. Tachyarrhythmias result from one of the three mechanisms described in Chapter 11: enhanced automaticity, reentry, or triggered activity. Tachyarrhythmias are categorized into those that arise *above* the ventricles (supraventricular) and those that arise *within* the ventricles.

SUPRAVENTRICULAR ARRHYTHMIAS

Figure 12-9 presents a schema to help organize the common supraventricular tachyarrhythmias presented in this section.

Sinus Tachycardia

Sinus tachycardia is characterized by an SA node discharge rate of >100 bpm with normal P waves and QRS complexes (Fig. 12-10). This rhythm most often results from increased sympathetic and/or decreased vagal tone. Sinus tachycardia is an appropriate physiologic response to exercise. However, it may also result from sympathetic stimulation in pathologic conditions, including fever, hypoxemia, hyperthyroidism, hypovolemia, and anemia. In disease states, sinus tachycardia is usually a sign of the severity of the primary pathophysiologic process, and treatment should be directed at the underlying cause.

Atrial Premature Beats

Atrial premature beats (APBs) are common in healthy as well as diseased hearts (Fig. 12-11). They originate from automaticity or reentry in an atrial focus outside the SA node and are often exacerbated by sympathetic stimulation. APBs are usually asymptomatic but may cause palpitations. On the ECG, an APB appears as an earlier-than-expected P wave with an *abnormal shape* (the impulse does not arise from the SA node, resulting in an abnormal sequence

Figure 12-9. Differentiation of common supraventricular tachyarrhythmias.

of conduction through the atria). The QRS complex that follows the P wave is usually normal, resembling the QRS during sinus rhythm, because ventricular conduction is not impaired. However, if the abnormal atrial focus fires very soon after the previous beat, the impulse may encounter an AV node that is still refractory to excitation, resulting in a blocked impulse that does not conduct to the ventricles. In that case, the premature P wave is *not* followed by a QRS complex and is termed a *blocked APB*. Similarly, if the ectopic focus fires just a bit later in diastole, it may conduct through the AV node but encounter portions of the His-Purkinje system (typically the right or left bundle branch) that are still refractory. As a result of failure of conduction in one of the bundle branches, the impulse is conducted through a portion of the ventricles more slowly than normal, producing QRS complexes that are abnormally wide (termed an APB with *aberrant conduction*).

Figure 12-10. Sinus tachycardia. The P wave and QRS complexes are normal, but the rate is >100 bpm.

Figure 12-11. Atrial premature beat (APB). The P wave occurs earlier than expected, and its shape is abnormal.

APBs require treatment only if they are symptomatic. Because caffeine, alcohol, and adrenergic stimulation (eg, emotional stress) can all predispose to APBs, it is important to address these factors. β-Blockers are the initial preferred pharmacologic treatment if needed.

Atrial Flutter

Atrial flutter is characterized by rapid, regular atrial activity at a rate of 180-350 bpm (Fig. 12-12). Many of these fast impulses reach the AV node during its refractory period and do not conduct to the ventricles, resulting in a slower ventricular rate, often an even fraction of the atrial rate. Thus, if the atrial rate is 300 bpm and 2:1 block occurs at the AV node (ie, every other atrial impulse finds the AV node refractory), the ventricular rate is 150 bpm. Because vagal maneuvers (eg, carotid sinus massage) decrease AV nodal conduction, they increase the degree of block, temporarily slowing the ventricular rate, which allows better visualization of the underlying atrial activity. In general, atrial flutter is caused by reentry over a large anatomically fixed circuit. In the common form of atrial flutter, this circuit is the atrial tissue along the tricuspid valve annulus: the circulating depolarization wave propagates up the interatrial septum, across the roof and down the free wall of the right atrium, and finally along the floor of the right atrium between the tricuspid valve annulus and inferior vena cava. Because large parts of the atrium are depolarized throughout the cycle, P waves often have a sinusoidal or "saw-tooth" appearance. Large flutter circuits can occur in other parts of the right or left atrium as well, usually associated with areas of atrial scarring from disease, prior heart surgery, or ablation procedures.

Atrial flutter generally occurs in patients with preexisting heart disease. It may be paroxysmal and transient, persistent (lasting for days or weeks), or permanent. Symptoms of atrial flutter depend on the accompanying ventricular rate. If the rate is <100 bpm, the patient may be asymptomatic. Conversely, faster rates often cause palpitations, dyspnea, or weakness. Paradoxically, antiarrhythmic medications that reduce the rate of atrial flutter by slowing conduction in the atrium may make the rhythm more dangerous by allowing the AV node more time to recover between impulses. In this situation, the AV node may begin to conduct in a 1:1 fashion, producing very rapid ventricular rates. For example, a patient with atrial flutter at a rate of

Figure 12-12. Atrial flutter is typified by rapid "saw-toothed" atrial activity (*arrows*).

280 bpm and 2:1 conduction block at the AV node would have a ventricular rate of 140 bpm. If the atrial rate then slows to 220 bpm, the AV node may be able to recover sufficiently between depolarizations to conduct every atrial impulse, causing the ventricular rate to *accelerate* to 220 bpm. In patients with limited cardiac reserve, this acceleration may result in a profound reduction of cardiac output and hypotension. Atrial flutter also predisposes to atrial thrombus formation, and anticoagulation therapy is often appropriate, as described below for AF.

Several approaches for the conversion of atrial flutter to sinus rhythm are available:

1. For symptomatic patients with recent-onset atrial flutter, the most expeditious therapy is electrical synchronized cardioversion to restore sinus rhythm. This technique is also used to revert chronic atrial flutter that has not responded to other approaches.
2. Flutter can be terminated by rapid atrial stimulation (burst pacing) using a temporary or permanent pacemaker (see Chapter 11). This procedure can be used when temporary atrial pacing wires are already present, as in the days following cardiac surgery. In addition, certain types of permanent pacemakers and implanted defibrillators can be programmed to perform burst pacing automatically when atrial flutter occurs.
3. Patients without an immediate need for cardioversion can begin pharmacologic therapy. First, the ventricular rate is slowed by drugs that increase AV block: β-blockers, certain calcium channel blockers (eg, verapamil, diltiazem), or digoxin. Once the rate is effectively slowed, attempts can be made to restore sinus rhythm using antiarrhythmic drugs that slow conduction or prolong the refractory period of the atrial myocardium (usually class IC or class III agents; see Chapter 17). Should these drugs fail to convert the rhythm, electrical cardioversion can be undertaken. Once sinus rhythm has been restored, antiarrhythmic drugs may be administered chronically to prevent recurrences.
4. When chronic therapy is required to prevent recurrences, catheter ablation is often a better alternative than pharmacologic approaches. In this method, an electrode catheter is inserted into the femoral vein, passed via the inferior vena cava to the right atrium, and used to localize and cauterize (ablate) part of the reentrant loop to permanently interrupt the flutter circuit.

Atrial Fibrillation

AF is a chaotic rhythm with an atrial rate so fast (350-600 discharges/min) that distinct P waves are not discernible on the ECG (Fig. 12-13). As with atrial flutter, many of the atrial impulses encounter refractory tissue at the AV node, allowing only some of the depolarizations to be conducted to the ventricles in a very irregular fashion (indicated by a characteristic "irregularly irregular" rhythm). The average ventricular rate in untreated AF is ~ 140-160 bpm. Because discrete P waves are not visible on the ECG, the baseline shows low-amplitude undulations punctuated by QRS complexes and T waves.

The mechanism of AF likely involves multiple wandering reentrant circuits within the atria, and in some patients, the rhythm repetitively shifts between fibrillation and atrial flutter. When fibrillation is paroxysmal (ie, sudden, unpredictable episodes), it is often initiated by rapid firing of foci in sleeves of atrial muscle that extend into the pulmonary veins. To sustain AF, a minimum number of reentrant circuits is needed, and an enlarged atrium increases the potential for this to occur. Thus, AF is often associated with right or left atrial enlargement. Accordingly, diseases that increase atrial pressure and size promote AF, including heart failure, mitral valve disease, hypertension, and pulmonary disease. Thyrotoxicosis and alcohol consumption can also precipitate AF in some individuals. In addition, AF is a common rhythm disturbance in the elderly.

As with atrial flutter, when the ventricular rate is <100 bpm, AF may be asymptomatic. When the rate is faster, as may occur before treatment is instituted and when AV nodal conduction is facilitated by elevated sympathetic tone during illness, the rapid ventricular rate may compromise cardiac output, resulting in hypotension and pulmonary congestion

Figure 12-13. Atrial fibrillation is characterized by chaotic atrial activity without organized P waves and by irregularity of the ventricular (QRS) rate.

(especially in patients with a hypertrophied or "stiff" left ventricle in whom the loss of normal atrial contraction can significantly reduce left ventricular filling and stroke volume). AF is also an important cause of embolic stroke and systemic thromboembolism. The absence of organized atrial contraction promotes blood stasis in the atria, increasing the risk of thrombus formation in the left atrial appendage (LAA), which can embolize to the cerebral circulation and other systemic sites. Thus, treatment of AF is directed at three aspects of the arrhythmia: (1) ventricular rate control, (2) assessment of the need for anticoagulation to prevent thromboembolism, and (3) consideration of methods to restore sinus rhythm.

Antiarrhythmic drug treatment of AF is similar to that of atrial flutter. β-Blockers or certain Ca^{++} channel antagonists (diltiazem, verapamil) are administered to promote block at the AV node so as to reduce the ventricular rate. Digitalis is less effective for this purpose, although it may be useful in patients with accompanying impairment of ventricular contractile function. For those who remain symptomatic despite adequate rate control, conversion to sinus rhythm is usually attempted, as described below.

AF that has been present for more than 48 hours may predispose to atrial thrombus formation, and systemic anticoagulation for at least 3 weeks is usually warranted prior to cardioversion to reduce the risk of thromboembolism (anticoagulant drugs are described in Chapter 17). Alternatively, a transesophageal echocardiogram can be performed to evaluate for the presence of thrombus; if none is found, cardioversion may proceed directly, with minimum thromboembolic risk, provided that anticoagulation is instituted for several weeks thereafter (since recovery of normal atrial contraction may be delayed for a period of time following cardioversion). Whether a patient with AF episodes should remain on anticoagulation for the long term is frequently based on the calculated CHA_2DS_2-VASc (pronounced "Chads-Vasc") score, in which points are assigned for the presence of **c**ongestive heart failure, **h**ypertension, **a**ge, **d**iabetes, prior **s**troke, **v**ascular disease, and **s**ex (see Table 12-2). Men with AF (persistent or intermittent) and a CHA_2DS_2-VASc score of ≥1, or women with a score of ≥2, are usually

TABLE 12-2 CHA_2DS_2-VASc Score

Characteristic	Points
Congestive heart failure	1
Hypertension	1
Age ≥ 75 years	2
Diabetes mellitus	1
Stroke history (or transient ischemic attack or thromboembolism)	2
Vascular disease (prior myocardial infarction or peripheral vascular disease)	1
Age 65-74	1
Sex: female gender	1

considered at sufficiently high risk of future thromboembolism to advise continued anticoagulation therapy.

Cardioversion to sinus rhythm can be attempted *chemically* by administration of class IC, IA, or III antiarrhythmic drugs (see Chapter 17 for descriptions of these classes). Alternatively, *electrical cardioversion* can be undertaken. Following successful conversion to sinus rhythm, antiarrhythmic drugs are often continued in an attempt to prevent recurrences. Note that these drugs have the capacity to cause serious, sometimes lethal, side effects (see Chapter 17). Thus, in patients with *asymptomatic* AF, it is often appropriate to simply control the ventricular rate and continue anticoagulation therapy chronically, rather than to pursue cardioversion. Such an approach is supported by clinical trials of AF that have assessed long-term clinical outcomes.

Because the efficacies and toxicities of antiarrhythmic drugs have been disappointing, nonpharmacologic options for the management of AF have been devised. For example, the surgical *maze procedure* places multiple incisions in the left and right atria to prevent the formation of reentry circuits and is sometimes performed in patients undergoing cardiac surgery for coronary artery or valve disease who also have AF. A less-invasive approach is the *percutaneous catheter ablation*. In this approach, areas of the left atrium around the pulmonary veins are subjected to radiofrequency or cryothermal (extreme cold) energy delivered by intracardiac catheters to interrupt potential reentry circuits and foci that initiate AF. Doing so requires extensive catheter manipulation and ablation in the left atrium, and risks of the procedure include stroke from systemic thromboembolism and cardiac perforation that could cause pericardial tamponade. Catheter ablation for AF is most appropriate for patients who have failed, or become intolerant to, antiarrhythmic drug therapy or for patients who prefer to avoid such medications.

When sinus rhythm cannot be maintained and the heart rate cannot be controlled adequately with medications, *catheter ablation of the AV node* is another available procedure. This method intentionally creates complete heart block as a means to permanently slow the ventricular rate. Permanent ventricular pacemaker placement is then also required to generate an adequate ventricular rate.

LAA ligation or occlusion, which can be performed through open surgical or percutaneous techniques, excludes the LAA from the circulation, removing it as a source of thromboembolism. The advantages and risks of such approaches are still being defined for patients with AF for whom it is unsafe to continue long-term anticoagulation therapy.

Paroxysmal Supraventricular Tachycardias

Paroxysmal supraventricular tachycardias (PSVTs) are manifested by (1) sudden onset and termination, (2) atrial rates between 140 and 250 bpm, and (3) narrow (normal) QRS complexes (Fig. 12-14), unless *aberrant conduction* is present, as summarized later. The mechanism of PSVTs is most often reentry involving the AV node, atrium, or an accessory pathway between an atrium and a ventricle. Enhanced automaticity and triggered activity in the atrium or AV node are less common causes.

Figure 12-14. Paroxysmal supraventricular tachycardia caused by AV nodal reentry. Retrograde P waves in this example occur simultaneously with, and are "hidden" in, the QRS complexes.

AV Nodal Reentrant Tachycardia

Atrioventricular nodal reentrant tachycardia (AVNRT) is the most common form of PSVT in adults. In the normal heart, the AV node is a lobulated structure that consists of a compact portion and several atrial extensions. The latter constitute two (or more) potential pathways for conduction through the AV node (Fig. 12-15). In some people, these extensions

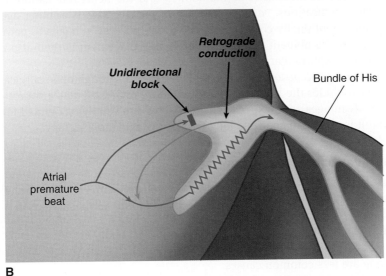

Figure 12-15. Common mechanism of AV nodal reentry. In most patients, the AV node is a lobulated structure consisting proximally of several atrial extensions and distally of a compact node portion. **A.** In patients with AV nodal reentry, two functionally distinct tracts exist within the AV node (termed the slow and fast pathways). The slow pathway conducts slowly and has a short refractory period, whereas the fast pathway conducts more rapidly but has a long refractory period. Impulses from above conduct down both pathways; because the fast pathway impulse reaches the distal common pathway first, it continues to the bundle of His. Conversely, the slow pathway impulse arrives later and encounters refractory tissue. **B.** An APB arrives at the entrance of the two pathways. The fast pathway is still refractory from the preceding beat, and the impulse is blocked, but the slow pathway has repolarized and is able to conduct. When the impulse reaches the distal portion of the fast pathway after traveling down the slower pathway, the fast pathway has repolarized and is able to conduct the impulse in a retrograde direction (exemplifying unidirectional block) as shown by the green route. The impulse can then travel back to the slow pathway, and a reentrant loop is initiated.

have different conduction times, providing both slow- and fast-conducting pathways. The fast pathway is characterized by a rapid conduction velocity, whereas the slow pathway demonstrates slower conduction but typically has a shorter refractory period than does the fast pathway. Thus, although the fast pathway conducts rapidly, it takes longer to recover between impulses compared with the slow pathway. Normally, a stimulus arriving at the AV node travels down both pathways, but the impulse traveling down the fast pathway reaches the bundle of His first. By the time the impulse traversing the slow pathway reaches the bundle of His, it encounters refractory tissue and is extinguished. Thus, under normal conditions, only the fast pathway impulse makes its way forward to the ventricles (see Fig. 12-15A).

In contrast, consider what happens when an APB spontaneously occurs (Fig. 12-15B). Because the refractory period of the fast pathway is relatively long, an APB would find that pathway unexcitable and unable to conduct the impulse. However, the impulse is able to conduct over the slow pathway (which *is* excitable because it has a shorter refractory period than does the fast pathway and has already repolarized when the APB arrives). By the time this impulse travels down the slowly conducting pathway and reaches the compact portion of the AV node, the distal end of the fast pathway may have had time to repolarize, and the impulse is able to propagate both distally (to the bundle of His and ventricles) *and* backward to the atria, up the fast pathway in a retrograde direction. On reaching the atria, the impulse can then circulate back down the slow pathway, completing the reentrant loop and initiating tachycardia as this sequence repeats. Thus, the fundamental conditions for reentry in AVNRT in this example are transient unidirectional block in the fast pathway (an APB encountering refractory tissue) and relatively slow conduction through the other pathway.

The ECG in AVNRT shows a regular tachycardia with normal-width QRS complexes. P waves may not be apparent, because retrograde atrial depolarization typically occurs simultaneously with ventricular depolarization (see Fig. 12-14). Thus, the retrograde P wave and QRS are inscribed at the same time, and the P is typically "hidden" in the QRS complex. When P waves *are* visible, they are superimposed on the terminal portion of the QRS complex and inverted (negative deflection) in limb leads II, III, and aVF, because of the caudocranial direction of atrial activation.

Rarely, the reentrant loop revolves in the reverse direction, with anterograde conduction down the fast pathway and retrograde conduction up the slow pathway. This is known as *atypical AVNRT*, and, unlike the more common rhythm, typically results in clearly visible retrograde P waves following the QRS complex on the ECG.

AVNRT often presents in teenagers or young adults. It is usually well tolerated but causes palpitations that many patients find frightening, and rapid tachycardias can cause light-headedness or shortness of breath. In elderly patients or those with underlying heart disease, more severe symptoms may result, such as syncope, angina, or pulmonary edema.

Acute treatment of AVNRT is aimed at terminating reentry by impairing conduction in the AV node. Transient increases in vagal tone produced by the Valsalva maneuver or carotid sinus massage (see Chapter 11) may block AV conduction, stopping the tachycardia. The most rapidly effective pharmacologic treatment is intravenous adenosine, which impairs AV nodal conduction and often aborts the reentrant rhythm (see Chapter 17). Other drug options include intravenous calcium channel antagonists (verapamil and diltiazem) or β-blockers.

Most patients with AVNRT have infrequent episodes that terminate with vagal maneuvers and do not require other specific interventions. Frequent symptomatic episodes, particularly when requiring visits to the emergency department for treatment, warrant preventive therapy: oral β-blockers, calcium channel blockers, or digoxin are often successful for this purpose. Catheter ablation of the slow AV nodal pathway is usually curative and recommended when pharmacologic therapy fails or is not desired by the patient, but has a small risk (<2%) of heart block owing to unintended damage to the fast AV nodal pathway, a complication that requires permanent pacemaker implantation. Chronic class IC or IA antiarrhythmic drugs are also effective but are often less desirable than catheter ablation, because of the associated potential drug toxicities.

Atrioventricular Reentrant Tachycardias

Atrioventricular reentrant tachycardias (AVRTs) are similar to AVNRTs except that in the former, one limb of the reentrant loop is constituted by an accessory pathway (*bypass tract*), rather than by separate fast and slow pathways within the AV node itself. As described in Chapter 11, an accessory pathway is an abnormal band of myocytes that spans the AV groove and connects atrial to ventricular tissue separately from the normal conduction system (see Fig. 11-10). Approximately 1 in 1500 people has such a pathway.

Accessory pathways allow an impulse to conduct from the atrium to ventricle (anterograde conduction), from the ventricle to atrium (retrograde conduction), or in both directions. Depending on the characteristics of the pathway, one of the two characteristic entities can result: (1) the ventricular preexcitation syndrome or (2) PSVT resulting from a concealed accessory pathway. Some pathways do not conduct impulses at rates sufficient to cause tachycardias and cause no symptoms at all.

Ventricular Preexcitation Syndrome

In patients with ventricular preexcitation (also termed Wolff-Parkinson-White [WPW] syndrome; see Chapter 11), atrial impulses can pass in an anterograde direction to the ventricles through both the AV node *and* the accessory pathway. Because conduction through the accessory pathway is usually faster than that via the AV node, the ventricles are stimulated *earlier* than by normal conduction over the AV node. During sinus rhythm, the activation of the ventricle from the accessory pathway causes a characteristic ECG appearance: (1) the PR interval is shortened (<0.12 seconds) because ventricular stimulation begins earlier than normal through the accessory pathway, (2) the QRS has a slurred rather than a sharp upstroke (referred to as a *delta wave*) because the initial ventricular activation by the accessory pathway is slower than activation over the Purkinje system, and (3) the QRS complex is widened because it represents fusion of two excitation wave fronts through the ventricles, one from the accessory pathway and one from the normal His-Purkinje system (Figs. 12-16 and 12-17).

Patients with WPW syndrome are predisposed to PSVTs because the accessory pathway provides a potential limb of a reentrant loop. The most common PSVT in these patients is **orthodromic** AVRT. During this tachycardia, an impulse travels *anterogradely* down the AV node to the ventricles and then *retrogradely* up the accessory tract back to the atria (see Fig. 12-17B). Because the ventricles in this situation are depolarized exclusively via the normal conduction system (through the AV node and the bundle of His), there is no delta wave during the tachycardia and the width of the QRS is usually normal. Retrograde P waves are often visible soon after each QRS complex because the atria are stimulated from below via retrograde conduction through the accessory pathway.

In fewer than 10% of patients with AVRT involving an accessory pathway, the reentrant arrhythmia travels in the opposite direction. Impulses travel *anterogradely* down the accessory pathway and *retrogradely* up the AV node (see Fig. 12-17C). Termed **antidromic** AVRT,

Figure 12-16. Wolff-Parkinson-White syndrome. The delta wave (*arrow*) indicates preexcitation of the ventricles. Note the shortened PR interval.

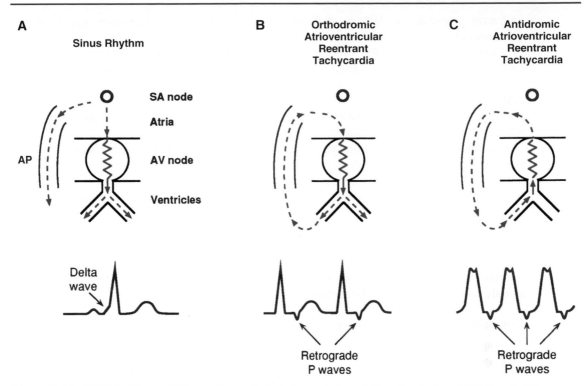

A Sinus Rhythm

B Orthodromic Atrioventricular Reentrant Tachycardia

C Antidromic Atrioventricular Reentrant Tachycardia

SA node

Atria

AP

AV node

Ventricles

Delta wave

Retrograde P waves

Retrograde P waves

Figure 12-17. Wolff-Parkinson-White syndrome. A. During normal sinus rhythm, the shortened PR interval, delta wave, and widened QRS complex indicate fusion of ventricular activation via the atrioventricular (AV) node and accessory pathway (AP). **B.** An APB can trigger an orthodromic atrioventricular reentrant tachycardia, in which impulses are conducted anterogradely down the AV node and retrogradely up the accessory pathway. Retrograde P waves are visible immediately after the QRS complex. There is no delta wave because anterograde ventricular stimulation passes exclusively through the AV node. **C.** Antidromic AV reentrant tachycardia in which impulses are conducted anterogradely down the accessory tract and retrogradely up the AV node. The QRS complex is greatly widened because the ventricles are stimulated by abnormal conduction through the accessory pathway rather than via the His-Purkinje system. SA, sinoatrial.

its ECG pattern is characterized by a *wide* QRS complex because the ventricles are activated entirely from anterograde conduction over the accessory pathway. From the ECG alone, such antidromic tachycardia is difficult to distinguish from ventricular tachycardia (described later in the chapter).

A third type of arrhythmia encountered in patients with WPW syndrome is anterograde conduction over the accessory pathway when AF or atrial flutter is present. Some accessory pathways have short refractory periods that allow faster rates of ventricular stimulation than does the AV node. Thus, during AF or atrial flutter, ventricular rates as fast as 300 bpm may result. Such rates are poorly tolerated and can lead to ventricular fibrillation and cardiac arrest, even in a young, otherwise healthy patient.

Pharmacologic management of arrhythmias in patients with the WPW syndrome requires greater caution than that of those with AVNRTs. Although digitalis, β-blockers, and certain calcium channel blockers are effective at blocking conduction through the AV node, they do not slow conduction over most accessory pathways. These drugs may actually *shorten* the refractory period of the accessory pathway, thus *speeding* conduction. Therefore, they could precipitate even faster ventricular rates (and hemodynamic collapse) when administered to patients with WPW syndrome who develop AF or flutter. In contrast, sodium channel blockers (specifically, class IA and IC antiarrhythmics) and some class III antiarrhythmic drugs (described in Chapter 17) slow conduction and prolong the refractory period of accessory pathways as well as the AV node; therefore, these are the preferred pharmacologic agents for this condition.

When a patient with WPW presents with a wide QRS tachycardia, acute therapy depends on the patient's tolerance of the arrhythmia. If accompanied by hemodynamic collapse, immediate cardioversion is required. Conversely, if the patient is hemodynamically stable, intravenous administration of procainamide (a class IA agent that slows conduction in the accessory pathway) or ibutilide (a class III agent that prolongs refractoriness in the accessory pathway) will often terminate the arrhythmia.

Patients who have WPW with symptomatic arrhythmias should generally undergo an invasive electrophysiologic study with radiofrequency ablation of the accessory pathway. Ablation abolishes conduction over the pathway, curing the condition. If this procedure is not an option, chronic oral therapy should include a drug that slows accessory pathway conduction (ie, a class IA, IC, or III agent).

The **Lown-Ganong-Levine syndrome** is also characterized by a short PR interval but a normal, narrow QRS complex (ie, no delta wave during sinus rhythm). It used to be considered a form of preexcitation, but most patients just have enhanced conduction through the normal AV node, thus shortening the PR interval. When PSVT occurs in these patients, it is usually simply due to AV nodal reentry.

Concealed Accessory Pathways

Accessory pathways do not always result in ECG findings of ventricular preexcitation (ie, short PR, delta wave). Many are capable of only *retrograde* conduction. In this case, during sinus rhythm, the ventricles are depolarized normally through the AV node alone, and the ECG appears normal (ie, the accessory pathway is *concealed*). However, because the accessory pathway is capable of retrograde conduction, it can form a limb of a reentrant circuit under appropriate circumstances and result in orthodromic AVRT.

Management of patients with tachycardia involving a concealed accessory pathway is the same as for patients with AVNRT. Because the reentrant circuit travels anterogradely down the AV node, vagal maneuvers and drugs that interrupt conduction over the AV node (eg, adenosine, verapamil, diltiazem, and β-blockers) can terminate the tachycardia. Another option for recurrent episodes is catheter ablation of the accessory pathway, which is curative in most patients.

Focal Atrial Tachycardia

Focal atrial tachycardia (AT) results from either automaticity of an atrial ectopic site or reentry. The ECG has the appearance of sinus tachycardia, with a P wave before each QRS complex, but the P-wave morphology is different from that of sinus rhythm, indicating depolarization of the atrium from an abnormal location. The arrhythmia can be paroxysmal and of limited duration, or it can persist. Short, asymptomatic bursts of AT are commonly observed on 24-hour ECG recordings, even in otherwise healthy people.

AT can be caused by digitalis toxicity and is also aggravated by elevated sympathetic tone (eg, during exertion or periods of illness). Initial treatment includes correction of any contributing factors. Unlike AVNRT or AVRT, vagal maneuvers (such as carotid sinus massage) may have no effect on atrial discharges from an ectopic pacemaker focus. However, β-blockers, calcium channel blockers, and class IC, IA, and III antiarrhythmic drugs can be effective. Catheter ablation is also a useful option for symptomatic patients.

Multifocal Atrial Tachycardia

In multifocal atrial tachycardia (MAT), the ECG shows an irregular rhythm with multiple (at least three different) P-wave morphologies, and the average atrial rate is >100 bpm (Fig. 12-18). An isoelectric (ie, "flat") baseline between P waves distinguishes MAT from the chaotic baseline

Figure 12-18. Multifocal atrial tachycardia. The rhythm is irregular, and each QRS is preceded by a P wave of varying morphology.

of AF. This rhythm is likely caused by either abnormal automaticity in several foci within the atria or triggered activity and occurs most often in the setting of severe pulmonary disease and hypoxemia. Because patients with this rhythm are often critically ill from the underlying disease, the mortality rate is high and treatment is aimed at the causative disorder. The calcium channel blocker verapamil is often effective at slowing the ventricular rate as a temporizing measure.

VENTRICULAR ARRHYTHMIAS

Ventricular arrhythmias include (1) ventricular premature beats (VPBs), (2) ventricular tachycardia (VT), and (3) ventricular fibrillation (VF). Ventricular arrhythmias are usually more dangerous than supraventricular rhythm disorders and are responsible for many of the ~ 300,000 sudden cardiac deaths that occur every year in the United States.

Ventricular Premature Beats

A VPB arises when an ectopic ventricular focus fires an action potential. On the ECG, a VPB appears as a *widened* QRS complex, because the impulse travels from its ectopic site through the ventricles via slow cell-to-cell connections rather than through the normal rapidly conducting His-Purkinje system (Fig. 12-19). Furthermore, the ectopic beat is not related to a preceding P wave.

VPBs can also occur in repeating patterns. When every alternate beat is a VPB, the rhythm is termed **bigeminy**. When two normal beats precede every VPB, **trigeminy** is present. Consecutive VPBs are referred to as **couplets** (two in a row) or **triplets** (three in a row).

Similar to APBs, VPBs are common even among healthy people and are often asymptomatic and benign. Specific precipitants of VPBs include medications (eg, β-adrenergic receptor agonists), caffeine, electrolyte abnormalities (eg, hypokalemia, hypomagnesemia), and hypoxia. VPBs are not dangerous by themselves, and in patients without heart disease, they confer no added risk of a life-threatening arrhythmia. They can, however, be an indication of an underlying cardiac disorder and take on added significance in that case. For example, in patients with structural heart disease, VPBs generally increase in frequency in relation to the severity of depressed ventricular contractility. They have been associated with an increased risk of sudden death in patients with heart failure or prior myocardial infarction.

Figure 12-19. Ventricular premature beats (*arrows*).

Figure 12-20. Monomorphic ventricular tachycardia.

In otherwise healthy persons, treatment of VPBs mainly involves reassurance and, if needed, symptomatic control using β-blockers. In patients with advanced structural heart disease with features that place them at risk of life-threatening ventricular arrhythmias, placement of an implantable cardioverter-defibrillator (ICD) is typically recommended.

Ventricular Tachycardia

VT is a series of three or more consecutive VPBs (Fig. 12-20). VT is divided arbitrarily into two categories. If it persists for more than 30 seconds, produces severe symptoms, such as syncope, or requires termination by cardioversion or administration of an antiarrhythmic drug, it is designated as **sustained VT**; shorter, self-terminating episodes are termed **nonsustained VT**. Both forms of VT are found most commonly in patients with structural heart disease, including myocardial ischemia and infarction, heart failure, ventricular hypertrophy, primary electrical diseases (eg, long-QT syndromes [LQTS]; see Box 12-1), valvular heart diseases, and congenital cardiac abnormalities.

The QRS complexes of VT are typically wide (>0.12 seconds) and occur at a rate of 100-200 bpm or sometimes faster. VT is further categorized according to its QRS morphology. When every QRS complex appears the same and the rate is regular, it is referred to as **monomorphic VT** (see Fig. 12-20). Sustained monomorphic VT usually indicates a structural abnormality that supports a reentry circuit, most commonly a region of myocardial scar from an old infarction or cardiomyopathy. Occasionally, sustained monomorphic VT occurs as a result of an ectopic ventricular focus in an otherwise healthy person (referred to as *idiopathic VT*).

Box 12-1	Genetic Mutations and Ventricular Arrhythmias

Genetic causes of arrhythmias occur either in association with forms of structural heart disease or as isolated conditions. Examples of inherited structural disease that can be complicated by life-threatening ventricular arrhythmias include **hypertrophic cardiomyopathy**, **familial dilated cardiomyopathies**, and **arrhythmogenic right ventricular cardiomyopathy** (**ARVC**), which are all described in Chapter 10. ARVC may be suspected on a standard ECG by the presence of inverted T waves in leads V_1 through V_3 and occasionally an *epsilon wave*, a terminal notch of the QRS complex in lead V_1 (see arrow in the adjacent figure), which reflects abnormal RV activation.

Several other inherited arrhythmic disorders occur in the absence of structural cardiac disease. They can cause life-threatening polymorphic VT or VF in young, otherwise healthy people without prior warning. The most common of these are (1) the Brugada syndrome, (2) the congenital long QT syndromes, and (3) familial catecholaminergic polymorphic VT.

| Box 12-1 | Genetic Mutations and Ventricular Arrhythmias (continued) |

The **Brugada syndrome** is inherited in an autosomal dominant fashion and has been linked in some families to mutations in a sodium channel subunit gene (*SCN5A*). A clue to the presence of this syndrome is a specific ECG finding of prominent ST elevation in leads V_1 through V_3 (see adjacent figure). This pattern may be present chronically or intermittently; in the latter case, the syndrome may be unmasked by administering sodium channel blocking antiarrhythmic drugs. Brugada syndrome is a potentially lethal condition, and ICD implantation is often required to prevent an arrhythmic death.

The **congenital long QT syndromes** (LQTS) are associated with prolonged ventricular repolarization, which can lead to life-threatening polymorphic VT (ie, torsades de pointes). Mutations in a number of different genes result in LQTS (the three most common are listed in the table below) by prolonging the action potential duration. Most mutations alter ion channel function to either *enhance* the depolarizing Na^+ current or *impair* the repolarizing K^+ current. Autosomal dominant and recessive patterns of inheritance occur.

Gene penetrance and symptomatology of patients with LQTS is highly variable, even for individuals with the same mutation. The degree of QT prolongation and, in some cases, the patient's gender are predictors of arrhythmic risk when a mutation is present. An affected patient may be asymptomatic and come to medical attention only as a result of the abnormal ECG or because of a family member who died suddenly. Others present with syncope or sudden death caused by torsades de pointes. The most common forms (LQT1 and LQT2) are associated with ventricular arrhythmias during physical exercise (particularly swimming) or emotional stress. Conversely, those with LQT3 are much more likely to experience cardiac events at rest or during sleep.

Other acquired conditions that further prolong the QT interval can trigger life-threatening arrhythmias in patients with LQTS, including hypokalemia, hypomagnesemia, hypocalcemia, and several medications (including many antiarrhythmic drugs). Conversely, β-blockers reduce the risk of arrhythmias in many forms of congenital LQTS, even though they do not shorten the QT interval. For patients at high risk of life-threatening arrhythmias, ICD implantation is warranted.

Familial catecholaminergic polymorphic VT, inherited in both autosomal dominant and recessive patterns, is marked by VT and/or VF during exercise or emotional arousal. The mechanism is thought to be triggered activity resulting from delayed afterdepolarizations (described in Chapter 11). Mutations in affected families have been demonstrated in at least two genes involved in intracellular calcium handling, including a missense mutation in the locus that codes for the cardiac ryanodine receptor (see Chapter 1). Treatment with a β-blocker, calcium channel blocker, and/or drug that inhibits ryanodine receptor–mediated calcium release (eg, the class IC antiarrhythmic flecainide has this additional attribute) may be effective; an ICD is also often recommended.

Genetic Basis of the Three Most Common Congenital Long QT Syndromes

Type	Gene (Location)	Protein	Mechanism of Prolonged Repolarization	Inheritance
LQT1	*KCNQ1* (11p15)	KvLQT1 (α subunit of I_{Ks} K^+ channel)	↓ Outward K^+ current	AD and AR
LQT2	*KCNH2* (7q35)	HERG (α subunit of I_{Kr} K^+ channel)	↓ Outward K^+ current	AD
LQT3	*SCN5A* (3p21)	Nav 1.5 (Na^+ channel)	↑ Inward Na^+ current	AD

AD, autosomal dominant; AR, autosomal recessive.

When the QRS complexes continually change in shape and the rate varies from beat to beat, the VT is referred to as **polymorphic**. Multiple ectopic foci or a continually changing reentry circuit is the cause. Torsades de pointes (discussed later in the chapter) and acute myocardial ischemia or infarction are the most common causes of polymorphic VT. Rare, inherited predispositions to polymorphic VT and sudden death arise from abnormalities of cardiac ion channels or calcium handling (eg, the long QT syndromes, the Brugada syndrome, familial catecholaminergic polymorphic VT), as described in Box 12-1. Sustained polymorphic VT usually degenerates to VF.

The symptoms of VT vary depending on the rate of the tachycardia, its duration, and the underlying condition of the heart. Sustained VT can cause low cardiac output resulting in loss of consciousness (syncope), pulmonary edema, or progress to cardiac arrest. These severe consequences of VT are most likely in patients who have underlying depressed contractile function. Conversely, if sustained VT is at a relatively slow rate (eg, <130 bpm), it may be well tolerated and cause only palpitations.

Distinguishing Monomorphic VT From Supraventricular Tachycardia

VT can usually be distinguished from SVT by the width of the QRS complex: it is routinely wide in the former and narrow (ie, normal) in the latter. However, under certain circumstances, arrhythmias that originate from sites above the ventricles *can* result in wide QRS complexes and may appear similar to monomorphic VT. This situation is termed *SVT with aberrant ventricular conduction*, or simply *SVT with aberrancy*, and may arise in three scenarios: (1) a patient has an underlying conduction abnormality (eg, a bundle-branch block), such that the QRS is abnormally wide even when in normal sinus rhythm; (2) repetitive rapid ventricular stimulation during SVT finds one of the bundle branches refractory (because of insufficient time to recover from the previous depolarization), such that the impulse propagates abnormally through the ventricles, causing the QRS to be distorted and wide; or (3) a patient develops antidromic tachycardia through an accessory pathway (described earlier).

Certain clinical and electrocardiographic features can help to distinguish wide QRS complexes of monomorphic VT from those of supraventricular rhythms with aberrant conduction. In patients with a history of prior myocardial infarction, congestive heart failure, or left ventricular dysfunction, a wide complex tachycardia is more likely to be VT rather than SVT with aberrancy. At the bedside, SVT is more probable if vagal maneuvers (such as the Valsalva maneuver or carotid sinus massage) affect the rhythm (see Fig. 12-9).

Electrocardiographically, a *supraventricular* tachyarrhythmia is more likely if the morphology of the QRS at the rapid rate is similar to that on the patient's ECG tracing obtained while in sinus rhythm (ie, the complex is widened because of an underlying bundle-branch block). Conversely, VT is more likely if (1) there is no relationship between the QRS complexes and any observed P waves (AV dissociation) or (2) the QRS complexes in each of the chest leads (V_1 through V_6) have a similar appearance, with a dominant positive or negative deflection (ie, there is "concordance" of the precordial QRS complexes). These features are summarized in Table 12-3. Other morphologic ECG features have been used to distinguish VT from SVT

TABLE 12-3 **Differentiation of Wide Complex Tachycardias**

Supports SVT With Aberrant Conduction	Supports Ventricular Tachycardia
QRS morphology same as when in sinus rhythm	History of prior MI or heart failure No relationship between P waves and QRS complexes
Rhythm responds to vagal maneuvers (see Fig. 12-9)	Concordance of QRS complexes in the chest leads (V_1-V_6)

MI, myocardial infarction; SVT, supraventricular tachycardia.

with aberrancy, but the distinction is often difficult. Most patients with wide QRS tachycardia should be managed as though they have VT until proven otherwise.

Management of Patients With VT

Sustained episodes of VT are dangerous because they can produce syncope or deteriorate into VF, which is fatal if not quickly corrected. Acute treatment usually consists of electrical cardioversion. Intravenous administration of certain antiarrhythmic drugs, such as amiodarone, procainamide, or lidocaine, can be considered if the patient is hemodynamically stable.

After sinus rhythm is restored, a patient who has had sustained VT requires careful evaluation to define whether underlying structural heart disease is present and to correct any aggravating factors, such as myocardial ischemia, electrolyte disturbances, or drug toxicities. Patients who have suffered VT in the setting of structural heart disease have a high risk of recurrence and sudden cardiac death; implantation of an ICD is usually warranted to automatically and promptly terminate future episodes.

Patients who experience VT in the absence of underlying structural heart disease are usually found to have idiopathic VT. This type of arrhythmia tends to originate from foci in the right ventricular outflow tract or in the septal portion of the left ventricle. It is rarely life threatening. β-Blockers, calcium channel blockers, or catheter ablation are commonly effective therapies to control symptomatic episodes of idiopathic VT.

Torsades de Pointes

Torsades de pointes ("twisting of the points") is a form of polymorphic VT that presents as varying amplitudes of the QRS, as if the complexes were "twisting" about the baseline (Fig. 12-21). It can result from early afterdepolarizations (triggered activity), particularly in patients who have a *prolonged QT interval*. QT prolongation (which indicates a lengthened action potential duration) can result from electrolyte disturbances (hypokalemia or hypomagnesemia), persistent bradycardia, and drugs that block cardiac potassium currents, including many antiarrhythmic agents (particularly the class III drugs sotalol, ibutilide, and dofetilide and some class I drugs, including quinidine, procainamide, and disopyramide). Many medications administered for noncardiac illnesses can also prolong the QT interval and predispose to torsades de pointes, including erythromycin, phenothiazines, haloperidol, and methadone. A rare group of hereditary ion channel abnormalities produces *congenital* QT prolongation, which can also lead to torsades de pointes (see Box 12-1).

Torsades de pointes is usually symptomatic, causing light-headedness or syncope, but is frequently self-limited. Its main danger results from degeneration into VF. When it is drug or electrolyte induced, correcting the underlying trigger abolishes recurrences, but measures to suppress episodes are required to allow time to address the cause. Administration of intravenous magnesium often suppresses repeated episodes. Additional preventive strategies are aimed at shortening the QT interval by increasing the underlying heart rate with intravenous

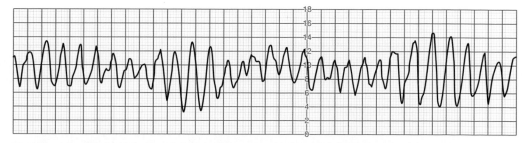

Figure 12-21. Torsade de pointes. The widened polymorphic QRS complexes demonstrate a waxing and waning pattern.

Figure 12-22. Ventricular fibrillation.

β-adrenergic–*stimulating* agents (eg, isoproterenol) or an artificial pacemaker. When torsades de pointes results from congenital prolongation of the QT interval, β-*blocking* drugs are the treatment of choice, because sympathetic stimulation may aggravate the arrhythmia in such patients.

Ventricular Fibrillation

VF is an immediately life-threatening arrhythmia (Fig. 12-22). It results in disordered, rapid stimulation of the ventricles with no coordinated contractions. The result is essentially cessation of cardiac output and death if not quickly reversed. This rhythm most often occurs in patients with severe underlying heart disease and is the major cause of mortality in acute myocardial infarction.

VF is often initiated by an episode of VT, which degenerates, it is believed, by the breakup of excitation waves into multiple smaller wavelets of reentry that wander through the myocardium. On the ECG, VF is characterized by a chaotic irregular appearance without discrete QRS waveforms.

Untreated, VF rapidly leads to death. The only effective therapy is prompt electrical defibrillation. As soon as the heart has been converted to a safe rhythm, the underlying precipitant of the arrhythmia (eg, myocardial ischemia, electrolyte imbalances, hypoxemia, or acidosis) should be sought and corrected to prevent further episodes. Intravenous antiarrhythmic drug therapy may be administered to prevent immediate recurrences. If no reversible inciting precipitant is found, survivors of VF usually receive an ICD.

Summary

- Disorders of impulse formation and conduction result in **bradyarrhythmias** (heart rate <60 bpm) and **tachyarrhythmias** (heart rate >100 bpm for three beats or more).

- The five basic considerations when confronted with a patient with an abnormal heart rhythm are (1) **identification**, (2) **pathogenesis**, (3) **precipitating factors**, (4) **clinical presentation**, and (5) **treatment**.

- When evaluating a patient with a slow heart rhythm, two key questions should be addressed: (1) "are P waves present?" and (2) "what is the relationship between the P waves and the QRS complexes?"

- Differentiation of tachyarrhythmias requires assessment of (1) the **width of the QRS** complex (normal or wide), (2) the **morphology and rate of the P waves**, (3) the **relationship between the P waves and the QRS complexes**, and (4) the **response to vagal maneuvers**.

- The ECG texts listed at the end of Chapter 4 provide multiple examples of arrhythmias and are suited for practicing the principles described in this chapter.

Review Questions

1. A 56-year-old woman presents to the emergency department because of light-headedness. An ECG rhythm strip is shown in the figure. What abnormality is present?

    a. First-degree AV block
    b. Type I second-degree AV block
    c. Type II second-degree AV block
    d. Third-degree (complete) heart block

2. A 68-year-old man with hypertension and diabetes mellitus presents to his primary physician for routine evaluation. On examination, his heart rate is noted to be irregular, though he is unaware of any cardiac irregularity. He does not describe chest discomfort or shortness of breath. He has no history of heart failure, coronary artery disease, stroke, or peripheral vascular disease. He drinks a glass of wine daily and his only source of caffeine intake is a cup of coffee 2 days per week. His medications include lisinopril (an angiotensin converting-enzyme inhibitor), metoprolol succinate (a beta-blocker), and metformin (a glucose-lowering agent). Earlier this year, blood tests to assess thyroid function were normal, and an echocardiogram showed mild left ventricular hypertrophy, normal left ventricular function, mild left atrial enlargement, and no other structural heart diseases. A rhythm strip from his ECG is shown in the figure. Which of the following interventions would be most appropriate for this patient?

    a. Immediate electrical cardioversion
    b. Transesophageal echocardiography followed by electrical cardioversion within the next week
    c. Add an antiarrhythmic drug to his medications (eg, amiodarone—described in Chapter 17) in an attempt to convert rhythm to sinus rhythm
    d. Initiate an oral anticoagulant and continue metoprolol

3. A 65-year-old with chronic obstructive airway disease presents with an exacerbation of pulmonary symptoms. He is admitted to the medical intensive care unit and is noted to be tachycardic. What is his heart rhythm in the figure?

   a. Sinus tachycardia
   b. Multifocal atrial tachycardia
   c. Atrial flutter
   d. Atrial fibrillation

Answers to Review Questions

1. **Choice c is correct.** This rhythm strip demonstrates type II second-degree AV block (see Fig. 12-6): there is intermittent absence of AV conduction (the fourth P wave is not followed by a QRS complex), without the preceding progressive prolongation of the PR interval that typifies type I second-degree AV block (see Fig. 12-5). In first-degree AV block, there would be constant prolongation of the PR interval without dropped QRS complexes (see Fig. 12-4). In third-degree AV block, there would be no relationship between the P waves and QRS complexes (see Fig. 12-8).

2. **Choice d is correct.** The electrocardiogram shows AF: there is chaotic atrial activity without organized P waves and an irregular ventricular rate. The ventricular rate is not excessive (~ 75 bpm) as a result of current beta-blocker therapy. The patient is asymptomatic and has no signs of hemodynamic compromise; thus, there is no urgency to proceed with electrical cardioversion. His CHA_2DS_2-VASc score is 3 (see Table 12-2: age 65-74, hypertension, diabetes), such that anticoagulation therapy is warranted. Choice c is not correct, because the addition of an antiarrhythmic drug could convert AF to sinus rhythm, and in the absence of anticoagulation therapy, such organization of atrial activity could dislodge a preformed atrial thrombus and result in thromboembolism. For that reason, elective electrical or pharmacological cardioversion should follow at least 3-4 weeks of anticoagulation therapy.

3. **Choice b is correct.** MAT is present, characterized by an irregular tachycardia, with each QRS preceded by a single P wave of varying morphologies (see also Fig. 12-18). MAT often reflects decompensated pulmonary disease, and its treatment is largely directed at improving the underlying pulmonary disorder.

Acknowledgments

Contributors to previous editions of this chapter were Morgan J. Prust, MD; Ranliang Hu, MD; Hillary K. Rolls, MD; Wendy Armstrong, MD; Nicholas Boulis, MD; Jennifer E. Ho, MD; Marc S. Sabatine, MD; Elliott M. Antman, MD; Leonard I. Ganz, MD; and William G. Stevenson, MD.

Additional Reading

Al-Khatib SM, Stevenson WG, Ackerman MJ, et al. 2017 AHA/ACC/HRS guideline for management of patients with ventricular arrhythmias and the prevention of sudden cardiac death: a report of the American College of Cardiology Foundation/American Heart Association Task Force on Clinical Practice Guidelines and the Heart Rhythm Society. *Circulation*. 2018;138:e272-e391.

January CT, Wann LS, Calkins H, et al. 2019 AHA/ACC/HRS focused update of the 2014 AHA/ACC/HRS guideline for the management of patients with atrial fibrillation: a report of the American College of Cardiology/American Heart Association Task Force on Practice Guidelines and the Heart Rhythm Society. *Circulation*. 2019;140:e125-e151.

Kusumoto FM, Schoenfeld MH, Barrett C, et al. 2018 ACC/AHA/HRS guideline on the evaluation and management of patients with bradycardia and cardiac conduction delay: a report of the American College of Cardiology/American Heart Association Task Force on Clinical Practice Guidelines and the Heart Rhythm Society. *Circulation*. 2019;140:e382-e482.

Link MS. Clinical practice. Evaluation and initial treatment of supraventricular tachycardia. *N Engl J Med*. 2012;367:1438-1448.

Nakano Y, Shimizu W. Genetics of long-QT syndrome. *J Hum Genet*. 2016;61:51-55.

13

Hypertension

Jenifer M. Brown | Gordon H. Williams |
Leonard S. Lilly

Over 70 million Americans, and 1 billion people throughout the world, have hypertension—a blood pressure (BP) high enough to be a danger to their well-being. This represents a great public health concern because hypertension is a major risk factor for coronary artery disease, stroke, heart failure, renal disease, and peripheral vascular disease. Moreover, because elevated BP is usually asymptomatic until an acute cardiovascular event strikes, screening for hypertension is a critical aspect of preventive medicine.

Hypertension is also a scientific problem of unexpected complexity. In ~90% of affected patients, the etiology of BP elevation is unknown, a condition termed primary or **essential hypertension (EH)**. Evidence suggests that the causes of EH are multiple and diverse, but considerable insight into those causes can be achieved by studying the normal physiology of BP control, as described in this chapter.

High BP attributed to a *definable* cause is termed **secondary hypertension**. Although far less common than EH, conditions that cause secondary hypertension are important because many are amenable to permanent cure and because they may carry excess risk beyond elevated BP. Notably, many of the conditions now understood to cause secondary hypertension were once unknown, and affected patients were therefore considered to have EH. As more is learned about the pathophysiology of high BP, fewer cases of hypertension will likely be considered to be of the essential type.

Following the descriptions of EH and secondary hypertension, this chapter considers the clinical consequences of elevated BP and approaches to treatment.

WHAT IS HYPERTENSION?

BP values vary widely in the population and tend to rise with age (Fig. 13-1). The risk of a vascular complication increases with higher values, so the cutoff points to delineate stages of hypertension are somewhat arbitrary. A recent guideline from the American Heart Association and American College of Cardiology defines categories of hypertension as listed in Table 13-1. By this classification, a normal BP is <120 mm Hg systolic and <80 mm Hg diastolic. A systolic BP ≥ 120 mm Hg is considered "elevated," and a systolic BP ≥130 mm Hg or diastolic BP ≥80 mm Hg establishes the diagnosis of **stage 1 hypertension**. More severe **stage 2 hypertension** is present if the systolic BP is ≥140 mm Hg or diastolic BP is ≥90 mm Hg. A person should not be labeled as hypertensive until obtaining ≥2 high readings on ≥ 2 separate occasions. Modern analyses confirm that both systolic and diastolic BP elevations contribute significantly to cardiovascular risk.

HOW IS BLOOD PRESSURE REGULATED?

HEMODYNAMIC FACTORS

BP is the product of cardiac output (CO) and total peripheral resistance (TPR):

$$BP = CO \times TPR$$

And CO is the product of cardiac stroke volume (SV) and heart rate (HR):

$$CO = SV \times HR$$

Figure 13-1. Relationship between blood pressure and age (*n* = 1029). Systolic (*upper curves*) and diastolic (*lower curves*) values are shown. Notice that by age 60, the average systolic pressure of women exceeds that of men. (Modified from Kotchen JM, McKean HE, Kotchen TA. Blood pressure trends with aging. *Hypertension*. 1982;4(suppl 3):111-129.)

As described in Chapter 9, SV is determined by (1) cardiac contractility; (2) the venous return to the heart (preload); and (3) the resistance the left ventricle must overcome to eject blood into the aorta (afterload).

It follows that at least four systems are directly responsible for BP regulation: the *heart*, which supplies the pumping pressure; the *blood vessel tone*, which largely determines systemic resistance; the *kidney*, which regulates intravascular volume; and *hormones*, which modulate the functions of the other three systems. Figure 13-2 shows how factors related to these systems contribute to CO and TPR.

The renal component of BP regulation deserves special mention, in light of the temptation to view hypertension simply as a cardiovascular problem. No matter how high the CO or TPR, renal excretion has the capacity to completely return BP to normal by reducing intravascular volume. Therefore, the maintenance of chronic hypertension requires renal participation.

TABLE 13-1 Classification of Blood Pressure in Adults
Normal Blood Pressure
<120 mm Hg systolic *and* ≤80 mm Hg diastolic
Elevated Blood Pressure
120-129 mm Hg systolic *and* ≤80 mm Hg diastolic
Hypertension
Stage 1: 130-139 mm Hg systolic *or* 80-89 mm Hg diastolic
Stage 2: ≥140 mm Hg systolic *or* ≥ 90 mm Hg diastolic

Modified from Whelton PK, Carey RM, Aronow WS, et al. 2017 ACC/AHA/AAPA/ABC/ACPM/AGS/APhA/ASH/ASPC/NMA/PCNA guideline for the prevention, detection, evaluation, and management of high blood pressure in adults: a report of the American College of Cardiology/American Heart Association Task Force on Clinical Practice Guidelines. *J Am Coll Cardiol*. 2018;71:e127-e248.

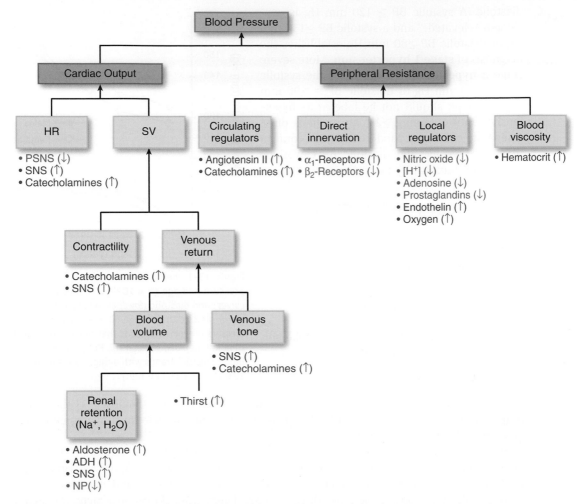

Figure 13-2. Regulation of systemic blood pressure. The *small arrows* indicate whether there is a stimulatory (↑) or inhibitory (↓) effect on the boxed parameters. ADH, antidiuretic hormone; HR, heart rate; NP, natriuretic peptides; PSNS, parasympathetic nervous system; SNS, sympathetic nervous system; SV, stroke volume.

Transplantation studies have confirmed this point: the implantation of a kidney from a normotensive person into a hypertensive one typically improves the BP. Similarly, surgical placement of a kidney from a genetically hypertensive rat into a previously normotensive one usually leads to hypertension.

In the presence of normally functioning kidneys, an increase in BP leads to augmented urine volume and sodium excretion, which then returns the BP to normal. This process, known as *pressure natriuresis*, is blunted in the kidneys of hypertensive patients; thus, higher pressures are required to excrete a given sodium and water load. There are at least two possible reasons for this blunted response. First, microvascular and tubulointerstitial injury within the kidneys of hypertensive patients impairs sodium excretion. Second, the defect may lie with hormonal factors critical to appropriate renal reactions to the sodium and intravascular volume environment (eg, the renin-angiotensin system, as described later in the chapter). In contrast to the first possibility, abnormalities of hormonal regulation are amenable to correction with appropriate therapy.

BLOOD PRESSURE REFLEXES

The cardiovascular system is endowed with feedback mechanisms that continuously monitor arterial pressure: when the pressure becomes excessively high or low, these mechanisms respond rapidly to maintain homeostasis. One such mechanism is the **baroreceptor reflex**, which is mediated by receptors in the walls of the aortic arch and the carotid sinuses. The baroreceptors monitor changes in pressure by sensing stretch and deformation of the arteries. If the arterial pressure rises, the baroreceptors are stimulated, increasing their transmission of impulses to the central nervous system (ie, the medulla). Negative feedback signals are then sent back to the circulation via the autonomic nervous system, causing the BP to fall back to its baseline level.

The higher the BP rises, the more the baroreceptors are stretched and the greater the impulse transmission rate to the medulla. Signals from the carotid sinus receptors are carried by the glossopharyngeal nerve (cranial nerve IX), whereas those from the aortic arch receptors are carried by the vagus nerve (cranial nerve X). These nerve fibers converge at the tractus solitarius in the medulla, where the baroreceptor impulses *inhibit* sympathetic nervous system outflow and *excite* parasympathetic effects. The net result is (1) a decline in peripheral vascular resistance (ie, vasodilation) and (2) a reduction in CO (because of a lower HR and reduced contractility). Each of these effects tends to lower arterial pressure back toward its baseline. Conversely, when a *fall* in systemic pressure is sensed by the baroreceptors, fewer impulses are transmitted to the medulla, leading to a reflexive *increase* in BP.

The main effect of the baroreceptor mechanism is to modulate moment-by-moment variations in systemic BP. However, the baroreceptor reflex is not involved in the long-term regulation of BP and does not prevent the development of chronic hypertension. The reason for this is that the baroreceptors constantly reset themselves. After a day or two of exposure to higher-than-baseline pressures, the baroreceptor-firing rate slows back to its control value, and a new set point is established.

ESSENTIAL HYPERTENSION

Approximately 90% of hypertensive patients have BPs that are elevated for no readily definable reason and are considered to have EH. The diagnosis of EH is one of exclusion; it is the option left to the clinician after considering the causes of secondary hypertension described later in this chapter.

EH is a description rather than a diagnosis, indicating only that a patient manifests a specific physical finding (high BP) for which no cause has been found. In all likelihood, different underlying defects are responsible for the elevated pressure in different subpopulations of patients. Because the exact nature of these defects is unknown, to understand EH is to understand the possibilities: what could go wrong with normal physiology to produce chronically elevated BP?

This description of EH therefore reflects what is currently known about its genetics and epidemiology, experimental findings, and natural history. The picture that emerges is that EH likely results from multiple defects of BP regulation that interact with environmental stressors. The regulatory defects may be acquired or genetically determined and may be independent of one another. As a result, EH patients exhibit varied combinations of abnormalities and, therefore, have various physiologic bases for their elevated BPs.

GENETICS AND EPIDEMIOLOGY

There is strong support for the role of heredity in EH. First-degree relatives of hypertensive patients have a higher rate of elevated BP than the general population. Further, concordance between identical twins is high and significantly greater than that between dizygotic twins. However, no singular, consistent genetic marker for hypertension has been identified. Instead, EH is likely a complex polygenic disorder, involving several loci.

While some autosomal dominant contributors to elevated BP have been discovered, such abnormalities are rare and are thought to represent only a small fraction of hypertensive patients. With respect to loci that affect hypertension in a polygenic way, genes regulating the renin-angiotensin-aldosterone axis have been most thoroughly studied because of the central role of this system in determining intravascular volume and vascular tone. Within this group, certain polymorphisms in the genes for *angiotensinogen*, *angiotensin-converting enzyme* (ACE), *the angiotensin type-1 receptor* and *aldosterone synthase* confer a small increase in the risk of developing hypertension. Additionally, polymorphisms in the gene for *alpha-adducin*, a cytoskeletal protein, may be involved in a subgroup of EH patients, possibly by increasing renal tubular sodium absorption. Finally, as described later in the chapter, significant associations exist among hypertension and obesity, insulin resistance, and diabetes. These conditions are all characterized by similar complex inheritance patterns, some of which may overlap with the genetic underpinnings of hypertension.

As genetics cannot explain the complete basis of hypertension, it stands to reason that the environment also plays a role. Indeed, hypertension has been epidemiologically linked to certain dietary and exercise patterns, poor access to health care, low socioeconomic status, and comorbid medical conditions such as obesity, diabetes, and kidney disease. Thus, the heritable traits described above most likely predispose individuals to develop hypertension after exposure to environmental triggers.

EXPERIMENTAL FINDINGS

Systemic Abnormalities

Multiple defects in BP regulation have been found in EH patients and their relatives. By themselves, or in conjunction with one another, these abnormalities may contribute to chronic BP elevation.

The *heart* can contribute to a high CO-based hypertension owing to sympathetic overactivity. For example, when tested under psychologically stressful conditions, hypertensive patients (and their first-degree relatives) often develop excessive HR acceleration compared with control subjects, suggesting an excessive sympathetic response.

The *blood vessels* may contribute to peripheral vascular resistance-based hypertension by constricting in response to (1) increased sympathetic activity; (2) abnormal regulation of vascular tone by local substances, including nitric oxide, endothelin, and natriuretic factors; or (3) ion channel defects in the contractile vascular smooth muscle.

The *kidney* can induce volume-based hypertension by retaining excessive sodium and water as a result of (1) failure to regulate renal blood flow appropriately; (2) ion channel defects (eg, reduced basolateral Na^+K^+-ATPase), which directly cause sodium retention; or (3) inappropriate hormonal regulation. For example, the renin-angiotensin-aldosterone axis is an important hormonal regulator of peripheral vascular resistance. Renin levels in EH patients (compared with those in normotensive persons) are subnormal in 25%, normal in ~60%, and high in 10%-15%. Because renin secretion should be *suppressed* by high BP, even "normal" levels are inappropriate in the context of hypertension. Thus, abnormalities of this system's regulation may play a role in some individuals with EH.

Figure 13-3 highlights these and other potential mechanisms of EH. Note that although the heart, blood vessels, and kidneys are the organs ultimately responsible for producing the pressure, primary defects may be located elsewhere as well (eg, the central nervous system,

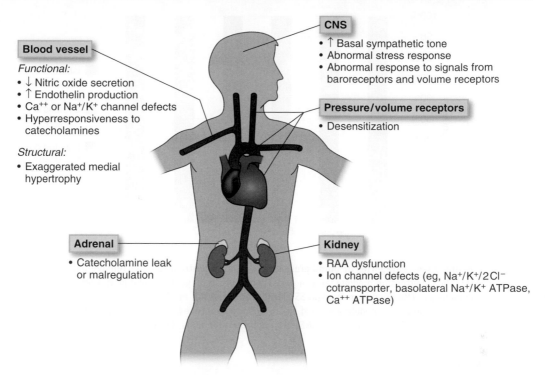

Figure 13-3. Potential primary abnormalities in essential hypertension (EH). These defects are supported by experimental evidence, but their specific contributions to EH remain unknown. CNS, central nervous system; RAA, renin-angiotensin-aldosterone system.

arterial baroreceptors, and adrenal hormone secretion). Yet, although abnormal regulation at these sites can contribute to elevated BP, it is important to remember that without renal complicity, malfunction of other systems would not produce sustained hypertension, since the normal kidney is capable of eliminating sufficient volume to return the BP to normal.

Insulin Resistance, Obesity, and the Metabolic Syndrome

Recent research has suggested that the hormone insulin may play a role in the development of EH. In many people with hypertension, especially those who are obese or have type 2 diabetes, there is impaired insulin-dependent transport of glucose into many tissues (termed *insulin resistance*). As a result, serum glucose levels rise, stimulating the pancreas to release additional insulin. Elevated insulin levels may contribute to hypertension via increased sympathetic activation or by stimulation of vascular smooth muscle cell hypertrophy, which increases vascular resistance. Smooth muscle cell hypertrophy may be caused by a direct mitogenic effect of insulin or through enhanced sensitivity to platelet-derived growth factor.

Obesity itself has been directly associated with hypertension. Possible explanations for this relationship include (1) the release of angiotensinogen from adipocytes as substrate for the renin-angiotensin system; (2) augmented blood volume related to increased body mass; and (3) increased blood viscosity caused by adipocyte release of profibrinogen and plasminogen activator inhibitor 1. The current epidemic of obesity has led to a dramatic increase in the number of people with *metabolic syndrome*. As described in Chapter 5, this condition represents a clustering of atherogenic risk factors, including hypertension, hypertriglyceridemia, low serum high-density lipoprotein (HDL), a tendency toward glucose intolerance, and truncal obesity. Current evidence suggests that insulin resistance is central to the pathogenesis of this clustering.

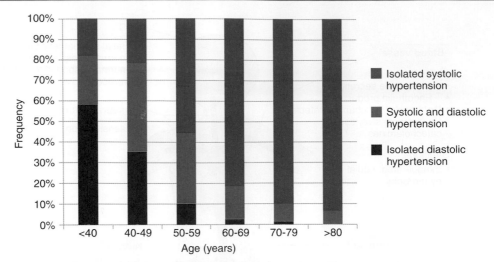

Figure 13-4. Categories of blood pressure elevation in untreated hypertensive patients. Isolated systolic hypertension predominates in patients older than 50 years, primarily as a result of decreased vascular compliance. (Modified from Franklin SS, Jacobs MJ, Wong ND, et al. Predominance of isolated systolic hypertension among middle-aged and elderly U.S. hypertensives: analysis based on National Health and Nutrition Examination Survey (NHANES III). *Hypertension*. 2001;37:869-874.)

NATURAL HISTORY

EH characteristically arises after young adulthood. Its prevalence increases with age, and more than 60% of Americans older than 60 years are hypertensive. In addition, the hemodynamic characteristics of BP elevation in EH tend to change over time. The systolic pressure increases throughout adult life, while the diastolic pressure rises until about the age of 50 and then declines slightly thereafter (see Fig. 13-1). Accordingly, diastolic hypertension is more common in young people, while a substantial number of hypertensive patients over age 50 have isolated systolic hypertension, with normal diastolic values (Fig. 13-4).

In younger persons with hypertension, elevated BP tends to be driven by high CO in the setting of relatively normal peripheral vascular resistance, termed the *hyperkinetic* phase of EH (Fig. 13-5). With advancing age, however, the effect of CO declines, perhaps because of the development of left ventricular hypertrophy (LVH) and its consequent reduced diastolic filling (which in turn reduces SV and CO). Conversely, vascular resistance increases with age due to medial hypertrophy as the vessels adapt to the prolonged pressure stress. Thus,

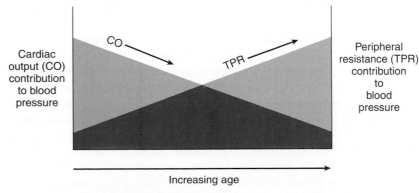

Figure 13-5. Hemodynamic progression of essential hypertension (EH). Schematic representation of the changing contribution of cardiac output (CO) and total peripheral resistance (TPR) as age increases in many patients with EH.

younger hypertensive patients often display augmented CO as the principal abnormality, and older patients tend to have elevated TPR as the major hemodynamic finding.

In summary, EH is a syndrome that may arise from many potential abnormalities, but it exhibits a characteristic hemodynamic profile and natural history. It is likely that multiple defects, separately inherited or acquired, act together to chronically raise BP.

SECONDARY HYPERTENSION

Although EH dominates the hypertensive population, a defined structural or hormonal cause for hypertension may be found in a small percentage of patients. Identification of such cases of secondary hypertension is important because the underlying conditions may require specific therapy different from that administered for EH, and these cases are often curable when identified early. If secondary hypertension is left uncontrolled, cardiovascular adaptations may develop, analogous to those of long-standing EH, that could cause the elevated pressures to persist even after the underlying cause is corrected.

Although secondary forms should be considered in the workup of all patients with hypertension, there are clues that a given patient may have one of the correctable conditions (Table 13-2):

1. *Age.* If a patient develops hypertension before age 20 or after age 50 (outside the usual range of EH), secondary hypertension is more likely.
2. *Severity.* Secondary hypertension often causes BP to rise dramatically, whereas most EH patients usually have mild-to-moderate hypertension.
3. *Onset.* Secondary forms of hypertension often present abruptly in a patient who was previously normotensive, rather than gradually progressing over years as is the usual case in EH.
4. *Associated signs and symptoms.* The process that induces hypertension may give rise to other characteristic abnormalities, identified by the history and physical examination. For

TABLE 13-2	Causes of Hypertension	
Type	Percent of Hypertensive Patients	Clinical Clues
Essential	~90%	• Age of onset: 20-50 y • Family history of hypertension • Normal serum K^+, urinalysis
Chronic renal disease	2%-4%	• ↑ Creatinine, abnormal urinalysis
Primary aldosteronism	<2%-15% (varies by sensitivity of screening)	• ↓ Serum K^+ • Severe or resistant hypertension • Adrenal mass on imaging studies
Renovascular	1%	• Abdominal bruit • Sudden onset (especially if age > 50 or <20) • ↓ Serum K^+
Pheochromocytoma	0.2%	• Paroxysms of palpitations, diaphoresis, and headache • Weight loss • Episodic hypertension in one third of patients
Coarctation of the aorta	0.1%	• Blood pressure in arms > legs or right arm > left arm • Midsystolic murmur between scapulae • Chest x-ray: aortic indentation, rib notching due to arterial collaterals
Cushing syndrome	0.1%	• "Cushingoid" appearance (eg, central obesity, hirsutism)

example, a renal artery *bruit* (swishing sound caused by turbulent blood flow through a stenotic artery) may be heard on abdominal examination in a patient with renal artery stenosis.

5. *Family history.* EH patients often have hypertensive first-degree relatives, whereas secondary hypertension more commonly occurs sporadically.

PATIENT EVALUATION

The clinical evaluation of a patient with recently diagnosed hypertension begins with a careful history and physical examination, including a search for clues to the secondary forms. For example, repeated urinary tract infections may suggest the presence of chronic pyelonephritis with renal damage as the cause of hypertension. Excessive weight loss may be an indicator of pheochromocytoma, whereas weight gain may point to the presence of Cushing syndrome (these conditions are described below). The history also should include an assessment of lifestyle behaviors that may contribute to hypertension, such as excessive alcohol consumption, and the medication list should be reviewed for drugs that may elevate BP (see next section). Obstructive sleep apnea is commonly associated with hypertension and should be considered particularly in patients who snore and have a history of hypertension refractory to medications.

Laboratory tests commonly performed in the initial evaluation of the hypertensive patient, including general screening for secondary causes, are (1) urinalysis and measurement of the serum concentration of creatinine and blood urea nitrogen to evaluate for renal abnormalities; (2) serum potassium level (often low in renovascular hypertension [RH] or primary aldosteronism); (3) blood glucose level (elevated in diabetes, which is strongly associated with hypertension and renal disease); (4) serum total and LDL cholesterol, HDL cholesterol, and triglyceride levels, as part of the global vascular risk screen; and (5) an electrocardiogram (for evidence of LVH caused by chronic hypertension).

If no abnormalities are found that suggest a secondary form of hypertension, the patient is presumed to have EH and treated accordingly. However, if the patient's BP remains elevated despite standard treatments, more detailed diagnostic testing for specific secondary causes may be undertaken.

EXOGENOUS CAUSES

Several medications can elevate BP. For example, oral contraceptives may cause secondary hypertension in some women. The mechanism is likely related to increased activity of the renin-angiotensin system. Estrogens increase the hepatic synthesis of angiotensinogen, leading to greater production of angiotensin II (AII) (Fig. 13-6). AII raises BP by several mechanisms, most notably by direct vasoconstriction and by stimulating the adrenal release of aldosterone. Aldosterone causes renal sodium retention and, therefore, increased intravascular volume.

Other medications that can raise BP include glucocorticoids, cyclosporine (an antirejection drug used in patients with organ transplants), erythropoietin (a hormone prescribed to increase bone marrow red blood cell formation, but also elevates BP by increasing blood viscosity and reversing local hypoxic vasodilatation), and sympathomimetic drugs (which are common in over-the-counter cold remedies). Nonsteroidal anti-inflammatory drugs can contribute to hypertension through dose-related augmentation of renal sodium and water retention.

Two other substances that may contribute to hypertension are alcohol (ie, chronic excessive consumption) and cocaine. Both of these are associated with increased sympathetic nervous system activity.

Figure 13-6. The renin-angiotensin-aldosterone system. Liver-derived angiotensinogen is cleaved in the circulation by renin (of kidney origin) to form angiotensin I (AI). AI is rapidly converted to the potent vasoconstrictor AII by angiotensin-converting enzyme. angiotensin II (AII) also modulates the release of aldosterone from the adrenal cortex. Aldosterone in turn acts to reabsorb Na^+ from the distal nephron, resulting in increased intravascular volume. The other listed effects of AII receptor stimulation may also contribute to the development and maintenance of hypertension.

ANGIOTENSINOGEN
(secreted by liver)

*RENIN
(secreted by kidney)*

ANGIOTENSIN I

ANGIOTENSIN-CONVERTING ENZYME

ANGIOTENSIN II

ANGIOTENSIN II RECEPTORS (AT_1 subtype)	
Arterial smooth muscle:	Vasoconstriction
Adrenal gland:	↑Aldosterone (↑renal Na^+ reabsorption)
Sympathetic nervous system:	Facilitates release of norepinephrine
Kidney:	↑Renal tubular Na^+ reabsorption
Brain:	Stimulates thirst and vasopressin secretion
Heart:	Enhances contractility and ventricular hypertrophy

RENAL CAUSES

Given the crucial role of the kidney in the control of BP, it is not surprising that renal dysfunction can lead to hypertension. In fact, renal disease contributes to two important endogenous causes of secondary hypertension: renal parenchymal disease, accounting for 2%-4% of hypertensive patients, and renovascular hypertension (renal arterial stenosis), which accounts for ~1%.

Renal Parenchymal Disease

Parenchymal damage to the kidney can result from diverse pathologic processes. The major mechanism by which injury leads to elevated BP is through increased intravascular volume. Damaged nephrons are unable to excrete normal amounts of sodium and water, leading to a rise in intravascular volume, elevated CO, and hence increased BP.

If renal function is only mildly impaired, BP may stabilize at a level at which the higher systemic pressure (and therefore renal perfusion pressure) enables sodium excretion to balance sodium intake. Conversely, if a patient has end-stage renal failure, the glomerular filtration rate may be so decreased that the kidneys simply cannot excrete sufficient volume, and malignant-range BP may follow. Renal parenchymal disease may further contribute to hypertension through the excessive elaboration of renin, even if the glomerular filtration rate is not severely reduced.

Renovascular Hypertension

Stenosis of one or both renal arteries leads to hypertension. Although emboli, vasculitis, and external compression of the renal arteries can be responsible, the two most common causes of RH are atherosclerosis and fibromuscular dysplasia. *Atherosclerotic* lesions arise from plaque formation either within the renal artery or in the aorta at the origin of the renal artery. This form accounts for about two-thirds of cases of RH and occurs most commonly in elderly men. In contrast, *fibromuscular* lesions consist of discrete regions of fibrous or muscular proliferation, generally within the arterial media. Fibromuscular dysplasia accounts for one-third of cases of RH and characteristically occurs in young women.

The elevated BP in RH arises from reduced renal blood flow to the affected kidney, which responds to the lower perfusion pressure by secreting renin. The latter raises the BP through the subsequent actions of AII (vasoconstriction) and aldosterone (sodium retention), as shown in Figure 13-6.

The diagnosis of RH is suggested by an abdominal bruit, which is found in 40%-60% of affected patients, or by the presence of unexplained hypokalemia (owing to excessive renal excretion of potassium as a result of an elevated aldosterone level). The diagnosis can be confirmed by duplex Doppler ultrasonography, computed tomographic angiography (CTA), or magnetic resonance angiography of the renal arteries.

Therapy of RH with antihypertensive drugs is often effective, particularly when an ACE inhibitor or angiotensin receptor blocker is included. These inhibitors of the renin-angiotensin system negate the hypertensive effects of elevated circulating renin in RH by impeding the formation or action of AII (see Chapter 17). However, these classes of drugs should be avoided, or used cautiously, in patients with *bilateral* renal artery stenosis. The inhibition of AII may excessively reduce intraglomerular pressure and filtration, thereby worsening renal function, in patients with bilateral disease who already have compromised perfusion to both kidneys. In select patients with RH (eg, those with recent onset hypertension due to RH, those whose BP remains elevated despite medical therapy, or those with progressive renal insufficiency due to renal artery stenosis), percutaneous catheter interventions or surgical reconstruction of the stenosed vessel may be more effective than continued medical antihypertensive therapy alone.

MECHANICAL CAUSES

Coarctation of the Aorta

Coarctation is an infrequently occurring congenital narrowing of the aorta, typically located just distal to the origin of the left subclavian artery (see Chapter 16). As a result of the relative obstruction to flow, the BP in the aortic arch, head, and arms is higher than that in the descending aorta, its branches, and the lower extremities. Sometimes the coarctation involves the origin of the left subclavian artery, causing lower pressure in the left arm compared with the right arm.

Hypertension in this condition arises by two mechanisms. First, reduced blood flow to the kidneys stimulates the renin-angiotensin system, resulting in vasoconstriction (via AII). Second, high pressures proximal to the coarctation stiffen the aortic arch through medial hyperplasia and accelerated atherosclerosis, blunting the normal baroreceptor response to elevated intravascular pressure.

Clinical clues to the presence of coarctation include symptoms of inadequate blood flow to the legs or left arm, such as claudication or fatigue, or the finding of weakened or absent femoral pulses. A midsystolic murmur associated with the stenotic segment of the aorta may be auscultated, especially over the back, between the scapulae. The chest radiograph may show indentation of the aorta at the level of the coarctation. It may also demonstrate a notched appearance of the ribs secondary to the enlargement of collateral intercostal arteries, which shunt blood around the aortic narrowing. Treatment options include angioplasty or surgical repair of the coarctation. However, hypertension may not abate completely after mechanical correction, in part because of persistent desensitization of the arterial baroreceptors.

ENDOCRINE CAUSES

Circulating hormones play an important role in the control of normal BP, so it should not be surprising that endocrine diseases may cause hypertension. When suspected, the presence of such conditions is evaluated in four ways:

1. Characteristic signs and symptoms
2. Measurement of hormone levels
3. Assessment of hormone secretion in response to stimulation or inhibition
4. Imaging studies to identify the source of excessive hormone secretion

Pheochromocytoma

Pheochromocytomas are catecholamine-secreting tumors of neuroendocrine cells (usually in the adrenal medulla) that account for ~0.2% of cases of hypertension. The release of epinephrine and norepinephrine by the tumor results in intermittent or chronic vasoconstriction, tachycardia, and other sympathetic-mediated effects. A characteristic presentation consists of paroxysmal rises in BP accompanied by "autonomic attacks" caused by the increased catecholamine levels: severe throbbing headaches, profuse sweating, palpitations, and tachycardia. Although some patients are actually normotensive between attacks, most have sustained hypertension. Ten percent of pheochromocytomas are malignant.

Determination of plasma catecholamine levels, or urine catecholamines and their metabolites (eg, vanillylmandelic acid and metanephrine), obtained under controlled circumstances, are used to identify this condition. Because some pheochromocytomas secrete only episodically, diagnosis may require measurement of catecholamines immediately following an attack.

Pharmacologic therapy of pheochromocytomas includes the combination of an α-receptor blocker (eg, phenoxybenzamine) combined with a β-blocker. However, once the tumor is localized by computed tomography, magnetic resonance imaging, or angiography, the definitive therapy is surgical resection. For patients with inoperable disease, treatment consists of α- and β-blockade as well as drugs that inhibit catecholamine biosynthesis (eg, α-methyltyrosine).

Adrenocortical Hormone Excess

Among the hormones produced by the adrenal cortex are mineralocorticoids and glucocorticoids. Excess of either of these can result in hypertension.

Mineralocorticoids, primarily aldosterone, increase blood volume by augmenting reabsorption of sodium into the circulation by the distal portions of the nephron. This occurs in exchange for potassium excretion into the urine, and resulting hypokalemia is an important marker of mineralocorticoid activity. *Primary aldosteronism* results either from an adrenal adenoma or from bilateral hyperplasia of the adrenal glands. While once considered rare, recent data suggest that the frequency of primary aldosteronism may be as high as 10%-15% among hypertensives, depending on the sensitivity of screening, with a substantial majority having the bilateral hyperplasia form. The diagnosis may be suspected by the presence of hypokalemia or severe resistant hypertension and is confirmed by the finding of excessive plasma aldosterone and a suppressed renin level. Therapy includes either surgical removal of the responsible adenoma (if present) or medical management with mineralocorticoid receptor antagonists.

Glucocorticoid-remediable aldosteronism (GRA), an uncommon hereditary (autosomal dominant) form of primary aldosteronism, results from a genetic rearrangement in which aldosterone synthesis abnormally comes under the regulatory control of adrenocorticotropic hormone (ACTH). This condition typically presents as severe hypertension in childhood or young adulthood, as opposed to the more common forms of primary aldosteronism, which are generally diagnosed in the third through sixth decades. Unlike other forms of hypertension, GRA-related BP elevation responds to glucocorticoid therapy, which suppresses ACTH release from the pituitary gland.

Secondary aldosteronism can result from increased AII production stimulated by rare renin-secreting tumors. More commonly, secondary elevation of aldosterone is a result of augmented circulating AII in women taking oral contraceptives (which stimulate hepatic production of angiotensinogen, as described earlier) or because of impaired AII degradation in chronic liver diseases.

Excess **glucocorticoids**, such as cortisol, elevate BP likely via blood volume expansion and synthesis of components of the renin-angiotensin system. In addition, though mineralocorticoids are more potent activators of mineralocorticoid receptors in the renal tubules, excess glucocorticoids may also activate them, promoting sodium retention and potassium excretion.

Nearly 80% of patients with *Cushing syndrome*, a disorder of glucocorticoid excess, have some degree of hypertension. These patients often present with classic "cushingoid" features: a characteristic rounded facial appearance, central obesity, proximal muscle weakness, and hirsutism. The cause of the excess glucocorticoids may be either a pituitary ACTH-secreting adenoma, a peripheral ACTH-secreting tumor (either of which causes adrenal cortical hyperplasia), or an adrenal cortisol-secreting adenoma. The diagnosis of Cushing syndrome is confirmed by a 24-hour urine collection for the measurement of cortisol or by a dexamethasone test, which evaluates whether exogenous glucocorticoids can suppress cortisol secretion.

Thyroid Hormone Abnormalities

Approximately one-third of *hyperthyroid* and one-fourth of *hypothyroid* patients have significant hypertension. Thyroid hormones exert their cardiovascular effects by (1) inducing sodium-potassium ATPases in the heart and vessels; (2) increasing blood volume; and (3) stimulating tissue metabolism and oxygen demand, with secondary accumulation of metabolites that modulate local vascular tone. Hyperthyroid patients develop hypertension through cardiac hyperactivity with an increase in blood volume. Hypothyroid patients demonstrate predominantly diastolic hypertension and an increase in peripheral vascular resistance. Though the precise mechanism is unclear, the latter effect appears to be mediated by sympathetic and adrenal activation in hypothyroidism.

CONSEQUENCES OF HYPERTENSION

Whatever the cause of BP elevation, the ultimate consequences are similar. High BP itself is generally asymptomatic but can result in devastating effects on many organs.

CLINICAL SIGNS AND SYMPTOMS

In the past, "classic" symptoms of hypertension were considered to include headache, epistaxis (nose bleeds), and dizziness. However, the usefulness of these symptoms has been called into question by studies that indicate that they are found no more frequently among hypertensive patients than in the general population. Other symptoms, such as flushing, sweating, and blurred vision, do appear to be more common in the hypertensive population. In general, however, most hypertensive patients are asymptomatic and are diagnosed simply by BP measurement during routine physical examination.

Several physical signs of hypertension discussed in the following sections result directly from elevated pressure, including LVH and retinopathy. In addition, when hypertension is complicated by atherosclerosis, arterial bruits may be present, particularly over the carotid and femoral arteries.

ORGAN DAMAGE CAUSED BY HYPERTENSION

Target organ complications of hypertension reflect the degree and duration of chronic BP elevation. Such organ damage can be attributed to (1) the increased workload of the heart and (2) arterial damage resulting from the combined effects of the elevated pressure itself (weakened vessel walls) and accelerated atherosclerosis (Fig. 13-7). Abnormalities of the

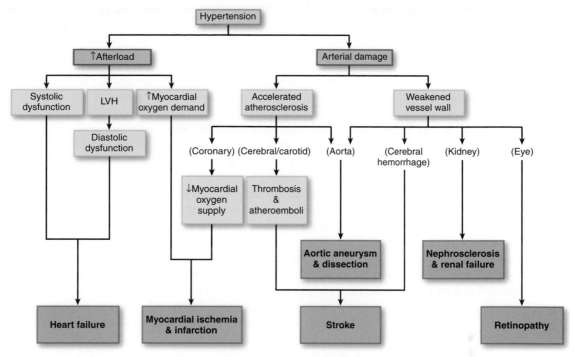

Figure 13-7. Pathogenesis of the major consequences of arterial hypertension. LVH, left ventricular hypertrophy.

vasculature that result from elevated pressure include smooth muscle hypertrophy, endothelial cell dysfunction, and fatigue of elastic fibers. Chronic hypertensive trauma to the endothelium promotes atherosclerosis, possibly by disrupting normal protective mechanisms, such as the secretion of nitric oxide. Arteries lined by atherosclerotic plaque may thrombose or may serve as a source of cholesterol emboli that occlude distal vessels, causing organ infarction (such as cerebrovascular occlusion, resulting in stroke). In addition, atherosclerosis of large arteries hinders their elasticity, resulting in systolic pressure spikes that can further traumatize endothelium or provoke events such as aneurysm rupture.

The major target organs for the destructive complications of chronic hypertension are the heart, the cerebrovascular system, the aorta and peripheral vascular system, the kidney, and the retina (Table 13-3). Left untreated, ~50% of hypertensive patients die of coronary artery

TABLE 13-3 Target Organ Damage in Hypertension	
Organ System	**Manifestations**
Heart	• Left ventricular hypertrophy • Heart failure • Myocardial ischemia and infarction
Cerebrovascular	• Stroke
Aorta and peripheral vascular	• Aortic aneurysm and/or dissection • Arteriosclerosis
Kidney	• Nephrosclerosis • Renal failure
Retina	• Arterial narrowing • Hemorrhages, exudates, papilledema

disease or congestive heart failure, about 33% succumb to stroke, and 10%-15% die from complications of renal failure.

Heart

The major cardiac effects of hypertension relate to the increased load against which the heart must contract and to accelerated atherosclerosis within the coronary arteries.

Left Ventricular Hypertrophy and Diastolic Dysfunction

The high arterial pressure (heightened afterload) increases the wall tension of the left ventricle, which compensates through hypertrophy. *Concentric hypertrophy* (without dilatation) is the normal pattern of compensation, although conditions that elevate BP via increased circulating volume (eg, primary aldosteronism) may instead cause *eccentric* hypertrophy with chamber dilatation (see Chapter 9). LVH results in increased stiffness of the left ventricle with diastolic dysfunction, manifested by elevation of LV filling pressures that can result in pulmonary congestion (ie, heart failure with preserved ejection fraction—see Chapter 9).

Physical findings of LVH may include a heaving LV impulse on chest palpation, indicative of the increased muscle mass. It is frequently accompanied by a fourth heart sound (S_4), as the left atrium contracts into the stiffened left ventricle (see Chapter 2).

LVH is one of the strongest predictors of cardiac morbidity in hypertensive patients. The degree of hypertrophy correlates with the development of congestive heart failure, angina, arrhythmias, myocardial infarction, and sudden cardiac death.

Systolic Dysfunction

Although LVH initially serves a compensatory role, later in the course of systemic hypertension, the increased LV mass may be insufficient to balance the high wall tension caused by the elevated pressure. As LV contractile capacity deteriorates, findings of systolic dysfunction become evident (ie, reduced CO and pulmonary congestion). Systolic dysfunction is also provoked by the accelerated development of coronary artery disease with resultant periods of myocardial ischemia.

Coronary Artery Disease

Chronic hypertension is a major contributor to the development of myocardial ischemia and infarction. These complications reflect the combination of accelerated coronary atherosclerosis (decreased myocardial oxygen supply) and the high systolic workload (increased oxygen demand). In addition, hypertensive patients have a higher incidence of post-myocardial infarction complications such as rupture of the ventricular wall, LV aneurysm formation, and congestive heart failure.

Cerebrovascular System

Hypertension is the major modifiable risk factor for strokes, also termed **cerebrovascular accidents (CVAs)**. Although diastolic pressure is important, it is the magnitude of the systolic pressure that has been most closely linked to CVAs. The presence of isolated systolic hypertension more than doubles a person's risk for stroke.

Hypertension-induced strokes can be hemorrhagic or, more commonly, atherothrombotic. *Hemorrhagic* CVAs result from rupture of microaneurysms in cerebral parenchymal vessels induced by long-standing hypertension. *Atherothrombotic* (also called *thromboembolic*) CVAs arise when portions of atherosclerotic plaque within the carotids or major cerebral arteries, or thrombi that form on those plaques, break off and embolize to smaller distal vessels. Thromboembolism to cerebral vessels from the heart may occur if atrial fibrillation (a cardiac arrhythmia for which there is a predisposition in hypertension) is present. Intracerebral vessels may also be directly occluded by local atherosclerotic plaque rupture and thrombosis.

Occlusion of small penetrating brain arteries can result in multiple tiny infarcts. As these lesions soften and are absorbed by phagocytic cells, small (≤3 mm diameter) cavities form, termed *lacunae*. These lacunar infarctions are seen almost exclusively in patients with long-standing hypertension and are usually localized to the penetrating branches of the middle and posterior circulation of the brain.

In addition, the generalized arterial narrowing found in hypertensive patients reduces collateral flow to ischemic tissues and imposes structural requirements for higher perfusion pressure to maintain adequate tissue flow. This leaves the hypertensive patient vulnerable to cerebral infarcts in areas supplied by the distal ends of arterial branches ("watershed" infarcts) if BP should fall suddenly.

Effective treatment of hypertension diminishes the risk of stroke and has contributed to a 50% reduction in deaths attributed to cerebrovascular events in recent decades.

Aorta and Peripheral Vasculature

The accelerated atherosclerosis associated with hypertension may result in plaque formation and narrowing throughout the arterial vasculature. In addition to the coronary arteries, lesions most commonly appear within the aorta and the major arteries that serve the lower extremities, neck, and brain.

Chronic hypertension may lead to the development of aneurysms, particularly of the abdominal aorta. An **abdominal aortic aneurysm** represents prominent dilatation of the vessel, usually located below the level of the renal arteries, contributed to by the mechanical stress of the high pressure on an arterial wall already weakened by medial damage and atherosclerosis (see Chapter 15). Aneurysms >6 cm in diameter have a very high likelihood of rupture within 2 years if not surgically corrected.

Another life-threatening vascular consequence of high BP is **aortic dissection** (described in Chapter 15). Elevated BP, especially in the highest ranges, accelerates degenerative changes in the media of the aorta. When the weakened wall is further exposed to high pressure, the intima may tear, allowing blood to dissect into the aortic media and propagate in either direction within the vessel wall, "clipping off" and obstructing major branch vessels along the way (including coronary or carotid arteries). The treatment of aortic dissection requires rigorous BP control and urgent surgical repair if the proximal aorta is involved.

Kidney

Hypertension-induced nephrosclerosis is a leading cause of kidney failure that results from damage to the renal vasculature. Histologically, the vessel walls become thickened with a hyaline infiltrate, known as *hyaline arteriolosclerosis* (Fig. 13-8). Greater levels of hypertension can induce smooth muscle hypertrophy and necrosis of capillary walls, termed *fibrinoid necrosis*. These changes result in reduced vascular supply and subsequent ischemic atrophy of tubules and, to a lesser extent, glomeruli. Because intact nephrons can usually compensate for those damaged by patchy ischemia, mild hypertension rarely leads to renal insufficiency in the absence of other insults to the kidney. However, malignant levels of hypertension can inflict permanent damage, leading to chronic renal failure.

One of the consequences of hypertensive renal failure is perpetuation of elevated BP. For example, progressive renal dysfunction compromises the ability of the kidney to regulate blood volume, which contributes further to chronic hypertension.

Retina

The retina is the only location where systemic arteries can be directly visualized by physical examination. High BP induces abnormalities that are collectively termed **hypertensive retinopathy**. Although vision may be compromised when the damage is extensive, more

Figure 13-8. Hypertension-associated kidney injury. The arteriolar walls are thickened by hyaline infiltrate (*short arrows*). The glomeruli (*long arrow*) appear sclerosed because of reduced vascular supply. (Courtesy of Dr. Helmut G. Rennke, Brigham and Women's Hospital, Boston, MA.)

commonly the changes serve as an asymptomatic clinical marker for the severity of hypertension and its duration.

Severe hypertension that is *acute* in onset (eg, uncontrolled and/or malignant hypertension) may burst small retinal vessels, causing *hemorrhages, exudation of plasma lipids*, and areas of *local infarction*. If ischemia of the optic nerve develops, patients may describe generalized blurred vision. Retinal ischemia caused by hemorrhage leads to more patchy loss of vision. *Papilledema*, or swelling of the optic disk with blurring of its margins, may arise from high intracranial pressure when the BP reaches malignant levels and cerebrovascular autoregulation fails.

Chronically elevated BP results in a different set of retinal findings. Papilledema is absent, but vasoconstriction results in *arterial narrowing*, and medial hypertrophy thickens the vessel wall, which "nicks" (indents) crossing veins. With more severe chronic hypertension, *arterial sclerosis* is evident as an increased reflection of light through the ophthalmoscope (termed "copper" or "silver" wiring). Although these changes are not in themselves of major functional importance, they indicate that the patient has had long-standing, poorly controlled hypertension.

HYPERTENSIVE CRISIS

Hypertensive crisis is a medical emergency characterized by a severe elevation of BP with the potential for acute end-organ injury. In the past, this type of elevation was usually a consequence of inadequate BP treatment. Now, a hypertensive crisis is more often caused by an acute hemodynamic insult (eg, acute renal disease) superimposed on a chronic hypertensive state. As a result of rapid pathologic changes (fibrinoid necrosis) within the blood vessels and kidneys, a spiraling increase in BP evolves. Further volume expansion and vasoconstriction occur as renal perfusion drops and serum renin and angiotensin levels rise.

Severe BP elevation results in increased intracranial pressure, and patients may present with **hypertensive encephalopathy** manifested by headache, blurred vision, confusion, somnolence, and sometimes coma. When hypertension results in acute damage to retinal vessels, **accelerated-malignant hypertension** is said to be present. Funduscopic examination shows the effects of the rapid pressure rise as hemorrhages, exudates, and sometimes papilledema, as described earlier. The increased load on the left ventricle during a hypertensive crisis may precipitate angina (because of increased myocardial oxygen demand) and/or pulmonary edema.

A hypertensive crisis requires rapid therapy to prevent permanent vascular complications. Correction of BP is generally followed by reversal of the acute pathologic changes, including papilledema and retinal exudation, although renal damage often persists.

TREATMENT OF HYPERTENSION

The therapeutic approach to the hypertensive patient should be influenced by two considerations. First, a single elevated BP measurement does not establish the diagnosis of hypertension because BP varies considerably from day to day. Moreover, BP measurement in the hospital, clinic, or medical office may be affected by the "white coat" effect resulting from patient anxiety. The average of multiple readings taken at two or more office visits and/or in the home provides a more reliable basis for labeling a patient as hypertensive. Indeed, current clinical guidelines recommend measuring BP outside of the medical setting to confirm the diagnosis of hypertension and to assist in properly adjusting medications. There is also evidence that automatic ambulatory BP measurements, taken over the course of 24 hours while the patient follows a daily routine, are more predictive of cardiovascular mortality than traditional in-clinic measurements.

Second, although even mild hypertension is a major public health problem because of its high prevalence, for the person with early hypertension, the near-term risks are small. For example, the additional risk of a stroke is ~1 in 850 per year. Hence, observation over time to determine whether the low-level hypertension persists, or whether lifestyle changes can reduce the pressure, is often a recommended alternative to immediate drug therapy. This is especially true in the absence of other cardiovascular risk factors such as smoking, diabetes, or high serum cholesterol. However, for patients with established cardiovascular disease or for those who have other major atherosclerotic risk factors, a more aggressive approach to pharmacologic therapy is usually warranted to reduce the risk burden.

For most hypertensive patients, the on-therapy BP goal is <130/80. Drug therapy is ultimately the most effective way to achieve this target and prevent future complications, but that should not deter consideration of other beneficial lifestyle changes.

NONPHARMACOLOGIC TREATMENT

Certain lifestyle modifications have been shown to be effective in lowering BP and should be considered in the treatment plan for any patient with hypertension.

Weight Reduction

Studies have consistently found obesity and hypertension to be highly correlated, especially when the obesity is of a central (abdominal) distribution. By some estimates, obesity accounts for 40%-60% of hypertension. BP reduction follows weight loss in a large portion of hypertensive patients who are more than 10% above their ideal weights. Each 10 kg of weight loss is associated with a 5-20 mm Hg fall in systolic BP.

Exercise

Sedentary normotensive people have a 20%-50% higher risk of developing hypertension than do their more active peers. Regular aerobic exercise, such as walking, jogging, or bicycling, has been shown to contribute to BP reduction over and above any resulting weight loss. A hypertensive patient who becomes physically conditioned manifests a lower resting HR and reduced levels of circulating catecholamines than before training, suggesting a fall in sympathetic tone.

Diet

In addition to caloric restriction for weight loss, changes in the composition of a patient's diet may be important for BP reduction. For example, a diet high in fruits, vegetables, and low-fat dairy products has been shown to significantly reduce BP.

Sodium

Salt restriction for people with high BP is a controversial issue, but there are several epidemiologic and clinical trials that support the benefit of moderating sodium intake in patients with hypertension. In normotensive persons, excess salt ingestion is simply excreted by the kidneys, but ~50% of patients with EH are found to have BPs that vary with sodium intake, suggesting a defect in natriuresis. Sensitivity to sodium levels is more common in African American and elderly hypertensive patients. Because low-salt diets tend to increase the effectiveness of antihypertensive medications in general, the current recommendation is to limit salt intake to <6 g of sodium chloride (<2.3 g sodium) per day, which is one-third less than the average U.S. consumption.

Potassium

Total body potassium content tends to decrease when a person eats a diet low in fruits and vegetables or takes potassium-wasting diuretics. Potassium deficiency has several theoretical effects that may raise BP and contribute to adverse cardiovascular outcomes, such that dietary supplements are routinely recommended to help replete low serum K^+ levels. There is no convincing evidence that prescribing potassium supplements to a normokalemic hypertensive patient will lower BP.

Alcohol

The chronic excessive intake of alcoholic beverages correlates with high BP and resistance to antihypertensive medications. Moreover, experimental evidence shows that BP (especially systolic) may rise acutely following alcohol consumption. The reason for this link remains incompletely understood, but decreasing chronic alcohol intake has been shown to lower BP.

Other

Low calcium intake and magnesium depletion have been associated with elevated BP, but the responsible mechanisms and the implications for therapy are unclear. Caffeine ingestion transiently increases BP (as much as 5-15 mm Hg after two cups of coffee), but routine use does not seem to produce chronic blood pressure elevation.

Smoking Cessation

Cigarette smoking transiently increases BP, likely because of the effect of nicotine on autonomic ganglia, and is a risk factor for the development of sustained hypertension. In addition, the atherogenic effect of smoking may contribute to the development of renovascular hypertension. Cigarette usage is associated with many other health hazards, and all patients should be discouraged from smoking.

Sleep Apnea

Obstructive sleep apnea is a risk factor for hypertension, especially in resistant cases. Treatment of sleep apnea with continuous positive airway pressure promotes small reductions in BP.

Relaxation Therapy

BP frequently rises under conditions of stress. In addition, essential hypertensive patients and their relatives often show higher-than-normal basal sympathetic tone and exaggerated autonomic responses to mental stress. Hence, relaxation techniques have been advocated as a method to control hypertension. Available methods include biofeedback and meditation. The effectiveness of such therapy has not been consistently demonstrated in clinical trials and seems to depend on the patient's attitude and long-term compliance.

In summary, there are a number of nonpharmacologic therapies for reducing elevated BP. The effectiveness of these should come as no surprise, given the extent to which environmental factors play a role in hypertension. Therefore, behavior-based interventions are recommended as first-line therapy in any patient whose hypertension is not an immediate danger.

PHARMACOLOGIC TREATMENT

Antihypertensive medications are the standard means to lower chronically elevated BP and are indicated if nonpharmacologic treatment proves inadequate to reach recommended targets. More than 100 drug preparations are available to treat hypertension, but fortunately the most commonly used medications fall into four classes: diuretics, sympatholytics, vasodilators, and drugs that interfere with the renin-angiotensin system (Table 13-4). The individual actions of these drug classes on the physiologic abnormalities in hypertension are shown in Figure 13-9. The pharmacology and use of antihypertensive drugs are described in greater detail in Chapter 17.

Diuretics have been in use for many decades to treat hypertension. They reduce circulatory volume, CO, and mean arterial pressure and are most effective in patients with mild-to-moderate hypertension who have normal renal function. They are especially effective in

TABLE 13-4 Classes of Antihypertensive Medications

Drug Class	Examples (See Chapter 17)	Physiologic Action
Diuretics	Thiazides	↓ Circulating volume
	Potassium-sparing diuretics	
	Loop diuretics	
Sympatholytics	β-Blockers	↓ Heart rate, cardiac contractility, and renin secretion
	Combined α- and β-blockers	Same as β-blocker plus vascular smooth muscle relaxation
	Central α_2-agonists	↓ Sympathetic tone
	Peripheral α_1-antagonists	Vascular smooth muscle relaxation
Vasodilators	Calcium channel blockers	↓ Peripheral vascular resistance
	Direct vasodilators (eg, hydralazine, minoxidil)	
Renin-angiotensin system antagonists	Angiotensin-converting enzyme inhibitors	↓ Peripheral vascular resistance and sodium retention
	AII receptor blockers	
	Direct renin inhibitors	

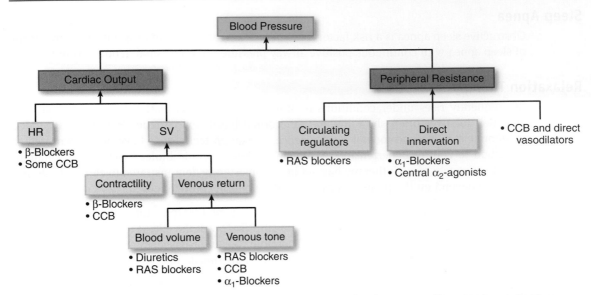

Figure 13-9. Physiologic effects of antihypertensive medications. Notice that some antihypertensive medications work at multiple sites. CCB, calcium channel blockers; HR, heart rate; RAS blockers, renin-angiotensin system blockers (ie, angiotensin-converting enzyme inhibitors and AII receptor blockers); SV, stroke volume.

African American or elderly persons, who tend to be salt sensitive. In clinical trials, diuretics have reduced the risk of strokes and cardiovascular events in hypertensive patients and are inexpensive compared with other agents. *Thiazide diuretics* (eg, hydrochlorothiazide, chlorthalidone [a thiazide-like diuretic]) and *potassium-sparing diuretics* (eg, spironolactone) promote Na^+ excretion in the distal nephron (see Chapter 17). *Loop diuretics* (eg, furosemide) are generally too potent, and their actions too short-lived, for use as antihypertensive agents; however, they are useful in lowering BP in patients with renal insufficiency, who often do not respond to other diuretics.

Thiazides, the most commonly used diuretics in hypertension, may result in adverse metabolic side effects, including elevation of serum glucose, cholesterol, and triglyceride levels. In addition, hypokalemia and hyperuricemia are potential side effects. However, when diuretics are prescribed in low dosages, it is often possible to accrue the desired antihypertensive effect while minimizing adverse complications.

Mineralocorticoid receptor antagonists (eg, spironolactone and eplerenone) have a mild diuretic effect via inhibition of aldosterone activity. While not first line therapies in EH, these agents *are* preferred medical therapy for patients with primary aldosteronism.

Sympatholytic agents include (1) β-blockers, (2) central α-adrenergic agonists, and (3) systemic α-adrenergic-blocking drugs. β-**Blockers** are believed to lower BP through several mechanisms, including (1) reducing CO through a decrease in HR and a mild decline in contractility and (2) decreasing the secretion of renin (and therefore levels of AII), which leads to a reduction in TPR. β-Blockers are less effective than diuretics in elderly and African American hypertensive patients. Adverse effects of β-blockers include bronchospasm (because of bronchiolar β_2-receptor blockade), fatigue, impotence, and hyperglycemia. They may also adversely alter lipid metabolism. Many β-blockers cause an increase in serum triglyceride levels and a decrease in HDL cholesterol levels.

Centrally acting α_2-**adrenergic agonists**, such as methyldopa and clonidine, reduce sympathetic outflow to the heart, blood vessels, and kidneys. These are now used only occasionally owing to a high frequency of side effects. Systemic α_1-**antagonists** (eg, prazosin, terazosin, doxazosin) cause a decrease in TPR through relaxation of vascular smooth muscle. They too are not often used for treatment of hypertension today because a major clinical trial showed that diuretic therapy is superior for prevention of adverse cardiovascular events. However, as drugs of this group are used primarily to relieve symptoms of prostatic enlargement in older men, a sometimes desired side benefit is BP lowering.

Peripheral **vasodilators** include calcium channel blockers, hydralazine, and minoxidil. **Calcium channel blockers** reduce the influx of Ca^{++} responsible for vascular smooth muscle contraction, thus reducing TPR (see Chapter 17). Clinical trials in patients with hypertension have shown that calcium channel blockers reduce the risk of myocardial infarction and stroke. Thus, once-daily sustained-release formulations of this group (eg, amlodipine, nifedipine, diltiazem) are frequently used to treat hypertension.

Hydralazine and *minoxidil* lower BP by directly relaxing vascular smooth muscle of precapillary resistance vessels. However, the resultant vasodilatation can result in a reflex increase in HR so that combined β-blocker therapy is frequently necessary. The use of these direct vasodilators has waned with the advent of newer agents with fewer side effects.

Drugs that interfere with the renin-angiotensin-aldosterone system include ACE inhibitors, AII receptor blockers (ARBs), and direct renin inhibitors. **ACE inhibitors** decrease BP by blocking the conversion of angiotensin I (AI) to AII (see Fig. 17-6), thereby reducing the vasopressor effect of AII and the secretion of aldosterone. As a result, peripheral vascular resistance falls, and sodium retention by the kidney declines. An additional antihypertensive effect of ACE inhibitors occurs via an *increase* in the concentration of the circulating vasodilator bradykinin (see Fig. 17-6). ACE inhibitors are important drugs that have been shown to reduce mortality rates in patients following an acute myocardial infarction and in patients with chronic heart failure with reduced ejection fraction (see Chapter 9). The drugs also slow the deterioration of renal function in patients with diabetic nephropathy. The most common side effect of ACE inhibitors is a reversible dry cough (likely related to the increased bradykinin effect); hyperkalemia and azotemia may also occur, as described in Chapter 17.

ARBs block the binding of AII to its receptors (ie, subtype AT_1 receptors) in blood vessels and other targets (see Fig. 17-6). By inhibiting the effects of AII (and thereby causing vasodilatation and reduced secretion of aldosterone), BP falls. In clinical trials, the antihypertensive efficacy of this group is similar to that of ACE inhibitors. They are very well-tolerated drugs, and unlike ACE inhibitors, cough is not a common side effect. Similar to ACE inhibitors, ARBs have been shown to reduce cardiovascular event rates (including myocardial infarction and stroke) in high-risk patients.

The oral **direct renin inhibitor** aliskiren reduces levels of AI and AII by binding to the proteolytic site of renin, thus inhibiting cleavage of angiotensinogen. Its antihypertensive effectiveness is no greater than that of other drugs that inhibit the renin-angiotensin-aldosterone axis, and it is rarely used.

Given the large number of effective antihypertensive medications that are available, the choice of which drug to use as initial therapy in an individual patient can seem daunting. Besides the exceptions noted above, clinical trial data reveal little difference between antihypertensive agents on cardiovascular outcomes in the average essential hypertensive subject, as long as equivalent decreases in BP are achieved. Current guidelines recommend the use of either a thiazide diuretic, calcium channel blocker, ACE inhibitor, or an ARB as equally effective first-line treatment options for EH. β-Blockers are no longer considered first-line therapy but are appropriate in certain circumstances.

Thiazide diuretics remain among the most popular choices by health care providers because of long-proven benefits and low cost. In certain circumstances, or if initial therapy with a single agent is not sufficient, another antihypertensive of a different class should be substituted or added (Table 13-5). For example, an ACE inhibitor would be given prime consideration in patients with hypertension who also have chronic heart failure, diabetes, or LV dysfunction following myocardial infarction. A β-blocker would be an appropriate choice in a patient with concurrent ischemic heart disease.

TABLE 13-5	Indications for Specific Antihypertensive Medications
Concurrent Condition	**Initial Therapy Drug Classes**
Heart failure	Diuretics β-Blockers ACE inhibitors AII receptor blockers Aldosterone antagonists
Postmyocardial infarction	β-Blockers ACE inhibitors AII receptor blockers Aldosterone antagonists
Diabetes	ACE inhibitors AII receptor blockers Calcium channel blockers
Chronic kidney disease	ACE inhibitors AII receptor blockers

ACE, angiotensin-converting enzyme.

There are other guiding principles. First, the chosen drug regimen should conform to the patient's specific needs. For example, an anxious young patient in the throes of the hyperkinetic phase of EH might be treated with a β-blocker, whereas a more effective choice for the same patient many years later, after the pressure becomes more dependent on peripheral vascular resistance, could be a vasodilator (eg, long-acting calcium channel blocker). Because therapy is likely to continue for many years, consideration of adverse effects and impact of drug therapy on the patient's quality of life are very important.

Another principle of antihypertensive drug therapy concerns the use of multiple agents. The effects of one drug, acting at one physiologic control point, can be defeated by natural compensatory mechanisms. For example, the drop in renal perfusion by a direct vasodilator can activate the renin-angiotensin system, prompting the kidney to retain volume, thereby blunting the antihypertensive benefit. Combination drug therapy is aimed at preventing such an action by using agents acting at different complementary sites. In this example, a direct vasodilator is often paired with a low-dose diuretic to avoid the undesired volume expansion effect.

In conclusion, hypertension emerges as a tremendously important clinical problem because of its high prevalence and potentially devastating consequences. The evaluation and treatment of a patient with hypertension require methodical consideration of the ways in which normal cardiovascular physiology may have gone awry. Since most patients fall into the category of EH, there is still much room for creative thought and research into underlying causes and targeted therapies for hypertension.

Summary

- **Elevated blood pressure** is present when the systolic reading is ≥120 mm Hg. **Stage 1 hypertension** indicates systolic BP ≥130 mm Hg or diastolic BP ≥80 mm Hg; **stage 2 hypertension** refers to systolic BP ≥140 mm Hg or diastolic BP ≥90 mm Hg.

- Hypertension is of unknown etiology in the majority of patients (termed **essential hypertension**).

- **Secondary hypertension** may arise from (1) renal conditions (eg, renal parenchymal disease and renal artery stenosis); (2) coarctation of the aorta; and (3) endocrine abnormalities (eg, pheochromocytoma, primary or secondary aldosteronism, Cushing syndrome, and thyroid dysfunction).
- Potential **complications** of hypertension include stroke, myocardial infarction, heart failure, aortic aneurysm and dissection, renal damage, and retinopathy.
- **Treatment of hypertension** includes lifestyle and dietary improvements and pharmacologic therapy.
- The most commonly recommended **antihypertensive drugs** include diuretics, ACE inhibitors, angiotensin receptor blockers, and calcium channel blockers.

Review Questions

1. A 45-year-old woman presents to her new primary care physician for an initial physical examination. She has no symptoms. Her blood pressure in the office is 152/90, but she reports she often has high readings in medical settings. She has tried checking her blood pressure at home, but measurements have been erratic and inconsistent. What is an appropriate next step?

    a. Prescribe a β-blocker and have her return for a blood pressure check in 6 weeks.
    b. Ignore the elevated pressure; this represents "white coat" hypertension.
    c. Order a 24-hour ambulatory blood pressure monitor.
    d. Order a series of tests to assess for secondary causes of hypertension.

2. A 35-year-old man presents to the primary care clinic for follow-up of elevated blood pressure readings at his last three appointments. He denies any symptoms or significant past medical history. His father had hypertension and suffered a stroke at age 38. On exam, his blood pressure is 150/90 in both arms and 160 systolic in his right calf; there are no murmurs or bruits. His laboratory evaluation is notable for a reduced serum potassium level of 3.3 mEq/L (normal = 3.5-5.0 mEq/L) with normal renal function testing. Which of the following secondary causes of hypertension is most likely?

    a. Cushing syndrome
    b. Coarctation of the aorta
    c. Pheochromocytoma
    d. Primary aldosteronism

3. A 68-year-old man presents to his physician for reevaluation of elevated readings on his home BP monitor over the past 6 months. His past medical history is notable for type 2 diabetes with microvascular complications including diabetic nephropathy. In clinic, his blood pressure is 165/80, a diagnosis of hypertension is confirmed, and a decision is made to initiate pharmacologic therapy. Which of the following would be a preferred choice of antihypertensive medication for this patient?

    a. Hydrochlorothiazide (a thiazide diuretic)
    b. Lisinopril (an angiotensin-converting enzyme inhibitor)
    c. Atenolol (a β-blocker)
    d. Doxazosin (a peripheral α1-receptor antagonist)

Answers to Review Questions

1. **Choice c is correct.** A single elevated blood pressure does not establish the diagnosis of hypertension, so commencing antihypertensive therapy would be premature in this asymptomatic patient. Although the patient attributes her elevated office blood pressure to anxiety, established hypertension cannot be excluded. Measurement of blood pressure while resting at home is often helpful to clarify whether hypertension is truly present, but this patient has had difficulty doing so. A 24-hour ambulatory monitor would therefore be a reasonable way to establish the diagnosis of hypertension. Assessment for secondary causes of hypertension is appropriate when elevated BP is resistant to drug therapy, when hypertension is of recent onset and severe, or when documented hypertension first develops at an uncommon age (eg, before age 20).

2. **Choice d is correct.** The presence of unprovoked hypokalemia raises suspicion for primary aldosteronism, in which excess aldosterone results in augmented renal sodium retention and potassium excretion. Cushing syndrome, a disorder of glucocorticoid excess, would be suggested by central obesity, proximal muscle weakness, and hirsutism, none of which are described in this patient. Coarctation of the aorta would result in elevated arm blood pressures and reduced pressure in the lower extremities, which is not the case here. Pheochromocytoma is more typically characterized by paroxysms of catecholamine excess, such as diaphoresis and tachycardia.

3. **Choice b is correct.** Thiazide diuretics and ACE inhibitors are among first-line therapies for established essential hypertension. In this patient, an ACE inhibitor would be optimal because of its benefits in slowing progression of diabetic nephropathy, whereas thiazide diuretics can worsen glycemic control. β-Blockers have a more limited role in treating isolated hypertension but may be preferred in patients with concurrent ischemic heart disease or chronic heart failure with preserved ejection fraction, for whom β-blockers have added cardiovascular benefit. Peripheral α1-receptor antagonists, such as doxazosin, are not first-line antihypertensives, but blood pressure lowering is an added benefit when such agents are prescribed for their primary use, symptomatic prostatic hypertrophy.

Acknowledgments

Contributors to previous editions of this chapter were Joshua Drago, MD; Christopher T. Lee, MD; Payman Zamani, MD; Rajeev Malhotra, MD; Rahul Deshmukh, MD; Allison McDonough, MD; Rajesh S. Mangrulkar, MD; Peter A. Nigrovic, MD; and Thomas J. Moore, MD.

Additional Reading

Flint AC, Conell C, Ren X, et al. Effect of systolic and diastolic blood pressure on cardiovascular outcomes. *N Engl J Med.* 2019;381:243-251.

Monticone S, D'Ascenzo F, Moretti C, et al. Cardiovascular events and target organ damage in primary aldosteronism compared with essential hypertension: a systemic review and meta-analysis. *Lancet Diabetes Endocrinol.* 2018;6:41-50.

Muntner P, Einhorn PT, Cushman WC, et al. Blood pressure assessment in adults in clinical practice and clinic-based research. *J Am Coll Cardiol.* 2019;73:317-335.

The SPRINT Research Group. A randomized trial of intensive versus standard blood-pressure control. *N Engl J Med.* 2015;373:2103-2116.

Whelton PK, Carey RM, Aronow WS, et al. 2017 ACC/AHA/AAPA/ABC/ACPM/AGS/APhA/ASH/ASPC/NMA/PCNA guideline for the prevention, detection, evaluation, and management of high blood pressure in adults: a report of the American College of Cardiology/American Heart Association Task Force on Clinical Practice Guidelines. *J Am Coll Cardiol.* 2018;71:e127-e248.

Williams B, Mancia G, Spiering W, et al. 2018 ESC/ESH Guidelines for the management of arterial hypertension. *Eur Heart J.* 2018;39:3021-3104.

Yang W-Y, Melgarejo JD, Thijs L, et al. Association of office and ambulatory blood pressure with mortality and cardiovascular outcomes. *JAMA.* 2019;322:409-420.

14 Diseases of the Pericardium

Mathew S. Lopes | Leonard S. Lilly

Diseases of the pericardium form a spectrum that ranges from benign, self-limited pericarditis to life-threatening cardiac tamponade. The clinical manifestations of these disorders and approaches to their management can be predicted from an understanding of pericardial anatomy and pathophysiology, as presented in this chapter.

ANATOMY AND FUNCTION

The pericardium is a two-layered sac that encircles the heart. The inner serosal layer (*visceral pericardium*) adheres to the outer wall of the heart and is reflected back on itself, at the level of the great vessels, to line the tough fibrous outer layer (*parietal pericardium*). A thin film of pericardial fluid slightly separates the two layers and decreases the friction between them.

The pericardium appears to serve three functions: (1) it fixes the heart within the mediastinum and limits its motion, (2) it prevents extreme dilatation of the heart during sudden rises of intracardiac volume, and (3) it may act as a barrier to limit the spread of infection from the adjacent lungs. However, patients with complete absence of the pericardium (either congenitally or after surgical removal) are generally asymptomatic, casting doubt on its actual importance in normal physiology. Yet, like the unnecessary appendix, the pericardium can become diseased and cause great harm.

In the healthy heart, intrapericardial pressure varies during the respiratory cycle from −5 mm Hg (during inspiration) to +5 mm Hg (during expiration) and nearly equals the pressure within the pleural space. However, pathologic changes in pericardial stiffness, or the accumulation of fluid within the pericardial sac, may profoundly increase this pressure.

ACUTE PERICARDITIS

The most common affliction of the pericardium is acute pericarditis, which refers to inflammation of its layers. Many disease states and etiologic agents can produce this syndrome (Table 14-1), the most frequent of which are described here.

TABLE 14-1	Causes of Acute Pericarditis

Infectious
  Viral
  Tuberculosis
  Pyogenic bacteria

Noninfectious
  Postmyocardial infarction or after cardiac surgery
  Uremia
  Neoplastic disease
  Radiation induced
  Connective tissue diseases
  Drug induced

ETIOLOGY

Infectious

Idiopathic and Viral Pericarditis

Acute pericarditis is most often of idiopathic origin, meaning that the actual cause is unknown. However, serologic studies have demonstrated that many such episodes are caused by viral infection, especially by echovirus or coxsackievirus group B. Although a viral origin could be confirmed in infected patients by comparing antiviral titers of acute and convalescent serum, this is rarely done in the clinical setting because the patient has usually recovered by the time those results would be available. Thus, idiopathic and viral pericarditis are considered similar clinical entities, and the terms are used interchangeably.

Other viruses known to cause pericarditis include those responsible for influenza, varicella, mumps, hepatitis B, and infectious mononucleosis. Pericarditis is the most common manifestation of cardiovascular disease in patients with HIV/AIDS, arising from viral infection itself or from superimposed tuberculous or other bacterial infections in this immunocompromised population.

Tuberculous Pericarditis

Although tuberculosis remains a worldwide problem, its incidence in the United States is low. It is, however, an important cause of pericarditis in immunosuppressed patients. Tuberculous pericarditis arises from reactivation of the organism in mediastinal lymph nodes, with spread into the pericardium. It can also extend directly from a site of tuberculosis within the lungs, or the organism can arrive at the pericardium by hematogenous dissemination.

Nontuberculous Bacterial Pericarditis (Purulent Pericarditis)

Bacterial pericarditis is a fulminant illness but is rare in otherwise healthy persons; it is most likely to occur in immunocompromised patients, including those with severe burns and malignancies. Pneumococci and staphylococci are responsible most frequently, whereas gram-negative infection occurs less often. Mechanisms by which bacterial invasion of the pericardium develops include (1) perforating trauma to the chest (eg, stab wound); (2) contamination during chest surgery; (3) extension of an intracardiac infection (ie, infective endocarditis); (4) extension of pneumonia or a subdiaphragmatic infection; and (5) hematogenous spread from a remote infection.

Noninfectious

Pericarditis Following Myocardial Infarction

There are two forms of pericarditis associated with acute myocardial infarction (MI). The early type occurs within the first few days after an MI. It likely results from inflammation extending from the epicardial surface of the injured myocardium to the adjacent pericardium; therefore, it is more common in patients with transmural (as opposed to subendocardial) infarctions. The prognosis following acute MI is not affected by the presence of pericarditis; its major importance is in distinguishing it from the pain of recurrent myocardial ischemia. This form of pericarditis occurs in fewer than 5% of patients with acute MI who are treated with acute reperfusion strategies (see Chapter 7), but it is more common in those who are not (and who, therefore, sustain larger infarctions).

The second form of post-MI pericarditis is known as *Dressler syndrome*, which can develop 2 weeks to several months following an acute infarction. Its cause is unknown, but it is thought to be of autoimmune origin, possibly directed against antigens released from necrotic myocardial cells. Dressler syndrome has become very rare since the advent of reperfusion therapies for acute MI. A clinically similar form of pericarditis may occur weeks to months following heart surgery, termed *postpericardiotomy pericarditis*.

Uremic Pericarditis

Pericarditis is a potentially serious complication of untreated chronic renal failure. While its pathogenesis in this setting is unknown, it has become uncommon with the widespread availability of dialysis. Pericarditis may also appear for the first time in patients already treated with chronic dialysis therapy and often responds to intensification of dialysis.

Neoplastic Pericarditis

Tumor involvement of the pericardium most commonly results from metastatic spread or local invasion by cancer of the lung, breast, or lymphoma. Primary tumors of the pericardium are rare. Neoplastic effusions are usually large and hemorrhagic and frequently lead to cardiac tamponade, a life-threatening complication described later in the chapter.

Radiation-Induced Pericarditis

Pericarditis may complicate radiation therapy to the thorax (eg, administered for the treatment of certain tumors), especially if the cumulative dose has exceeded 4000 cGy. Radiation-induced damage causes a local inflammatory response that can result in pericardial effusions and ultimately fibrosis. Cytologic examination of the pericardial fluid helps to distinguish radiation-induced pericardial damage from that of tumor invasion.

Pericarditis Associated With Connective Tissue Diseases

Pericardial involvement is common in many connective tissue diseases, including systemic lupus erythematosus (SLE), rheumatoid arthritis, and progressive systemic sclerosis. For example, 20%-40% of patients with SLE experience clinically detectable pericarditis during the course of the disease. Customary treatment of the underlying connective tissue disease usually ameliorates the pericarditis as well.

Drug-Induced Pericarditis

Several pharmaceutical agents can cause pericarditis as a side effect, often by inducing a systemic lupus-like syndrome (Table 14-2). These drugs include the antiarrhythmic *procainamide* and the vasodilator *hydralazine*. Pericarditis is also an infrequent side effect of *immune checkpoint inhibitors*, which are used to treat some types of cancer. Drug-induced pericarditis usually abates when the causative agent is discontinued.

Pathogenesis

Similar to other inflammatory processes, pericarditis is characterized by three stages: (1) local *vasodilation* with transudation of protein-poor, cell-free fluid into the pericardial

TABLE 14-2	Examples of Drug-Induced Pericarditis

Related to drug-induced SLE-like syndrome
   Procainamide
   Hydralazine
   Methyldopa
   Isoniazid
   Phenytoin

Not related to drug-induced SLE-like syndrome
   Anthracycline antineoplastic agents (eg, doxorubicin, daunorubicin)
   Minoxidil
   Immune checkpoint inhibitors (eg, ipilimumab, pembrolizumab, nivolumab)

SLE, systemic lupus erythematosus.

space; (2) *increased vascular permeability*, with leak of protein into the pericardial space; and (3) *leukocyte exudation*, initially by neutrophils, followed later by mononuclear cells.

The leukocytes are of critical importance because they help contain or eliminate the offending infectious or autoimmune agent. However, metabolic products released by these cells may prolong inflammation, cause pain and local cellular damage, and mediate somatic symptoms such as fever. Therefore, the immune response to pericardial injury may significantly contribute to tissue damage and symptomatology.

PATHOLOGY

The pathologic appearance of the pericardium depends on the underlying cause and severity of inflammation. **Serous pericarditis** is characterized by scant polymorphonuclear leukocytes, lymphocytes, and histiocytes. The exudate is a thin fluid secreted by the mesothelial cells lining the serosal surface of the pericardium. This likely represents the early inflammatory response common to all types of acute pericarditis.

Serofibrinous pericarditis is the most commonly observed morphologic pattern in patients with pericarditis. The pericardial exudate contains plasma proteins, including fibrinogen, yielding a grossly rough and shaggy appearance (termed "bread and butter" pericarditis). Portions of the visceral and parietal pericardium may become thickened and fused. Occasionally, this process leads to a dense scar that restricts movement and diastolic filling of the cardiac chambers, as described later in the chapter.

Suppurative (or purulent) pericarditis is an intense inflammatory response associated most commonly with bacterial infection. The serosal surfaces are erythematous and coated with purulent exudate. **Hemorrhagic pericarditis** refers to a grossly bloody form of pericardial inflammation and is most often caused by tuberculosis or malignancy.

CLINICAL FEATURES

History

The most frequent symptoms of acute pericarditis are *chest pain* and *fever* (Table 14-3). The pain may be severe and usually localizes to the retrosternal area and left precordium; it may also radiate to the back and to the ridge of the left trapezius muscle. What differentiates it from myocardial ischemia or infarction is that the pain of pericarditis is typically sharp, *pleuritic* (it is aggravated by inspiration and coughing), and *positional* (eg, sitting and leaning forward often lessen the discomfort). *Dyspnea* is common during acute pericarditis but is not exertional and probably results from a reluctance of the patient to breathe deeply because of pleuritic pain.

TABLE 14-3	Clinical Features of Acute Pericarditis
Pleuritic and/or positional chest pain	
Fever	
Pericardial friction rub	
ECG abnormalities	
New pericardial effusion (not in all patients)	

ECG, electrocardiogram.

Patients with idiopathic or viral pericarditis are typically young and previously healthy. Pericarditis of other causes should be suspected in patients with the underlying conditions listed in Table 14-1 who develop typical sharp, pleuritic chest pain.

Physical Examination

A scratchy pericardial *friction rub* is common in acute pericarditis and is believed to be produced by the movement of the inflamed pericardial layers against one another. Auscultation of the rub is best heard using the diaphragm of the stethoscope with the patient leaning forward while exhaling (which brings the pericardium closer to the chest wall and stethoscope). In its full form, the rub consists of three components, corresponding to the phases of greatest cardiac movement: ventricular contraction, ventricular relaxation, and atrial contraction. Characteristically, the pericardial rub is evanescent, coming and going from one examination to the next.

DIAGNOSTIC STUDIES

The presence of pleuritic, positional chest pain and the characteristic pericardial friction rub implicate the presence of acute pericarditis. However, certain laboratory studies are helpful to confirm the diagnosis and to assess for impending complications.

The *electrocardiogram* (ECG) is abnormal in 90% of patients with acute pericarditis and helps to distinguish it from other forms of cardiac disease, such as an acute coronary syndrome. The most important ECG pattern, which reflects inflammation of the adjacent myocardium, consists of *diffuse ST-segment elevation* in most of the ECG leads, usually with the exception of aVR and V_1 (Fig. 14-1). In addition, *PR-segment depression* in several leads is often evident, reflecting abnormal atrial repolarization related to atrial epicardial inflammation. These abnormalities are in contrast to the ECG of acute ST-segment elevation MI, in which the ST segments are elevated only in the leads overlying the region of infarction, and PR depression is not expected.

Blood studies typically reveal signs of acute inflammation, including an increased white blood cell count (usually a mild lymphocytosis in acute viral/idiopathic pericarditis) and elevation of serum inflammatory markers (eg, erythrocyte sedimentation rate and C-reactive protein). Some patients with acute pericarditis also demonstrate elevated serum cardiac biomarkers (eg, cardiac troponins), suggesting inflammation of the neighboring myocardium.

Further testing in acute pericarditis often includes *echocardiography* to evaluate for the presence and hemodynamic significance of a pericardial effusion. Additional studies that may be useful in individual cases to help define the cause of pericarditis include (1) testing for tuberculosis (tuberculin skin test or interferon-gamma release assay blood test), (2) serologic tests (antinuclear antibodies and rheumatoid factor) to screen for connective tissue diseases, and (3) a careful search for malignancy, especially of the lung and breast (physical

Figure 14-1. Electrocardiogram in acute pericarditis. Diffuse ST-segment elevation is present. Also notice depression of the PR segment (*arrow*).

examination supplemented by chest imaging and mammography). The yield of diagnostic *pericardiocentesis* (removal of pericardial fluid through a needle) in uncomplicated acute pericarditis is low and should be reserved for patients with very large effusions or evidence of cardiac chamber compression, as described below.

TREATMENT

Idiopathic or viral pericarditis is a self-limited disease that usually runs its course in 1-3 weeks. Management consists of *rest*, to reduce the interaction of the inflamed pericardial layers, and *pain relief* by analgesic and anti-inflammatory drugs (aspirin, ibuprofen, and other nonsteroidal anti-inflammatory agents). Colchicine, a drug with anti-inflammatory properties usually used to treat gout, may be useful as an additional agent in acute pericarditis. It has been shown to decrease the recurrence rate after an initial episode. Oral corticosteroids are effective for severe or recurrent pericardial pain but should *not* be used in uncomplicated cases because of potentially significant side effects and because steroid use is associated with an increased rate of recurrent episodes of pericarditis.

The forms of pericarditis related to MI are treated in a similar fashion, with rest and aspirin. Other nonsteroidal anti-inflammatory agents are often avoided immediately following an MI because of experimental evidence linking them to delayed healing of the infarct.

Purulent pericarditis requires more aggressive treatment, including catheter drainage of the pericardium and intensive antibiotic therapy. Nevertheless, even with such therapy, the mortality rate is very high. Tuberculous pericarditis requires prolonged multidrug antituberculous therapy. Pericarditis in the setting of uremia often resolves following intensive dialysis. Neoplastic pericardial disease usually indicates widely metastatic cancer, and therapy is unfortunately only palliative.

PERICARDIAL EFFUSION

ETIOLOGY

The normal pericardial space contains 15-50 mL of pericardial fluid, a plasma ultrafiltrate secreted by the mesothelial cells that line the serosal surface. A larger volume of fluid may accumulate in association with any of the forms of acute pericarditis previously described.

In addition, noninflammatory serous effusions may result from conditions of (1) increased capillary permeability (eg, severe hypothyroidism), (2) increased capillary hydrostatic pressure (eg, congestive heart failure), or (3) decreased plasma oncotic pressure (eg, cirrhosis or the nephrotic syndrome). Chylous effusions may occur in the presence of lymphatic obstruction of pericardial drainage, most commonly caused by neoplasms and tuberculosis.

PATHOPHYSIOLOGY

Because the pericardium is a relatively stiff structure, the relationship between its internal volume and pressure is not linear, as shown in curve A in Figure 14-2. Notice that the initial portion of the curve is nearly flat, indicating that at the low volumes normally present within the pericardium, a small increase in volume leads to only a small rise in pressure. However, when the intrapericardial volume expands beyond a critical level (see Fig. 14-2, *arrow*), a dramatic increase in pressure is incited by the nondistensible sac. At that point, even a minor increase in volume can translate into an enormous compressive force on the heart.

Three factors determine whether a pericardial effusion remains clinically silent or whether symptoms of cardiac compression ensue: (1) the *volume* of fluid, (2) the *rate* at which the fluid accumulates, and (3) the *compliance* characteristics of the pericardium.

A *sudden* increase of pericardial volume, as may occur in chest trauma with intrapericardial hemorrhage, results in marked elevation of pericardial pressure (see Fig. 14-2, steep portion of curve A) and the potential for severe cardiac chamber compression. Even lesser amounts of fluid may cause significant elevation of pressure if the pericardium is pathologically noncompliant and stiff, as may occur in the presence of tumor or fibrosis of the sac. In contrast, if the pericardial effusion accumulates *slowly*, over weeks to months, the pericardium gradually stretches, such that the volume-pressure relationship

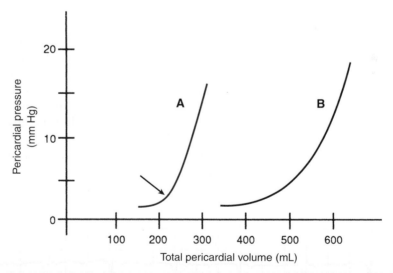

Figure 14-2. Schematic representation of the volume-pressure relationship of normal pericardium. A. At the lowest levels, a small rise in volume results in a small rise in pressure. However, when the limits of pericardial stretch are reached (*arrow*), the curve becomes very steep, and a further small rise in intrapericardial volume results in significantly increased pressure. **B.** Chronic slow accumulation of volume allows the pericardium to gradually stretch over time; thus, the curve shifts to the right, and much larger volumes are accommodated at lower pressures. (Modified from Freeman GL, LeWinter MM. Pericardial adaptations during chronic dilation in dogs. *Circ Res.* 1984;54:294.)

TABLE 14-4	Clinical Features of Large Pericardial Effusion
Soft heart sounds	
Reduced intensity of friction rub	
Ewart sign (dullness over posterior left lung)	

curve shifts toward the right (see Fig. 14-2, curve B). With this adaptation, the pericardium can accommodate larger volumes without marked elevation of intrapericardial pressure.

CLINICAL FEATURES

A spectrum of possible symptoms is associated with pericardial effusions. For example, the patient with a large effusion may be asymptomatic, may complain of a dull constant ache in the left side of the chest, or may present with findings of cardiac tamponade, as described later in the chapter. In addition, the effusion may cause symptoms resulting from compression of adjacent structures, such as dysphagia (difficulty swallowing because of esophageal compression), dyspnea (shortness of breath resulting from lung compression), hoarseness (due to recurrent laryngeal nerve compression), or hiccups (resulting from phrenic nerve stimulation).

On examination (Table 14-4), a large pericardial fluid "insulates" the heart from the chest wall, and the heart sounds may be muffled. In fact, a friction rub that had been present during the acute phase of pericarditis may disappear if a large effusion develops and separates the inflamed layers from one another. Dullness to percussion of the left lung over the angle of the scapula may be present (known as the *Ewart sign*) owing to compressive atelectasis by the enlarged pericardial sac.

DIAGNOSTIC STUDIES

The *chest radiograph* may be normal if only a small pericardial effusion is present. However, if more than ~250 mL has accumulated, the cardiac silhouette enlarges in a globular, symmetric fashion. In large effusions, the ECG may demonstrate reduced voltage of the complexes. In the presence of very large effusions, the height of the QRS complex may vary from beat to beat (*electrical alternans*), a result of a constantly changing electrical axis as the heart swings from side to side within the large pericardial volume (Fig. 14-3).

One of the most useful laboratory tests in the evaluation of an effusion is *echocardiography* (Fig. 14-4), which can identify pericardial collections as small as 20 mL. This noninvasive technique can quantify the volume of pericardial fluid, determine whether

Figure 14-3. Electrical alternans. Rhythm strip of lead V_1 showing alternating height of the QRS complex from beat to beat, due to shifting of the cardiac axis as the heart swings within a large pericardial effusion.

ventricular filling is compromised, and, when necessary, help direct the placement of a pericardiocentesis needle.

TREATMENT

If the cause of the effusion is known, therapy is directed toward the underlying disorder (eg, intensive dialysis for uremic effusion). If the cause is not evident, the clinical state of the patient determines whether pericardiocentesis (removal of pericardial fluid) should be undertaken. An asymptomatic effusion, even of large volume, can be observed for long periods without specific intervention. However, if serial examination demonstrates a precipitous rise in pericardial volume or if hemodynamic compression of the cardiac chambers becomes evident, then pericardiocentesis should be performed for therapeutic drainage and for analysis of the fluid.

Figure 14-4. Two-dimensional echocardiogram (parasternal short-axis view) of a pericardial effusion (PE) surrounding the heart. LV, left ventricle.

CARDIAC TAMPONADE

At the opposite end of the spectrum from the asymptomatic pericardial effusion is cardiac tamponade. In this condition, pericardial fluid accumulates under high pressure, compresses the cardiac chambers, and severely limits filling of the heart. As a result, ventricular stroke volume and cardiac output decline, potentially leading to hypotension, shock, and death.

ETIOLOGY

Any etiology of acute pericarditis (see Table 14-1) can progress to cardiac tamponade, but the most common causes are neoplastic, postviral, and uremic pericarditis. Acute hemorrhage into the pericardium is also an important cause of tamponade, which can result (1) from blunt or penetrating chest trauma, (2) from rupture of the left ventricular (LV) free wall following MI (see Chapter 7), or (3) as a complication of a dissecting aortic aneurysm (see Chapter 15).

PATHOPHYSIOLOGY

As a result of the surrounding tense pericardial fluid, the heart is compressed, and *the diastolic pressure within each chamber becomes elevated and equal to the pericardial pressure*. The pathophysiologic consequences of this are illustrated in Figure 14-5. Because the compromised cardiac chambers cannot accommodate normal venous return, the systemic and pulmonary venous pressures rise. The increase of systemic venous pressure results in signs of right-sided heart failure (eg, jugular venous distention), whereas elevated pulmonary venous pressure leads to pulmonary congestion. In addition, reduced filling of the ventricles during diastole decreases the systolic stroke volume, and the cardiac output declines.

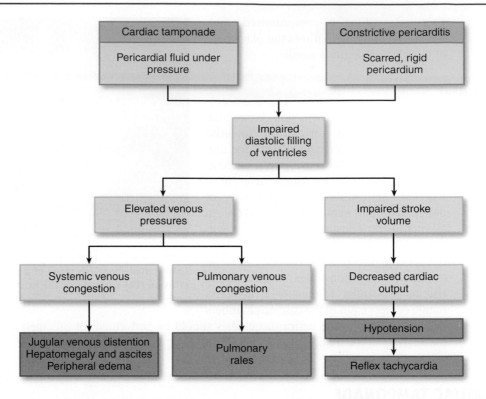

Figure 14-5. Pathophysiology of cardiac tamponade and constrictive pericarditis. The symptoms and signs (*orange boxes*) arise from impaired diastolic filling of the ventricles in both conditions.

These derangements trigger compensatory mechanisms aimed at maintaining tissue perfusion, initially through activation of the sympathetic nervous system (eg, increased heart rate and contractility). Nonetheless, failure to evacuate the effusion leads to inadequate perfusion of vital organs, shock, and ultimately death.

CLINICAL FEATURES

Cardiac tamponade should be suspected in any patient with known pericarditis, pericardial effusion, or chest trauma who develops signs and symptoms of systemic vascular congestion and decreased cardiac output (Table 14-5). The key physical findings include (1) jugular venous distention, (2) systemic hypotension, and (3) a "small, quiet heart" on physical examination, a result of the insulating effects of the effusion. Other signs include sinus tachycardia and pulsus paradoxus (described later). Dyspnea and tachypnea reflect pulmonary congestion and decreased oxygen delivery to peripheral tissues.

If tamponade develops suddenly, symptoms of profound hypotension are evident, including confusion and agitation. However, if the effusion develops more slowly, over a period of

TABLE 14-5 Clinical Features of Cardiac Tamponade
Jugular venous distention
Hypotension with pulsus paradoxus
Quiet precordium on palpation
Sinus tachycardia

Box 14-1	Measurement of Pulsus Paradoxus at the Bedside

Pulsus paradoxus is an exaggeration of the normal decline in systolic blood pressure that occurs with inspiration. It can be measured at the bedside using a manual sphygmomanometer. First, inflate the sphygmomanometer to a level greater than the patient's systolic pressure. As the cuff is slowly deflated, carefully listen for the appearance of the first Korotkoff sounds. This level marks the maximum systolic pressure and occurs during expiration. If the pressure is held at that level (ie, if you stop deflating the cuff) in a patient with pulsus paradoxus, the Korotkoff sounds will drift in and out, audible with expiration, and absent with inspiration. That is, the systolic pressure will fall during inspiration to a level below the cuff's pressure, and no sound will be heard during that time. Next, slowly deflate the cuff and continue listening. When the cuff pressure falls to the level just below the patient's systolic pressure during inspiration, the Korotkoff sounds stop drifting in and out (ie, they are audible during both inspiration and expiration). Pulsus paradoxus is calculated as the difference between the initial systolic pressure (when the intermittent Korotkoff sounds are first heard) and this pressure (when the sounds are first audible throughout the respiratory cycle). In the presence of cardiac tamponade, this pressure difference is >10 mm Hg.

weeks, then fatigue (caused by low cardiac output) and peripheral edema (owing to right-sided heart failure) may be the presenting complaints.

Pulsus paradoxus is an important physical sign in cardiac tamponade that can be recognized at the bedside using a standard blood pressure cuff. It refers to a *decrease of systolic blood pressure >10 mm Hg during normal inspiration* (see Box 14-1).

Pulsus paradoxus is not really "paradoxical"; it is just an exaggeration of appropriate cardiac physiology. Normally, expansion of the thorax during inspiration causes the intrathoracic pressure to become more negative compared with the expiratory phase. This facilitates systemic venous return of blood to the chest and augments filling of the right ventricle (RV). The transient increase in RV size shifts the interventricular septum toward the left, which diminishes LV filling. As a result, in normal persons, LV stroke volume and systolic blood pressure decline slightly following inspiration.

In cardiac tamponade, this situation is exaggerated because both ventricles share a reduced, fixed volume as a result of external compression by the tense pericardial fluid. In this case, the inspiratory increase of RV volume and bulging of the interventricular septum toward the left have a proportionally greater effect on the limitation of LV filling. Thus, in tamponade, there is a more substantial reduction of LV stroke volume (and therefore systolic blood pressure) following inspiration.

Pulsus paradoxus may also be manifested by other conditions in which inspiration is exaggerated, including severe asthma and chronic obstructive airway disease.

DIAGNOSTIC STUDIES

Echocardiography is highly useful to evaluate whether pericardial effusion has led to cardiac tamponade physiology. A very important indicator of high-pressure pericardial fluid is compression and collapse of the RV during diastole (see Fig. 3-12). In addition, echocardiography can differentiate between cardiac tamponade and other causes of low cardiac output, such as ventricular contractile dysfunction. The definitive diagnostic procedure for cardiac tamponade is *cardiac catheterization* with measurement of intracardiac and intrapericardial pressures, usually combined with therapeutic *pericardiocentesis*, as described in the next section.

TREATMENT

Removal of the high-pressure pericardial fluid is the only intervention that reverses the life-threatening physiology of this condition. Pericardiocentesis is best performed in the cardiac catheterization laboratory, where the hemodynamic effect of fluid removal can be assessed. The patient is positioned head up at a 45-degree angle to promote pooling of the effusion, and a needle is inserted into the pericardial space through the skin, usually just below the xiphoid process (which is the safest location to avoid piercing a coronary artery). A catheter is then threaded into the pericardial space and connected to a transducer for pressure measurement. Another catheter is passed through a systemic vein into the right side of the heart, and simultaneous recordings of intracardiac and intrapericardial pressures are compared. In tamponade, the pericardial pressure is elevated and is equal to the diastolic pressures within all of the cardiac chambers, reflecting the compressive force of the surrounding effusion.

In addition, the right atrial pressure tracing, which is equivalent to the jugular venous pulsation observed on physical examination, displays a characteristic abnormality (Fig. 14-6). During early diastole in a normal person, as the RV pressure falls and the tricuspid valve opens, blood quickly flows from the right atrium into the RV, leading to a rapid decline in the right atrial pressure (the y descent). In tamponade, however, the pericardial fluid compresses the RV and prevents its rapid expansion. Thus, the right atrium cannot empty quickly, and the y descent is blunted.

Following successful pericardiocentesis, the pericardial pressure falls to normal and is no longer equal to the diastolic pressures within the heart chambers, which also decline to their appropriate levels. After initial aspiration of fluid, the pericardial catheter may be left in place for 1-2 days to allow more complete drainage.

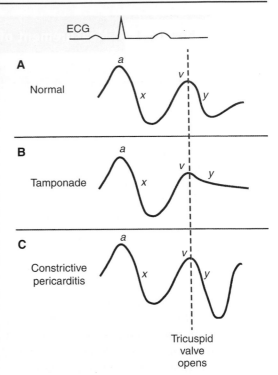

Figure 14-6. Schematic diagrams of right atrial (or jugular venous) pressure recordings. A. Normal. The initial a wave represents atrial contraction. The v wave reflects passive filling of the atrium during systole, when the tricuspid valve is closed. After the tricuspid valve opens, the right atrial pressure falls (y descent) as blood empties into the right ventricle. B. Cardiac tamponade. High-pressure pericardial fluid compresses the heart, impairing right ventricular filling, so that the y descent is blunted. C. Constrictive pericarditis. The *earliest* phase of diastolic filling is not impaired so that the y descent is not blunted. The y descent appears accentuated because it descends from a higher-than-normal right atrial pressure. The right atrial c wave (described in Chapter 2) is not shown.

When peripardial fluid is obtained for diagnostic purposes, it should be stained and cultured for bacteria, fungi, and acid-fast bacilli (tuberculosis), and cytologic examination should be performed to evaluate for malignancy. Other common measurements of pericardial fluid include cell counts (eg, white cell count is elevated in bacterial infections and other inflammatory conditions) and protein and lactate dehydrogenase levels. If the concentration ratio of pericardial protein to serum protein is >0.5, or that of pericardial LDH to serum LDH is >0.6, then the fluid is consistent with an exudate; otherwise, it is more likely a transudate. When tuberculosis is suspected, it is also useful to measure the level of adenosine deaminase in the pericardial fluid. Studies have indicated that an elevated level is highly sensitive and specific for tuberculosis.

If cardiac tamponade recurs following pericardiocentesis, the procedure can be repeated. In some cases, more definitive surgical treatment (removal of part or all of the pericardium) is required to prevent reaccumulation of the effusion.

CONSTRICTIVE PERICARDITIS

The other major potential complication of pericardial diseases is constrictive pericarditis. This is a condition not frequently encountered but is important to understand, because it can masquerade as other more common disorders. In addition, it is an affliction that may cause profound symptoms yet is often fully correctable if recognized.

ETIOLOGY AND PATHOGENESIS

In the early part of the 20th century, tuberculosis was the major cause of constrictive pericarditis but that is much less common today in industrialized societies. The most frequent cause now is "idiopathic" (ie, months to years following presumed idiopathic or viral acute pericarditis). However, any etiology of pericarditis can lead to this complication, including prior radiation therapy to the left side of the chest.

PATHOLOGY

Following an episode of acute pericarditis, any pericardial effusion that has accumulated usually undergoes gradual resorption. However, in patients who later develop constrictive pericarditis, the fluid undergoes organization, with subsequent fusion of the pericardial layers, followed by fibrous scar formation. In some patients, calcification of the adherent layers ensues, further stiffening the pericardium.

PATHOPHYSIOLOGY

The pathophysiologic abnormalities in constrictive pericarditis occur during diastole; systolic contraction of the ventricles is usually normal. In this condition, a rigid, scarred pericardium encircles the heart and *inhibits normal filling of the cardiac chambers*. For example, as blood passes from the right atrium into the RV during diastole, the RV size expands and quickly reaches the limit imposed by the constricting pericardium. At that point, further filling is suddenly arrested, and venous return to the right heart ceases. Thus, systemic venous pressure rises, and signs of right-sided heart failure ensue. In addition, the impaired filling of the left ventricle causes a reduction in stroke volume and cardiac output, which leads to lower blood pressure.

CLINICAL FEATURES

The symptoms and signs of constrictive pericarditis usually develop over months to years. They result from (1) elevated systemic venous pressure (jugular venous distention, hepatomegaly with ascites, and peripheral edema) and (2) reduced cardiac output (fatigue, hypotension, and reflex tachycardia). Because the most impressive physical findings are often the insidious development of hepatomegaly and ascites, patients may be mistakenly suspected of having hepatic cirrhosis or an intra-abdominal tumor. However, careful inspection of the elevated jugular veins can point to the correct diagnosis of constrictive pericarditis.

On cardiac examination, an early diastolic "knock" may follow the second heart in patients with severe calcific constriction. It represents the sudden cessation of ventricular diastolic filling imposed by the rigid pericardial sac.

In contrast to cardiac tamponade, pericardial constriction results in pulsus paradoxus less frequently. Recall that in tamponade, this finding reflects inspiratory augmentation of RV filling, at the expense of LV filling. However, in constrictive pericarditis, the negative intrathoracic pressure generated by inspiration is not easily transmitted through the rigid pericardial shell to the right-sided heart chambers; therefore, inspiratory augmentation of RV filling is more limited. Rather, when a patient with severe pericardial constriction inhales, the negative intrathoracic pressure draws blood toward the thorax, where it cannot be accommodated by the constricted right-sided cardiac chambers. As a result, the increased venous return accumulates in the intrathoracic systemic veins, causing the jugular veins to become more distended during inspiration (**Kussmaul sign**). This is the opposite of normal physiology, in which inspiration results in a *decline* in jugular venous pressure, as venous return is drawn into the heart. Thus, typical findings in pericardial disease can be summarized as follows:

	Constrictive Pericarditis	Cardiac Tamponade
Pulsus paradoxus	+	+++
Kussmaul sign	+++	−

DIAGNOSTIC STUDIES

The *chest radiograph* in constrictive pericarditis shows a normal or mildly enlarged cardiac silhouette. Calcification of the pericardium can be detected in some patients with severe chronic constriction. The ECG generally shows nonspecific ST and T-wave abnormalities; atrial arrhythmias are common.

Echocardiographic evidence of constriction is subtle. The pericardium, if well imaged, is thickened. The ventricular cavities are small and contract vigorously, but ventricular filling terminates abruptly in early diastole, as the chambers reach the limit imposed by the surrounding rigid shell. Aberrant diastolic motion of the interventricular septum, and alterations of LV inflow velocities during respiration assessed by Doppler, also reflect the abnormal pattern of diastolic filling.

Computed tomography or *magnetic resonance imaging* is superior to echocardiography in the assessment of pericardial anatomy and thickness. The presence of normal pericardial thickness (<2 mm) by these modalities makes constrictive pericarditis a much less likely diagnosis.

The diagnosis of constrictive pericarditis can be confirmed by *cardiac catheterization*, which reveals four key features:

1. Elevation and equalization of the diastolic pressures in each of the cardiac chambers.
2. An early diastolic "dip and plateau" configuration in the RV and LV tracings (Fig. 14-7). This pattern reflects blood flow into the ventricles at the very onset of diastole, just after the tricuspid and mitral valves open, followed by sudden cessation of filling as further expansion of the ventricles is arrested by the surrounding rigid pericardium.

Figure 14-7. Schematic tracings of left ventricular (LV) and right ventricular (RV) pressures in a normal heart (A) and in constrictive pericarditis (B). In the latter situation, early diastolic ventricular filling abruptly halts as the volume in each ventricle quickly reaches the limit imposed by the constricting pericardium. Throughout most of diastole, the LV and RV pressures are abnormally elevated and equal.

3. A prominent *y* descent in the right atrial pressure tracing (see Fig. 14-6). After the tricuspid valve opens, the right atrium quickly empties into the RV (and its pressure rapidly falls) during the very brief period before filling is arrested. This is in contrast to cardiac tamponade, in which the external compressive force throughout the cardiac cycle *prevents* rapid ventricular filling, even in early diastole, such that the *y* descent is blunted.

4. During the respiratory cycle, there is discordance in the RV and LV *systolic* pressures (the RV systolic pressure rises with inspiration, while that of the LV declines). This is explained as follows: in normal persons, the negative intrathoracic pressure induced by inspiration causes the systolic pressure of both ventricles to decline slightly. In contrast, in constrictive pericarditis, the heart is isolated from the rest of the thorax by the surrounding rigid shell. In this circumstance, negative intrathoracic pressure induced by inspiration decreases the pressure in the pulmonary veins but not in the left-sided cardiac chambers. This causes a decline in the pressure gradient driving blood back to the left side of the heart from the pulmonary veins, such that left ventricle filling is diminished. Less ventricular filling reduces the stroke volume and results in a *lower* LV systolic pressure (and is the likely mechanism of pulsus paradoxus in some patients with constrictive pericarditis). Simultaneously, because the two ventricles share a fixed space limited by the rigid pericardium, the reduced LV volume allows the interventricular septum to shift toward the left, which enlarges the RV (this reciprocal behavior is termed *ventricular interdependence*). The subsequent increase in RV filling *augments* RV systolic pressure during inspiration. During expiration, the situation is reversed, with the RV systolic pressure declining and that of the LV increasing.

The clinical and hemodynamic findings of constrictive pericarditis are similar to those of the restrictive cardiomyopathies (described in Chapter 10), and features that distinguish these syndromes are summarized in Table 14-6. A transvenous myocardial biopsy is sometimes necessary to differentiate between these conditions (biopsy results are normal in constriction but usually abnormal in restrictive cardiomyopathies; see Chapter 10).

TABLE 14-6 Constrictive Pericarditis vs Restrictive Cardiomyopathy

Feature	Constrictive Pericarditis	Restrictive Cardiomyopathy
Chest radiography • Pericardial calcifications	Yes (25%-30% of patients)	Absent
CT or MRI • Thickened pericardium	Yes	No
Echocardiography • Thickened pericardium	Yes (but difficult to visualize)	No
• Respiratory cycle effect on transvalvular Doppler velocities	Exaggerated variations	Normal
Cardiac catheterization • Equalized LV and RV diastolic pressures	Yes	Often, LV > RV
• Elevated PA systolic pressure	Uncommon	Common
• Effect of inspiration on systolic pressures	Discordant: LV↓, RV↑	Concordant: LV↓, RV↓
Endomyocardial biopsy	Normal	Abnormal (eg, amyloid)

CT, computed tomography; LV, left ventricle; MRI, magnetic resonance imaging; PA, pulmonary artery; RV, right ventricle.

TREATMENT

The only effective treatment of severe constrictive pericarditis is surgical removal of the pericardium. Symptoms and signs of constriction may not resolve immediately after surgery because of the associated stiffness of the neighboring outer wall of the heart, but subsequent clinical improvement is the rule in patients with otherwise intact cardiac function. The degree of improvement depends on the underlying etiology, with the most favorable outcomes in patients with an idiopathic/postviral pericarditis origin, and the least favorable benefit when prior radiation therapy is the cause.

Summary

- **Acute pericarditis** is characterized by three stages: (1) local vasodilation with transudation of protein-poor, cell-free fluid into the pericardial space; (2) increased vascular permeability, with leak of protein into the pericardial space; and (3) leukocyte exudation, initially by neutrophils, followed later by mononuclear cells.
- Acute pericarditis is most often of **idiopathic or viral cause** and is usually a self-limited illness.
- Common **clinical findings in acute pericarditis** include pleuritic chest pain, fever, pericardial friction rub, and diffuse ST-segment elevation on the ECG, often accompanied by PR-segment depression.
- **Treatment of common acute pericarditis** (ie, viral or idiopathic pericarditis) consists of a nonsteroidal anti-inflammatory drug; the addition of colchicine may reduce the frequency of recurrences and shorten the duration of the acute illness.
- **Glucocorticoid drugs should not be used as initial therapy** for acute pericarditis as they increase the likelihood of recurrences.
- Complications of pericarditis include **cardiac tamponade** (accumulation of pericardial fluid under high pressure, which compresses the cardiac chambers) and **constrictive pericarditis** (restricted filling of the heart because of the surrounding rigid pericardium).

Review Questions

1. A 45-year-old previously healthy woman presents to the emergency department with fever and pleuritic anterior chest pain. Her blood pressure is 120/78 and the heart rate is 104 and regular. There is no jugular venous distention. The lungs are clear to auscultation. On cardiac auscultation there is a pericardial friction rub. The electrocardiogram shows sinus tachycardia and ST elevation in most of the leads. Echocardiography demonstrates a small posterior pericardial effusion without cardiac chamber compression. Which of the following is correct?

   a. A bacterial etiology is most likely responsible for this condition.
   b. Kussmaul sign is an expected physical finding.
   c. Corticosteroid therapy is indicated to prevent progression of the effusion.
   d. Depression of the PR segment in several ECG leads would support the diagnosis of acute pericarditis.

2. Which of the following physical findings is typical in a patient with acute pericarditis who has developed cardiac tamponade?

a. Marked hypertension
b. Pericardial knock
c. Inspiratory fall in systolic blood pressure >10 mm Hg
d. Louder pericardial friction rub

3. A 56-year-old man presents for evaluation because of progressive exertional dyspnea in recent weeks. He is found to have marked jugular venous distention with Kussmaul sign, clear lungs, and bilateral ankle edema. His blood pressure is 110/74 without pulsus paradoxus. Echocardiography shows normal left and right ventricular contractile function and no pericardial effusion. He has a history of Hodgkin lymphoma 25 years ago, treated with chemotherapy and mediastinal radiation therapy. Which of the following statements is correct?

a. Prior chemotherapy is likely responsible for these findings.
b. CT imaging will likely demonstrate increased pericardial thickness.
c. Treatment should consist of an angiotensin converting-enzyme inhibitor and beta-blocker.
d. Cardiac catheterization would show much higher left ventricular diastolic pressures than right ventricular diastolic pressures.

Answers to Review Questions

1. Choice d is correct. This patient presents with symptoms, signs, and ECG findings of acute pericarditis. In addition to the typical finding of diffuse ST-segment elevation on the ECG, deviation of the PR segment is also often present, reflecting atrial epicardial inflammation. The most common infectious causes of acute pericarditis are viral, not bacterial. Kussmaul sign (abnormal inspiratory augmentation of the jugular venous pressure) is characteristic of pericardial constriction, not acute pericarditis. Appropriate therapies for acute idiopathic or viral pericarditis include nonsteroidal anti-inflammatory therapy and colchicine. Corticosteroids should be avoided in uncomplicated cases, as such therapy is associated with an increased frequency of pericarditis recurrences.

2. Choice c is correct. Pulsus paradoxus, an inspiratory fall in systolic blood pressure >10 mm Hg, is a helpful diagnostic feature in patients with cardiac tamponade. It is thought to arise from exaggerated inspiratory augmentation of right ventricular filling at the expense of LV filling. Patients with tamponade are often hypotensive. Any prior pericardial friction rub may soften, as the typically large pericardial effusion in cardiac tamponade separates the inflamed pericardial layers from one another, reducing their rub-producing interaction.

3. Choice b is correct. The history and examination are consistent with constrictive pericarditis, including jugular venous distention with Kussmaul sign (abnormal inspiratory augmentation of jugular venous pressure), and prior mediastinal radiation therapy is the likely cause. While imaging of the pericardium is often difficult by echocardiography, CT or magnetic resonance imaging shows increased pericardial thickening in a large majority of patients with this condition. Cardiac catheterization would show elevation and equalization of the right and left ventricular diastolic pressures. Angiotensin converting-enzyme inhibition and beta-blocker therapies improve symptoms and outcomes in patients with heart failure with reduced ejection fraction, but that is not present by echocardiography in this patient.

Acknowledgments

Contributors to previous editions of this chapter were Yin Ren, MD; Yanerys Ramos, MD; Thomas G. Roberts, MD; Angela Fowler, MD; Kathy Glatter, MD; and Alan Braverman, MD.

Additional Reading

Adler Y, Charron P, Imazio M, et al. 2015 ESC Guidelines for the diagnosis and management of pericardial diseases: the task force for the Diagnosis and Management of Pericardial Diseases of the European Society of Cardiology (ESC). *Eur Heart J.* 2015;36:2921-2964.

Altan M, Toki MI, Gettinger SN, et al. Immune checkpoint inhibitor-associated pericarditis. *J Thorac Oncol.* 2019;14:1102-1108.

Chiabrando JG, Bonaventura A, Vecchié A, et al. Management of acute and recurrent pericarditis. JACC state of the art review. *J Am Coll Cardiol.* 2020; 75:76-92.

Garcia MJ. Constrictive pericarditis versus restrictive cardiomyopathy? *J Am Coll Cardiol.* 2016;67:2061-2076.

Herzog E, ed. *Management of Pericardial Disease.* London, UK: Springer-Verlag; 2014.

Imazio M, Gaita F, LeWinter M. Evaluation and treatment of pericarditis: a systematic review. *JAMA.* 2015;314:1498-1506.

Klein AL, Abbara S, Agler DA, et al. American Society of Echocardiography clinical recommendations for multimodality cardiovascular imaging of patients with pericardial disease. *J Am Soc Echocardiogr.* 2013;26:965-1012.

Lilly LS. Treatment of acute and recurrent idiopathic pericarditis. *Circulation.* 2013;127:1723-1726.

15

Diseases of the Peripheral Vasculature

Stanislav Henkin | Mark A. Creager

Peripheral vascular disease is an umbrella term that includes a number of diverse pathologic entities that affect the arteries, veins, and lymphatics. Although this terminology makes a distinction between the "central" coronary and "peripheral" systemic vessels, the vasculature as a whole constitutes a dynamic, integrated, and multifunctional organ system that does not naturally comply with this semantic division.

Blood vessels serve many critical functions. First, they regulate the differential distribution of blood and delivery of nutrients and oxygen to tissues. Second, blood vessels actively synthesize and secrete vasoactive substances that regulate vascular tone, as well as antithrombotic substances that maintain the fluidity of blood and vessel patency (see Chapters 6 and 7). Third, the vessels play an integral role in the transport and distribution of immune cells to traumatized or infected tissues. Disease states of the peripheral vasculature interfere with these essential functions.

Peripheral vascular diseases result from processes that can be grouped into three categories: (1) *structural changes in the vessel wall* secondary to degenerative conditions, infection, or inflammation that lead to dilatation, aneurysm, dissection, or rupture; (2) *narrowing of the vascular lumen* caused by atherosclerosis, thrombosis, or inflammation; and (3) *spasm of* vascular smooth muscle. These processes can occur in isolation or in combination.

DISEASES OF THE AORTA

The aorta is the largest conductance vessel of the vascular system. In adults, its diameter is ~3 cm at its origin at the base of the heart. The **ascending aorta**, 5-6 cm in length, leads to the **aortic arch**, from which arise three major branches: the brachiocephalic trunk (which bifurcates into the right common carotid and subclavian arteries), the left common carotid, and the left subclavian arteries. In about 10% of people, there is variation in the anatomy of the aortic arch (eg, the left common carotid artery originates from the brachiocephalic trunk). As the **descending aorta** continues beyond the arch, its diameter narrows to ~2-2.5 cm in healthy adults. As the aorta pierces the diaphragm, it becomes the **abdominal aorta**, providing arteries to the abdominal viscera before bifurcating into the left and right common iliac arteries, which supply the pelvic organs and lower extremities.

The aorta, like other arteries, is composed of three layers (see Fig. 5-1). At the luminal surface, the *intima* consists of endothelial cells overlying the internal elastic lamina. The endothelial layer is a functional interface between the vasculature and circulating blood cells and plasma. The *media* is composed of smooth muscle cells and a matrix that includes collagen and elastic fibers. Collagen provides tensile strength that enables the vessels to withstand high-pressure loads. Elastin is capable of stretching to 250% of its original length and confers a distensible quality on vessels that allows them to recoil under pressure. The *adventitia* is composed primarily of collagen fibers, perivascular nerves, and vasa vasorum, a rich vascular network that supplies oxygenated blood to the aorta.

The aorta is subject to injury from mechanical trauma because it is continuously exposed to high pulsatile pressure and shear stress. The predominance of elastin in the media (2:1 over collagen) allows the aorta to expand during systole and recoil during diastole. The recoil of the aorta against the closed aortic valve contributes to the distal propagation of blood flow during the phase of left ventricular relaxation. With advancing age, the elastic component of the aorta and its branches degenerates, and as collagen becomes more prominent, the arteries stiffen. Systolic blood pressure (SBP), therefore, tends to rise with age because less energy is dissipated into the aorta during left ventricular contraction.

Diseases of the aorta most commonly appear as one of three clinical conditions: aneurysm, dissection, or obstruction.

Aortic Aneurysms

An aneurysm is an abnormal localized dilatation of an artery. In the aorta, aneurysms are distinguished from *diffuse ectasia*, which is a generalized and lesser increase of the aortic diameter. Ectasia develops in older patients as elastic fiber fragments, smooth muscle cells decrease in number, and acid mucopolysaccharide ground substance accumulates within the vessel wall.

The term *aneurysm* is applied when the diameter of a portion of the aorta has increased by at least 50% compared with normal. A **true aneurysm** represents a dilatation of all three layers of the aorta, creating a large bulge of the vessel wall. True aneurysms are characterized as either fusiform or saccular, depending on the extent of the vessel's circumference within the aneurysm. A *fusiform* aneurysm, the more common type, is characterized by symmetrical dilation of the entire circumference of a segment of the aorta. A *saccular* aneurysm is a localized outpouching involving only a portion of the circumference.

In contrast, a **pseudoaneurysm** (also termed **false aneurysm**) is a contained *rupture* of the vessel wall that develops when blood leaks out of the vessel lumen through a hole in the intimal and medial layers and is contained by a layer of adventitia or perivascular organized thrombus. Pseudoaneurysms develop at sites of vessel injury caused by infection or trauma, such as puncture of the vessel during surgery or percutaneous catheterization. They are very unstable and are prone to rupture completely.

Aneurysms may be confined to the abdominal aorta (most common) or the thoracic aorta or involve both locations. They may also appear in peripheral and cerebral arteries.

Etiology and Pathogenesis of True Aortic Aneurysms

The etiologies of aortic aneurysm formation include inherited genetic conditions, degenerative disorders, infections, vasculitis, aortic dissection, and trauma (Table 15-1). Aortic aneurysms caused by inherited disorders of connective tissue typically affect the *ascending thoracic aorta* and are characterized histologically by **medial degeneration**, a condition of degeneration and fragmentation of elastic fibers, with subsequent accumulation of collagenous and mucoid material within the medial layer. These genetic disorders include Marfan syndrome, Loeys-Dietz syndrome, the vascular form of Ehlers-Danlos syndrome (type IV), and familial thoracic

TABLE 15-1	**Conditions Associated with True Aortic Aneurysms**

1. Medial degeneration (usually affects ascending thoracic aorta)
   - Marfan syndrome
   - Loeys-Dietz syndrome
   - Ehlers-Danlos syndrome (type IV)
   - Bicuspid aortic valve
   - Familial
2. Atherosclerosis/degenerative (usually affects descending thoracic and abdominal aorta)
3. Infections of arterial wall
4. Vasculitis
   - Takayasu arteritis
   - Giant cell arteritis
5. Aortic dissection
6. Trauma

aortic aneurysms. *Marfan syndrome* is caused by missense mutations of the fibrillin-1 gene (FBN1), which impair formation of functional microfibrils in elastin. Abnormal fibrillin-1 also limits the binding and inactivation of transforming growth factor β (TGF-β), a signaling molecule that regulates cellular proliferation and differentiation. *Loeys-Dietz syndrome* is an autosomal dominant disorder caused by genetic mutations of TGF-β receptors. While thoracic aortic aneurysms have been associated with both increased activity of TGF-β and mutations of its receptors, the mechanism by which aberrant TGF-β signaling alters vascular integrity is not yet known. *Ehlers-Danlos type IV* syndrome results from mutations encoding type III procollagen. *Familial thoracic aortic aneurysms* may be caused by mutations of the TGF-β receptor or SMAD3 (gene that encodes a protein involved in TGF-β binding), as well as of genes encoding the smooth muscle–specific alpha-actin (ACTA2), the beta-myosin heavy chain (MYH11), and myosin light chain kinase (MYLK), which are essential components of the contractile complex in vascular smooth muscle cells. Medial degeneration also characterizes the form of thoracic aortic aneurysm associated with bicuspid aortic valves.

Aneurysms of the *descending thoracic* and *abdominal aorta* are usually associated with degenerative disorders including **atherosclerosis** and its risk factors (smoking, hypertension, dyslipidemia, male gender, advanced age). However, it is unlikely that atherosclerosis alone is responsible for such aneurysm development. Rather, other important pathophysiologic mechanisms include a genetic predisposition, local vessel inflammation, and an imbalance between synthesis and degradation of extracellular matrix proteins. For example, specific proteases (eg, elastase, collagenase) and matrix metalloproteinases derived from inflammatory cells and vascular endothelial and smooth muscle cells may contribute to the breakdown of elastin and collagen. Aneurysm formation is also associated with markers of inflammation, including C-reactive protein (CRP) and cytokines such as interleukin-6 (IL-6). Levels of both CRP and IL-6 have been shown to correlate with the size of aneurysms and inflammatory cells such as B and T lymphocytes and macrophages are frequently found on histologic examination. Angiotensin II, via its effect on inflammation and oxidative stress, has also been implicated in experimental models of abdominal aortic aneurysms.

Infrequent causes of aortic aneurysms include weakness of the media from infections of the vessel wall by *Salmonella* species, staphylococci, streptococci, tuberculosis, syphilis, or fungi. Inflammatory diseases such as Takayasu arteritis or giant cell arteritis (both described later in the chapter) may similarly weaken the vessel and result in aneurysm formation. Aortic dissection (described below) and traumatic injury may each weaken the aortic wall and cause aneurysm formation.

Clinical Presentation and Diagnosis

Most aneurysms are asymptomatic, though some patients, especially those with abdominal aortic aneurysms, may be aware of a pulsatile mass. Others present with symptoms related to compression of neighboring structures by an expanding aneurysm. Thoracic aortic aneurysms may compress the trachea or mainstem bronchus, resulting in cough, dyspnea, or pneumonia. Compression of the esophagus can result in dysphagia, and involvement of the recurrent laryngeal nerve may lead to hoarseness. Aneurysms of the ascending aorta may dilate the aortic ring, resulting in aortic regurgitation and symptoms of congestive heart failure. Abdominal aortic aneurysms may cause abdominal or back pain or nonspecific gastrointestinal symptoms.

Aortic aneurysms are often first suspected when dilatation of the vessel is observed on chest or abdominal radiographs, particularly if the wall is calcified. Aneurysms of the abdominal aorta or of the large peripheral arteries may also be discovered by careful palpation during physical examination. The diagnosis is confirmed by ultrasonography, contrast-enhanced computed tomography (CT), or magnetic resonance (MR) imaging (Fig. 15-1).

The most devastating consequence of an aortic aneurysm is rupture, which can be fatal. An aneurysm may leak slowly or burst suddenly, resulting in profound blood loss and hypotension. Thoracic aortic aneurysms may rupture into the pleural space, mediastinum, or bronchi. Abdominal aortic aneurysms may rupture into the retroperitoneal space or abdominal cavity or erode into the intestines, resulting in massive gastrointestinal bleeding.

Natural history studies have shown that the risk of rupture is related to the size of the aneurysm, as predicted by the Laplace relationship (ie, wall tension is proportional to the product of pressure and radius). The mean rates of thoracic and abdominal aortic aneurysms expansion

Figure 15-1. Abdominal aortic aneurysm. Computed tomographic angiogram (CTA) of an abdominal aortic aneurysm, indicated by the *green arrow*. (Courtesy of Frank Rybicki, MD, Brigham and Women's Hospital, Boston, MA.)

are 0.1 and 0.4 cm/year, respectively. Thoracic aneurysms rupture at an annual rate of 2% for aneurysms <5 cm in diameter, 3% for aneurysms 5-5.9 cm, and 7% for aneurysms >6 cm. Abdominal aneurysms <4, 4-4.9, and 5-5.9 cm have annual rates of rupture of 0.3%, 1.5%, and 6.5%, respectively. Abdominal aneurysms >6 cm have a markedly higher risk of rupture.

To identify abdominal aortic aneurysms among those at highest risk for its occurrence, the U.S. Preventive Services Task Force (USPSTF) recommends a one-time ultrasound screening for men between the ages of 65 and 75, if they have ever smoked. There is less evidence to recommend similar screening for women or men who have never smoked.

Treatment

Treatment of an aortic aneurysm is based on its size and the patient's overall medical condition and comorbidities. Once an aneurysm is identified, its dimensions should be closely monitored through repeated imaging, typically every 6-12 months depending on size and rate of growth. In general, surgical treatment is considered for ascending aortic aneurysms >5.5-6.0 cm. Ascending aortic aneurysms in patients with Marfan and Loeys-Dietz syndromes (in whom the risk of rupture is greater) should be considered for surgical repair if the diameter is ≥5 and ≥4.5 cm, respectively. Surgical or endovascular repair is generally recommended for descending thoracic and abdominal aortic aneurysms measuring 5.5 cm or more and for smaller aneurysms that enlarge at a rate >1.0 cm/year.

The mortality associated with elective surgical repair of thoracic aortic aneurysms is 3%-5%. Patients are maintained on cardiopulmonary bypass as the aneurysm is resected and replaced with a prosthetic Dacron graft. Patients with aneurysms involving multiple aortic segments have staged repairs, in which one segment is corrected at a time. Some patients with descending thoracic and thoracoabdominal (involving both thoracic and abdominal aortic segments) aortic aneurysms may be candidates for minimally invasive repair, in which an endovascular stent graft is positioned across the aneurysm. Although there are no randomized trials that compare surgical vs endovascular repair for descending thoracic and thoracoabdominal aortic aneurysms, observational data suggests lower short-term morbidity and mortality, but higher risk of future reinterventions, in the endovascular group.

Surgical repair of abdominal aortic aneurysms involves placement of a prosthetic graft. The operative mortality for such procedures at high-volume institutions is 1%-2%. Percutaneous endovascular repair of infrarenal abdominal aortic aneurysms with stent grafts can be performed in selected patients with less acute morbidity and mortality, and long-term results are similar to that of surgical repair.

Medical management, including risk factor reduction (eg, smoking cessation, treatment of hypertension), is recommended for patients with aneurysms of any size. Given that abdominal aortic aneurysm is considered an atherosclerotic coronary heart disease equivalent, initiation of aspirin and statin therapy is generally recommended. β-Blockers and angiotensin II receptor antagonists (which lower blood pressure and also inhibit TGF-β), may reduce the expansion rate of thoracic aortic aneurysms in patients with Marfan syndrome; it is not clear whether they are effective for other causes or types of aneurysms.

AORTIC DISSECTION

Aortic dissection is a life-threatening condition in which blood from the vessel lumen passes through a tear in the intima into the medial layer and spreads along the artery. Other related acute syndromes include aortic intramural hematoma, penetrating aortic ulcer, and aortic rupture. *Acute intramural hematoma* is a variant of aortic dissection characterized by a hemorrhage in the wall of the aorta without evidence of an intimal tear. A *penetrating atherosclerotic ulcer* results from erosion of a plaque into the aortic wall. *Aortic rupture* may be a complication of aortic dissection, intramural hematoma, penetrating atherosclerotic ulcer, or result from trauma.

Etiology, Pathogenesis, and Classification

Aortic dissection arises from a circumferential or transverse tear in the intimal layer of the vessel wall that allows blood from the lumen, under the driving force of systemic pressure, to enter into the media and propagate along the plane of the muscle layer. Another potential origin of aortic dissection is rupture of vasa vasorum with hemorrhage into the media, forming a hematoma in the arterial wall that subsequently tears through the intima and into the vessel's lumen.

Any condition that interferes with the normal integrity of the elastic or muscular components of the medial layer can predispose to aortic dissection. Such degeneration may arise from chronic hypertension, aging, and/or medial degeneration (which, as described earlier, is a feature of certain hereditary connective tissue disorders, such as Marfan syndrome and Ehlers-Danlos syndrome). In addition, traumatic insult to the aorta (eg, blunt chest trauma or accidental vessel damage during intra-arterial catheterization or cardiac surgery) can also initiate dissection.

Aortic dissection is most common in the sixth and seventh decades and occurs more frequently in men. More than two-thirds of patients have a history of hypertension. Dissection most commonly involves the ascending thoracic aorta (65%) and descending thoracic aorta (20%), while the aortic arch (10%) and abdominal aortic (5%) segments are less commonly affected.

Dissections are commonly classified into two categories (Stanford types A and B), depending on their location and extent (Fig. 15-2). In *type A dissection* (proximal dissection), the ascending aorta and/or aortic arch is involved, regardless of the site of the primary tear. A *type B dissection* (distal dissection) does not involve the ascending aorta or arch and is, therefore, confined to the descending thoracic and abdominal aorta. This distinction is important because treatment strategies and prognoses are determined by location. Proximal aortic involvement tends to be more devastating because of the potential for extension into the coronary and arch vessels, the support structures of the aortic valve, or the pericardial space. Approximately two-thirds of dissections are type A and one-third are type B. Dissections may also be classified as acute or chronic, with acute dissections presenting with symptoms of <2 weeks' duration.

Clinical Presentation and Diagnosis

The most common symptom of aortic dissection is sudden, severe pain with a "tearing" or "ripping" quality in the anterior chest (typical of type A dissections) or between the scapulae (type B dissections). The pain travels as the dissection propagates along the aorta and can radiate anywhere in the thorax or abdomen. Painless dissection is possible but uncommon (6.4% of cases).

Other symptoms relate to the catastrophic complications that can occur at the time of presentation or thereafter (Table 15-2) and include (1) rupture through the adventitia anywhere

TYPE A   **TYPE B**

Figure 15-2. Aortic dissection. Type A involves the ascending aorta, whereas type B does not. (Reprinted from Braverman AC, Thompson R, Sanchez L. Diseases of the aorta. In: Bonow RO, Mann DL, Zipes DP, et al., eds. *Braunwald's Heart Disease: A Textbook of Cardiovascular Medicine*. 9th ed. Philadelphia, PA: Elsevier; 2012.)

TABLE 15-2	**Complications of Aortic Dissection**

Rupture
    Pericardial tamponade
    Hemomediastinum
    Hemothorax (usually left-sided)

Occlusion of aortic branch vessels
    Carotid (stroke)
    Coronary (myocardial infarction)
    Splanchnic (visceral infarction)
    Renal (acute renal failure)
    Iliac, brachiocephalic, subclavian (limb ischemia)

Distortion of aortic annulus
    Aortic regurgitation

along the aorta (often into the left pleural space or pericardium); (2) occlusion of major branches of the aorta by the propagating hematoma within the vessel wall, which compresses the lumen and can result in myocardial infarction (coronary artery involvement), stroke (carotid artery involvement), visceral ischemia, renal failure, or loss of pulse in an extremity; and (3) extension into the aortic root, with disruption of the aortic valve support apparatus causing aortic regurgitation.

Several important physical findings may be present. Hypertension is frequently detected, either as an underlying cause of dissection, a result of the sympathetic nervous system response to the severe pain, or because of diminished renal vascular flow, with activation of the renin-angiotensin system. If the dissection has occluded one of the subclavian arteries, a difference in SBP between the arms is noted. Neurologic deficits may accompany dissection into the carotid vessels. If a type A dissection results in aortic regurgitation, an early diastolic murmur can be detected on auscultation. Leakage from a type A dissection into the pericardial sac may produce signs of cardiac tamponade (see Chapter 14).

The diagnosis of aortic dissection must not be delayed, because catastrophic complications or death may rapidly ensue. The confirmatory imaging techniques most useful in detecting dissection include contrast-enhanced CT, transesophageal echocardiography (TEE), MR angiography, and contrast angiography. Each of these techniques has specific advantages and disadvantages, and the decision of which to employ is guided by a hospital's local expertise. In emergency situations, CT scanning or TEE can generally be obtained rapidly and offer excellent sensitivity and specificity for the diagnosis.

Treatment

The goal of acute treatment is to arrest progression of the dissecting channel. Suspicion of acute aortic dissection warrants immediate medical therapy to reduce blood pressure (aiming for a systolic pressure of 100-120 mm Hg) and to decrease the force of left ventricular contraction and thus minimize aortic wall shear stress. Useful pharmacologic agents in this regard include β-blockers (to reduce the force of contraction and heart rate as well as to lower blood pressure) and vasodilators such as sodium nitroprusside (to rapidly reduce blood pressure). In proximal (type A) dissections, early surgical correction has been shown to improve outcomes compared with medical therapy alone. Surgical therapy involves repairing the intimal tear, suturing the edges of the false channel, and if necessary, inserting a synthetic aortic graft.

In contrast, patients with uncomplicated type B dissections are initially managed with aggressive medical therapy alone; early surgical intervention does not further improve the outcome in these patients. Surgery is indicated, however, if there is clinical evidence of propagation of the dissection, compromise of major branches of the aorta (eg, causing mesenteric ischemia), impending rupture, or ongoing pain despite control of hypertension. Percutaneous catheter-based repair with endovascular stent grafts has been used successfully in selected patients with type B dissections. The graft seals the entry site of the dissection, resulting in thrombosis of the false lumen.

PERIPHERAL ARTERY DISEASES

Peripheral artery disease (PAD) is defined by the presence of a flow-limiting lesion in an artery that provides blood supply to the limbs. The major causes of such arterial stenosis or occlusion are atherosclerosis, thromboembolism, and vasculitis. The clinical presentation of these disorders results from decreased perfusion to the affected extremity.

PERIPHERAL ATHEROSCLEROTIC VASCULAR DISEASE

Etiology and Pathogenesis

The most common cause of PAD is atherosclerosis. It is a prevalent vascular disorder, affecting ~4% of persons over the age of 40 and 15%-20% of those over the age of 70. The pathology of atherosclerotic PAD is identical to that of coronary artery disease (CAD), and the major coronary risk factors (eg, cigarette smoking, diabetes mellitus, dyslipidemia, and hypertension) are also associated with PAD. Approximately 40% of patients with PAD actually have clinically significant CAD. As a consequence of the systemic nature of atherosclerosis, patients with PAD have a twofold to fivefold increased risk of cardiovascular death compared with patients without this condition. Thus, detection of PAD is useful in identifying patients at increased risk of adverse cardiovascular events.

The pathophysiology of atherosclerotic PAD is also similar to that of CAD. Ischemia of the affected region occurs when the balance between oxygen supply and demand is upset; exercise raises the demand for blood flow in the limbs' skeletal muscle, and a stenosed or obstructed artery cannot provide an adequate supply. Rest improves symptoms as the balance between oxygen supply and demand is restored.

Recall from Chapter 6 that the degree of blood flow reduction relates closely to the extent of vessel narrowing, the length of the stenosis, and blood viscosity. The Poiseuille equation describes this relationship:

$$Q = \frac{\Delta P \pi r^4}{8 \eta L}$$

in which Q = flow, ΔP = pressure drop across the stenosis, r = vessel radius, η = blood viscosity, and L = length of stenosis. Thus, the degree of vessel narrowing by the stenosis (ie, the change in r) has the greatest impact on flow. For example, if the radius is reduced by one-half, the flow will be reduced to 1/16th of its baseline. The equation also indicates that for stenoses of the same length and radius, higher flow rates correspond to greater pressure drops across the stenoses. That is, as the flow velocity increases across a stenotic vessel, the blood turbulence results in a loss of kinetic energy. The result is a decline in perfusion pressure distal to the stenosis.

During exercise, products of skeletal muscle metabolism (eg, adenosine) act locally to dilate arterioles. The resulting decrease in vascular resistance serves to increase blood flow to the active muscle (recall that flow = pressure/resistance). In turn, the increased flow stimulates healthy arterial endothelium to release vasodilating factors such as nitric oxide, thereby increasing the radii of upstream conduit vessels. However, in PAD, obstructed arteries cannot respond to the vasodilating stimuli, thereby limiting flow increases. In addition, dysfunctional atherosclerotic endothelium does not release normal amounts of vasodilating substances (see Chapter 6). Thus, the physical properties of a stenosis and the reduced vasodilator activity imposed by diseased endothelium prevent adequate blood flow from reaching distal tissues and contribute to ischemia.

Hemodynamic changes alone cannot account for the dramatic reduction in exercise capacity experienced by PAD patients; alterations in muscle structure and function are also present. One such change is the denervation and dropout of muscle fibers, which is thought to occur as an adaptation to intermittent ischemia. The loss of such fibers can explain the reduced muscle strength and atrophy that occur in PAD patients. Even viable muscle fibers in affected limbs may show abnormalities of mitochondrial oxidative metabolism.

In summary, atherosclerotic lesions produce stenoses in peripheral conduit vessels and limit blood flow to the affected extremity. Mechanisms normally in place to compensate for increased demand, such as endogenous release of vasodilators during exercise and recruitment of microvessels, fail in the face of endothelial dysfunction and diminished flow velocity. Thus, states of increased oxygen demand are not met with adequate supply, producing limb ischemia. Adaptations to ischemia include changes in muscle fiber metabolism and muscle fiber dropout. Together, these physical and biochemical changes result in weak lower limbs that suffer ischemic discomfort during exercise. Severe peripheral atherosclerosis may reduce limb blood flow to such an extent that it cannot satisfy *resting* metabolic requirements. This results in critical limb ischemia, which may progress to tissue necrosis and gangrene that may threaten viability of the extremity.

Clinical Presentation and Diagnosis

PAD may affect the aorta or the iliac, femoral, popliteal, and tibioperoneal arteries (Fig. 15-3). Patients with PAD may therefore develop buttock, thigh, or calf discomfort precipitated by walking and relieved by rest. This classic symptom of exertional limb fatigue and pain is known as **intermittent claudication.** However, intermittent claudication occurs in only about a third of patients with PAD. Another third of patients have atypical symptoms, and the rest are asymptomatic. In severe PAD, patients may experience pain at rest, usually affecting the feet or toes. The chronically reduced blood flow in this case predisposes the extremity to ulceration, infection, and skin necrosis (Fig. 15-4). Patients who smoke or have diabetes mellitus are at high risk of these complications.

The location of claudication corresponds to the diseased artery, with the femoral and popliteal arteries being the most common sites (Table 15-3). The arteries of the upper extremities are less frequently affected, but brachiocephalic or subclavian artery disease can cause arm claudication.

Figure 15-3. An angiogram demonstrating peripheral artery disease. There is occlusion of the left femoral artery (*blue arrow*) and stenosis of the right popliteal artery (*green arrow*). Collateral vessels that circumvent areas of stenosis and occlusion are present (*red arrows*). (Courtesy of Michael L. Steigner, MD, Brigham and Women's Hospital, Boston, MA.)

A   B

Figure 15-4. Leg ulcers. A. Ulceration affecting the foot in a patient with diabetes and peripheral artery disease. (Courtesy of Christian E. Sampson, MD, Brigham and Women's Hospital, Boston, MA.) **B.** Venous insufficiency ulcer near the medial malleolus of the right leg. Notice the venous stasis pigmentation of the surrounding skin. (Courtesy of Lauren R. Bayer, PA, Brigham and Women's Hospital, Boston, MA.)

Due to the variety of symptoms in patients with PAD, a careful physical examination is of great importance. Femoral, popliteal, and pedal pulses should be palpated. Pulses are graded on a 0-2 scale (0, absent; 1, diminished; 2, normal). Reduced pulses are typically found distal to the stenotic segment. Bruits (swishing sounds auscultated over a region of turbulent blood flow) may be audible in the abdomen (because of stenoses within the mesenteric or renal arteries) or over iliac, femoral, or subclavian arterial stenoses. In patients with chronic severe ischemia, the lack of blood perfusion results in muscle atrophy, pallor, cyanotic discoloration, hair loss, and occasionally gangrene and necrosis of the foot and digits.

Ischemic ulcers resulting from PAD often begin as small traumatic wounds in areas of increased pressure or in regions prone to injury, such as the tips of the toes and the volar (bottom) surface of the foot (see Fig. 15-4A). These often painful ulcers fail to heal owing to the inadequate blood supply. Diabetic patients with peripheral sensory neuropathies are particularly susceptible to ulcers at sites of trauma or pressure from ill-fitting footwear. Ischemic ulcers can be distinguished from venous insufficiency ulcers, which develop more proximally and on the medial portion of the leg. Venous ulcers are also associated with reddish-brown pigmentation and varicose veins (see Fig. 15-4B).

TABLE 15-3 Relation of Stenotic Site to Claudication Symptoms	
Site	**Location of Claudication Symptoms**
Distal aorta or iliac arteries	Buttocks, hips, thighs, or calves
Femoral or popliteal arteries	Calves
Subclavian or axillary arteries	Arms

Box 15-1 | Measurement and Interpretation of the Ankle-Brachial Index

The ABI is the ratio of the SBP measured at the ankle to that measured at the brachial artery. To determine the ABI, the patient should lie supine for 10 minutes with the head and heels fully supported. A Doppler ultrasound probe is used to detect flow in the brachial, posterior tibial (PT), and dorsalis pedis (DP) arteries. A blood pressure cuff is placed on each arm to measure the SBP at the brachial arteries and on each of the lower calves, just above the malleoli, to measure the SBP at the PT and DP arteries. Use the higher of the PT and DP values on each side as the ankle pressure measurement. Finally, divide the ankle pressure measurement by the higher of the two brachial artery pressure measurements to determine the ABI.

A normal ABI is ≥1.0. An index ≤0.9 is diagnostic of PAD. Patients with PAD may be asymptomatic or have symptoms of intermittent claudication or rest pain. An index <0.5 is found in patients with severe PAD and critical limb ischemia.

Ankle pressure measurement using a Doppler probe at the right dorsalis pedis artery.

In the evaluation of PAD, it is helpful to measure the ratio of blood pressure in the ankles to that in the arms (termed the *ankle-brachial index* [*ABI*]) using a blood pressure cuff and a Doppler instrument to detect blood flow (Box 15-1). Other testing to assess peripheral perfusion includes limb *segmental systolic pressure measurements* (using pneumatic cuffs placed along the extremity) and *pulse volume recordings* (ie, graphical measurement of volume changes in segments of the extremity with each pulse). *Duplex ultrasonography* is a commonly used noninvasive method to visualize and assess the extent of arterial stenoses and the corresponding reductions in blood flow. Other more advanced imaging studies (eg, *MR angiography*, *CT angiography*, or intra-arterial *contrast angiography*) are obtained when revascularization procedures are planned.

Treatment

Atherosclerosis risk factor modification (eg, smoking cessation, LDL cholesterol lowering, and control of diabetes and hypertension) is important in reducing the likelihood of *coronary* events. Platelet inhibitors, such as aspirin and clopidogrel, reduce cardiovascular morbidity and mortality in patients with PAD. Low-dose rivaroxaban (an oral anticoagulant that inhibits factor Xa) in combination with aspirin reduces cardiovascular and limb events compared to aspirin alone, though is also associated with increased bleeding complications.

Specific treatment of PAD includes supportive care of the feet to prevent trauma and ulceration. Exercise, particularly walking, improves endurance in part by increasing metabolic efficiency in the skeletal muscle of the legs. A formal exercise program is considered first-line therapy in the management of PAD.

Pharmacologic therapies are sometimes useful in the treatment of claudication. For example, *cilostazol* is a selective phosphodiesterase inhibitor that increases cyclic adenosine monophosphate and has vasodilator and platelet-inhibiting properties; it has been shown to improve exercise capacity in patients with PAD. Conversely, most vasodilator drugs (see Chapter 17) are not helpful in relieving claudication. To date, clinical trials examining angiogenic growth factors and stem cell therapies have failed to show efficacy in patients with PAD.

Mechanical revascularization is indicated when medical therapy has failed for patients with disabling claudication and as first-line therapy in cases of critical limb ischemia. In advanced cases, therapy is directed at healing ischemic ulcerations and preventing limb loss. Catheter-based interventions, such as percutaneous transluminal angioplasty and stent implantation, can be performed on selected patients whose vascular anatomy is conducive to these procedures. Surgical approaches include bypass operations to circumvent the occluded arteries using saphenous vein or prosthetic grafts. However, amputation may be necessary if blood flow cannot be satisfactorily reestablished to maintain limb viability.

ACUTE ARTERIAL OCCLUSION

Acute arterial occlusion is caused either by embolization from a proximal vascular site or by thrombus formation *in situ*. The origin of arterial emboli is most often the heart, usually resulting from disorders that cause intracardiac stasis of flow, such as atrial fibrillation (Table 15-4). Emboli may also originate from thrombus or atheromatous material overlying a segment of the aorta. Rarely, arterial emboli originate from the *venous* circulation. If a venous clot travels to the right-heart chambers and is able to pass through an abnormal intracardiac communication (eg, an atrial septal defect or patent foramen ovale), it then enters the systemic arterial circulation (a condition known as **paradoxical embolism**). Primary arterial thrombus formation may appear at sites of endothelial damage or atherosclerotic stenoses, or within bypass grafts.

The extent of tissue damage from thromboembolism depends on the site of the occluded artery, the duration of occlusion, and the degree of collateral circulation serving the tissue beyond the obstruction. Common symptoms and signs that may develop from abrupt reduction in blood supply include pain, pallor, paralysis, paresthesia, and pulselessness (termed the "five *P*s"). A sixth *P*, poikilothermia (coolness), is also often manifested.

Patients with a proven acute arterial occlusion should be treated with a parenteral anticoagulant such as heparin (followed by an oral anticoagulant) to prevent propagation of the clot and to reduce the likelihood of additional embolic events. A revascularization procedure (catheter-based thrombolysis or thrombectomy, surgical embolectomy, or bypass surgery) is indicated if limb viability is at risk.

TABLE 15-4 Origins of Arterial Emboli

Cardiac origin
Stagnant left atrial flow (eg, atrial fibrillation, mitral stenosis)
Left ventricular mural thrombus (eg, dilated cardiomyopathy, myocardial infarction, ventricular aneurysm)
Valvular lesions (endocarditis, thrombus on prosthetic valve)
Left atrial myxoma (mobile tumor in left atrium)

Aortic origin
Thrombus material overlying atherosclerotic segment

Venous origin
Paradoxical embolism travels through intracardiac shunt

Atheroembolism is the condition of peripheral arterial occlusion by atheromatous material (ie, cholesterol, platelets, and fibrin) derived from more proximal vascular sites, such as atherosclerotic lesions or aneurysms. The emboli lodge distally, resulting in occlusion of small arteries in the muscle and skin. Patients typically present with acute pain and tenderness at the involved site. Occlusion of digital vessels may result in the "blue toe" syndrome, culminating in gangrene and necrosis. Other findings may include livedo reticularis (purplish mottling of involved skin), kidney failure (caused by renal atheroembolism), and intestinal ischemia. Although an estimated 50%-60% of cases are spontaneous, atheroembolism may occur after intra-arterial procedures (eg, cardiac catheterization) when atherosclerotic material is unintentionally dislodged from the proximal vasculature. Ischemia resulting from atheroemboli is difficult to manage because the heterogeneous composition and distribution of emboli often preclude surgical removal or thrombolytic therapy. Surgical intervention to remove or bypass the source of emboli may be necessary to prevent recurrences.

VASCULITIC SYNDROMES

Vasculitis (vessel wall inflammation) results from immune complex deposition or cell-mediated immune reactions directed against the vessel wall. Immune complexes activate the complement cascade with subsequent release of chemoattractants and anaphylatoxins that direct neutrophil migration to the vessel wall and increase vascular permeability. Neutrophils injure the vessel by releasing lysosomal contents and producing toxic oxygen-derived free radicals. In cell-mediated immune reactions, T lymphocytes bind to vascular antigens and release lymphokines that attract additional lymphocytes and macrophages to the vessel wall. These inflammatory processes can cause end-organ ischemia through vascular necrosis or local thrombosis.

The cause of most of the vasculitic syndromes is unknown, but they often can be distinguished from one another by the pattern of involved vessels and by histologic characteristics. Three important examples of vasculitic syndromes are Takayasu arteritis, giant cell arteritis, and thromboangiitis obliterans.

Takayasu arteritis is a chronic vasculitis of unknown etiology that targets the aorta and its major branches. The estimated annual incidence is 1.2-2.6 cases per million. Between 80% and 90% of affected persons are women, with onset typically between the ages of 10 and 40. Most reported cases have been from Asia and Africa, but it is a worldwide disease. Patients typically present with systemic complaints such as malaise and fever; focal symptoms are related to inflammation of the affected vessel and include cerebrovascular ischemia (brachiocephalic or carotid artery involvement), myocardial ischemia (coronary artery), arm claudication (brachiocephalic or subclavian artery), or hypertension (renal artery). The carotid and limb pulses are diminished or absent in nearly 85% of patients at the time of diagnosis; hence, this condition is often termed "pulseless" disease. Takayasu arteritis is also an uncommon cause of aortic aneurysm or aortic dissection. Histologic examination of affected vessels reveals continuous or patchy granulomatous inflammation with lymphocytes, histiocytes, and multinucleated giant cells, resulting in intimal proliferation, disruption of the elastic lamina, and fibrosis. Antiendothelial antibodies may also play a role in the disease. Steroid and cytotoxic drugs can reduce vascular inflammation and alleviate symptoms of Takayasu arteritis. Surgical bypass of obstructed vessels may be helpful in severe cases, after active inflammation has subsided. The 5-year survival rate is 80%-90%. Prognosis is adversely affected by end-organ complications and when there is progression of disease despite therapeutic medications.

Giant cell arteritis (also termed **temporal arteritis**) is a chronic vasculitis of medium-sized to large arteries that most commonly involves the cranial vessels or the aortic arch and its branches. It is an uncommon disease, with an incidence of 24 per 100,000, and the typical onset is after age 50; 65% of patients are female. Giant cell arteritis may be associated with the inflammatory condition known as polymyalgia rheumatica. Histologic findings in affected vessels include lymphocyte and macrophage infiltration, intimal fibrosis, and focal necrosis, with granulomas containing multinucleated giant cells.

Symptoms and signs of giant cell arteritis depend on the distribution of affected arteries and may include diminished temporal pulses, prominent headache (temporal artery involvement), or facial pain and claudication of the jaw while chewing (facial artery involvement). Ophthalmic artery arteritis leads to impaired vision, with permanent partial or complete loss in 15%-20% of patients. Serum markers of inflammation (eg, erythrocyte sedimentation rate and CRP) are invariably elevated in patients with giant cell arteritis. Ultrasound examination supports the diagnosis by demonstrating a hypoechoic halo around the involved arterial lumen with vessel stenosis and/or occlusion. The diagnosis can be confirmed by biopsy of an involved vessel, usually a temporal artery, but treatment should not wait for biopsy results. High-dose systemic steroids are first-line therapy in treatment of giant cell arteritis, followed by a gradual tapering of the dose. Disease activity is monitored by following serum inflammatory markers and symptoms. Glucocorticoid-sparing agents (ie, methotrexate or tocilizumab) may be used in cases of relapsing giant cell arteritis or if glucocorticoid-induced complications occur. Giant cell arteritis usually has a self-limited course of 1-5 years.

Thromboangiitis obliterans (Buerger disease) is a segmental inflammatory disease of small and medium-sized arteries, veins, and nerves involving the distal vessels of the upper and lower extremities. It is most prevalent in the Far and Middle East and has a very strong association with cigarette smoking. It is most common in men younger than age 45; only 10%-25% of patients are female. There is an increased incidence of human leukocyte antigen A9 (HLA-A9) and HLA-B5 in affected persons.

Thromboangiitis obliterans presents with a triad of symptoms and signs: distal arterial occlusion, Raynaud phenomenon (described in the next section), and migrating superficial vein thrombophlebitis. Arterial occlusion results in arm and foot claudication as well as ischemia of the digits. Traditional laboratory markers of inflammation and autoimmune disease are usually not detected. Arteriographic features of involved arteries include areas of stenosis interspersed with normal-appearing vessels with more severe disease distally, collateral vessels with a "corkscrew" appearance around the stenotic regions, and lack of atherosclerosis in proximal arteries. The diagnosis can be established by tissue biopsy, although this is rarely needed. Biopsy specimens of affected vessels reveal an occlusive, highly cellular, inflammatory thrombus, with limited involvement of the vessel wall and preservation of the internal elastic lamina (Fig. 15-5). The most important treatment for thromboangiitis obliterans is

Acute phase: Thrombus including neutrophils and giant cells occludes the vessel lumen but spares the wall.

Subacute phase: Progressive organization of the thrombus takes place.

Chronic phase: Inflammation is no longer present and organized thrombus and vascular fibrosis remain.

Platelets   Erythrocyte

Figure 15-5. Pathophysiologic phases of thromboangiitis obliterans. (Reprinted from Piazza G, Creager MA. Thromboangiitis obliterans. *Circulation*. 2010;121(16):1858-1861.)

smoking cessation, which usually prevents progression of the disease and its complications. Debridement of necrotic tissue and wound care may be necessary in advanced cases. Revascularization is not usually an option because of the distal location of the arterial lesions.

VASOSPASM: RAYNAUD PHENOMENON

Raynaud phenomenon is a vasospastic disease of the digital arteries that occurs in susceptible people when exposed to cool temperatures or sometimes during emotional stress. Vasospasm is an extreme vasoconstrictor response that temporarily obliterates the vascular lumen, inhibiting blood flow. Typically, such episodes are characterized by a triphasic color response. First, the fingers and/or toes blanch to a distinct white as blood flow is interrupted (Fig. 15-6). The second phase is characterized by cyanosis, related to local accumulation of desaturated hemoglobin, followed by a third phase of ruddy color as blood flow resumes. The color response may be accompanied by numbness, paresthesias, or pain of the affected digits.

This condition may occur as an isolated disorder, termed *primary Raynaud phenomenon* or *Raynaud disease*. Patients are predominantly women between the ages of 20 and 40. Primary Raynaud phenomenon most often manifests in the fingers in a symmetric manner, but 40% of patients also have involvement of the toes. The prognosis of primary Raynaud phenomenon is generally benign, with only a minority reporting a worsening of symptoms over time.

Secondary Raynaud phenomenon may appear as a component of other conditions. Common causes include connective tissue diseases (eg, scleroderma and systemic lupus erythematosus) and arterial occlusive disorders. Other causes of secondary Raynaud phenomenon include carpal tunnel syndrome, thoracic outlet syndrome, blood dyscrasias, certain drugs, and thermal or vibration injury. Suspicion for secondary Raynaud phenomenon should be raised if there is asymmetry of affected digits, initial symptoms develop after age 40, or if digital ulceration occurs.

Even in healthy vessels, cold exposure normally produces a vasoconstrictor response. Cooling stimulates the sympathetic nervous system, resulting in local discharge of norepinephrine, which binds to vascular adrenergic receptors. In the fingers and toes, only vasoconstricting α-receptors are present; other regional circulations have both constrictor and dilator adrenergic responses. Thus, a modest vasoconstriction of the digits results when healthy people are exposed to cooling. In contrast, in Raynaud phenomenon, cold exposure induces *severe* vasoconstriction.

A variety of mechanisms have been proposed to explain the vasospastic response to cold and stress in patients with primary Raynaud phenomenon, including an exaggerated sympathetic discharge in response to cold, heightened vascular sensitivity to adrenergic stimuli, or excessive release of vasoconstrictor stimuli, such as serotonin, thromboxane, and endothelin. In patients with secondary Raynaud phenomenon caused by connective tissue diseases or arterial occlusive disease, the digital vascular lumen is largely obliterated by sclerosis or inflammation, resulting in lower intraluminal pressure and greater susceptibility to sympathetically mediated vasoconstriction.

Figure 15-6. Raynaud phenomenon. Blanching of the fourth digit (*red arrow*) is evident (phase 1 of the tricolor response).

Treatment of Raynaud phenomenon involves avoiding cold environments, dressing in warm clothes, and wearing insulated gloves or footwear. There has also been some success in preventing vasospasm with pharmacologic agents that relax vascular tone, including calcium channel blockers, α-adrenergic blockers, and phosphodiesterase type 5 inhibitors such as sildenafil (see Chapter 17); these measures are employed when conservative therapies do not control symptoms.

VENOUS DISEASE

Veins are high-capacitance vessels that contain more than 70% of the total blood volume. In contrast to the muscular structure of arteries, the subendothelial layer of veins is thin, and the tunica media comprises fewer, smaller bundles of smooth muscle cells intermixed with reticular and elastic fibers. While veins of the extremities possess intrinsic vasomotor activity, transport of blood back to the heart relies greatly on external compression by the surrounding skeletal muscles and on a series of one-way endothelial valves.

Veins of the extremities are classified as either deep or superficial. In the lower extremities, where most peripheral venous disorders occur, the deep veins generally course along the arteries, whereas the superficial veins are located subcutaneously. The superficial vessels drain into deeper veins through a series of perforating connectors, ultimately returning blood to the heart.

VARICOSE VEINS

Varicose veins (Fig. 15-7) are dilated, tortuous superficial vessels that often develop in the lower extremities. Clinically apparent varicose veins occur in 10%-20% of the general population. They affect women two to three times more frequently than men, and roughly half of patients have a family history of this condition. Varicosities can occur in any vein in the body but are most common in the saphenous veins of the leg and their tributaries. They may also develop in the anorectal area (hemorrhoids), in the lower esophageal veins (esophageal varices), and in the spermatic cord (varicocele).

Varicosity is thought to result from intrinsic weakness of the vessel wall, from increased intraluminal pressure, or from congenital defects in the structure and function of venous valves. Varicose veins in the lower extremities are classified as either primary or secondary. *Primary* varicose veins originate in the superficial system and factors that lead to their development include pregnancy, prolonged standing, and obesity. During pregnancy or prolonged standing, the high venous pressure within the legs contributes to varicosities when there is underlying weakness of the vessel walls. In obese patients, the adipose tissue surrounding vessel walls offers less structural support to veins than does lean mass. *Secondary* varicose veins occur when an abnormality

Figure 15-7. A patient with varicose veins of the left leg (*arrow*). (Courtesy of Marie Gerhard-Herman, MD, Brigham and Women's Hospital, Boston, MA.)

in the deep venous system is the cause of superficial varicosities. These may develop in the setting of deep venous insufficiency or occlusion or when the perforating veins (which connect the deep and superficial veins) are incompetent. In such cases, deep venous blood is shunted retrograde through perforating channels into superficial veins, increasing intraluminal pressure and volume and causing dilatation and varicosity formation.

Many people with varicose veins are asymptomatic but seek treatment for cosmetic reasons. When symptoms do develop, they include a dull ache, "heaviness," or a pressure sensation in the legs after prolonged standing. Superficial venous insufficiency may result when venous valves are unable to function normally in the dilated veins. This can cause swelling and skin ulceration that is particularly severe near the ankle. Stasis of blood within varicose veins can promote superficial vein thrombosis, and varicosities can also rupture, causing a localized hematoma.

Varicose veins are usually treated conservatively. Patients should elevate their legs while supine, avoid prolonged standing, and wear external compression stockings that counterbalance the increased venous hydrostatic pressure. Varicose veins that are symptomatic, or associated with signs of venous insufficiency, may be treated with more advanced techniques, including sclerotherapy, thermal ablation, or surgery. Sclerotherapy involves the localized intravenous administration of an irritating chemical agent to fibrose varicose veins. Endovenous thermal ablation procedures use laser or radiofrequency catheters to deliver heat energy, which induces thromboses and is used to obliterate varicose great saphenous veins. Surgical therapy involves direct vein ligation and removal.

Chronic Venous Insufficiency

Chronic venous insufficiency (CVI) is characterized by elevated venous pressure with extravasation of edema into the tissues of the lower extremities. CVI develops when venous blood return to the heart is impaired by mechanisms that include valvular incompetence of deep or superficial veins, venous obstruction, and calf muscle pump dysfunction. A secondary form of CVI is *postphlebitic syndrome*, resulting from venous valvular damage or persistent venous occlusion after deep vein thrombosis (described below).

Patients with CVI may experience pain or achiness in the legs, particularly when standing for prolonged periods. Physical findings include varicose veins, edema, skin inflammation and hyperpigmentation, and ulcerations. Noninvasive testing with duplex ultrasound is useful to detect the cause of CVI, such as venous obstruction. Compression stockings are the mainstay of treatment. Associated venous ulcerations are treated with compression bandages and absorbent dressings. Venous ablation techniques as described in the previous section are used to treat varicose veins that contribute to CVI.

Venous Thromboembolism

The term *venous thrombosis* or *thrombophlebitis* is used to describe thrombus formation within a superficial or deep vein and the inflammatory response in the vessel wall that it incites. Thrombi in the lower extremities are classified by location as either deep venous thrombi or superficial venous thrombi.

Initially, the venous thrombus is composed principally of platelets and fibrin. Later, red blood cells become interspersed within the fibrin, and the thrombus tends to propagate in the direction of blood flow. The changes in the vessel wall can be minimal or can include granulocyte infiltration, loss of endothelium, and edema. Thrombi may diminish or obstruct vascular flow, or they may dislodge and form thromboemboli.

Deep Venous Thrombosis
Epidemiology, Etiology, and Pathophysiology
Deep venous thrombosis (DVT) occurs most commonly in the veins of the calves but may also develop initially in more proximal veins such as the popliteal, femoral, and iliac vessels. If

left untreated, a third of DVTs that arise in the calves propagate to these proximal veins. The two major consequences of DVT are pulmonary embolism (PE) and postphlebitic syndrome.

In 1856, Virchow described a triad of factors that predispose to venous thrombosis: (1) stasis of blood flow, (2) hypercoagulability, and (3) vascular damage. Stasis disrupts laminar flow and brings platelets into contact with the endothelium. This allows coagulation factors to accumulate and retards the influx of clotting inhibitors. Factors that slow venous flow and induce stasis include immobilization (eg, prolonged bed rest after surgery or sitting in a car or an airplane for a long trip), cardiac failure, and hyperviscosity syndromes (Table 15-5).

Various clinical disorders cause systemic hypercoagulability, including resistance of coagulation factor V to activated protein C, a prothrombin gene mutation, and inherited deficiencies of antithrombin, protein C, and protein S. Pancreatic, lung, stomach, breast, and genitourinary tract adenocarcinomas are associated with a high prevalence of venous thrombosis. This is thought to occur in part because necrotic tumor cells release thrombogenic factors. Other conditions that contribute to hypercoagulability are listed in Table 15-5.

Vascular damage, either by external injury or by intravenous catheters, can denude the endothelium and expose subendothelial collagen. Exposed collagen acts as a substrate for the binding of von Willebrand factor and platelets and initiates the clotting cascade, leading to clot formation. Less severe damage can cause endothelial *dysfunction* that contributes to thrombosis by disrupting the production of vasodilating and antiplatelet substances (eg, nitric oxide and prostacyclin, as explained in Chapter 6) and antithrombotic molecules such as thrombomodulin and heparan sulfate (described in Chapter 7). Recent evidence indicates that atherosclerotic risk factors, such as hyperlipidemia and diabetes, are also associated with DVT formation.

The risk of venous thrombosis is particularly high after fractures of the spine, pelvis, and bones of the lower extremities. The risk following bone fracture may be related to stasis of blood flow, increased coagulability, and possibly traumatic endothelial damage. In addition, venous thrombosis may arise in patients following surgical procedures, particularly major orthopedic operations.

Women have a severalfold increase in the incidence of venous thrombus formation during late pregnancy and the early postpartum period. In the third trimester, the fetus compresses

TABLE 15-5 **Conditions that Predispose to DVT and Pulmonary Embolism**

Stasis of blood flow
    Prolonged inactivity (following surgery, prolonged travel)
    Immobilized extremity (following bone fracture)
    Heart failure (with systemic venous congestion)
    Hyperviscosity syndromes (eg, polycythemia vera)

Hypercoagulable states
    Inherited disorders of coagulation
        Resistance to activated protein C (factor V Leiden)
        Prothrombin gene mutation (PT G20210A)
        Antithrombin deficiency
        Deficiency of protein C or protein S
    Antiphospholipid antibodies/lupus anticoagulant
    Neoplastic disease (eg, pancreatic, lung, stomach, or breast cancers)
    Pregnancy and oral contraceptive use
    Myeloproliferative diseases
    Smoking

Vascular damage
    Instrumentation (eg, intravenous catheters)
    Trauma

the inferior vena cava and can cause stasis of blood flow, and high levels of circulating estrogen may induce a hypercoagulable state. Oral contraceptives and other pharmacologic estrogen products also predispose to thrombus formation.

Clinical Presentation

Patients with DVT may be asymptomatic, may describe calf or thigh discomfort when standing or walking, or may report unilateral leg swelling. The physical signs of proximal DVT include edema of the involved leg and occasionally localized warmth and erythema. Tenderness may be present over the course of the phlebitic vein, and a deep venous cord (induration along the thrombosed vessel) is occasionally palpable. Calf pain produced by dorsiflexion of the foot (the Homan sign) is a nonspecific and unreliable marker of DVT.

Diagnosis

The primary laboratory tests for the diagnosis of DVT include measurement of the serum D-dimer level and venous compression ultrasonography. *D-Dimer*, a by-product of fibrin degradation that can be measured in a peripheral blood sample, is highly sensitive for the diagnosis of DVT and/or acute PE. Because D-dimer may also be elevated in many other conditions (such as cancer, inflammation, infection, and necrosis), a positive test result is *not specific* for DVT. Thus, a normal D-dimer value helps exclude the presence of DVT, but an elevated level does not definitively confirm the diagnosis.

Venous compression duplex ultrasonography is a readily available noninvasive technique that is 95% sensitive for the diagnosis of symptomatic DVT in a proximal vein but only 75% sensitive for diagnosing symptomatic calf vein thrombi. This technique uses real-time ultrasound scanning to image the vein and pulsed Doppler ultrasound to assess blood flow within it (Fig. 15-8). Criteria used for diagnosis of DVT with duplex ultrasonography include the inability to compress the vein with direct pressure (suggesting the presence of an intraluminal thrombus), direct visualization of the thrombus, and absence of blood flow within the vessel.

Other diagnostic techniques are sometimes used. For example, *MR venography* can aid in the diagnosis of proximal DVT, particularly pelvic vein thrombi, which are difficult to detect by ultrasound. *Contrast venography* is now a rarely used invasive imaging technique that can provide a definitive diagnosis. Radiocontrast material is injected into a foot vein, and images are obtained as the contrast ascends through the venous system of the leg. DVT is diagnosed by the presence of a filling defect (see Fig. 15-8).

Treatment

In patients with proximal DVT, elevation of the affected extremity above the level of the heart helps reduce edema and tenderness, and anticoagulation prevents extension of the thrombus and PE. Choices for initial anticoagulation include subcutaneous low molecular weight heparin (LMWH), intravenous unfractionated heparin, and certain direct oral anticoagulants (eg, rivaroxaban or apixaban). Long-term management consists of an oral anticoagulant, and treatment duration depends on the underlying cause of DVT. Available choices for long-term oral anticoagulation include warfarin (a vitamin K antagonist), the direct thrombin inhibitor dabigatran, and the factor Xa inhibitors rivaroxaban, apixaban, and edoxaban (see Chapter 17). Catheter-based thrombolysis may be useful for selected patients with iliofemoral deep vein thrombosis to lower the risk of postphlebitic syndrome.

Treatment of patients with calf DVT is more controversial because pulmonary emboli from that site are uncommon. Some experts advocate serial noninvasive monitoring to determine if the thrombus propagates into proximal veins, whereas others treat such thrombosis with an oral anticoagulant for 3-6 months. If the risk of proximal propagation is high (as in patients with cancer), anticoagulant treatment rather than surveillance is recommended.

Prophylaxis against DVT is appropriate in clinical situations in which the risk of developing the condition is high, such as immobilization following surgery. Prophylactic measures may

Figure 15-8. Diagnostic imaging of deep venous thrombosis. A. Normal venogram. Contrast material was injected into a foot vein and fills the leg veins in this radiograph. **B.** Venogram demonstrating extensive thrombosis of the deep calf veins, popliteal vein, and femoral vein. *Arrow* indicates a filling defect in the femoral vein due to the presence of thrombus. The deep calf veins are filled with thrombus and cannot be visualized. **C.** Ultrasound indicating deep venous thrombosis. The thrombus appears as an echogenic area (*arrows*) within the femoral vein (V). A healthy vein would be easily compressible by the ultrasound transducer. This vein, however, has the same diameter at baseline (*top panel*) and after compression (*bottom panel*), confirming the presence of thrombus within it. Art, artery.

include subcutaneous unfractionated heparin, LMWH, low-dose oral warfarin, or low doses of one of the direct oral anticoagulants, as well as compression stockings, and/or intermittent external pneumatic compression of the legs to prevent venous stasis.

Pulmonary Embolism

Epidemiology, Etiology, and Pathophysiology

PE supervenes when a clot, most often derived from DVT in a proximal vein of the lower extremities, dislodges and travels through the inferior vena cava and right heart chambers, finally reaching and obstructing a portion of the pulmonary vasculature. PE is common (incidence of ~600 000 per year in the United States) and can be fatal, with an untreated mortality rate of 30%-40%. In patients with PE, gas exchange is often impaired because of the associated anatomic dead space and ventilation-perfusion mismatches that ensue in the lungs. As a result, the alveolar-arterial oxygen gradient increases and hypoxemia may occur. Pulmonary vascular resistance may rise as a consequence of the mechanical obstruction and because vasoactive and bronchoconstrictive mediators released by platelets within emboli induce constriction of the pulmonary vasculature and bronchospasm, respectively. The increased pulmonary vascular resistance may lead to elevated right ventricular (RV) wall stress, RV dilatation, and impaired contraction, compromising cardiac output. Recurrent and chronic PE can cause remodeling of the pulmonary vasculature with pulmonary hypertension leading to right-sided heart failure.

Clinical Presentation

Patients with PE may experience dyspnea, pleuritic chest pain (due to pleural irritation), hemoptysis, cough, or syncope (due to reduced cardiac output). Signs may include tachypnea, bronchospasm, and evidence of elevated pulmonary artery pressure, including an accentuated pulmonic component of the second heart sound and jugular venous distention.

Diagnosis

Many of the diagnostic tests used for DVT are also helpful in evaluating for PE. In addition, the most common *electrocardiographic* abnormality is sinus tachycardia; there may be evidence of RV strain (eg, inverted T waves in leads V_1-V_4 or an "S1-Q3-T3" pattern: a prominent S wave in lead I, Q wave in lead III, and inverted T wave in lead III). RV strain may also produce elevated serum levels of cardiac-specific troponins or B-type natriuretic peptide (described in Chapters 7 and 9, respectively). *Arterial blood gas* analysis may show decreased arterial oxygenation but is insensitive in the diagnosis of PE. The preferred test to confirm the diagnosis is *computed tomographic angiography* (CTA; Fig. 15-9). For patients who cannot tolerate CTA, such as those with renal insufficiency or hypersensitivity to radioiodinated contrast agents, radionuclide *ventilation-perfusion (V/Q) lung scanning* may be obtained instead but is less precise for the diagnosis of PE. Catheter-based *pulmonary angiography* is rarely necessary for confirmation.

Treatment

In patients with established PE, urgent anticoagulation is instituted to prevent recurrent embolism. Anticoagulation measures are similar to those used for DVT. In patients with PE and hemodynamic compromise including hypotension (termed *massive PE*), systemic thrombolytic therapy is recommended. Occasionally, surgical pulmonary embolectomy is performed. Patients with submassive PE, characterized by RV dysfunction but without hypotension, may be considered for systemic or catheter-directed thrombolytics (infusion of low-dose thrombolytic directly into the pulmonary artery). In patients with proximal DVT or established PE who cannot be treated with anticoagulants (eg, because of a bleeding disorder), an

Figure 15-9. CT angiogram displaying a massive pulmonary embolism. There is a large filling defect in the main pulmonary artery that extends into branches of both left and right pulmonary arteries (*blue arrow*). (Courtesy of Andetta Hunsaker, MD, Brigham and Women's Hospital, Boston, MA.)

intravascular filter can be percutaneously inserted into the inferior vena cava to prevent subsequent emboli from reaching the lungs.

Superficial Thrombophlebitis

Superficial thrombophlebitis is a benign disorder associated with inflammation and thrombosis of a superficial vein, just below the skin. It may occur, for example, as a complication of an in-dwelling intravenous catheter. It is characterized by erythema, tenderness, and edema over the involved vein. Treatment consists of local heat and rest of the involved extremity. Aspirin or other anti-inflammatory medications may relieve the associated discomfort. Unlike DVT, superficial thrombophlebitis does not lead to PE.

Summary

- **True aneurysms** are caused by degenerative changes in the aortic wall; medial degeneration is associated with ascending thoracic aortic aneurysms, and atherosclerosis is commonly found in descending thoracic and abdominal aortic aneurysms.

- A **false aneurysm** (pseudoaneurysm) represents a hole in the arterial intima and media contained by a layer of adventitia or perivascular clot.

- **Symptoms of aortic aneurysms** relate to compression of adjacent structures (back pain, dysphagia, respiratory symptoms) or blood leakage, with the most severe consequence being aneurysm rupture.

- **Aortic dissection** results from a tear in the intima that allows blood to enter into the medial layer, often in the setting of advanced age, hypertension, or cystic medial degeneration.

- **Type A (proximal) aortic dissections** involve the ascending aorta, are life threatening, and require surgical repair.

- **Type B dissections** are confined to the descending aorta and often are managed by pharmacologic therapy alone.

- **PAD** is a common atherosclerotic disease of large and medium-sized arteries, resulting in claudication of the limbs.

- **PAD is treated** by risk factor modification, exercise, antiplatelet agents, and sometimes cilostazol, a selective phosphodiesterase inhibitor.

- **Arterial embolism** arises from thrombus within the heart, from proximal arterial sites, or paradoxically from the systemic veins in the presence of an intracardiac shunt (eg, atrial septal defect or patent foramen ovale).

- **Therapeutic options for acute arterial occlusion** include anticoagulation, thrombolysis, and surgical or endovascular interventions.

- **Vasculitic syndromes** are inflammatory diseases of blood vessels that impair arterial flow and result in localized and systemic symptoms; such syndromes are distinguished from one another by the pattern of vessel involvement and morphologic findings.

- **Raynaud phenomenon** is an episodic vasospasm of arteries that supply the digits of the upper and lower extremities; it may be a primary condition (Raynaud disease) or may appear in association with other disorders such as connective tissue diseases or blood dyscrasias.

- **Varicose veins** are dilated tortuous vessels that may present cosmetic problems; they may cause discomfort, become thrombosed, or lead to venous insufficiency.

- Initial **management of varicose veins** is conservative, with periodic leg elevation and compression stockings; severe symptomatic varicose veins can be treated with sclerotherapy, radiofrequency or laser ablation, or surgical ligation and removal.

- **Chronic venous insufficiency** develops when venous pressure is increased and return of blood flow is impaired by venous valvular reflux, resulting in chronic lower extremity edema, varicosities, and skin ulceration.

- **Venous thrombosis** results from stasis of blood flow, hypercoagulability, and vascular damage; the major complication is PE.

- **Venous compression ultrasonography** is the primary tool used to diagnose DVT.

- PE can be confirmed by **CT angiography or ventilation-perfusion scintigraphy**.

- **Anticoagulation therapy** with LMWH or unfractionated intravenous heparin (UFH), or a direct oral anticoagulant, such as rivaroxaban or apixaban, constitutes usual initial treatment for DVT and PE; one of the direct oral anticoagulants or warfarin are used for long-term management.

Review Questions

1. A 66-year-old carpenter presents for routine evaluation by his primary care physician. He has no symptoms. He has been smoking a pack of cigarettes per day for the past 50 years, and drinks 1 beer nightly. His vital signs reveal a regular heart rate at 65 bpm, blood pressure 155/90, and normal oxygen saturation on room air. His body mass index is elevated at 35 kg/m^2. Examination is remarkable for a palpable and dilated abdominal aorta. Laboratory results are significant for elevated low-density lipoprotein cholesterol of 180 mg/dL. The patient is counseled on the importance of smoking cessation and medications are prescribed to treat his elevated blood pressure and cholesterol. Ultrasound imaging shows a 4.9-cm fusiform abdominal aortic aneurysm (AAA) inferior to the origin of the renal arteries. Which of the following statements regarding AAA is true?

   a. High alcohol intake is a significant risk factor for the development of abdominal aortic aneurysms.
   b. Medial degeneration would be seen on histopathology examination of his aortic aneurysm.
   c. A repeat abdominal aortic ultrasound in 6 months should be recommended.
   d. Endovascular and open surgical repair of abdominal aortic aneurysms have similar short- and long-term mortality rates.

2. A 57-year-old woman with hypertension, hyperlipidemia, former smoking history, and coronary artery disease presents for evaluation of left-sided leg pain. She reports that when she walks more than 2 blocks, she experiences a cramp in her left calf; it resolves after 2 minutes of rest. Her vital signs show a regular pulse of 60 bpm and blood pressure 125/70. Physical examination reveals absence of lower extremity edema. There are normal right

femoral, popliteal, and pedal pulses, and a normal left femoral pulse, but absence of left popliteal and pedal pulses. Neurological examination is normal. What is the next step in diagnosis?

a. Venous duplex ultrasonography of lower extremities
b. Arterial duplex ultrasonography of lower extremities
c. Computed tomography angiography of lower extremities
d. Ankle-brachial index measurement

3. A 27-year-old woman with leukemia presents to the emergency department for evaluation of the sudden onset of shortness of breath and chest discomfort 6 hours earlier. She has been very sedentary since recent hospitalization, spending most of the day in bed. Other than chemotherapy, her only other medication is oral contraception for prevention of pregnancy. Her vital signs show a reduced body mass index (BMI) of 17.5 kg/m²; heart rate 115, in a regular rhythm; blood pressure 135/65; and oxygen saturation 91% on room air. Physical examination reveals an anxious woman who appears short of breath. Her right calf appears swollen. The electrocardiogram shows sinus tachycardia. CT angiography of the chest shows pulmonary emboli in the right and left pulmonary arteries with extension to segmental and subsegmental branches. Which one of the following factors did *not* contribute to venous thromboembolism?

a. Low BMI
b. Acute leukemia
c. Oral contraception
d. Prolonged bed rest

Answers to Review Questions

1. **Answer c is correct.** This 66-year-old man has a moderate-size abdominal aortic aneurysm (AAA). His risk factors for AAA include hypertension, hyperlipidemia, and smoking. Given the size of the aneurysm, repeat abdominal aortic ultrasonography in 6 months is indicated to evaluate for rate of growth. Repair would be indicated if the diameter increases to >5.5 cm or grows by >1.0 cm/year. Although cigarette smoking, hypertension, and hyperlipidemia are significant risk factors for AAA, high alcohol intake is not. Medial degeneration is typically found in ascending thoracic aortic aneurysms, while atherosclerosis is more common in AAA. Although long-term mortality of endovascular and open repair of AAAs are similar, short-term mortality with endovascular repair is lower.

2. **Answer d is correct.** This woman has symptoms and signs of peripheral artery disease (PAD). Her risk factors for PAD include prior cigarette smoking, hypertension, hyperlipidemia, and coronary artery disease. The next step in diagnosis is measuring the ankle-brachial indices (ABI). An ABI ≤ 0.9 is diagnostic of PAD. Arterial duplex ultrasonography of the lower extremities, CT angiography, and MR angiography are additional tools for further investigation of PAD anatomy, used in preparation for invasive treatment. Venous duplex ultrasonography is utilized for the diagnosis of deep and superficial venous thrombosis, not PAD.

3. **Answer a is correct.** This 27-year-old woman presents with deep venous thrombosis and pulmonary embolism. She has multiple risk factors for developing venous thromboembolism including malignancy (acute leukemia), prolonged bed rest, and oral contraceptive usage. Low BMI is not a risk factor for venous thromboembolism (VTE). In distinction, obesity *is* a risk factor for VTE.

Acknowledgments

Contributors to previous editions of this chapter were Sruthi Renati, MD; Fan Liang, MD; Arash Mostaghimi, MD; Mary Beth Gordon, MD; Geoffrey McDonough, MD; Michael Diminick, MD; Stuart Kaplan, MD; and Jesse Salmeron, MD.

Additional Reading

Creager MA, Beckman JA, Loscalzo J, eds. *Vascular Medicine: A Companion to Braunwald's Heart Disease*. Philadelphia, PA: Elsevier Saunders; 2019.

Creager MA, Loscalzo J. Diseases of the aorta. In: Jameson JL, Kasper DL, Longo DL, et al., eds. *Harrison's Principles of Internal Medicine*. 20th ed. New York, NY: McGraw-Hill; 2018:1917-1922.

Creager MA, Loscalzo J. Arterial diseases of the extremities. In: Jameson JL, Kasper DL, Longo DL, et al., eds. *Harrison's Principles of Internal Medicine*. 19th ed. New York, NY: McGraw-Hill; 2018:1923-1929.

Gerhard-Herman MD, Gornik HL, Barrett C, et al. 2016 AHA/ACC guideline on the management of patient with lower extremity peripheral artery disease: executive summary: a report of the American College of Cardiology/American Heart Association Task Force on Clinical Practice Guidelines. *Circulation*. 2017;135:e686-e725.

Goldhaber SZ, Bounzameaux H. Pulmonary embolism and deep vein thrombosis. *Lancet*. 2012;379:1835-1846.

Hess CN, Norgren L, Ansel GM, et al. A structured review of antithrombotic therapy in peripheral artery disease with a focus on revascularization; a TASC (InterSociety Consensus for the Management of Peripheral Artery Disease) initiative. *Circulation*. 2017;135:2534-2555.

Nienaber CA, et al. Aortic dissection. *Nat Rev Dis Primers*. 2016;2:1-18.

Tritschler T, Kraaijpoel N, LeGal G, et al. Venous thromboembolism: advances in diagnosis and treatment. *JAMA*. 2018;320:1583-1594.

Verma S, Siu SC. Aortic dilatation in patients with bicuspid aortic valve. *N Engl J Med*. 2014;370:1920-1929.

16

Congenital Heart Disease

Jonathan W. Cunningham | David W. Brown

Congenital heart disorders are the most common form of birth defects and are the leading cause of death from birth abnormalities in the first year of life. These conditions affect ~8 of 1000 live births, and an estimated 1 million people in the United States today were born with congenital heart lesions. Some abnormalities are severe and require immediate medical attention, whereas many are less pronounced and have minimal clinical consequences. Although congenital heart defects are present at birth, milder defects may remain inapparent for weeks, months, or years and may even escape detection until adulthood.

The past half-century has witnessed tremendous advances in the understanding of the pathophysiology of congenital heart diseases and substantial improvements in the ability to evaluate and treat those afflicted. Research has shown that genetic mutations, environmental factors, maternal illness, or ingestion of toxins during pregnancy can contribute to cardiac malformations.

The survival of children with congenital heart disease has also improved dramatically in recent decades, largely because of better diagnostic and interventional techniques. However, the lifelong needs of affected patients include guidance regarding physical activity, pregnancy, and employment.

Formation of the cardiovascular system begins during the 3rd week of embryonic development. Soon after, a unique circulation develops that allows the fetus to mature in the uterus, using the placenta as the primary organ of gas, nutrient, and waste exchange. At birth, the fetal lungs inflate and become functional, making the placenta unnecessary and dramatically altering circulation patterns to allow the neonate to adjust to life outside the womb. Given the remarkable complexity of these processes, it is easy to envision that cardiovascular malfunctions could arise.

This chapter begins with an overview of fetal cardiovascular development and then describes the most common forms of congenital heart disease.

NORMAL DEVELOPMENT OF THE CARDIOVASCULAR SYSTEM

By the 3rd week of gestation, the nutrient and gas exchange needs of the rapidly growing embryo can no longer be met by diffusion alone, and the tissues begin to rely on a developing cardiovascular system.

DEVELOPMENT OF THE HEART TUBE

In the middle of the 3rd week of embryogenesis, mesodermal cells proliferate at the cranial end of the early embryonic disc. They eventually form two longitudinal cell clusters known as angioblastic cords. These cords canalize and become paired endothelial heart tubes (Fig. 16-1). Lateral embryonic folding gradually causes these two tubes to oppose one another and allows them to fuse in the ventral midline, forming a single endocardial tube by day 22. From inside to outside, the layers of this primitive heart tube are an endothelial lining that becomes the endocardium, a layer of gelatinous connective tissue (cardiac jelly), and a thick muscular layer that is derived from the splanchnic mesoderm and develops into the myocardium. The endocardial tube is continuous with the aortic arch system rostrally and with the venous system caudally. The primitive heart begins to beat around day 22 or 23, causing blood to circulate by the beginning of the 4th week. The space overlying the developing cardiac area eventually becomes the pericardial cavity, housing the future heart.

FORMATION OF THE HEART LOOP

As the tubular heart grows and elongates, it develops a series of alternate constrictions and dilations, creating the first sign of the primitive heart chambers—the truncus arteriosus, the bulbus cordis, the primitive ventricle, the primitive atrium, and the sinus venosus (Fig. 16-2). Continued growth and elongation within the confined pericardial cavity force the heart tube to bend on itself on day 23, eventually forming a U-shaped loop with the round end pointing ventrally and to the right by day 28. The result of this looping is placement of the atrium and sinus venosus above and behind the truncus arteriosus, bulbus cordis, and ventricle (Fig. 16-3). At this point, neither definitive septa between the developing chambers nor definitive valvular tissue have formed. The connection between the primitive atrium and ventricle is termed the **atrioventricular (AV) canal**. In time, the AV canal becomes two separate canals, one

A Endocardial heart tube

B Fusing endocardial heart tubes

C Endocardial heart tube

Figure 16-1. Embryonic transverse sections illustrating fusion of the two heart tubes into a single endocardial heart tube. A. 18 days. **B.** 21 days. **C.** 22 days.

To aortic arches

— Truncus arteriosus   [Aorta, pulmonary artery]

— Bulbus cordis   [Outlet of ventricles]

— Primitive ventricle   [Inlet of ventricles]

Atrioventricular
canal →

— Primitive atrium   [Right and left atria]

— Sinus venosus   [Part of right atrium]

Figure 16-2. The straight heart tube at ~22 days. The structures that will ultimately form from each segment are listed in *brackets*.

housing the tricuspid valve and the other the mitral valve. The sinus venosus is eventually incorporated into the right atrium, forming both the coronary sinus and a portion of the right atrial wall. The bulbus cordis and truncus arteriosus contribute to the future ventricular outflow tracts, forming parts of the proximal aorta and pulmonary artery.

SEPTATION

Septation of the developing atrium, AV canal, and ventricle occurs between the 4th and 6th weeks. Although these events are described separately here, they actually occur simultaneously.

Septation of the Atria

The primary atrial septum, also known as the **septum primum**, begins as a ridge of tissue on the roof of the common atrium that grows downward into the atrial cavity (Fig. 16-4). As the septum primum advances, it leaves a large opening known as the **ostium primum** between the crescent-shaped leading edge of the septum and the endocardial cushions sur-

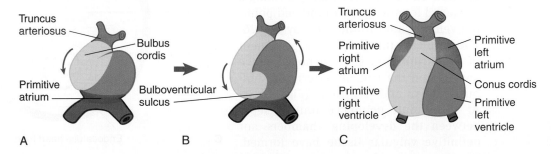

Figure 16-3. Formation of the heart loop. A, B. By day 23, continued growth and elongation within the confined pericardial space necessitate bending of the heart tube on itself, forming a U-shaped loop that points ventrally and to the right. **C.** Looping eventually places the atria above and behind the primitive ventricles.

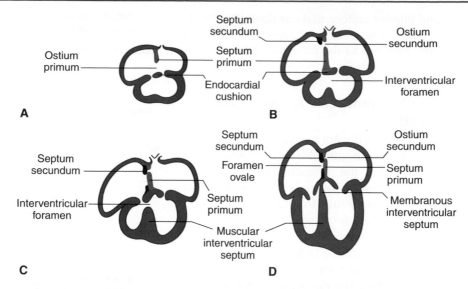

Figure 16-4. Atrial septal formation at 30 days (A), 33 days (B), and 37 days (C) of development as well as in the newborn (D). As the septum primum grows toward the ventricles, the opening between it and the AV canal is the ostium primum. Before the ostium primum completely closes, perforations within the upper portion of the septum primum form the ostium secundum. A second ridge of tissue, the septum secundum, grows downward to the right of the septum primum, partially covering the ostium secundum. The foramen ovale is an opening of the septum secundum that is covered by the "flap valve" of the lower septum primum. (Modified from Moss AJ, Adams FH. *Heart Disease in Infants, Children, and Adolescents.* Baltimore, MD: Williams & Wilkins; 1968:16.)

rounding the AV canal. The ostium primum allows passage of blood between the forming atria. Eventually, the septum primum fuses with the superior aspect of the endocardial cushions (described in more detail in the next section), obliterating the ostium primum. However, before closure of the ostium primum is complete, small perforations appear in the center of the septum primum that ultimately coalesce to form the **ostium secundum**, preserving a pathway for blood flow between the atria (see Fig. 16-4). Following closure of the ostium primum, a second, more muscular membrane, the **septum secundum**, begins to develop immediately to the right of the superior aspect of the septum primum. This septum grows downward and overlaps the ostium secundum. The septum secundum eventually fuses with the endocardial cushions, although only in a partial fashion, leaving an oval-shaped opening known as the **foramen ovale**. The superior edge of the septum primum then gradually regresses, leaving the lower edge to act as a "flaplike" valve that allows only right-to-left flow through the foramen ovale (Fig. 16-5). During gestation, blood passes from the right atrium to the left atrium because the pressure in the fetal right atrium is greater than that in the left atrium. This pressure gradient changes direction postnatally, causing the valve to close, as described later.

Septation of the Atrioventricular Canal

Growth of the **endocardial cushions** contributes to atrial septation and, as described later, to the membranous portion of the interventricular septum. Endocardial cushions initially begin as swellings of the gelatinous connective tissue layer within the AV canal. They are then populated by migrating cells from the primitive endocardium and subsequently transform into mesenchymal tissue. Tissue growth occurs primarily in the horizontal plane, resulting in septation of the AV canal through the continued growth of the lateral, superior, and inferior endocardial cushions (Fig. 16-6). Septation creates the right and left canals that later give rise to the tricuspid and mitral orifices, respectively.

Septation of the Ventricles and Ventricular Outflow Tracts

At the end of the 4th week, the primitive ventricle begins to grow, leaving a median muscular ridge, the primitive interventricular septum. Most of the early increase in height of the septum results from dilation of the two new ventricles forming on either side of it. Only later does new cell growth in the septum itself contribute to its size. The free edge of the muscular interventricular septum does not fuse with the endocardial cushions; the opening that remains and allows communication between the right ventricle (RV) and left ventricle (LV) is the **interventricular foramen** (Fig. 16-7). This remains open until the end of the 7th week of gestation, when the fusion of tissue from the right and left bulbar ridges and the endocardial cushions forms the membranous portion of the interventricular septum.

During the 5th week, neural crest–derived mesenchymal proliferation occurring in the bulbus cordis and truncus arteriosus creates a pair of protrusions known as the bulbar ridges (Fig. 16-8). These ridges fuse in the midline and undergo a 180-degree spiraling process, forming the aorticopulmonary septum. This

Figure 16-5. Diagrammatic depiction of the flap-type valve of the foramen ovale. A. Before birth, the valve permits only right-to-left flow of blood from the higher-pressured right atrium (RA) to the lower-pressured left atrium (LA). **B.** Following birth, the pressure in the LA becomes greater than that in the RA, causing the septum primum to close firmly against the septum secundum. (Derived from Moore KL, Persaud TVN. *The Developing Human*. Philadelphia, PA: WB Saunders; 1993:318.)

septum divides the bulbus cordis and the truncus arteriosus into two arterial channels, the pulmonary artery and the aorta, the former continuous with the RV and the latter with the LV.

Figure 16-6. The progression of septal formation in the atrioventricular canal through successive stages. The septum forms through growth of the superior, inferior, and lateral endocardial cushions. The endocardial cushions are masses of mesenchymal tissue that surround the atrioventricular canal and aid in the formation of the orifices of the mitral and tricuspid valves, as well as the upper interventricular septum and lower interatrial septum.

Development of the Cardiac Valves

Semilunar Valve Development (Aortic and Pulmonary Valves)

The semilunar valves start to develop just before the completion of the aorticopulmonary septum. The process begins when three outgrowths of subendocardial mesenchymal tissue form around both the aortic and pulmonary orifices. These growths are ultimately shaped and excavated by the joint action of programmed cell death and blood flow to create the three thin-walled cusps of both the aortic and pulmonary valves.

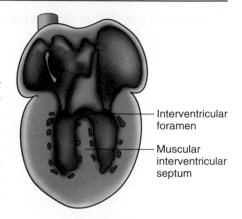

Figure 16-7. The interventricular septum and the interventricular foramen. (Derived from Moore KL, Persaud TVN. *The Developing Human*. Philadelphia, PA: WB Saunders; 1993:325.)

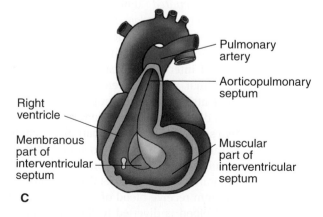

Figure 16-8. Formation of the aorticopulmonary septum occurs via fusion of the bulbar ridges, resulting in division of the bulbus cordis and truncus arteriosus into the aorta and pulmonary artery (A, 5 weeks; B, 6 weeks; C, 7 weeks). The bulbus cordis becomes the right ventricular outflow tract. Fusion of tissue from the endocardial cushions, the aorticopulmonary septum, and the muscular interventricular septum creates the membranous interventricular septum. (Derived from Moore KL, Persaud TVN. *The Developing Human*. Philadelphia, PA: WB Saunders; 1993:322.)

Atrioventricular Valve Development (Mitral and Tricuspid Valves)

After the endocardial cushions fuse to form the septa between the right and left AV canals, the surrounding subendocardial mesenchymal tissue proliferates and develops outgrowths similar to those of the semilunar valves. These are also sculpted by programmed cell death that occurs within the inferior surface of the nascent leaflets and in the ventricular wall. This process leaves behind only a few fine muscular strands to connect the valves to the ventricular wall (Fig. 16-9). The superior portions of these strands eventually degenerate and are replaced by strings of dense connective tissue, becoming the chordae tendineae.

FETAL AND TRANSITIONAL CIRCULATIONS

The fetal circulation elegantly serves the needs of *in utero* development. At birth, the circulation automatically undergoes modifications that establish the normal blood flow pattern of a newborn infant.

FETAL CIRCULATION

In fetal life, oxygenated blood leaves the placenta through the umbilical vein (Fig. 16-10). The majority of this blood is shunted through the fetal **ductus venosus**, bypassing the hepatic vasculature and proceeding directly into the inferior vena cava (IVC). IVC blood is therefore a mixture of *well-oxygenated* umbilical venous blood and the blood of *low oxygen tension* returning from the systemic veins of the fetus. Because of this mixture, the oxygen tension of inferior vena caval blood is higher than that of blood returning to the fetal right atrium from the superior vena cava. This distinction is important because these two streams of blood are partially separated within the right atrium to follow different circulatory paths. The consequence of this separation is that the fetal brain and myocardium receive blood of relatively higher oxygen content, whereas the more poorly oxygenated blood is diverted to the placenta (via the descending aorta and umbilical arteries) for subsequent oxygenation.

A

Interventricular foramen

Lumen of left ventricle

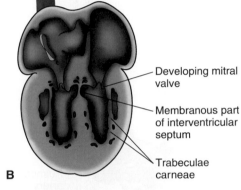

B

Developing mitral valve

Membranous part of interventricular septum

Trabeculae carneae

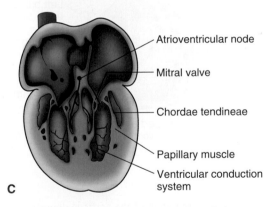

C

Atrioventricular node

Mitral valve

Chordae tendineae

Papillary muscle

Ventricular conduction system

Figure 16-9. Proliferation of mesenchymal tissue surrounding the atrioventricular canals forms the atrioventricular valves. A–C. Progression of the process, including degeneration of myocardium and replacement by connective tissue that forms the chordae tendineae; their muscular attachments to the ventricular wall are the papillary muscles. (Derived from Moore KL, Persaud TVN. *The Developing Human.* Philadelphia, PA: WB Saunders; 1993:325.)

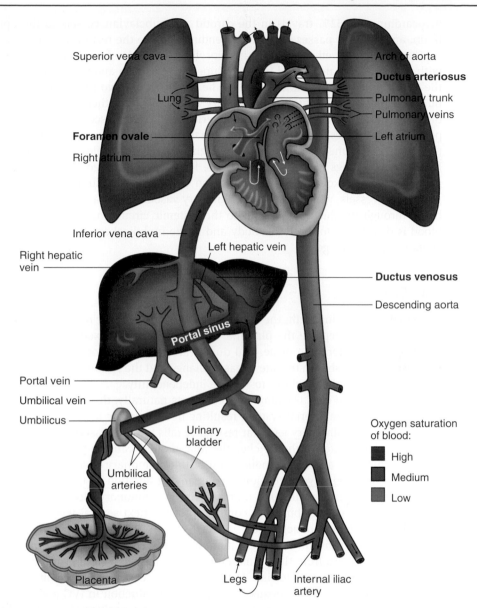

Figure 16-10. The fetal circulation. *Arrows* indicate the direction of blood flow. Three shunts (ductus venosus, foramen ovale, and ductus arteriosus) allow most of the blood to bypass the liver and lungs during fetal life but cease to function shortly after birth. (Modified from Moore KL, Persaud TVN. *The Developing Human*. Philadelphia, PA: WB Saunders; 1993:344.)

Most IVC blood entering the right atrium is directed to the left atrium through the foramen ovale. This intracardiac shunt of relatively well-oxygenated blood is facilitated by the inferior border of the septum secundum, termed the crista dividens, which is positioned such that it overrides the opening of the IVC into the right atrium. This shunted blood then mixes with the small amount of poorly oxygenated blood returning to the left atrium through the fetal pulmonary veins (remember that the lungs are not ventilated *in utero*; the developing pulmonary tissues actually *remove* oxygen from the blood). From the left atrium, blood flows into the LV and is then pumped into the ascending aorta. This well-oxygenated blood is distributed primarily to three territories: (1) ~9% enters the coronary arteries and perfuses the myocardium, (2) 62% travels in the carotid and subclavian vessels to the upper body and brain, and (3) 29% passes into the descending aorta to the rest of the fetal body.

The remaining well-oxygenated inferior vena caval blood entering the right atrium mixes with poorly oxygenated blood from the superior vena cava and passes to the RV. In the fetus, the RV is the actual "workhorse" of the heart, providing two-thirds of the total cardiac output. This output flows into the pulmonary artery and from there either into the lungs (12% of RV output), or through the **ductus arteriosus** into the descending aorta (88% of RV output), where it mixes with the better oxygenated blood from the LV described in the previous paragraph. This unequal distribution of right ventricular outflow is actually quite efficient. Bypassing the lungs is desired because the fetal lungs are filled with amniotic fluid and are incapable of gas exchange. The low oxygen tension of this fluid causes constriction of the pulmonary vessels, which increases pulmonary vascular resistance and facilitates shunting of blood through the ductus arteriosus to the systemic circulation. From the descending aorta, blood is distributed to the lower body and to the umbilical arteries, leading back to the placenta for gas exchange.

TRANSITIONAL CIRCULATION

Immediately following birth, the neonate rapidly adjusts to life outside the womb. The newly functioning lungs replace the placenta as the organ of gas exchange, and the three shunts (ductus venosus, foramen ovale, and ductus arteriosus) that operated during gestation ultimately close. This shift in the site of gas exchange and the resulting changes in cardiovascular architecture allow the newborn to survive independently.

As the umbilical cord is clamped or constricts naturally, the low-resistance placental flow is removed from the arterial system, resulting in an increase in systemic vascular resistance. Simultaneously, pulmonary vascular resistance falls for two reasons: (1) the mechanical inflation of the lungs after birth stretches the lung tissues, causing pulmonary artery expansion and wall thinning, and (2) vasodilatation of the pulmonary vasculature occurs in response to the rise in blood oxygen tension accompanying aeration of the lungs. This reduction in pulmonary resistance results in a dramatic rise in pulmonary blood flow. It is most marked within the first day after birth but continues for the next several weeks until adult levels of pulmonary resistance are achieved.

As pulmonary resistance falls and more blood travels to the lungs through the pulmonary artery, venous return from the pulmonary veins to the left atrium also increases, causing left atrial volume and pressure to rise. At the same time, cessation of umbilical venous flow and constriction of the ductus venosus cause a relative reduction in IVC and right atrial volume. As a result, the flap valve of the foramen ovale becomes positioned more midline against the septum secundum, eliminating the previous flow between the atria (see Fig. 16-5). Failure of the valve to permanently fuse to the septum secundum results in a *patent foramen ovale (PFO)*, as described later in this chapter.

With oxygenation now occurring in the newborn lungs, the ductus arteriosus becomes superfluous and closes. During fetal life, a high circulating level of prostaglandin E_1 (PGE_1) is generated in response to relative hypoxia, which causes the smooth muscle of the ductus arteriosus to relax, keeping it patent. After birth, PGE_1 levels decline as the oxygen tension rises and the ductus therefore constricts. In a healthy full-term infant, this occurs during the first hours to days after delivery. The responsiveness of the ductus to vasoactive substances depends on the gestational age of the fetus, and it often fails to constrict in premature infants. This results in the congenital anomaly known as *patent ductus arteriosus (PDA)* (described below).

With the anatomic separation of the circulatory paths of the right and left sides of the heart now complete, the stroke volume of the LV increases and that of the RV decreases, equalizing the cardiac output from both ventricles. The augmented pressure and volume load placed on the LV induces the myocardial cells of that chamber to hypertrophy, while the decreased pressure and volume loads on the RV result in gradual regression of RV wall thickness.

COMMON CONGENITAL HEART LESIONS

Congenital heart defects are generally well tolerated before birth. The fetus benefits from shunting of blood through the ductus arteriosus and the foramen ovale, allowing the bypass of most defects. It is only after birth, when the neonate has been separated from the maternal circulation and the oxygenation it provides, and the fetal shunts have closed, that congenital heart defects usually become manifest.

Congenital heart lesions can be categorized as *cyanotic* or *acyanotic*. Cyanosis refers to a blue-purple discoloration of the skin and mucous membranes caused by an elevated blood concentration of deoxygenated hemoglobin (usually >4 g/dL, which corresponds to an arterial O_2 saturation of $\sim 80\%$-85% in a neonate with a normal total hemoglobin level). In congenital heart disease, cyanosis results from defects that allow poorly oxygenated blood from the right side of the heart to be shunted to the left side, bypassing the lungs.

Acyanotic lesions include intracardiac or vascular stenoses, valvular regurgitation, and defects that result in *left-to-right* shunting of blood. Large left-to-right shunts at the atrial, ventricular, or great vessel level (all described in the following sections) cause the pulmonary artery volume and pressure to increase and can be associated with the later development of pulmonary arteriolar hypertrophy and subsequently increased resistance to flow. Over time, the elevated pulmonary resistance may force the direction of the original shunt to reverse, causing *right-to-left* flow to supervene, accompanied by the physical findings of hypoxemia and cyanosis. The development of pulmonary vascular disease as a result of a chronic large left-to-right shunt is known as *Eisenmenger syndrome* and is described later in the chapter.

Patients with congenital heart disease are susceptible to infective endocarditis. Chapter 8 describes the pathophysiology of endocarditis and summarizes the appropriate selection of patients for antibiotic prophylaxis prior to procedures that can result in bacteremia.

ACYANOTIC LESIONS

Atrial Septal Defect

An atrial septal defect (ASD) is a persistent opening in the interatrial septum after birth that allows direct communication between the left and right atria. ASDs are relatively common, occurring with an incidence of 1 in 1500 live births. They can occur anywhere along the atrial septum, but the most common site is at the region of the foramen ovale, termed an *ostium secundum* ASD (Fig. 16-11). This defect arises from inadequate formation of the septum secundum, excessive resorption of the septum primum, or a combination.

Less commonly, an ASD appears in the inferior portion of the interatrial septum, adjacent to the AV valves. Named as *ostium primum* defect, this abnormality results from the failure of the septum primum to fuse with the endocardial cushions.

A third type of atrial septal abnormality is termed a *sinus venosus defect* and is closely related to ASDs but is morphologically distinct. This condition represents an "unroofing" defect with absence of normal tissue between the right pulmonary vein(s) and the right atrium but is technically not a deficiency of the anatomic atrial septum (ie, frequently the atrial septum itself is fully intact). As sinus venosus defects are often large and result in flow from the right pulmonary veins and left atrium into the right atrium, the pathophysiology is similar to that of a true ASD.

A   **B**

Figure 16-11. Atrial septal defect (ASD), ostium secundum type. A. The *arrow* indicates shunted flow from the left atrium (LA) into the right atrium (RA). **B.** Schematic representation of blood flow through an uncomplicated ASD, resulting in enlargement of the RA, right ventricle (RV), and pulmonary artery (PA). Ao, aorta; IVC, inferior vena cava; LV, left ventricle; SVC, superior vena cava.

Another distinct condition related to ASDs is *patent foramen ovale* which is present in ~20% of the general population. It too is not a true ASD (ie, no atrial septal tissue is "missing") but represents persistence of normal fetal anatomy. As described earlier, the foramen ovale typically functionally closes in the days after birth, and it is permanently sealed by the age of 6 months through fusion of the atrial septa. A PFO remains when this fusion fails to occur.

A PFO is usually clinically silent because the one-way valve, though not sealed, remains functionally closed since the left atrial pressure is higher than that in the right atrium. However, a PFO takes on significance if the right atrial pressure becomes elevated (eg, in states of pulmonary hypertension or right-heart failure), resulting in pathologic *right-to-left* intracardiac shunting. In that case, deoxygenated blood passes directly into the arterial circulation. Occasionally, a PFO can be implicated in a patient who has suffered a systemic embolism (eg, a stroke). This situation, termed *paradoxical embolism*, occurs when thrombus in a systemic vein breaks loose, travels to the right atrium, then passes across the PFO to the left atrium *if* right-heart pressures are elevated, at least transiently (eg, during a cough, sneeze, or Valsalva type maneuver), and then into the systemic arterial circulation.

Pathophysiology

In the case of an uncomplicated ASD, oxygenated blood from the left atrium is shunted into the right atrium, but not vice versa. Flow through the defect is a function of its size and the filling properties (compliance) of the ventricles into which the atria pass their contents. Normally after birth, the RV becomes more compliant than does the LV, owing to the regression of right ventricular wall thickness and an increase in LV thickness, facilitating the left-to-right directed shunt at the atrial level. The result is volume overload and enlargement of the right atrium and RV (see Fig. 16-11B). If right ventricular compliance diminishes over time (because of the excessive load), the left-to-right shunt may lessen. Occasionally, if severe pulmonary vascular disease develops (eg, Eisenmenger syndrome), the direction of the shunt may actually reverse (causing right-to-left flow), such that desaturated blood enters the systemic circulation, resulting in hypoxemia and cyanosis.

Symptoms

Most infants with ASDs are asymptomatic. The condition may be detected by the presence of a murmur on routine physical examination during childhood or adolescence, but the exam findings are subtle and 25% of ASDs are not diagnosed until adulthood. If symptoms do occur, they include dyspnea on exertion, fatigue, and recurrent lower respiratory tract infections. The most common symptoms in adults are decreased stamina and palpitations due to atrial tachyarrhythmias resulting from right atrial enlargement.

Physical Examination

A prominent systolic impulse may be palpated along the lower left sternal border, representing contraction of the dilated RV (termed an *RV heave*). The second heart sound (S_2) demonstrates a widened, fixed splitting pattern (see Chapter 2). This occurs because the normal respiratory variation in systemic venous return is countered by reciprocal changes in the volume of blood shunted across the ASD. In addition, the increased volume of blood flowing across the pulmonary valve often creates a systolic murmur at the upper-left sternal border. A middiastolic murmur may also be present at the lower left sternal border owing to the increased flow across the tricuspid valve. Blood traversing the ASD itself does not produce a murmur because of the absence of a significant pressure gradient between the atria.

Diagnostic Studies

On *chest radiograph*, the heart may be enlarged because of right atrial and right ventricular dilatation, with prominence of the pulmonary artery and increased pulmonary vascular markings. The *electrocardiogram (ECG)* may show right ventricular hypertrophy and right atrial enlargement and incomplete or complete right bundle branch block are common. In patients with the ostium primum type of ASD, left axis deviation is common and is thought to be a result of displacement and hypoplasia of the left bundle branch's anterior fascicle. *Echocardiography* reveals right atrial and right ventricular enlargement when present; the ASD may be visualized directly, or its presence may be implied by the demonstration of a transatrial shunt by Doppler flow assessment. The magnitude and direction of shunt flow and an estimation of right ventricular systolic pressure can also be determined by echo Doppler measurements.

Given the high sensitivity of echocardiography, it is rarely necessary to perform *cardiac catheterization* to confirm the presence of an ASD. However, catheterization may be useful to assess pulmonary vascular resistance and to diagnose concurrent coronary artery disease in older adults. In a normal person undergoing cardiac catheterization, the oxygen saturation measured in the right atrium is similar to that in the superior vena cava. However, an ASD with left-to-right shunting of well-oxygenated blood causes the saturation in the right atrium to be much greater than that of the superior vena cava.

Treatment

Most patients with ASDs remain asymptomatic. However, if the volume of shunted blood is hemodynamically significant (even in the absence of symptoms), elective surgical repair is recommended to prevent the development of heart failure or chronic pulmonary vascular disease. The defect is repaired by direct suture closure or with a pericardial or synthetic patch. In children and young adults, morphologic changes in the right heart often return to normal after repair. Percutaneous ASD repair, using a closure device deployed via an intravenous catheter, is a less invasive alternative to surgery in selected patients with secundum ASDs.

Ventricular Septal Defect

A ventricular septal defect (VSD) is an abnormal opening in the interventricular septum (Fig. 16-12). VSDs are relatively common, with an incidence of 1.5-3.5 per 1000 live births. They are most often located in the membranous (70%) and muscular (20%) portions of the septum. Rare VSDs occur just below the aortic valve or adjacent to the AV valves.

Pathophysiology

The hemodynamic changes and magnitude of the shunt that accompany VSDs depend on the size of the defect and the relative resistances of the pulmonary and systemic vasculatures. In small VSDs, the defect itself offers more resistance to flow than the pulmonary or systemic vasculature, thereby preventing a significant quantity of left-to-right shunting. Conversely, with larger "nonrestrictive" defects, the volume of the shunt is determined by the relative pulmonary and systemic vascular resistances. In the perinatal period, the pulmonary vascular resistance approximates the systemic vascular resistance, and minimal shunting occurs between the two ventricles. After birth, however, as the pulmonary vascular resistance falls, an increasing left-to-right shunt through the defect develops. When this shunt is large, the RV, pulmonary circulation, left atrium, and LV experience relative volume overload. Initially, the increased blood return to the LV augments stroke volume (via the Frank–Starling mechanism); but over time, the increased volume load can result in progressive chamber dilatation,

A   **B**

Figure 16-12. Ventricular septal defect (VSD). A. The *arrow* indicates shunted flow from the left ventricle (LV) toward the right ventricular (RV) outflow tract. **B.** Schematic representation of blood flow through an uncomplicated VSD. The *dashed lines* represent increased blood return to the left side of the heart as a result of the shunt, which causes enlargement primarily of the left atrium (LA) and LV. Ao, aorta; IVC, inferior vena cava; PA, pulmonary artery; RA, right atrium; SVC, superior vena cava.

systolic dysfunction, and symptoms of heart failure. In addition, the augmented circulation through the pulmonary vasculature can cause pulmonary vascular disease as early as 2 years of age. If pulmonary vascular resistance eventually approaches or exceeds systemic resistance, the intracardiac shunt may reverse its direction (ie, Eisenmenger syndrome), leading to systemic hypoxemia and cyanosis.

Symptoms

Patients with small VSDs typically remain symptom free. Conversely, 10% of infants with VSDs have large defects and develop early symptoms of heart failure, including tachypnea, poor feeding, failure to thrive, and frequent lower respiratory tract infections. Patients with VSDs complicated by pulmonary vascular disease and reversed shunts may present with dyspnea and cyanosis. Bacterial endocarditis (see Chapter 8) can develop, regardless of the size of the VSD.

Physical Examination

The most common physical finding is a harsh holosystolic murmur that is best heard at the left sternal border. Smaller defects tend to have the loudest murmurs because of the great turbulence of flow that they cause. A systolic thrill can commonly be palpated over the region of the murmur. In addition, a middiastolic rumbling murmur is often present at the apex owing to the increased flow across the mitral valve. If pulmonary vascular disease develops, the holosystolic murmur diminishes as the pressure gradient across the defect decreases. In such patients, an RV heave, a loud pulmonic closure sound (P_2), and cyanosis may be evident.

Diagnostic Studies

On *chest radiographs*, the cardiac silhouette may be normal in patients with small defects, but in those with large shunts, cardiomegaly and prominent pulmonary vascular markings are present. If pulmonary vascular disease has developed, enlarged pulmonary arteries with peripheral tapering may be evident. The *ECG* shows left atrial enlargement and left ventricular hypertrophy in those with a large shunt, and right ventricular hypertrophy is usually evident if pulmonary vascular disease has developed. *Echocardiography* with Doppler studies can accurately determine the location of the VSD, identify the direction and magnitude of the shunt, and provide an estimate of right ventricular systolic pressure. *Cardiac catheterization* demonstrates increased oxygen saturation in the RV compared with the right atrium, the result of shunting of highly oxygenated blood from the LV into the RV.

Treatment

By age 2, at least 50% of small and moderate-sized VSDs undergo sufficient partial or complete spontaneous closure to make intervention unnecessary. Surgical correction of the defect is recommended in the first few months of life for children with accompanying heart failure or pulmonary vascular hypertension. Moderate-sized defects without pulmonary vascular disease but with significant left-to-right shunting can be corrected later in childhood. Less-invasive catheter-based treatments are also used in selected patients.

Patent Ductus Arteriosus

The ductus arteriosus is the vessel that connects the pulmonary artery to the descending aorta during fetal life. PDA results when the ductus fails to close after birth, resulting in a persistent connection between the great vessels (Fig. 16-13). It has an overall incidence of about 1 in 2500-5000 live term births. Risk factors for its presence include first trimester maternal rubella infection, prematurity, and birth at a high altitude.

Figure 16-13. Patent ductus arteriosus (PDA). A. The *arrow* indicates shunted flow from the descending aorta (Ao) toward the pulmonary artery (PA). **B.** Schematic representation of blood flow through an uncomplicated PDA. The *dashed lines* represent increased blood return to the left side of the heart as a result of the shunt, which causes enlargement of the left atrium (LA), left ventricle (LV), and Ao. IVC, inferior vena cava; RA, right atrium; RV, right ventricle; SVC, superior vena cava.

Pathophysiology

As described earlier, the smooth muscle of the ductus arteriosus usually constricts after birth owing to the sudden rise in blood oxygen tension and a reduction in the level of circulating prostaglandins. Over the next several weeks, intimal proliferation and fibrosis result in permanent closure. Failure of the ductus to close results in a persistent shunt between the descending aorta and the left pulmonary artery. The magnitude of flow through the shunt depends on the cross-sectional area and length of the ductus itself as well as the relative resistances of the systemic and pulmonary vasculatures. Prenatally, when the pulmonary vascular resistance is high, blood is diverted away from the immature lungs to the aorta. As the pulmonary resistance drops postnatally, the shunt reverses direction, and blood flows from the aorta into the pulmonary circulation instead. Because of this left-to-right shunt, the pulmonary circulation, left atrium, and LV become volume overloaded. Persistent PDA can thus lead to left ventricular dilatation and left-sided heart failure, whereas the right heart remains normal unless pulmonary vascular disease ensues. If the latter does develop, Eisenmenger syndrome results, with reversal of the shunt causing blood to flow from the pulmonary artery, through the ductus, to the descending aorta. In this case, the resulting flow of desaturated blood to the lower extremities causes cyanosis of the feet; the upper extremities are not cyanotic, because they receive normally saturated blood from the aorta proximal to the ductus.

Symptoms

Children with small PDAs are generally asymptomatic. Those with large left-to-right shunts develop early congestive heart failure with tachycardia, poor feeding, slow growth, and recurrent lower respiratory tract infections. Moderate-sized lesions can present with fatigue, dyspnea, and palpitations in adolescence and adult life. Atrial fibrillation may occur owing to left atrial dilatation. Turbulent blood flow across the defect can set the stage for endovascular infection, similar to endocarditis but more accurately termed *endarteritis*.

Physical Examination

The most common finding in a patient with a left-to-right shunt through a PDA is a *continuous, machinelike* murmur (see Fig. 2-10), heard best at the left subclavicular region. The murmur is present throughout the cardiac cycle because a pressure gradient exists between the aorta and pulmonary artery in both systole and diastole. However, if pulmonary vascular disease develops, the gradient between the aorta and the pulmonary artery decreases, leading to diminished flow through the PDA, and the murmur becomes shorter (the diastolic component may disappear). If Eisenmenger syndrome develops, lower extremity cyanosis and clubbing may be present as poorly oxygenated blood is shunted to the descending aorta.

Diagnostic Studies

With a large PDA, the *chest radiograph* shows an enlarged cardiac silhouette (left atrial and left ventricular enlargement) with prominent pulmonary vascular markings. In adults, calcification of the ductus may be visualized. The *ECG* shows left atrial enlargement and left ventricular hypertrophy when a large shunt is present. *Echocardiography* with Doppler imaging can visualize the defect, demonstrate flow through it, and estimate right-sided systolic pressures. *Cardiac catheterization* is usually unnecessary for diagnostic purposes. When performed in patients with a left-to-right shunt, it demonstrates a step up in oxygen saturation in the pulmonary artery compared with the RV, and angiography shows the abnormal flow of blood through the PDA.

Treatment

In the absence of other congenital cardiac abnormalities or severe pulmonary vascular disease, a PDA should generally be therapeutically occluded. Although many spontaneously close during the first months after birth, this rarely occurs later. Given the constant risk of endarteritis and the minimal complications of corrective procedures, even a small asymptomatic PDA is commonly referred for closure. For neonates and premature infants with congestive heart failure, a trial of prostaglandin synthesis inhibitors (eg, indomethacin) can be administered in an attempt to constrict the ductus. Definitive closure can be accomplished by surgical division or ligation of the ductus or by transcatheter techniques in which an occluding device is placed.

Congenital Aortic Stenosis

Congenital aortic stenosis (AS) is most often caused by abnormal structural development of the valve leaflets. It occurs in 5 of 10,000 live births and is four times as common in males as in females. Twenty percent of patients have an additional abnormality, most commonly coarctation of the aorta (discussed later). The aortic valve in congenital AS usually has a **bicuspid** leaflet structure instead of the normal three-leaflet configuration, causing an eccentric stenotic opening through which blood is ejected. Most bicuspid aortic valves are actually nonobstructive at birth and therefore only rarely result in congenital AS. More often, bicuspid valves become progressively stenotic over a great many years, as the leaflets progressively fibrose and calcify, and represent a common cause of AS in adults (see Chapter 8).

Pathophysiology

Because the valvular orifice is significantly narrowed, left ventricular systolic pressure must increase to pump blood across the valve into the aorta. In response to this increased pressure load, the LV hypertrophies (Fig. 16-14). The high-velocity jet of blood that passes through the stenotic valve may impact the proximal aortic wall and contribute to dilatation of that vessel.

Symptoms

The clinical picture of AS depends on the severity of the lesion. Fewer than 10% of infants experience symptoms of heart failure before age 1, but if they do, they manifest tachycardia, tachypnea, failure to thrive, and poor feeding. Most older children with congenital AS are asymptomatic and develop normally. When symptoms do occur, they are similar to those of adult AS and include fatigue, exertional dyspnea, angina pectoris, and syncope (see Chapter 8).

Physical Examination

Auscultation reveals a harsh crescendo–decrescendo systolic murmur, loudest at the base of the heart with radiation toward the neck. It is often preceded by a systolic ejection click (see Chapter 2), especially when a bicuspid valve is present. Unlike the murmurs of ASD, VSD, or PDA, the murmur of congenital AS is characteristically present from birth because it does not depend on the postnatal decline in pulmonary vascular resistance. With advanced disease, the ejection time becomes longer, causing the peak of the murmur to occur later in systole. In advanced disease, the markedly prolonged ejection time causes a delay in closure of the aortic valve such that A_2 occurs *after* P_2—a phenomenon known as reversed splitting (also termed "paradoxical splitting") of S_2 (see Chapter 2).

Figure 16-14. Congenital aortic valve stenosis. A. The *jagged arrow* traverses the narrowed aortic valve. **B.** Schematic representation of obstructed flow through the narrowed aortic valve (*jagged arrow*). Left ventricular (LV) hypertrophy results from the chronically increased pressure load. Poststenotic dilatation of the aorta (Ao) is common. IVC, inferior vena cava; LA, left atrium; PA, pulmonary artery; RA, right atrium; RV, right ventricle; SVC, superior vena cava.

Diagnostic Studies

The *chest radiograph* of an infant with AS may show an enlarged LV and a dilated ascending aorta. The *ECG* often shows left ventricular hypertrophy. *Echocardiography* identifies the abnormal structure of the aortic valve and the degree of left ventricular hypertrophy. Doppler assessment allows calculation of the pressure gradient across the stenotic valve and valve area. *Cardiac catheterization*, if necessary, confirms the pressure gradient across the valve.

Treatment

In milder forms, congenital AS does not require correction but should be followed closely as the degree of stenosis may worsen over time. Severe obstruction of the aortic valve during infancy may mandate immediate repair. Transcatheter balloon valvuloplasty is the first line of intervention at that age, but surgical repair may be necessary if valvuloplasty fails to relieve the obstruction or if significant aortic regurgitation results from balloon dilation. Often, valvuloplasty in infancy is only palliative, and repeat catheter balloon dilation or surgical revision is needed later.

Pulmonic Valve Stenosis

Obstruction to right ventricular outflow may occur at the level of the pulmonic valve (eg, from congenitally fused valve commissures), within the body of the RV (ie, in the RV outflow tract), or in the pulmonary artery. *Valvular* pulmonic stenosis is the most frequent form (Fig. 16-15).

A   **B**

Figure 16-15. Congenital pulmonary valve stenosis. A. The *jagged arrow* traverses the narrowed pulmonary valve. **B.** Schematic representation of obstructed flow through the narrowed pulmonary valve (*jagged arrow*). Right ventricular hypertrophy results from the chronically increased pressure load. Ao, aorta; IVC, inferior vena cava; LA, left atrium; LV, left ventricle; PA, pulmonary artery; RA, right atrium; RV, right ventricle; SVC, superior vena cava.

Pathophysiology

The consequence of pulmonic stenosis is impairment of right ventricular outflow, which leads to increased RV pressure and chamber hypertrophy. The clinical course is determined by the severity of the obstruction. Although mild pulmonic stenosis rarely progresses and is unlikely to affect RV function, untreated severe pulmonic stenosis typically results in right-sided heart failure.

Symptoms

Children with mild or moderate pulmonic stenosis are asymptomatic. The diagnosis is often first made on discovery of a murmur during physical examination. Severe stenosis may cause manifestations such as dyspnea with exertion, exercise intolerance, and with decompensation, symptoms of right-sided heart failure, including abdominal fullness and pedal edema.

Physical Examination

The physical findings in pulmonic stenosis depend on the severity of the obstruction. If the stenosis is severe with accompanying right ventricular hypertrophy, a prominent jugular venous a wave can be observed (see Chapter 2) and an RV heave is palpated over the sternum. A loud, late-peaking, crescendo–decrescendo systolic ejection murmur is heard at the upper left sternal border, often associated with a palpable thrill. Widened splitting of the S_2 with a soft P_2 component is caused by the delayed closure of the stenotic pulmonary valve.

In more moderate stenosis, a pulmonic ejection sound (a high-pitched "click") follows S_1 and precedes the systolic murmur. It occurs during the early phase of right ventricular contraction as the stenotic valve leaflets suddenly reach their maximum level of ascent into the pulmonary artery, just before blood ejection. Unlike other sounds and murmurs produced by the right side of the heart, the pulmonic ejection sound *diminishes* in intensity during inspiration. This occurs because with inspiration, the augmented right-sided filling elevates the leaflets into the pulmonary artery prior to RV contraction, preempting the rapid tensing in early systole that is thought to produce the sound.

Diagnostic Studies

The *chest radiograph* may demonstrate an enlarged right atrium and ventricle with poststenotic pulmonary artery dilation (thought to be caused by the impact of the high-velocity jet of blood against the wall of the pulmonary artery). The *ECG* shows right ventricular hypertrophy with right axis deviation. *Echocardiography* with Doppler imaging assesses the pulmonic valve morphology, determines the presence of right ventricular hypertrophy, and accurately measures the pressure gradient across the obstruction.

Treatment

Mild pulmonic stenosis usually does not progress or require treatment. Moderate or severe valvular obstruction at the valvular level can be relieved by dilating the stenotic valve by means of transcatheter balloon valvuloplasty. Long-term results of this procedure have been uniformly excellent, and right ventricular hypertrophy usually regresses subsequently.

Coarctation of the Aorta

Coarctation of the aorta typically consists of a discrete narrowing of the aortic lumen (Fig. 16-16). This anomaly has an incidence of 1 in 6000 live births, and the most common associated cardiac abnormality is a bicuspid aortic valve. Aortic coarctation often occurs in patients with Turner syndrome (45, XO).

In the past, coarctations were described as either "preductal" (infantile) or "postductal" (adult-type) based on the location of the aortic narrowing in relation to the ductus arteriosus. These terms have been largely abandoned because the vast majority of coarctations are actually juxtaductal (ie, "next to" the ductus), and etiologic differences between the preductal and postductal categories have not been substantiated.

While the actual pathogenesis of aortic coarctation has not been defined, one theory contends that reduced antegrade blood flow through the left side of the heart and ascending aorta during fetal life leads to hypoplastic development of the aorta ("no flow, no grow"). Another theory is that ectopic muscular ductus arteriosus tissue extends into the aorta during fetal life and constricts following birth at the same time the ductus is caused to close. More recent evidence suggests that aortic coarctation may be just one manifestation of a more diffuse aortic disease.

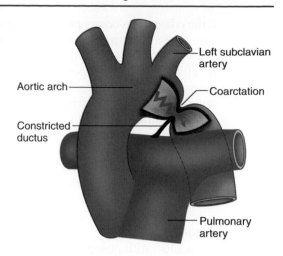

Figure 16-16. Coarctation of the aorta. A pressure gradient is present across the narrowed lumen of the aorta.

Pathophysiology

Because of the impedance of aortic narrowing in coarctation, the LV faces increased afterload. Blood flow to the head and upper extremities is preserved because the vessels supplying these areas usually branch off the aorta proximal to the obstruction, but flow to the descending aorta and lower extremities may be diminished. If coarctation is not corrected, compensatory alterations include (1) development of left ventricular hypertrophy and (2) dilatation of collateral blood vessels from the intercostal arteries that bypass the coarctation and provide blood to the more distal descending aorta. Eventually, these collateral vessels enlarge and can erode the undersurface of the ribs.

Symptoms

Patients with severe coarctation usually present very shortly after birth with symptoms of heart failure. Infants may also exhibit *differential cyanosis* if the ductus arteriosus fails to constrict and remains patent. The upper half of the body, supplied by the LV and the ascending aorta, is perfused with well-oxygenated blood; however, the lower half appears cyanotic because it is largely supplied by right-to-left flow of poorly oxygenated blood from the pulmonary artery, across the PDA, and into the descending aorta, beyond the coarctation.

When the coarctation is less severe, a patient may be asymptomatic or experience only mild weakness or pain in the lower extremities following exercise (ie, *claudication*). In asymptomatic cases, coarctation may be suspected by the finding of upper extremity hypertension later in life (see Chapter 13).

Physical Examination

On examination, the femoral pulses are weak and delayed. An elevated blood pressure in the upper body is the most common finding. If the coarctation occurs *distal* to the takeoff of the left subclavian artery, the systolic pressure in the arms is greater than that in the legs.

If the coarctation occurs *proximal* to the takeoff of the left subclavian artery, the systolic pressure in the right arm may exceed that in the left arm. A systolic pressure in the right arm that is 15-20 mm Hg greater than that in a leg is sufficient to suspect coarctation, because normally the systolic pressure in the legs is *higher* than that in the arms. A midsystolic ejection murmur (caused by turbulent flow through the coarctation) may be audible over the chest and/or back. A prominent tortuous collateral arterial circulation may create continuous murmurs over the chest in adults.

Diagnostic Studies

In adults with uncorrected coarctation of the aorta, *chest radiography* generally reveals notching of the inferior surface of the posterior ribs owing to enlarged intercostal vessels supplying collateral circulation to the descending aorta. An indented aorta at the site of coarctation may also be visualized. The *ECG* shows left ventricular hypertrophy resulting from the pressure load placed on that chamber. *Doppler echocardiography* confirms the diagnosis of coarctation and assesses the pressure gradient across the lesion. *Magnetic resonance (or CT) imaging* demonstrates in detail the length and severity of coarctation (see Fig. 16-17). Diagnostic *catheterization* and angiography are rarely necessary.

Figure 16-17. Magnetic resonance imaging of coarctation of the aorta. This lateral view demonstrates coarctation, manifest as a focal aortic narrowing (*white arrow*). AA, ascending aorta; DA, descending aorta; LA, left atrium; RA, right atrium; TAA, transverse aortic arch.

Treatment

In neonates with severe obstruction, prostaglandin infusion is administered to keep the ductus arteriosus patent, thus maintaining blood flow to the descending aorta before surgery is undertaken. In children, elective repair is usually performed to prevent systemic hypertension. Several effective surgical procedures are available, including excision of the narrowed aortic segment with end-to-end reanastomosis and direct repair of the coarctation, sometimes using synthetic patch material. For older children, adults, and patients with recurrent coarctation after previous repair, transcatheter interventions (balloon dilatation with or without stent placement) are usually successful.

CYANOTIC LESIONS

Tetralogy of Fallot

Tetralogy of Fallot results from a single developmental defect: an abnormal anterior and cephalad displacement of the infundibular (outflow tract) portion of the interventricular septum. As a consequence, four anomalies arise that characterize this condition, as shown in Figure 16-18: (1) a VSD caused by anterior malalignment of the interventricular septum, (2) subvalvular pulmonic stenosis because of obstruction from the displaced infundibular septum (often with valvular pulmonic stenosis), (3) an overriding aorta that receives blood from both ventricles, and (4) right ventricular hypertrophy owing to the high-pressure load placed on the RV by the pulmonic stenosis. Tetralogy of Fallot is the most common form of cyanotic con-

Figure 16-18. Tetralogy of Fallot is characterized by four associated anomalies. (1) A ventricular septal defect, (2) obstruction to right ventricular outflow (*jagged arrow*), (3) an overriding aorta that receives blood from both ventricles, and (4) right ventricular hypertrophy. Ao, aorta; IVC, inferior vena cava; LA, left atrium; LV, left ventricle; PA, pulmonary artery; RA, right atrium; RV, right ventricle; SVC, superior vena cava.

genital heart disease after infancy, occurring in 5 of 10,000 live births and is often associated with other cardiac defects, including a right-sided aortic arch (25% of patients), ASD (10% of patients), and less often, an anomalous origin of the left coronary artery. A microdeletion in chromosome 22 (22q11) has been identified in patients with a syndrome that includes tetralogy of Fallot as one of the cardiovascular manifestations (see Box 16-1).

Box 16-1   Genetics of Congenital Heart Disease

Progress in the understanding of genetic influences on cardiac development and congenital heart disease is proceeding rapidly. Although nearly all cardiac congenital anomalies can occur as isolated findings, the clustering of certain forms with heritable syndromes and known genetic abnormalities provides clues to the underlying basis of certain defects.

Among infants with **Down syndrome** (trisomy 21), the incidence of congenital heart defects is nearly 40%. Many of these are common abnormalities such as ASDs, VSDs, and PDAs. There is also a high incidence of a rare condition known as common AV canal, which consists of a large primum ASD and VSD and a common (undivided) AV valve. These central heart structures are usually formed by the endocardial cushions and cells of neural crest origin, which are known to have abnormal migration patterns in patients with trisomy 21.

Turner syndrome (45, XO) is associated with left-sided obstructive congenital heart lesions, including bicuspid aortic valve, coarctation of the aorta, and occasionally hypoplastic left heart syndrome (underdevelopment of the LV and aorta). The specific genes responsible for these abnormalities have not yet been elucidated.

In contrast, discrete gene abnormalities *have* been identified in other syndrome-associated forms of congenital heart disease. Many patients with **Williams syndrome** (characterized by mental retardation, hypercalcemia, renovascular hypertension, facial abnormalities, and short stature) have supravalvular AS, and some have a more diffuse arteriopathy of the aorta as well as pulmonary artery obstruction. The genetic abnormality in Williams syndrome is a deletion on

| Box 16-1 | Genetics of Congenital Heart Disease (continued) |

chromosome 7 (7q11.23), a region that includes the elastin gene. Abnormalities in the production of elastin, a critical component of the arterial wall, may be responsible for the observed arteriopathy.

DiGeorge syndrome (characterized by pharyngeal defects, hypocalcemia due to absent parathyroid glands, and T-cell dysfunction secondary to hypoplasia of the thymus) is associated with congenital abnormalities of the cardiac outflow tracts, including tetralogy of Fallot, truncus arteriosus (a large VSD over which a single large outflow vessel arises), and interrupted aortic arch. Most patients with DiGeorge syndrome have a microdeletion within chromosome 22 (22q11), a region that contains the *TBX1* gene. This gene encodes a transcription factor that appears to play a critical role in developmental patterning of the cardiac outflow tracts.

CHARGE syndrome (the acronym for **c**oloboma [congenital absence of portions of eye structures], **h**eart defects, choanal **a**tresia [nasal passage obstruction], **r**etardation of growth and development, **g**enitourinary malformation, **e**ar abnormalities) is an autosomal dominant disorder that includes some or all of the listed components. Associated cardiac abnormalities include interrupted aortic arch, tetralogy of Fallot, double outlet RV, and AV septal defects. The incidence of the syndrome is ~1:10,000 children, and most are found to have a mutation or microdeletion in the *CHD7* gene, the protein product of which is a transcription regulator associated with several tissue-specific target genes.

Several other transcription factors involved in heart development likely contribute to congenital heart disease. Some families with heritable forms of ASDs have mutations in the transcription factor gene *Nkx2.5*. An associated transcription factor gene *GATA4* appears to collaborate with *Nkx2.5* and has also been implicated in familial septal defect syndromes. Mutations in *TBX5*, yet another transcription factor gene, are responsible for **Holt–Oram syndrome** (also known as the heart–hand syndrome), an autosomal dominant disorder whose characteristic cardiac defects include secundum ASDs and VSDs.

Pathophysiology

Increased resistance by the subvalvular pulmonic stenosis causes deoxygenated blood returning from the systemic veins to be diverted from the RV, through the VSD to the LV, and into the systemic circulation, resulting in systemic hypoxemia and cyanosis. The magnitude of shunt flow across the VSD is primarily a function of the severity of the pulmonary stenosis, but acute changes in systemic and pulmonary vascular resistances can affect it as well.

Symptoms

Children with tetralogy of Fallot often experience dyspnea on exertion. "Spells" may occur following exertion, feeding, or crying when systemic vasodilatation results in an increased right-to-left shunt. Manifestations of such spells include irritability, cyanosis, hyperventilation, and occasionally syncope or convulsions. Children learn to alleviate their symptoms by squatting down, which is thought to increase systemic vascular resistance by "kinking" the femoral arteries, thereby decreasing the right-to-left shunt and directing more blood from the RV to the lungs.

Physical Examination

Children with tetralogy of Fallot and moderate pulmonary stenosis often have mild cyanosis, most notably of the lips, mucous membranes, and digits. Infants with severe pulmonary stenosis may present with profound cyanosis in the first few days of life. Chronic hypoxemia caused by the right-to-left shunt commonly results in clubbing of the fingers and toes. Right ventricular hypertrophy may be appreciated on physical examination as a palpable heave along the left sternal border. The second heart sound is single, composed of a normal aortic component; the pulmonary component is soft and usually inaudible. A systolic ejection murmur at the upper left sternal border is created by turbulent blood flow through the stenotic right ventricular outflow tract. There is usually no distinct murmur related to the VSD, because it is typically large and thus generates little turbulence.

Diagnostic Studies

Chest radiography demonstrates prominence of the RV and decreased size of the main pulmonary artery segment, giving the appearance of a "boot-shaped" heart. Pulmonary vascular markings are typically diminished because of decreased flow through the pulmonary circulation. The *ECG* shows right ventricular hypertrophy with right axis deviation. *Echocardiography* details the right ventricular outflow tract anatomy, the malaligned VSD, right ventricular hypertrophy, and other associated defects, as does *cardiac catheterization.*

Treatment

Before definitive surgical correction of tetralogy of Fallot was developed, several forms of palliative therapy were undertaken. These involved creating anatomic communications between the aorta (or one of its major branches) to the pulmonary artery, establishing a left-to-right shunt to increase pulmonary blood flow. Such procedures are occasionally used today in infants for whom definitive repair is planned at an older age. Complete surgical correction of tetralogy of Fallot involves closure of the VSD and enlargement of the subpulmonary infundibulum with the use of a pericardial patch; pulmonic valve repair is required in some patients. Elective repair is usually recommended at 3-6 months of age to decrease the likelihood of future complications. Most patients who have undergone successful repair grow to become asymptomatic adults, although lifelong monitoring is necessary to follow the status of the pulmonary valve, right ventricular function and surveillance for atrial and ventricular arrhythmias. Antibiotic prophylaxis to prevent endocarditis is required in some patients (see Chapter 8).

Transposition of the Great Arteries

In transposition of the great arteries (TGA), each great vessel inappropriately arises from the opposite ventricle; that is, the aorta originates from the RV and the pulmonary artery originates from the LV (Fig. 16-19). This anomaly accounts for ~7% of congenital heart defects, affecting 40 of 100,000 live births. Whereas tetralogy of Fallot is the most common etiology of cyanosis after infancy, TGA is the most common cause of cyanosis in the neonatal period.

The precise cause of transposition remains unknown. One theory contends that failure of the aorticopulmonary septum to spiral in a normal fashion during

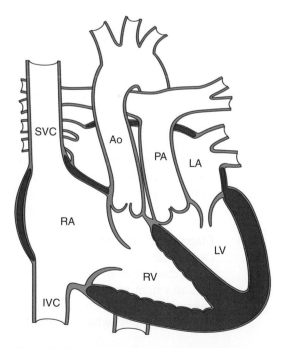

Figure 16-19. Transposition of the great arteries. The aorta (Ao) and pulmonary artery (PA) arise abnormally from the right ventricle (RV) and left ventricle (LV), respectively. IVC, inferior vena cava; LA, left atrium; RA, right atrium; SVC, superior vena cava.

fetal development is the underlying problem. It has also been suggested that the defect may be the result of abnormal growth and absorption of the subpulmonary and subaortic infundibuli during the division of the truncus arteriosus. Normally, reabsorption of the subaortic infundibulum places the forming aortic valve posterior and inferior to the pulmonary valve and in continuity with the LV. In TGA, the process of infundibular reabsorption may be reversed, placing the pulmonary valve over the LV instead.

Pathophysiology

TGA separates the pulmonary and systemic circulations by placing the two circuits in parallel rather than in series. This arrangement forces desaturated blood from the systemic venous system to pass through the RV and then return to the systemic circulation through the aorta without undergoing normal oxygenation in the lungs. Similarly, oxygenated pulmonary venous return passes through the LV and then back through the pulmonary artery to the lungs without imparting oxygen to the systemic circulation. The result is an extremely hypoxic, cyanotic neonate. Without intervention to create mixing between the two circulations, TGA is a lethal condition.

TGA is compatible with life *in utero* because flow through the ductus arteriosus and foramen ovale allows communication between the two circulations. Oxygenated fetal blood flows from the placenta through the umbilical vein to the right atrium, and then most of it travels into the left atrium through the foramen ovale. The oxygenated blood in the left atrium passes into the LV and is pumped out the pulmonary artery. Most of the pulmonary artery flow travels through the ductus arteriosus into the aorta, instead of the high-resistance pulmonary vessels, such that oxygen is provided to the developing tissues.

After birth, normal physiologic closure of the ductus and the foramen ovale eliminates the shunt between the parallel circulations and, without intervention, would result in death because oxygenated blood does not reach the systemic tissues. However, if the ductus arteriosus and foramen ovale remain patent (either naturally or with exogenous prostaglandins or surgical intervention), communication between the parallel circuits is maintained, and sufficiently oxygenated blood may be provided to the brain and other vital organs.

Symptoms and Physical Examination

Infants with transposition appear blue, with the intensity of the cyanosis dependent on the degree of intermixing between the parallel circuits. In most cases, generalized cyanosis is apparent on the first day of life and progresses rapidly as the ductus arteriosus closes. Palpation of the chest reveals a right ventricular impulse at the lower sternal border as the RV faces systemic pressures. Auscultation may reveal an accentuated S_2, which reflects closure of the anteriorly placed aortic valve just under the chest wall. Prominent murmurs are uncommon and may signal an additional defect.

Diagnostic Studies

Chest radiography is usually normal, although the base of the heart may be narrow owing to the more anterior–posterior orientation of the aorta and pulmonary artery. The *ECG* demonstrates right ventricular hypertrophy, reflecting the fact that the RV is the systemic "high-pressure" pumping chamber. The definitive diagnosis of transposition can be made by *echocardiography*, which demonstrates the abnormal orientation of the great vessels.

Treatment

TGA is a medical emergency. Initial treatment includes maintenance of the ductus arteriosus by prostaglandin infusion and mechanical creation of an interatrial communication using a balloon catheter (termed the Rashkind procedure). Such intervention allows adequate mixing of the two circulations until definitive corrective surgery can be performed. The current corrective procedure of choice is the "arterial switch" operation (Jatene procedure), which involves transection of the great vessels above the semilunar valves and origin of the coronary arteries. The great vessels are then reversed to the natural configuration, so the aorta arises from the LV and the pulmonary artery arises from the RV. The coronary arteries are then relocated to the new aorta.

EISENMENGER SYNDROME

Eisenmenger syndrome is the condition of severe pulmonary vascular obstruction that results from chronic left-to-right shunting through a congenital cardiac defect. The elevated pulmonary vascular resistance causes reversal of the original shunt (to the right-to-left direction) and systemic cyanosis.

The mechanism by which increased pulmonary flow causes this condition is unknown. Histologically, the pulmonary arteriolar media hypertrophies and the intima proliferates, reducing the cross-sectional area of the pulmonary vascular bed. Over time, the vessels become thrombosed, and the resistance of the pulmonary vasculature rises, causing the original left-to-right shunt to decrease. Eventually, if the resistance of the pulmonary circulation exceeds that of the systemic vasculature, the direction of shunt flow reverses.

With reversal of the shunt to the right-to-left direction, symptoms arise from hypoxemia, including exertional dyspnea and fatigue. Reduced hemoglobin saturation stimulates the bone marrow to produce more red blood cells (erythrocytosis), which can lead to hyperviscosity, symptoms of which include fatigue, headaches, and stroke (caused by cerebrovascular occlusion). Infarction or rupture of the pulmonary vessels can result in hemoptysis.

On examination, a patient with Eisenmenger syndrome appears cyanotic with digital clubbing. A prominent *a* wave in the jugular venous pulsation reflects elevated right-sided pressure during atrial contraction. A loud P_2 is common. The murmur of the inciting left-to-right shunt is usually *absent*, because the original pressure gradient across the lesion is negated by the elevated right-heart pressures.

Chest radiography in Eisenmenger syndrome is notable for proximal pulmonary artery dilatation with peripheral tapering. Calcification of the pulmonary vasculature may be seen. The *ECG* demonstrates right ventricular hypertrophy and right atrial enlargement. *Echocardiography* with Doppler studies can usually identify the underlying cardiac defect and quantitate the pulmonary artery systolic pressure.

Treatment includes the avoidance of activities that can exacerbate the right-to-left shunt. These include strenuous physical activity, high altitude, and the use of peripheral vasodilator drugs. Pregnancy is especially dangerous; the rate of spontaneous abortion is 20%-40%, and maternal mortality is ∼45%. Supportive measures for Eisenmenger syndrome include prompt treatment of infections, management of rhythm disturbances, and phlebotomy for patients with symptomatic erythrocytosis.

Although there are no remedies that reverse the disease process in Eisenmenger syndrome, pulmonary vasodilator therapy can provide symptomatic relief and improve the patient's quality of life. Effective agents include endothelin receptor antagonists, prostacyclin analogs, and phosphodiesterase inhibitors (see Chapter 17). Surgical or transcatheter device closure of the anatomic shunt permitting the reversed right to left flow is generally contraindicated. That is, shunt closure eliminates a pathway for blood to exit the RV in the face of high pulmonary vascular resistance and could precipitate acute right ventricular failure. The only effective long-term strategy for severely affected patients is lung or heart-lung transplantation. Fortunately, with the dramatic advances that have been made in the detection and early correction of severe congenital heart defects, Eisenmenger syndrome has become less common.

Summary

- **Formation of the cardiovascular system** begins during the 3rd week of embryonic development; the fetal circulation uses the placenta as the primary organ of gas, nutrient, and waste exchange. At birth, the fetal lungs inflate, and the circulation is altered to allow the neonate to adjust to life outside the womb.

- **Cardiac malformations occur in 0.8% of live births**, representing the most common form of birth defects and the leading cause of death from birth abnormalities in the first year of life.

- Congenital heart lesions can be grouped into **cyanotic or acyanotic** defects, depending on whether the abnormality results in right-to-left shunting of blood.

- **Acyanotic defects** often result in either volume overload (ASD, VSD, PDA) or pressure overload (AS, pulmonic stenosis, coarctation of the aorta).

- Chronic volume overload resulting from a large left-to-right shunt can ultimately result in increased pulmonary vascular resistance, reversal of the direction of shunt flow, and subsequent cyanosis (**Eisenmenger syndrome**).

- Among the most common **cyanotic defects** are tetralogy of Fallot and transposition of the great arteries.

Review Questions

1. A 35-year-old woman is found to have fixed splitting of the second heart sound. Which congenital cardiac abnormality is likely present?

   a. Patent ductus arteriosus
   b. Atrial septal defect
   c. Ventricular septal defect
   d. Coarctation of the aorta

2. An 18-year-old student presents for evaluation of palpitations. Cardiac examination reveals a continuous, machinelike murmur that is loudest inferior to the left clavicle. This finding is suggestive of which congenital cardiac abnormality?

   a. Patent ductus arteriosus
   b. Ventricular septal defect
   c. Tetralogy of Fallot
   d. Transposition of the great arteries

3. A systolic ejection click is associated with which congenital cardiac abnormality?

   a. Patent ductus arteriosus
   b. Coarctation of the aorta
   c. Atrial septal defect
   d. Bicuspid aortic valve

4. An asymptomatic 19-year-old college student is found to have a harsh holosystolic murmur at the lower left sternal border, which does not increase in intensity with inspiration. Which congenital cardiac abnormality is likely present?

a. Patent ductus arteriosus
b. Patent foramen ovale
c. Ventricular septal defect
d. Pulmonic stenosis

5. Which congenital heart lesion is associated with Turner syndrome (45, XO)?

a. Atrial septal defect
b. Ventricular septal defect
c. Coarctation of the aorta
d. Patent ductus arteriosus

6. Children with which congenital cardiac lesion learn to alleviate their symptoms by squatting?

a. Coarctation of the aorta
b. Tetralogy of Fallot
c. Patent ductus arteriosus
d. Transposition of the great arteries

Answers to Review Questions

1. Choice b is correct. Fixed splitting of the second heart sound (S₂) is typical of an atrial septal defect (ASD). This is thought to occur in part because the normal respiratory variation in systemic venous return is countered by reciprocal changes in the volume of blood shunted across the ASD.

2. Choice a is correct. The most common finding in a patient with a left-to-right shunt through a patent ductus arteriosus is a continuous, machinelike murmur (see Fig. 2-10), heard best at the left subclavicular region. The murmur is present throughout the cardiac cycle because a pressure gradient exists between the aorta and pulmonary artery in both systole and diastole. However, if pulmonary vascular disease develops, the gradient between the aorta and the pulmonary artery decreases, leading to diminished flow through the PDA, and the murmur becomes shorter (the diastolic component may disappear).

3. Choice d is correct. In congenital aortic stenosis, auscultation reveals a harsh crescendo–decrescendo systolic murmur, loudest at the base of the heart with radiation toward the neck. The murmur is often preceded by a systolic ejection click, especially when a bicuspid valve is present.

4. Choice c is correct. Ventricular septal defects (VSDs) are a cause of harsh holosystolic murmurs at the mid-to-lower left sternal border. Small VSDs tend to cause the loudest murmurs because of the greater turbulence of flow that they cause compared to larger defects. A systolic thrill can sometimes be palpated over the region of the murmur. Tricuspid regurgitation causes a holosystolic murmur at the left lower sternal border, but in distinction to VSDs, that murmur increases with inspiration.

5. **Choice c is correct.** Turner syndrome (45, XO) is a heritable condition associated with left-sided obstructive congenital heart lesion, including bicuspid aortic valve, coarctation of the aorta, and occasionally hypoplastic left heart syndrome (underdevelopment of the LV and aorta).

6. **Choice b is correct.** Children with tetralogy of Fallot often experience "spells" following exertion, feeding, or crying, when systemic vasodilatation results in an increased right-to-left shunt. Manifestations include irritability, cyanosis, hyperventilation, and occasionally syncope or convulsions. Squatting increases systemic venous return to the right heart and systemic vascular resistance, therefore increasing pulmonary blood flow by increased right ventricular filling and decreased right to left shunt across the VSD.

Acknowledgments

Contributors to previous editions of this chapter were Zena L. Knight, MD; David D. Berg, MD; Vijay G. Sankaran, MD; Yi-Bin Chen, MD; Douglas W. Green, MD; Raymond Tabibiazar, MD; Lakshmi Halasyamani, MD; Andrew Karson, MD; Michael D. Freed, MD; and Richard Liberthson, MD.

Additional Reading

Allen HD, Shaddy RE, Penny DJ, et al., eds. *Moss and Adams' Heart Disease in Infants, Children, and Adolescents: Including the Fetus and Young Adult*. 9th ed. Philadelphia, PA: Lippincott Williams & Wilkins; 2016.

Ashworth MT. *Pathology of Heart Disease in the Fetus, Infant and Child*. Cambridge, UK: Cambridge University Press; 2019.

Moore KL, Persaud TVN, Torchia MG. *The Developing Human: Clinically Oriented Embryology*. 11th ed. Edinburgh, UK: Elsevier; 2020.

Park MK. *Pediatric Cardiology for Practitioners*. 6th ed. Philadelphia, PA: Saunders; 2014.

Perloff JK. *The Clinical Recognition of Congenital Heart Disease*. 6th ed. Philadelphia, PA: Saunders; 2012.

Pierpoint ME, Brueckner M, Chung WK, et al. Genetic basis of congenital heart disease: revisited: a scientific statement from the American Heart Association. *Circulation*. 2018;138:e653-e711.

Sadler TW. *Langman's Medical Embryology*. 14th ed. Philadelphia, PA: Lippincott Williams & Wilkins; 2018.

Stout KK, Daniels CJ, Aboulhosn JA, et al. 2018 AHA/ACC Guideline for the management of adults with congenital heart disease: executive summary. *J Am Coll Cardiol*. 2019;73:1494-563.

Zaidi S, Brueckner M. Genetics and genomics of congenital heart disease. *Circ Res*. 2017;120:923-940.

17

Cardiovascular Drugs

Ankeet S. Bhatt | Victor Nauffal | Leonard S. Lilly

Chapter Outline

Inotropic Drugs and Vasopressors
Cardiac Glycosides (Digitalis)
Sympathomimetic Amines
Phosphodiesterase-3 Inhibitors
Vasopressin

Vasodilator Drugs
Angiotensin-Converting Enzyme
Inhibitors
Angiotensin II Type 1 Receptor
Antagonists
Angiotensin Receptor–Neprilysin
Inhibitor
Direct-Acting Vasodilators
Calcium Channel Blockers
Organic Nitrates
Natriuretic Peptides
Phosphodiesterase-5 Inhibitors
Endothelin Receptor Antagonists

Antiadrenergic Drugs
Central Adrenergic Inhibitors
(CNS α_2-Agonists)
Sympathetic Nerve-Ending
Antagonists
Peripheral α-Adrenergic Receptor
Antagonists
β-Adrenergic Receptor Antagonists

Antiarrhythmic Drugs
Class IA Antiarrhythmics
Class IB Antiarrhythmics
Class IC Antiarrhythmics
Class II Antiarrhythmics
Class III Antiarrhythmics
Class IV Antiarrhythmics
Adenosine

Diuretics
Loop Diuretics
Thiazide Diuretics
Potassium-Sparing Diuretics

Antithrombotic Drugs
Platelet Inhibitors
Anticoagulant Drugs: Parenteral
Agents
Anticoagulant Drugs: Oral Agents

Lipid-Regulating Drugs
HMG-CoA Reductase Inhibitors
Cholesterol Absorption Inhibitor
Proprotein Convertase Subtilisin/
Kexin Type 9 (PCSK9) Inhibitors
n-3 Fatty Acids
Bile Acid–Binding Agents
Niacin
Fibrates

This chapter reviews the physiologic basis and clinical use of cardiovascular drugs. Although a multitude of drugs are available to treat cardiac disorders, these agents can be grouped by their pharmacologic actions into a small number of categories. Additionally, many drugs are useful in more than one form of heart disease.

INOTROPIC DRUGS AND VASOPRESSORS

Inotropic drugs are used to increase the force of ventricular contraction when myocardial systolic function is impaired. The pharmacologic agents in this category include the cardiac glycosides, sympathomimetic amines, and phosphodiesterase-3 inhibitors (Table 17-1). Although they work through different mechanisms, they are all thought to enhance

TABLE 17-1	Inotropic Drugs	
Class	**Examples**
Cardiac glycosides	Digoxin
Sympathomimetic amines	Dopamine
	Dobutamine
	Norepinephrine
	Epinephrine
	Isoproterenol
Phosphodiesterase-3 inhibitors	Milrinone

cardiac contraction by increasing the intracellular calcium concentration, thus augmenting actin and myosin interaction. The hemodynamic effect is to shift a depressed ventricular performance curve (Frank-Starling curve) in an upward direction (Fig. 17-1), so that for a given ventricular filling pressure, stroke volume and cardiac output (CO) are increased.

Cardiac Glycosides (Digitalis)

The cardiac glycosides are called "digitalis" because the drugs of this class are based on extracts of the foxglove plant, *Digitalis purpurea*. The most commonly used member of this group is **digoxin**.

Mechanism of Action

The two desired effects of digoxin are (1) to improve contractility of the failing heart (mechanical effect) and (2) to prolong the refractory period of the atrioventricular (AV) node in patients with supraventricular arrhythmias (electrical effect).

Mechanical Effect

The action by which digoxin improves contractility is attributed to inhibition of sarcolemmal Na^+K^+-ATPase, which is normally responsible for maintaining transmembrane Na^+ and K^+ gradients. By inhibiting this transporter, digitalis causes the intracellular $[Na^+]$ to rise. As

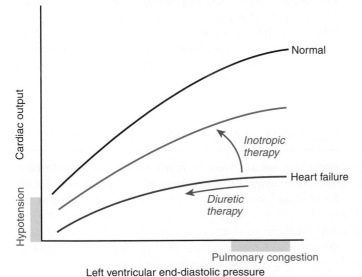

Figure 17-1. **Ventricular performance (Frank-Starling) curve.** In systolic heart failure, the curve is displaced downward, so that at a given left ventricular end-diastolic pressure (LVEDP), the cardiac output is lower than in a normal heart. Diuretics reduce LVEDP but do not change the position of the curve; thus, pulmonary congestion improves but cardiac output may fall. Inotropic drugs shift the curve upward, toward normal, so that at any LVEDP, the cardiac output is greater.

shown in Figure 17-2, an increase in intracellular sodium content reduces Ca^{++} extrusion from the cell via the Na^+/Ca^{++} exchanger. Consequently, more Ca^{++} is pumped into the sarcoplasmic reticulum, and when subsequent action potentials excite the cell, a greater-than-normal amount of Ca^{++} is released to the myofilaments, thereby enhancing the force of contraction.

Electrical Effect

The major therapeutic electrical effect of digoxin occurs at the AV node, where it slows conduction and increases refractoriness by modulation of autonomic nervous system output (Table 17-2). Digoxin enhances vagal tone and reduces sympathetic activity, thus decreasing the frequency of transmission of atrial impulses through the AV node.

Clinical Uses

Digoxin has been used historically as an inotropic agent to treat heart failure with reduced ejection fraction (see Chapter 9). Although no longer a mainstay of therapy in heart failure, digitalis is sometimes useful in treating patients with heart failure complicated by atrial fibrillation. Unlike ACE inhibitors, β-blockers, and mineralocorticoid receptor antagonists, digoxin does not prolong the life expectancy of patients with chronic heart failure. Thus, its use has declined in recent years.

Digoxin is also occasionally prescribed as an antiarrhythmic agent, although other agents are more effective, safer, and used more frequently. By impairing AV nodal conduction, digitalis reduces the rate of ventricular stimulation in patients with rapid atrial fibrillation or atrial flutter. Digitalis may also terminate supraventricular reentrant tachycardias (eg, AVNRT—see Chapter 12), likely through enhancement of vagal tone, which slows impulse conduction and prolongs the effective refractory period of the AV node.

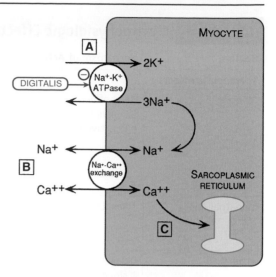

Figure 17-2. Mechanism of action of digitalis (inotropic effect). A. Digitalis inhibits the sarcolemmal Na^+K^+-ATPase, causing intracellular $[Na^+]$ to rise. **B.** Increased cytosolic $[Na^+]$ reduces the transmembrane Na^+ gradient; thus, the Na^+/Ca^+ exchanger drives less Ca^{++} out of the cell. **C.** The increased intracellular $[Ca^{++}]$ is stored in the sarcoplasmic reticulum, such that with subsequent action potentials, greater-than-normal Ca^{++} is released to the contractile elements in the cytoplasm, intensifying the force of contraction.

Pharmacokinetics and Toxicity

Digoxin is administered orally or intravenously and is excreted by the kidney. A series of loading doses is necessary to raise the drug's concentration into the therapeutic range. The subsequent maintenance dosage depends on the patient's renal function.

The potential for digitalis toxicity is significant because of a narrow therapeutic window. Many factors contribute to digitalis intoxication, the most common of which is hypokalemia, often caused by concurrent administration of diuretics. Hypokalemia exacerbates digitalis toxicity because it further inhibits Na^+K^+-ATPase. Other conditions that promote digitalis toxicity include hypomagnesemia and hypercalcemia. In addition, the administration of other drugs (eg, amiodarone) may raise the serum digoxin concentration by altering its clearance or volume of distribution.

Extracardiac signs of acute digitalis toxicity are often gastrointestinal (eg, nausea, vomiting, anorexia). Cardiac toxicity includes several types of arrhythmias, some of which may be life threatening (Table 17-2). In atrial tissue and ventricular Purkinje fibers, a high digoxin concentration results in three consequences that may lead to dangerous arrhythmias (Fig. 17-3):

TABLE 17-2	Electrophysiologic Effects of Digitalis	
Region	**Mechanism of Action**	**Clinical Effect**
Therapeutic effects		
AV node	Vagal effect ↓ Conduction velocity ↑ Effective refractory period	↓ Rate of transmission of atrial impulses to the ventricles in supraventricular tachyarrhythmias
		May interrupt reentrant circuits passing through the AV node
Toxic effects		
Sinoatrial node	↑ Vagal effect and direct suppression	Sinus bradycardia
		Sinoatrial block (impulse not transmitted from SA node to atrium)
Atrium	Delayed afterdepolarizations (triggered activity), ↑ slope of phase 4 depolarization (↑ automaticity)	Atrial premature beats
		Nonreentrant SVT (ectopic rhythm)
	Variable effects on conduction velocity and ↑ refractory period (can fragment conduction and lead to re-entry)	Reentrant PSVT
AV node	Direct and vagal-mediated conduction block	AV block (first, second, or third degree)
AV junction (between AV node and His bundle)	Delayed afterdepolarizations (triggered activity), ↑ slope of phase 4 depolarization (↑ automaticity)	Accelerated junctional rhythm
Purkinje fibers and ventricular muscle	Delayed afterdepolarizations (triggered activity), ↓ conduction velocity and ↑ refractory period (can lead to reentry)	Ventricular premature beats
	↑ Slope of phase 4 depolarization (↑ automaticity)	Ventricular tachycardia

AV, atrioventricular; PSVT, paroxysmal supraventricular tachycardia; SA, sinoatrial; SVT, supraventricular tachycardia.

Figure 17-3. Direct effects of digitalis on the Purkinje cell action potential. The *solid tracing* represents depolarization and repolarization of a normal cell; the *dashed tracing* demonstrates the effects of digitalis. **A.** The maximum diastolic potential is less negative, and there is an increase in the slope of phase 4 depolarization, endowing the cell with intrinsic automaticity, and the potential for ectopic rhythms. **B.** Because depolarization of the cell occurs at a more positive voltage, there is partial inactivation of fast sodium channels, the rate of rise of phase 0 is decreased, and conduction velocity is slowed, which, if present heterogeneously among neighboring cells, produces conditions for reentry. **C.** Delayed afterdepolarizations may develop at high concentrations of digitalis in association with the increased intracellular calcium concentration and can result in triggered tachyarrhythmias.

1. *Less negative resting potential.* Inhibition of Na^+K^+-ATPase causes the resting potential to become less negative. Consequently, there is a voltage-dependent partial inactivation of the fast Na^+ channels, which leads to a slower rise of phase 0 depolarization and a reduction in conduction velocity (Fig. 1-16). The slowed conduction, if present heterogeneously among neighboring cells, enhances the possibility of reentrant arrhythmias.

2. *Decreased action potential duration.* Digitalis-induced elevated intracellular $[Ca^{++}]$ increases the activity of a Ca^{++}-dependent K^+ channel. The opening of this channel promotes K^+ efflux and more rapid *repolarization*. In addition, high intracellular $[Ca^{++}]$ inactivates Ca^{++} channels, decreasing the inward *depolarizing* Ca^{++} current. These effects decrease the action potential duration and shorten the refractory period, increasing the time during which cardiac fibers are responsive to external stimulation and allowing greater opportunity for propagation of arrhythmic impulses.

3. *Enhanced automaticity.* Digoxin enhances automaticity and may generate ectopic rhythms by two mechanisms:

   a. The less negative membrane resting potential can induce phase 4 gradual depolarization, even in nonpacemaker cells (see Chapter 11), and an action potential is triggered each time that threshold voltage is reached.

   b. The digoxin-induced increase in intracellular $[Ca^{++}]$ may trigger delayed afterdepolarizations (Fig. 17-3 and Chapter 11). If an afterdepolarization reaches the threshold voltage, an action potential (ectopic beat) is generated. Ectopic beats may lead to additional afterdepolarizations and self-sustaining arrhythmias such as ventricular tachycardia.

In addition, the augmented direct and indirect vagal effects of toxic doses of digitalis slow conduction through the AV node, such that various degrees of AV block, including complete heart block, can occur.

The treatment of digitalis-induced tachyarrhythmias may include administration of potassium (if hypokalemia is present), intravenous atropine for bradyarrhythmias, or lidocaine (discussed later in the chapter) for ventricular ectopy. High-grade AV block may require temporary pacemaker therapy. In patients with severe intoxication, administration of digoxin-specific antibodies may be lifesaving.

SYMPATHOMIMETIC AMINES

Sympathomimetic amines are inotropic drugs that bind to cardiac β_1-receptors leading to increased activity of adenylate cyclase and increased formation of cyclic adenosine monophosphate (cAMP) (Fig. 17-4). Increased cAMP activates specific protein kinases, which promote intracellular calcium influx by phosphorylating L-type calcium channels. The increased calcium entry triggers a corresponding rise in Ca^{++} release from the sarcoplasmic reticulum, which enhances the force of contraction. Intravenous dopamine and dobutamine are commonly used sympathomimetic amines in the treatment of acute heart failure. Table 17-3 summarizes the receptor actions and major hemodynamic effects of these agents.

Dopamine is an endogenous catecholamine and the precursor of norepinephrine. It possesses a combination of actions that makes it attractive in the treatment of heart failure associated with hypotension and poor renal perfusion. There are various types of receptors with different affinities for dopamine. At *low dosages*, <2 μg/kg/min, dopamine interacts primarily with dopaminergic receptors distributed in the renal and mesenteric vascular beds. Stimulation of these receptors causes local vasodilation and increases renal blood flow and glomerular filtration, facilitating diuresis.

Intermediate dosages of dopamine, 2-10 μg/kg/min, increase inotropy directly by stimulating cardiac β_1-receptors and indirectly by promoting norepinephrine release from sympathetic nerve terminals. These actions increase heart rate, cardiac contractility, and stroke volume, all of which augment CO.

Figure 17-4. Mechanism by which β-adrenergic stimulation increases contractility. β_1-Receptor stimulation acts through G proteins (guanine nucleotide regulatory proteins), the alpha subunit (α) of which activates adenylate cyclase. The latter increases cyclic adenosine monophosphate (cAMP) production, which mediates protein kinase phosphorylation of cellular proteins, including ion channels. Phosphorylation of the slow Ca^{++} channel increases calcium influx, which augments the force of contraction. cAMP is degraded by phosphodiesterase (PD). ATP, adenosine triphosphate.

At *high dosages*, >10 μg/kg/min, dopamine also stimulates systemic α-receptors, thereby causing vasoconstriction and elevating systemic resistance. High-dose dopamine is indicated in hypotensive states such as shock. However, these doses are inappropriate in most patients with cardiac failure because the peripheral vasoconstriction increases the resistance against which the heart contracts (ie, higher afterload), which could impair left ventricular output.

The most important side effect of dopamine is provocation of tachyarrhythmias.

Dobutamine is a synthetic analog of dopamine that stimulates β_1-, β_2-, and α-receptors. It increases cardiac contractility by virtue of the β_1 effect but does not increase peripheral resistance because of the balance between α-mediated vasoconstriction and β_2-mediated vasodilation. Thus, it is useful in the treatment of heart failure not accompanied by hypotension. Unlike dopamine, dobutamine does not stimulate dopaminergic receptors (ie, no renal vasodilating effect), nor does it facilitate the release of norepinephrine from peripheral nerve endings. Like dopamine, it is useful for short-term therapy (<1 week), after which time it loses its efficacy, presumably because of down-regulation of adrenergic receptors. The major adverse effect is the provocation of tachyarrhythmias.

Norepinephrine is an endogenous catecholamine synthesized from dopamine in adrenergic postganglionic nerves and in adrenal medullary cells (where it is both secreted and serves as

TABLE 17-3 Sympathomimetic Drug Effects

Drug	Receptor Stimulation			
	D_1 (↑ Renal Perfusion)	α (Vasoconstriction)	β_1 (↑ Contractility)	β_2 (Vasodilation)
Dopamine	+[a]	++++[b]	++++	++
Dobutamine	0	+	++++	+
Norepinephrine	0	++++	++++	0
Epinephrine	0	++++[b]	++++	++
Isoproterenol	0	0	++++	++++

[a]Low dosage.
[b]High dosage.

a precursor of epinephrine). Through its β_1-activity, norepinephrine has positive inotropic and chronotropic effects. Acting at peripheral α-receptors, it is also a potent vasoconstrictor. The increase in total peripheral resistance causes the mean arterial blood pressure to rise.

Norepinephrine's side effects include tachyarrhythmias, though less so than dopamine.

Epinephrine, formed by the addition of a methyl group to norepinephrine, is the predominant endogenous catecholamine produced in the adrenal medulla. Administered as an intravenous infusion at low dosages, its stimulation of β_1-receptors enhances ventricular contractility and speeds impulse generation, thus increasing stroke volume, heart rate, and CO. However, at this dosage range, β_2-mediated vasodilation may reduce total peripheral resistance and blood pressure.

At higher dosages, epinephrine is a potent vasopressor because α-mediated constriction dominates over β_2-mediated vasodilation. In this case, the effects of positive inotropy, positive chronotropy, and vasoconstriction act together to raise systemic blood pressure.

Epinephrine is used most often when the combination of inotropic and chronotropic stimulation is desired. The most common toxic effect is the precipitation of tachyarrhythmias. Epinephrine should be avoided in patients receiving β-blocker therapy, because unopposed α-mediated vasoconstriction could produce significant hypertension.

Isoproterenol is a synthetic epinephrine analog. Unlike norepinephrine and epinephrine, it is a "pure" β-agonist, having activity almost exclusively at β_1- and β_2-receptors, with almost no α-receptor effect. In the heart, isoproterenol has positive inotropic and chronotropic effects, thereby increasing CO. In peripheral vessels, stimulation of β_2-receptors results in vasodilation and reduced peripheral resistance, which may cause blood pressure to fall.

Isoproterenol is sometimes used in emergency circumstances to increase the heart rate in patients with bradycardia or heart block (eg, as a temporizing measure before pacemaker implantation). Isoproterenol should be avoided in patients with myocardial ischemia, in whom the increased heart rate and inotropic stimulation would further increase myocardial oxygen consumption.

PHOSPHODIESTERASE-3 INHIBITORS

Milrinone, a nondigitalis, noncatecholamine agent, exerts its positive inotropic actions by inhibiting phosphodiesterase type 3 in cardiac myocytes (Fig. 17-4). This inhibition slows the breakdown of intracellular cAMP, the ultimate result of which is enhanced Ca^{++} entry into the cell and increased force of contraction. Additionally, in vascular smooth muscle, milrinone-induced augmentation of cAMP results in beneficial vasodilation (in vascular tissue, cAMP inhibits myosin light chain kinase and cross-bridge formation between myosin heads and actin filaments).

Milrinone is sometimes used in the treatment of acute heart failure when there has been insufficient improvement with conventional vasodilators, inotropic agents, and diuretics. It has the potential for serious adverse effects, including provocation of ventricular arrhythmias, and chronic milrinone therapy is associated with *increased* mortality. Its use is therefore limited to hospitalized patients for short-term therapy or in patients with end-stage heart failure as palliative therapy to facilitate hospital discharge.

Table 17-4 summarizes the actions and toxicities of commonly used inotropic drugs.

VASOPRESSIN

Vasopressin, the endogenous antidiuretic hormone secreted by the posterior pituitary, primarily functions to maintain water balance (see Chapter 9). It also acts as a potent nonadrenergic vasoconstrictor when administered intravenously at supraphysiologic doses, by directly stimulating vascular smooth muscle V_1 receptors. It is useful for supporting blood pressure in patients with vasodilatory shock, as may occur in sepsis.

TABLE 17-4	Summary of Actions and Adverse Effects of Selected Inotropic Drugs	
Drug	**Mechanism of Action**	**Major Adverse Effects**
Cardiac glycosides		
Digoxin	Inhibition of sarcolemmal Na$^+$K$^+$-ATPase	**Gastrointestinal:** nausea, vomiting
	Enhanced vagal tone	**Cardiac:** atrial, nodal, and ventricular tachyarrhythmias; high-degree AV block
Sympathomimetic amines		
Dopamine	Low dosage (<2 µg/kg/min): D$_1$ receptor stimulation results in mesenteric and renal arterial dilation (facilitates diuresis)	Tachycardia, arrhythmias, hypertension
	Medium dosage (2-10 µg/kg/min): β$_1$-receptor stimulation and release of norepinephrine from sympathetic nerve terminals (inotropic effect)	
	High dosage (>10 µg/kg/min): α-receptor stimulation (peripheral vasoconstriction)	
Dobutamine	β$_1$-, β$_2$-, and α-receptor stimulation	Tachyarrhythmias
Phosphodiesterase-3 inhibitors		
Milrinone	Increased intracellular cAMP due to inhibition of its breakdown by phosphodiesterase	**Gastrointestinal:** nausea, vomiting
		Cardiac: arrhythmias

AV, atrioventricular; cAMP, cyclic adenosine monophosphate; D$_1$, dopamine 1.

VASODILATOR DRUGS

Vasodilator drugs play a central role in the treatment of heart failure and hypertension. As described in Chapter 9, the fall in CO in heart failure triggers important compensatory pathways, including the adrenergic nervous system and the renin-angiotensin-aldosterone system (see Fig. 9-9). As a result of activation of these pathways, two potent natural vasoconstrictors are released into the circulation: norepinephrine and angiotensin II (AII). These hormones bind to receptors in arterioles and veins, causing vascular smooth muscle contraction. Initially, vasoconstriction is beneficial in heart failure because it maximizes left ventricular preload (venous constriction enhances venous return) and helps to maintain mean arterial pressure (because of arteriolar constriction).

However, over time, persistent activation of these systems may become maladaptive. The elevated venous return to the heart resulting from venous constriction may ultimately lead to a rise in the pulmonary capillary hydrostatic pressure and pulmonary congestion. Excessive arteriolar constriction increases the resistance against which the left ventricle must contract (ie, increased afterload) and therefore ultimately impedes stroke volume and CO. Vasodilator therapy is directed at modulating such excessive constriction of veins and arterioles, thus reducing pulmonary congestion and augmenting forward CO (see Fig. 9-10).

Vasodilators are also useful antihypertensive drugs. Recall from Chapter 13 that mean arterial blood pressure is the product of CO and total peripheral resistance (MAP = CO × TPR). Vasodilator drugs decrease arteriolar resistance and therefore lower blood pressure.

Individual vasodilator drug classes act at specific vascular sites (Fig. 17-5). Nitrates, for example, are primarily venodilators, whereas hydralazine is a pure arteriolar dilator. Some drugs, such as ACE inhibitors, α-blockers, sodium nitroprusside, and nesiritide, are balanced vasodilators that act on both sides of the systemic circulation. Agents that act as pulmonary arteriolar vasodilators are described later in this section.

Figure 17-5. Examples of systemic vasodilator drugs and their sites of action: the venous bed, the arteriolar bed, or both. ACE, angiotensin-converting enzyme; ARB, angiotensin receptor blocker; ARNI, angiotensin receptor–neprilysin inhibitor.

ANGIOTENSIN-CONVERTING ENZYME INHIBITORS

The renin-angiotensin system plays a critical role in cardiovascular homeostasis. The major effector of this pathway (Fig. 17-6) is AII, which is formed by the cleavage of angiotensin I by ACE. All the actions of AII known to affect blood pressure are mediated by its binding to the angiotensin II type 1 (AT_1) receptor (see Fig. 13-6). Interaction with this receptor generates a

Figure 17-6. The renin-angiotensin system. Angiotensin-converting enzyme (ACE) generates angiotensin II, which results in actions that include vasoconstriction, sodium retention, and increased sympathetic activity. ACE inhibitors and angiotensin II type 1 (AT_1) receptor antagonists impair these effects. ACE also promotes the degradation of the natural vasodilator bradykinin; thus, ACE inhibition—but not AT_1 receptor inhibition—results in accumulation of bradykinin and enhanced vasodilation.

series of intracellular reactions that cause arteriolar vasoconstriction and the adrenal release of aldosterone, which promotes Na^+ reabsorption from the distal nephron. As a result of these actions on vascular tone and sodium homeostasis, AII plays a major role in blood pressure and blood volume regulation. By blocking the formation of AII, ACE inhibitors decrease systemic arterial pressure, facilitate natriuresis (by decreasing aldosterone production, thus reducing Na^+ reabsorption), and limit adverse ventricular remodeling (see Chapter 9).

Another action of ACE inhibitors, which likely contributes to their hemodynamic effects, is related to bradykinin (BK) metabolism (Fig. 17-6). The natural vasodilator BK is normally degraded to inactive metabolites by ACE. Because ACE inhibitors impede that degradation, BK accumulates and contributes to the antihypertensive effect, likely by stimulating the endothelial release of nitric oxide and biosynthesis of vasodilating prostaglandins.

Clinical Uses

Hypertension

In hypertensive patients, ACE inhibitors lower blood pressure. They also increase renal blood flow, usually without altering the glomerular filtration rate (GFR), because of dilation of both the afferent and efferent glomerular arterioles. Used alone, ACE inhibitors show similar antihypertensive efficacy as diuretics and calcium channel blockers (CCBs). ACE inhibitors are often recommended therapy in diabetic hypertensive patients and those with chronic renal insufficiency, because the drugs slow the development of diabetic nephropathy (a syndrome of progressive renal deterioration, proteinuria, and hypertension) and progression of renal dysfunction through favorable effects on intraglomerular pressure.

Heart Failure

In heart failure, ACE inhibitors reduce peripheral vascular resistance ($\downarrow$afterload), reduce cardiac filling pressures ($\downarrow$preload), and increase CO. The augmented CO reduces the drive for compensatory neurohormonal stimulation in heart failure, such that elevated levels of norepinephrine fall. In addition, clinical trials have shown that ACE inhibitors improve survival in patients with chronic heart failure and following myocardial infarction. Some studies have shown that ACE inhibition also reduces the risk of myocardial infarction and death in patients with chronic vascular disease, including coronary artery disease (CAD), even if left ventricular function is not impaired.

The primary excretory pathway of most ACE inhibitors is via the kidney (Table 17-5), so dosages should generally be reduced in patients with renal dysfunction.

Adverse Effects

Cough

Irritation of the upper airways resulting in a dry cough occurs in up to 20% of patients receiving ACE inhibitor therapy. Its mechanism may relate to the increased BK concentration provoked by ACE inhibitors. This side effect may last weeks after the drug is discontinued.

Hypotension

This is a rare side effect when ACE inhibitors are used to treat hypertension. It is more likely to occur in heart failure patients in whom intravascular volume depletion has resulted from vigorous diuretic use. As such, patients have significant activation of the renin-angiotensin system, and blood pressure is largely maintained by AII-mediated vasoconstriction; the administration of an ACE inhibitor can result in hypotension because of the sudden reduction of circulating AII. This side effect is avoided by temporarily reducing the diuretic regimen and starting ACE inhibitor therapy at low dosage.

TABLE 17-5 Drugs that Interfere with the Renin-Angiotensin System	
Drug	**Major Elimination Pathway**
ACE inhibitors	
Benazepril	Renal
Captopril	Renal
Enalapril	Renal
Fosinopril	Hepatic/renal
Lisinopril	Renal
Moexipril	Hepatic/renal
Perindopril	Renal
Quinapril	Renal
Ramipril	Renal
Trandolapril	Hepatic/renal
Angiotensin II receptor antagonists	
Candesartan	Hepatic/renal
Eprosartan	Hepatic/renal
Irbesartan	Hepatic/renal
Losartan	Hepatic/renal
Olmesartan	Hepatic/renal
Telmisartan	Hepatic
Valsartan	Hepatic/renal
Angiotensin receptor-neprilysin inhibitor	
Sacubitril/valsartan	Hepatic/renal

Renal Insufficiency

Administration of an ACE inhibitor to patients with intravascular volume depletion may result in hypotension, decreased renal perfusion, and azotemia. ACE inhibitor therapy can also precipitate renal failure in patients with *bilateral renal artery stenosis* because such patients rely on high efferent glomerular arteriolar resistance (which is highly dependent on AII) to maintain glomerular filtration. Administering an ACE inhibitor decreases efferent arteriolar tone and glomerular hydrostatic pressure and may therefore worsen GFR in this setting.

Hyperkalemia

ACE inhibitors indirectly reduce the serum aldosterone concentration, such that the serum potassium concentration may rise. Conditions that may further increase serum potassium levels and can result in dangerous hyperkalemia during ACE inhibitor use include renal insufficiency, diabetes (owing to hyporeninemic hypoaldosteronism), and concomitant use of potassium-sparing diuretics.

Other Effects

Very rare adverse reactions to ACE inhibitors include angioedema and agranulocytosis. ACE inhibitors should not be used in pregnancy because they have been shown to cause fetal injury.

Angiotensin II Type 1 Receptor Antagonists

AT_1 receptor antagonists, also termed angiotensin receptor blockers (ARBs), are a second group of drugs that interfere with the renin-angiotensin system. There are at least two distinct subtypes of AII receptors: AT_1 and AT_2. All the actions of AII known to affect blood pressure (eg, vasoconstriction, aldosterone release, renal Na^+ reabsorption, and sympathetic nervous system stimulation) are mediated by its binding to receptors of the AT_1 subtype. The AT_2 receptor subtype is abundant during fetal development and has been located in some adult tissues, but its precise role in normal physiology is unknown.

ARBs compete with AII for AT_1 receptors and therefore inhibit AII-mediated effects (Fig. 17-6), thus lowering the blood pressure of hypertensive patients. Unlike ACE inhibitors, ARBs do not raise serum BK levels.

Each of the available ARBs (listed in Table 17-5) is excreted primarily in the bile, but most are also partly excreted in the urine. Trials have demonstrated that ARBs are as effective as ACE inhibitors in treating hypertension, and they are among the best tolerated antihypertensive drugs. As with ACE inhibitors, the blood pressure–lowering effect of ARBs is enhanced by concurrent use of a thiazide diuretic. Also, like ACE inhibitors, ARBs have the potential side effects of hypotension and hyperkalemia (owing to reduced aldosterone levels). Unlike ACE inhibitors, ARBs typically do not commonly cause cough or angioedema.

In heart failure with reduced ejection fraction, ARBs display hemodynamic benefits similar to those of ACE inhibitors (see Chapter 9). Thus, ARBs are generally recommended for heart failure patients who are intolerant of ACE inhibitors (eg, because of ACE inhibitor–induced cough). Studies in patients with type 2 diabetes have demonstrated that ARBs (like ACE inhibitors) slow the progression of diabetic nephropathy and renal insufficiency.

Angiotensin Receptor-Neprilysin Inhibitor

Angiotensin receptor-neprilysin inhibition (ARNI) represents an extension of ARB therapy for the treatment of HFrEF. The currently available drug of this class combines the ARB valsartan with sacubitril, a drug whose active metabolite inhibits the enzyme neprilysin (Fig. 17-7). Neprilysin normally degrades several natural vasodilating peptides (including BK, atrial natriuretic peptide, and B-type natriuretic peptide [BNP]), and inhibition of neprilysin by sacubitril augments these substances that are beneficial for HFrEF patients.

A large clinical trial of patients with chronic symptomatic HFrEF showed that compared with an ACE inhibitor, valsartan/sacubitril significantly reduced mortality rates and heart failure hospitalizations. As a result, current US guidelines recommend that for symptomatic chronic heart failure patients with reduced ejection fraction, who are not acutely decompensated and have previously tolerated an ACE inhibitor or ARB, that valsartan/sacubitril be substituted for those drugs (see Chapter 9).

The main potential side effects of ARNI therapy are hypotension, hyperkalemia, and worsening renal function, such that it should not be prescribed concurrently with an ACE inhibitor,

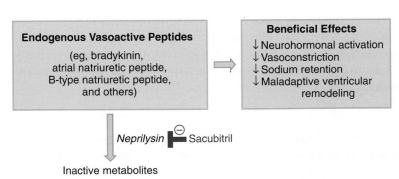

Figure 17-7. Mechanism of action of sacubitril. Several beneficial endogenous vasodilating peptides are degraded to inactive metabolites by the enzyme neprilysin. Inhibition of neprilysin by sacubitril reduces their degradation and enhances the beneficial hemodynamic effects.

additional ARB, or potassium-sparing diuretic, which can also contribute to these adverse effects. Similar to ACE inhibitors, sacubitril/valsartan can rarely cause angioedema. Thus, it is recommended that prior ACE inhibitor therapy be withheld for at least 36 hours prior to initiating sacubitril/valsartan.

As described in Chapter 9, blood levels of BNP and NT-proBNP correlate with the severity of heart failure and typically decline as a patient's symptoms improve. However, since sacubitril blocks the degradation of BNP by neprilysin, the BNP level may actually *rise* on this drug, despite clinical improvement. In distinction, NT-proBNP is *not* metabolized by neprilysin, and its blood level does decline as expected as heart failure is treated.

DIRECT-ACTING VASODILATORS

Hydralazine, minoxidil, sodium nitroprusside, and fenoldopam are examples of direct-acting vasodilators (Table 17-6). Hydralazine and minoxidil are used primarily as long-term oral vasodilators, whereas nitroprusside and fenoldopam are administered intravenously in acute settings.

Hydralazine is a potent and direct arteriolar dilator that acts at the level of precapillary arterioles and has no effect on systemic veins. The fall in blood pressure following arteriolar dilation results in a baroreceptor-mediated increase in sympathetic outflow and cardiac stimulation (eg, reflex tachycardia), which could precipitate myocardial ischemia in patients with underlying CAD. Therefore, hydralazine is often combined with a β-blocker to blunt this undesired response.

As newer drugs have emerged, hydralazine is now used only occasionally as an antihypertensive. It is sometimes prescribed concurrently with the venodilator isosorbide dinitrate to treat heart failure in patients with systolic dysfunction. This combination improves symptoms in patients with mild-to-moderate heart failure and has been shown to reduce morbidity and mortality rates (see Chapter 9).

Hydralazine possesses low bioavailability because of extensive first-pass hepatic metabolism. It has a short half-life (2-4 hours) in the circulation, but its effect persists as long as 12 hours because the drug binds avidly to vascular tissues.

The most common side effects of hydralazine include headache (owing to cerebral vasodilation), palpitations (reflex tachycardia), and flushing (increased systemic vasodilation). In addition, a syndrome similar to systemic lupus (characterized by arthralgias, myalgia, skin rashes, and fever) may develop.

TABLE 17-6	**Direct Vasodilators**		
Drug	**Clinical Use**	**Route of Administration**	**Major Adverse Effects**
Hydralazine	• Hypertension (chronic and acute therapy) • HFrEF	Oral, intravenous bolus, intramuscular	• Hypotension, tachycardia • Headache, flushing • Angina • Drug-induced lupus
Minoxidil	• Chronic therapy of hypertension	Oral	• Reflex tachycardia • Na$^+$ retention • Hypertrichosis
Nitroprusside	• Hypertensive emergencies • Acute heart failure	Intravenous infusion	• Hypotension • Thiocyanate and cyanide toxicity
Fenoldopam	• Hypertensive emergencies	Intravenous infusion	• Hypotension • Increased intraocular pressure

HFrEF, heart failure with reduced ejection fraction.

Minoxidil also results in arteriolar vasodilation without significant venodilation. Its mechanism of action involves an increase in potassium channel permeability, which results in smooth muscle cell hyperpolarization and relaxation. Given the availability of newer antihypertensive agents, minoxidil is now used rarely, and its primary clinical use is in the treatment of intractable hypertension. For example, it may occasionally be prescribed to patients with renal failure who are refractory to other antihypertensive regimens. It is well absorbed from the gastrointestinal tract and is metabolized primarily by hepatic glucuronidation. Although it has a short half-life, its pharmacologic effects persist even after serum drug concentration falls, probably because, like hydralazine, the drug binds avidly to vascular tissues. Side effects of minoxidil include reflex sympathetic stimulation and fluid retention, hypertrichosis (excessive hair growth) and occasional pericardial effusions (unknown mechanism).

Sodium nitroprusside, a potent dilator of both arterioles and veins, is administered intravenously to treat hypertensive emergencies and for preload and afterload modulation in severe heart failure. Sodium nitroprusside is a complex of iron, cyanide groups, and a nitroso moiety, and its metabolism by red blood cells results in the liberation of nitric oxide (Fig. 17-8). Nitric oxide causes vasodilation through activation of guanylate cyclase in vascular smooth muscle (as described later in this chapter; see also Chapter 6).

Sodium nitroprusside's hemodynamic effects result from its ability to decrease arterial resistance and to increase venous capacitance. In a patient with impaired left ventricular contractile function, the decreased systemic resistance induced by sodium nitroprusside (ie, decreased afterload) augments forward CO, while venous dilation reduces return of blood to the heart. The latter decreases pulmonary capillary hydrostatic pressure and improves symptoms of pulmonary congestion.

Sodium nitroprusside is often the treatment of choice for hypertensive emergencies because of its great potency, rapid action, and short half-life. A β-blocker is often administered concurrently to counteract the reflex increase in sympathetic outflow that may occur with this drug.

Sodium nitroprusside is administered by continuous intravenous infusion. Its onset of action begins within 30 seconds, and its peak effect is achieved in 2 minutes. Its effectiveness dissipates within minutes of discontinuation. After sodium nitroprusside is metabolized into nitric oxide and cyanide, the liver, in the presence of a sulfhydryl donor, transforms cyanide into thiocyanate; the thiocyanate, in turn, is excreted by the kidney. *Thiocyanate accumulation and toxicity*, manifested by blurred vision, tinnitus, disorientation, and/or nausea, may occur with continued use, especially in the setting of renal impairment. Thus, it is important to monitor serum levels of thiocyanate if sodium nitroprusside is administered for more than 24 hours. In addition, excessive infusion rates of sodium nitroprusside, or a deficiency in hepatic thiosulfate stores, can result in lethal *cyanide toxicity*, the early signs of which include metabolic acidosis, headache, and nausea, followed by loss of consciousness.

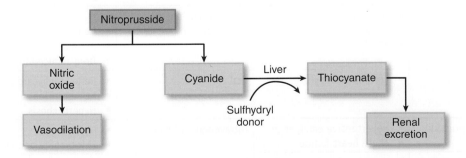

Figure 17-8. Sodium nitroprusside is a complex of iron, cyanide, and a nitroso group. Erythrocyte metabolism liberates cyanide and the active vasodilator nitric oxide. The cyanide is metabolized in the liver to thiocyanate, which is eliminated by the kidneys.

Fenoldopam is a rapidly acting intravenous arteriolar vasodilator used to treat severe hypertension. It is a selective agonist of peripheral dopamine 1 (D_1) receptors, the activation of which results in arteriolar vasodilation through a cAMP-dependent mechanism. Unlike other intravenous antihypertensive agents, it maintains or enhances renal perfusion, and its activation of renal tubular D_1 receptors facilitates natriuresis. Unlike dopamine, fenoldopam does not stimulate α- or β-adrenergic receptors.

Fenoldopam is administered by continuous intravenous infusion. Its onset of action is rapid, achieving 50% of its maximal effect within 15 minutes and a steady state in 30-60 minutes. It has a rapid offset of action after discontinuation (an elimination half-life of <10 minutes), which is a desirable effect that minimizes the risk of excessive blood pressure reduction during treatment of hypertensive emergencies. However, nitroprusside works even faster and is used more often for this purpose. The most common side effects are headache, dizziness, and tachycardia. Fenoldopam also increases intraocular pressure (probably by slowing aqueous humor drainage) and should therefore be avoided in patients with glaucoma.

Calcium Channel Blockers

The CCBs are described here as a group, but differences exist among the drugs of this class. The common property of CCBs is their ability to impede the influx of Ca^{++} through membrane channels in cardiac and smooth muscle cells. Two principal types of voltage-gated Ca^{++} channels have been identified in cardiac tissue, termed L and T. The L-type channel is responsible for the Ca^{++} entry that maintains phase 2 of the action potential (the "plateau" in Fig. 1-13). The T-type Ca^{++} channel likely plays a role in the initial depolarization of nodal tissues. It is the L-type channel that is antagonized by available CCBs.

Mechanism of Action

Intracellular calcium modulates contractile force in the myocardium and in vascular smooth muscle. At both sites, the effect of Ca^{++} channel blockade is to decrease the amount of Ca^{++} available to the contractile proteins within these cells, which results in vasodilation of vascular smooth muscle and a negative inotropic effect in cardiac muscle.

Vascular Smooth Muscle

Contraction of vascular smooth muscle depends on the cytoplasmic Ca^{++} concentration, which is regulated by the transmembrane flow of Ca^{++} through voltage-gated channels during depolarization. Intracellular Ca^{++} interacts with calmodulin to form a Ca^{++}-calmodulin complex. This complex stimulates myosin light chain kinase, which phosphorylates myosin light chains and leads to cross-bridge formation between myosin heads and actin, causing smooth muscle contraction. CCBs promote relaxation of vascular smooth muscle by inhibiting Ca^{++} entry through the voltage-gated channels. Other organs possessing smooth muscle (including gastrointestinal, uterine, and bronchiolar tissues) are also susceptible to this relaxing effect.

Cardiac Cells

As described in Chapter 1, cardiac muscle also depends on Ca^{++} influx during depolarization for contractile protein interactions, but by a different mechanism than that in vascular smooth muscle. Ca^{++} entry into the cardiac cell during depolarization triggers additional intracellular Ca^{++} release from the sarcoplasmic reticulum, leading to contraction. By blocking Ca^{++} entry, CCBs interfere with excitation-contraction coupling and decrease the force of contraction. Because the pacemaker tissues of the heart (eg, sinoatrial [SA] and AV node) are the most dependent on the inward Ca^{++} current for phase 0 depolarization, some CCBs

TABLE 17-7	Calcium Channel Blockers			
Drug	**Vasodilation**	**Negative Inotropic Effect**	**Suppress AV Node Conduction**	**Major Adverse Effects**
Verapamil	+	+++	+++	• Hypotension • Bradycardia, AV block • Constipation • Peripheral edema
Diltiazem	++	++	++	• Hypotension • Bradycardia, AV block • Peripheral edema

Dihydropyridines
  Amlodipine
  Felodipine
  Isradipine
  Nicardipine
  Nifedipine
  Nisoldipine
	+++	0 to +	0	• Hypotension
				• Headache, flushing
				• Peripheral edema

AV, atrioventricular.

reduce the rate of sinus firing and AV nodal conduction (Table 17-7). The effect on cardiac conduction appears to depend not only on whether the specific CCB reduces the inward Ca^{++} current but also on whether it delays recovery of the Ca^{++} channel to its preactivated state. **Verapamil** and **diltiazem** have this property, whereas **nifedipine** and the other dihydropyridine CCBs do not.

Clinical Uses

As a result of their actions on vascular smooth muscle and cardiac cells, CCBs are useful in several cardiovascular disorders through the mechanisms summarized in Table 17-8. In angina pectoris, they exert beneficial effects by reducing myocardial oxygen consumption as well as by potentially increasing oxygen supply through coronary dilation. The latter effect is also useful in the management of coronary artery vasospasm.

TABLE 17-8	Clinical Effects of Calcium Channel Blockers
Condition	**Mechanism**

Angina pectoris	↓ Myocardial oxygen consumption
	  ↓ Blood pressure (↓ afterload)
	  ↓ Contractility
	  ↓ Heart rate (verapamil and diltiazem)
	↑ Myocardial oxygen supply
	  ↑ Coronary dilation

Coronary artery spasm	Coronary artery vasodilation
Hypertension	Arteriolar smooth muscle relaxation
Supraventricular arrhythmias	(Verapamil and diltiazem): decrease conduction velocity and increase refractoriness of atrioventricular node

CCBs are often used to treat hypertension. More so than β-blockers or ACE inhibitors, CCBs are particularly effective in elderly patients. Nifedipine and the other dihydropyridines are the most potent vasodilators of this class.

CCBs are usually administered orally as long-acting once-a-day formulations. Routes of excretion vary. For example, nifedipine and verapamil are eliminated primarily in the urine, whereas diltiazem is excreted through the liver. Common side effects (Table 17-7) include hypotension (owing to excessive vasodilation) and ankle edema (caused by local vasodilation of peripheral vascular beds). Since verapamil and diltiazem may result in bradyarrhythmias, they should be used with caution in patients already receiving β-blocker therapy and those with underlying conduction disease. Long-acting versions of CCBs should be prescribed for extended use to prevent rapid fluctuations in blood pressure that can occur with short-acting agents. Also, recall from Chapter 6 that β-blockers and/or nitrates are generally preferred over CCBs for initial therapy in patients with chronic CAD.

ORGANIC NITRATES

Nitrates constitute one of the oldest treatments of angina pectoris. They are also used in acute ischemic syndromes and in heart failure. The main physiologic action of nitrates is vasodilation, particularly of systemic veins.

Mechanism of Action

Nitrates produce vascular smooth muscle relaxation. The proposed mechanism involves the conversion of the administered drug to nitric oxide at or near the plasma membrane of vascular smooth muscle cells (Fig. 17-9). Nitric oxide activates guanylate cyclase to produce cyclic guanosine monophosphate (cGMP) leading to smooth muscle relaxation (see Chapter 6). This mechanism of vascular smooth muscle relaxation is similar to that associated with nitroprusside and endogenous endothelial-derived nitric oxide.

Hemodynamic Effects and Clinical Uses

At low doses, nitroglycerin, the prototypical organic nitrate, produces greater dilation of veins than of arterioles. The venodilation results in venous pooling, diminished venous return,

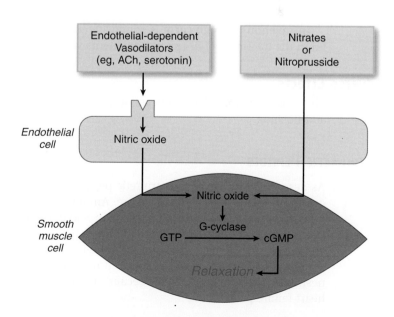

Figure 17-9. Organic nitrates incite vascular smooth muscle (SM) relaxation by conversion to nitric oxide (NO) at or near the cell membrane. Nitroprusside and endothelial-dependent vasodilators also promote NO delivery to vascular smooth muscle and cause relaxation. In the SM, NO stimulates formation of cyclic guanosine monophosphate (cGMP), which mediates relaxation.

and hence decreased right and left ventricular filling. Systemic arterial resistance is generally unaffected, but CO may fall because of the diminished preload, especially in patients with intravascular volume depletion (see Fig. 9-10). *Arterial* dilation occurs to some extent in the coronary arteries and may also occur in the facial vessels and the meningeal arterioles, giving rise to the side effects of flushing and headache, respectively.

At *high* doses, nitrates can result in widespread arteriolar dilation, which may cause systemic hypotension and reflex tachycardia.

The major use of nitrates is in the treatment of angina pectoris through venodilation, leading to reduced left ventricular preload. The smaller left ventricular size lowers ventricular wall stress and myocardial oxygen consumption, which alleviates the oxygen imbalance in ischemic states. Nitrates are also useful in patients with coronary artery spasm (Prinzmetal variant angina) by dilating the coronary arterioles.

Agents and Pharmacokinetics

Many formulations of nitrates are available. When the relief of acute angina is the objective, rapid onset of action is essential. However, in the long-term prevention of anginal attacks in a patient with chronic CAD, duration of action and predictability of effect are more crucial than the speed of drug effect.

Sublingual **nitroglycerin tablets** or **sprays** are used for treatment of acute angina attacks. The peak action of these agents occurs within 3 minutes, because they are rapidly absorbed into the bloodstream via the oral mucosa. Their effect, however, diminishes rapidly, falling off within 15-30 minutes, as the drug is deactivated in the liver. These forms of nitroglycerin are also effective when taken prophylactically, immediately before situations known by the patient to produce angina (eg, before walking up a hill).

Long-acting nitrates are used to prevent chest discomfort in the chronic management of CAD and must be given in sufficient dosage to saturate the liver's deactivating capacity. For this purpose, oral doses of **sustained-release nitroglycerin, isosorbide dinitrate**, or **isosorbide mononitrate** are used. These agents have a duration of action of 2-14 hours. **Transdermal nitroglycerin patches** applied to the skin also delivers a sustained release of nitroglycerin. Of note, the efficacy of long-acting nitrate therapy is attenuated by the development of drug tolerance with continuous use. For this reason, it is important that dosing regimens allow a drug-free interval of several hours each day to maintain efficacy.

Intravenous nitroglycerin is administered by continuous infusion. This form is most useful in the treatment of hospitalized patients with persistent angina or acute heart failure.

Adverse Effects

The most common adverse effects of nitrates are hypotension, reflex tachycardia, headache, and flushing.

NATRIURETIC PEPTIDES

As described in Chapter 9, natriuretic peptides are secreted from atrial and ventricular myocardium in patients with heart failure. Among their beneficial physiologic effects, these peptides promote vasodilation and result in sodium and water excretion. The pharmacologic agent **nesiritide** (human recombinant BNP) replicates these effects. It results in vasodilation, augmented CO, reduction of the undesired activation of the renin-angiotensin and sympathetic nervous systems, and augmented natriuresis. Despite these effects, the clinical role of nesiritide is still being defined, because its use has not been shown to improve survival in heart failure patients.

PHOSPHODIESTERASE-5 INHIBITORS

Sildenafil and tadalafil, phosphodiesterase type 5 (PDE5) inhibitors used to treat erectile dysfunction, have also been shown to improve exercise capacity in patients with a form (WHO group I) of pulmonary arterial hypertension (PAH), a condition associated with increased pulmonary vascular resistance. These drugs inhibit the breakdown of cGMP in the pulmonary vasculature, which enhances vasodilation. However, if administered concurrently with a nitrate, PDE5 inhibitors can cause severe hypotension and that combination of drugs is contraindicated.

ENDOTHELIN RECEPTOR ANTAGONISTS

Endothelin-1 (ET-1) is a vasoactive peptide that is synthesized and released primarily by endothelial cells. ET-1 binds to two types of receptors: ET_A and ET_B. Both receptor types are present on vascular smooth muscle cells, where their activation results in *vasoconstriction* (Fig. 17-10). This effect is mediated by G protein–coupled activation of phospholipase C, which promotes formation of inositol triphosphate (IP_3). IP_3 stimulates Ca^{++} release from intracellular stores, resulting in smooth muscle contraction and therefore vasoconstriction. ET_B receptors are also located on endothelial cells, where their stimulation promotes *vasodilation* instead, via increased production of nitric oxide (Fig. 17-10). In the intact blood vessel, smooth muscle vasoconstriction by ET-1 dominates over the vasodilator effect in both systemic and pulmonary arteries.

Drugs that antagonize ET-1 receptors act as vasodilators, and the main therapeutic use of this class is in the treatment of PAH, which is associated with activation of the ET-1 system. Among agents in this group, **bosentan** and **macitentan** antagonize both ET_A and ET_B receptors. **Ambrisentan** selectively inhibits the ET_A receptor. Each of these orally administered drugs reduces pulmonary vascular resistance and pulmonary artery pressure and improves exertional capacity and dyspnea in patients with PAH.

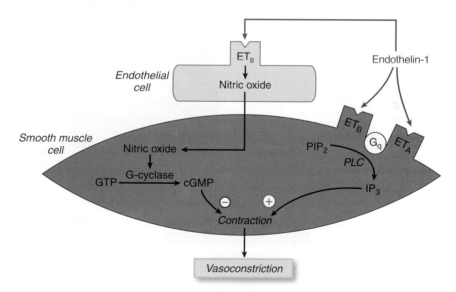

Figure 17-10. Endothelin-1 receptors and modulation of vascular tone. Endothelin-1 (ET-1) binds to ET_B and ET_A receptors on vascular smooth muscle, which are coupled to Gq protein, activating phospholipase C (PLC) and catalyzing the hydrolysis of phosphatidylinositol bisphosphate (PIP_2) to inositol triphosphate (IP_3). IP_3 stimulates the release of calcium from intracellular stores, resulting in smooth muscle cell contraction and vasoconstriction. Conversely, ET-1 activation of the ET_B receptor on *endothelial cells* promotes vasodilation via increased production of nitric oxide. The vasoconstrictive effect predominates in the intact blood vessel. Therefore, ET-1 receptor blockade with currently available pharmaceuticals (either nonselective blockade of both receptors or selective ET_A receptor blockade) results in vasodilation.

Endothelin receptor antagonists are generally well tolerated. The main adverse effects are a reversible elevation of hepatic transaminases and peripheral edema. These agents are also teratogenic and should not be prescribed to pregnant women.

ANTIADRENERGIC DRUGS

Drugs that interfere with the sympathetic nervous system act at various sites, including the central nervous system (CNS), postganglionic sympathetic nerve endings, and peripheral α- and β-receptors (Fig. 17-11).

Normally, when a sympathetic nerve is stimulated, norepinephrine is released, traverses the synapse, and stimulates postsynaptic α- and β-receptors. Norepinephrine within the synapse can also bind to *presynaptic* β- and α_2-receptors, providing a feedback mechanism that

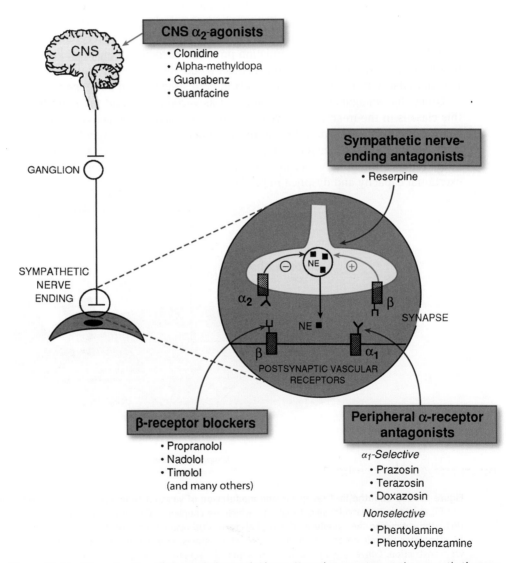

Figure 17-11. Sites of action of the antiadrenergic drugs. Note that receptors at the sympathetic nerve ending bind norepinephrine (NE) and provide feedback: the β-receptor stimulates, and the α_2-receptor inhibits, further NE release. CNS, central nervous system.

TABLE 17-9	Responses to Adrenergic Receptor Stimulation	
Receptor Type	**Distribution**	**Response**
α_1	Vascular smooth muscle (arterioles and veins)	Vasoconstriction
α_2	Presynaptic adrenergic nerve terminals	Inhibition of NE release
	Vascular smooth muscle (coronary and renal arterioles)	Vasoconstriction
β_1	Heart	Increases heart rate
		Increases contractility
		Speeds AV node conduction
	Kidney (JG cells)	Increases renin release
	Presynaptic adrenergic nerve terminals	Increases NE release
	Adipose tissue	Stimulates lipolysis
β_2	Vascular smooth muscle (arterioles, except skin and cerebral)	Vasodilation
	Bronchial smooth muscle	Bronchodilation
	Liver	Stimulates glycogenolysis

AV, atrioventricular; JG, juxtaglomerular; NE, norepinephrine.

modulates further release of the hormone. The presynaptic β-receptors increase, and the α_2-receptors inhibit, further norepinephrine release.

The consequences of receptor stimulation depend on the organ involved (Table 17-9). The effect of α_1-receptor stimulation on vascular smooth muscle is vasoconstriction, whereas β_2-stimulation causes vasodilation. In the CNS, α_2-stimulation *inhibits* sympathetic outflow to the periphery, thereby contributing to vasodilation.

CENTRAL ADRENERGIC INHIBITORS (CNS α_2-AGONISTS)

α_2-Receptors are located in the presynaptic neurons of the CNS. When stimulated by an α_2-agonist, *diminished* sympathetic outflow from the medulla results. This action reduces peripheral vascular resistance and decreases cardiac stimulation, resulting in a fall in blood pressure and heart rate. CNS α_2-agonists were once among the most commonly used antihypertensive drugs but have largely given way to better tolerated agents with fewer side effects and greater cardioprotective benefits.

The drugs in this group are listed in Figure 17-11. They are all available as oral preparations, and clonidine can also be prescribed as a skin patch that is applied and left in place for 1 week at a time, facilitating drug compliance. Side effects of CNS α_2-agonists include sedation, dry mouth, bradycardia, and, if the drug is stopped suddenly, the possibility of rebound hypertension.

SYMPATHETIC NERVE-ENDING ANTAGONISTS

Reserpine was the first drug found to interfere with the sympathetic nervous system. It inhibits the uptake of norepinephrine into storage vesicles in postganglionic and central neurons, leading to norepinephrine degradation. The antihypertensive effect results from the depletion of catecholamines, which decreases myocardial contractility and total peripheral vascular resistance.

Reserpine's CNS toxicity represents its chief drawback. It often produces sedation, and the most serious potential toxicity is psychotic depression. Newer, better-tolerated antihypertensive agents have largely supplanted the use of reserpine and other sympathetic nerve-ending antagonists.

PERIPHERAL α-ADRENERGIC RECEPTOR ANTAGONISTS

Peripheral α-antagonists (Table 17-10) are divided into those that act on both α_1- and α_2-receptors and those that inhibit α_1 alone. α_1-Selective receptor antagonists (**prazosin, terazosin, doxazosin**) are occasionally prescribed for the treatment of hypertension. Their selectivity for the α_1-receptor explains their ability to produce less reflex tachycardia than nonselective agents. Normally, drug-induced vasodilation results in baroreceptor-mediated stimulation of the sympathetic nervous system and an undesired increase in heart rate. This effect is amplified by drugs that block the presynaptic α_2-receptor, because feedback inhibition of norepinephrine release is prevented. However, α_1-selective agents do not block the negative feedback on the α_2-receptor. Thus, further norepinephrine release and reflex sympathetic side effects are blunted.

Historically, the principal indication for α_1-antagonists was for treatment of hypertension. However, in a large prospective, randomized trial, patients treated with the α_1-antagonist doxazosin experienced more adverse cardiac outcomes than those treated with a thiazide diuretic. Thus, α_1-antagonists have fallen out of favor in the management of hypertension. Terazosin and doxazosin are mainly used today to treat the symptoms of benign prostatic hyperplasia, because the drugs also beneficially relax prostatic smooth muscle.

Phentolamine and **phenoxybenzamine** are nonselective α-blockers. They are used in the treatment of pheochromocytoma, a tumor that abnormally secretes catecholamines into the circulation (see Chapter 13). Otherwise, these drugs are rarely used because the α_2-blockade impairs the normal feedback inhibition of norepinephrine release, an undesired effect, as indicated earlier.

β-ADRENERGIC RECEPTOR ANTAGONISTS

The β-adrenergic antagonists ("β-blockers") are used for a number of cardiovascular conditions, including ischemic heart disease, hypertension, heart failure, and tachyarrhythmias.

Because catecholamines increase inotropy, chronotropy, and conduction velocity in the heart, it follows that β-receptor antagonists decrease inotropy, slow the heart rate, and decrease conduction velocity. When the sympathetic nervous system is activated (eg, during exercise), these antagonists can substantially diminish catecholamine-mediated effects.

β-Blockers can be distinguished from one another by specific properties (Table 17-11): (1) the relative affinity of the drug for β_1- and β_2-receptors, (2) whether partial β-*agonist* activity is present, (3) whether the drug also has vasodilator properties (eg, via α_1-receptor blockade), and (4) differences in pharmacokinetic properties. The goal of β_1-*selective* agents is to achieve myocardial receptor blockade, with less effect on bronchial and vascular smooth muscle

TABLE 17-10 α-Receptor Antagonists		
Mechanism/Drug	**Indications**	**Major Adverse Effects**
Selective peripheral α_1-blockade Prazosin Terazosin Doxazosin	• Hypertension • Benign prostatic hyperplasia	• Postural hypotension • Headache, dizziness
Nonselective α-blockade Phentolamine Phenoxybenzamine	• Pheochromocytoma	• Postural hypotension • Reflex tachycardia

TABLE 17-11	β-Adrenergic Blockers	
Activity	**Nonselective β-Blockers**	**β$_1$-Selective β-Blockers**
No β-agonist activity	Carvedilol[a]	Atenolol
	Labetalol[a]	Betaxolol
	Propranolol	Bisoprolol
	Nadolol	Esmolol[b]
	Timolol	Metoprolol
		Nebivolol[c]
β-Agonist activity	Carteolol	Acebutolol
	Penbutolol	
	Pindolol	

[a]Also has α$_1$-adrenergic–blocking properties.
[b]Administered intravenously only.
[c]Also has vasodilating properties, likely mediated by nitric oxide.

(tissues that exhibit β$_2$-receptors), thus producing less bronchospasm and vasoconstriction in susceptible patients. Agents with partial β-agonist effects (termed *intrinsic sympathomimetic activity*) slow the heart rate less than other β-blockers and may be better tolerated by patients with resting bradycardia.

During short-term use, nonselective β-antagonists tend to reduce cardiac output because they decrease heart rate and contractility as well as slightly increase peripheral resistance (via β$_2$-receptor blockade). β-Antagonists that have partial agonist activity (such as pindolol) or those that possess some α-blocking activity (such as labetalol) can actually lower peripheral resistance by interacting with their respective β$_2$- and α-receptors.

Clinical Uses
Ischemic Heart Disease
The beneficial effects of β-blockers in ischemic heart disease are related to their ability to decrease myocardial oxygen demand. They reduce heart rate, blood pressure (afterload), and contractility. The negative inotropic effect is directly related to blockade of the cardiac β-receptor, which results in decreased calcium influx into the myocyte (see Fig. 17-4). β-Blockers are effective in treating angina in individuals with chronic CAD and also improve survival following acute myocardial infarction. Agents with intrinsic sympathomimetic activity are less beneficial in this regard than β-blockers without it.

Hypertension
β-Blockers are sometimes used as antihypertensive agents, though the mechanisms responsible for blood pressure lowering are not completely understood. With initial use, the antihypertensive action is thought to result from a decrease in cardiac output, in association with slowing of the heart rate and mild decrease in contractility. However, with chronic administration, other mechanisms are likely at work, including reduced renal secretion of renin and possibly CNS effects. β-Blockers that also manifest α$_1$-receptor blocking properties are more effective at lowering blood pressure.

Heart Failure
The negative inotropic effect of β-blockade would be expected to worsen heart failure symptoms in patients with underlying left ventricular systolic dysfunction. However, trials in

patients with all classes of clinically stable chronic heart failure have actually shown a survival *benefit* with long-term β-blocker administration using specific agents of this class (carvedilol, metoprolol succinate, and bisoprolol [see Chapter 9]). The mechanism may relate to blunting of the cardiotoxic effects of excessive circulating catecholamines. Because of the potential risk of transiently *worsening* heart failure in tenuous patients, β-blocker therapy should be started at low dosage, augmented slowly, and carefully monitored.

Other conditions that benefit from β-blocker therapy include tachyarrhythmias (as discussed later in the chapter) and hypertrophic cardiomyopathy (see Chapter 10).

Adverse Effects

Fatigue may occur during β-blocker therapy and is most likely a CNS side effect. β-Blockers with less lipid solubility (eg, nadolol) penetrate the blood-brain barrier poorly and may have fewer CNS adverse effects than more lipid-soluble drugs, such as propranolol. Other potential adverse effects relate to the predictable consequences of β-blockade:

1. β_2-Blockade associated with use of nonselective agents (or large doses of β_1-selective blockers) can exacerbate *bronchospasm*, worsening preexisting asthma or chronic obstructive lung disease.
2. The impairment of AV nodal conduction by β_1-blockade can cause conduction blocks.
3. β_2-Blockade can precipitate arterial *vasospasm*, which could result in Raynaud phenomenon (see Chapter 15) or worsen symptoms of peripheral vascular disease.
4. Abrupt withdrawal of a β-antagonist after chronic use could precipitate myocardial ischemia in patients with CAD.
5. β_2-Blockade may impair recovery from hypoglycemia in diabetics suffering an insulin reaction. In addition, β-blockers may mask the sympathetic warning signs of hypoglycemia, such as tachycardia. If β-blockers are used in diabetics, β_1-selective agents are generally preferred.

Other potential side effects include insomnia, depression, and impotence. Finally, β-antagonists should be used with caution in combination with nondihydropyridine CCBs (verapamil or diltiazem), because both types of drugs can impair myocardial contractility and AV nodal conduction, possibly precipitating heart failure or AV conduction blocks.

ANTIARRHYTHMIC DRUGS

Drug therapy is a common approach to treat cardiac tachyarrhythmias. However, antiarrhythmic drugs must be prescribed with care because of potential serious adverse effects. A thorough understanding of the mechanisms of action, indications, and toxicities of these drugs is of particular importance.

Although a number of classification systems exist, the Vaughan-Williams grouping is most widely used. It divides antiarrhythmic drugs into four classes based on their main electrophysiologic mechanisms of action (Table 17-12):

1. *Class I* drugs primarily block the fast sodium channel responsible for phase 0 depolarization of the action potential in cardiac muscle cells and Purkinje fibers (see Chapter 1). These drugs are further divided into three subtypes based on the degree of sodium channel blockade and the effect on the cell's action potential duration.
2. *Class II* drugs are β-adrenergic receptor antagonists (β-blockers).
3. *Class III* drugs prolong the action potential duration, predominantly by blocking potassium channels responsible for repolarization, with little effect on the rise of phase 0 depolarization.
4. *Class IV* drugs block the L-type calcium channel.

Drugs that do not conveniently fit into these classes (and are described separately) include adenosine and digitalis glycosides.

TABLE 17-12 Classification of Antiarrhythmic Drugs

Class	General Mechanism	Examples
I	**Na⁺ channel blockade**	
IA	Moderate block ($\downarrow\downarrow$ phase 0 upstroke rate; prolonged AP duration)	Quinidine Procainamide Disopyramide
IB	Mild block ($\downarrow$phase 0 upstroke rate; shortened AP duration)	Lidocaine Mexiletine
IC	Marked block ($\downarrow\downarrow\downarrow$ phase 0 upstroke rate; no change in AP duration)	Flecainide Propafenone
II	**β-Adrenergic receptor blockade**	Propranolol Esmolol Metoprolol
III	**K⁺ channel blockade** (prolongation of AP duration)	Amiodarone Dronedarone Sotalol Dofetilide Ibutilide
IV	**Ca⁺⁺ channel antagonists**	Verapamil Diltiazem

AP, action potential.

Regardless of the class, the goal of antiarrhythmic drugs is to abolish the mechanisms by which tachyarrhythmias occur. As described in Chapter 11, these mechanisms are (1) increased automaticity of pacemaker or nonpacemaker cells, (2) reentrant circuits, and (3) triggered activity.

In the case of arrhythmias caused by *increased automaticity*, treatment is aimed at lowering the maximum frequency at which cardiac action potentials can occur by (1) reducing the slope of spontaneous phase 4 diastolic depolarization and/or (2) prolonging the effective refractory period.

Antiarrhythmic drugs inhibit *reentrant* rhythms by a different mechanism. The initiation of a reentrant circuit relies on a region of unidirectional block and slowed conduction (Fig. 17-12). For a reentrant rhythm to sustain itself, the length of time it takes for an impulse to propagate around the circuit must exceed the effective refractory period of the tissue. If an impulse returns to an area of myocardium that was depolarized moments earlier but has not yet recovered excitability, it cannot restimulate that tissue. Thus, one strategy to stop reentry is to lengthen the tissue's refractory period. When the refractory period is pharmacologically prolonged, a propagating impulse confronts inactive sodium channels, cannot conduct further, and is extinguished.

A second means to interrupt reentrant circuits is to *additionally impair* impulse propagation within the already slowed retrograde limb. This is accomplished via pharmacologic blockade of the Na⁺ chan-

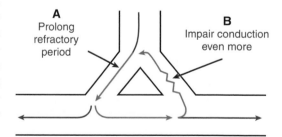

Figure 17-12. Two strategies to interrupt reentry.
A. Prolonging the tissue refractory period causes returning impulses to find the tissue unexcitable.
B. Further impairing conduction causes the impulse to "die out" in the slow retrograde limb of the circuit.

nels responsible for phase 0 depolarization. Such blockade fully abolishes the compromised impulse conduction within the retrograde limb and breaks the self-sustaining loop.

The elimination of the third type of tachyarrhythmia, *triggered activity*, requires suppression of early and delayed afterdepolarizations.

An ideal pharmacologic agent would suppress ectopic foci and interrupt reentrant loops without affecting normal conduction pathways. Unfortunately, when the concentrations of antiarrhythmic drugs exceed their narrow therapeutic ranges, even normal electrical activity may become suppressed. In addition, most antiarrhythmic drugs have the potential to aggravate rhythm disturbances (termed *proarrhythmic effect*). For example, this may occur when an antiarrhythmic drug prolongs the action potential duration and induces early afterdepolarizations, resulting in a triggered type of arrhythmia, such as life-threatening torsades de pointes (see Chapter 12). Drug-induced proarrhythmia occurs most often in patients with left ventricular dysfunction or in those with an increased QT interval (a sign that the action potential is already prolonged).

Class IA Antiarrhythmics

Mechanism of Action

Effect on Reentrant Arrhythmias

Class IA agents produce moderate blockade of the fast sodium channels, thus slowing the rate of phase 0 depolarization and reducing tissue conduction velocities (Fig. 17-13). If impaired sufficiently within a reentrant circuit, the impulse will die out within the already slowed retrograde limb, aborting the rhythm. In addition, class IA agents prolong the cell's action potential and the refractory period (largely via blockade of potassium channels responsible for repolarization). Thus, an impulse traveling in the reentrant loop encounters unexcitable tissue and is extinguished.

Effect on Arrhythmias Caused by Increased Automaticity

In atrial and ventricular ectopic pacemaker cells, class IA agents depress the slope of phase 4 depolarization (through inhibition of pacemaker channels) and raise the threshold to a less negative voltage (by blocking excitable sodium channels). As a result, it takes longer to reach threshold and fire the action potential, thus suppressing automatic activity.

Effect on the Electrocardiogram

Because the conduction velocity is decreased and the action potential duration and repolarization are prolonged, the effect of class IA agents is to mildly prolong the QRS duration in some patients and the QT interval in most patients (Table 17-13). At higher dosages, the drugs

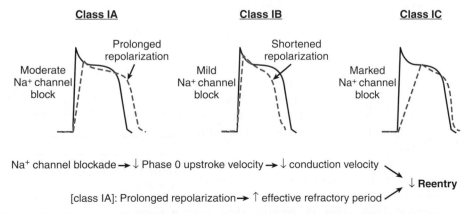

Figure 17-13. Electrophysiologic effects of the class I antiarrhythmic drugs on the Purkinje cell action potential.

TABLE 17-13	Effect of Antiarrhythmic Drugs on Electrocardiographic Intervals[a]			
Class	**PR**	**QRS**	**QT**	**ECG Appearance** Normal ECG
IA	0	↑	↑	
IB	0	0	0 or ↓	
IC	↑	↑	0 or ↑	
II	0 or ↑	0	0	
III	0 or ↑	0 or ↑	↑	
IV	↑	0	0	

[a]The predominant effects on the electrocardiographic segments are shown in red.

may substantially lengthen these intervals, potentially setting the stage for afterdepolarizations (described in Chapter 11) and drug-induced arrhythmias.

Clinical Uses

Class IA drugs are effective in treating reentrant and ectopic supraventricular and ventricular tachycardias (Table 17-14). However, their use has declined because of the development of more effective and less proarrhythmic strategies.

TABLE 17-14	Common Clinical Uses of Antiarrhythmic Drugs
Class	**Use**
IA	• Atrial fibrillation and flutter • PSVT • Ventricular tachycardia
IB	• Ventricular tachycardia • Digitalis-induced arrhythmias
IC	• Atrial fibrillation and PSVT
II	• Atrial or ventricular premature beats • PSVT • Atrial fibrillation and flutter • Ventricular tachycardia
III	• Ventricular tachycardia (amiodarone and sotalol) • Atrial fibrillation and flutter • Bypass tract–mediated PSVT
IV	• PSVT • Atrial fibrillation and flutter (↓ VR) • Multifocal atrial tachycardia (↓ VR)

PSVT, paroxysmal supraventricular tachycardia (eg, AV nodal re-entrant tachycardia); VR, ventricular rate.

Specific Class IA Drugs

Quinidine displays the electrophysiologic effects inherent to class IA agents but also has anti-cholinergic properties that may *augment* conduction at the AV node, thus antagonizing its direct suppressant effect. Because quinidine is metabolized primarily by the liver, its dosage must be reduced in patients with hepatic dysfunction.

Noncardiac and cardiac side effects occur frequently during quinidine therapy. The most common are related to the gastrointestinal tract, including nausea, vomiting, and diarrhea. *Cinchonism* refers to CNS toxicity by quinidine manifested by tinnitus, confusion, hearing loss, and visual disturbances. Since quinidine can cause excessive prolongation of the QT interval, it may lead to torsades de pointes.

Procainamide has similar electrophysiologic effects as quinidine, but does not prolong the action potential (and therefore QT interval) as much. It is available for oral or parenteral administration and is primarily used when intravenous delivery of a class IA drug is desired. More than 50% of the drug is excreted unchanged in the urine; the remainder undergoes acetylation by the liver to form *N*-acetyl procainamide (NAPA), which is subsequently excreted by the kidneys. In renal failure, or in patients who are rapid acetylators, high serum levels of NAPA may accumulate. NAPA shares procainamide's ability to prolong the action potential and refractory period, but it does not alter the rate of phase 4 depolarization or the slope of phase 0 upstroke of the action potential.

Noncardiac side effects of procainamide are common and include fever, myalgias, and gastrointestinal upset (less frequently than with quinidine). Approximately one-third of patients develop a systemic lupus–like syndrome after 6 months of therapy, manifested by arthralgias, rash, and connective tissue inflammation. It most often occurs among patients who are slow acetylators and is reversible on cessation of drug therapy. As a result of these side effects, procainamide is generally reserved for short-term use.

Disopyramide's electrophysiologic and antiarrhythmic effects are similar to those of quinidine, but it has a greater anticholinergic effect. More so than quinidine or procainamide, disopyramide also has a pronounced negative inotropic effect and must be used with caution in patients with left ventricular systolic dysfunction. However, its negative inotropic property renders it a useful antiarrhythmic agent for patients who also have hypertrophic cardiomyopathy with dynamic outflow tract obstruction, for whom a reduced force of contraction is desired (see Chapter 10).

Disopyramide is administered orally. The primary excretory pathway is via the kidneys, and toxic levels may accumulate in patients with renal insufficiency. QT prolongation and precipitation of ventricular arrhythmias (including torsades de pointes) can occur, and anticholinergic side effects, such as constipation, urinary retention, and glaucoma exacerbation, are common.

CLASS IB ANTIARRHYTHMICS

Mechanism of Action

Class IB drugs inhibit the fast sodium channel, but unlike IA agents, they typically *shorten* the action potential duration and the refractory period. Such shortening is attributed to blockade of small sodium currents that normally continue through phase 2 of the action potential.

Class IB drugs at therapeutic concentrations do not substantially alter the electrical activity of normal tissue; rather, they preferentially act on diseased or ischemic cells (Box 17-1). Conditions present during ischemia—acidosis, faster rates of cell stimulation, and increased extracellular potassium concentration (and consequently a less negative diastolic membrane potential)—increase the ability of class IB drugs to block the sodium channel. This blockade reduces the slope of phase 0 depolarization and slows the conduction velocity, thus impairing conduction in ischemic cells and inhibiting reentrant arrhythmias (see Fig. 17-13). The automaticity of ectopic

Box 17-1	Use Dependence of Class I Antiarrhythmic Drugs

An important characteristic of class I antiarrhythmic drugs is their "state-dependent" (also termed "use-dependent") binding to the Na^+ channel. Conformational differences in the channel's states result in a relatively low affinity of these drugs for resting closed channels, and a higher affinity, and therefore greater blocking potency, for channels in their open or inactivated states (refer to Chapter 1 for a description of channel states). Therefore, class I drugs exhibit their greatest effect in cardiac cells that are depolarized. There are two therapeutic consequences:

1. In injured or ischemic tissue, there is constant partial depolarization of cells, which shifts some of the Na^+ channels persistently into the inactivated state. The associated slowed conduction in such tissue may set the stage for reentrant types of arrhythmias (see Chapter 11). By preferentially binding and blocking Na^+ channels in the persistently depolarized, injured membrane, class I drugs prevent their participation in such slow conduction and thus have the capacity to suppress reentrant rhythms.
2. During normal rhythmic depolarizations, a class I agent binds avidly to the inactivated Na^+ channels that develop during phase 2 of the action potential. Subsequently, the drug dissociates from the channel in diastole, as inactivated channels revert to the resting closed state upon repolarization. However, during fast heart rates (ie, tachyarrhythmias), the interval between depolarizations becomes shorter, and drug dissociation is therefore less complete. This results in an accumulating fraction of drug-blocked channels, and the potential for too few available unblocked channels to support a subsequent action potential, thus accentuating the antiarrhythmic effect of the drug at faster heart rates.

pacemakers is also suppressed by decreasing phase 4 spontaneous depolarization and (in the case of some drugs of this class) by raising the threshold potential. In addition, intravenous lidocaine, a member of this class, suppresses delayed after depolarizations.

Because the QT interval is not prolonged by class IB drugs, and may actually be shortened (Table 17-13), early afterdepolarizations do not occur, and torsades de pointes is not an expected complication.

Clinical Uses

The most common use of class IB drugs is in the suppression of ventricular arrhythmias, especially those that appear in association with ischemia or digitalis toxicity. Conversely, they have little effect on *atrial* tissue at therapeutic concentrations because of the shorter action potential duration of atrial cells, which allows less time for the drug to bind and block the Na^+ channel.

Specific Class IB Drugs

Lidocaine, administered intravenously, is used to suppress some ventricular arrhythmias in hospitalized patients. As a result of rapid distribution and hepatic metabolism, lidocaine must be administered as a continuous infusion following a loading bolus. Because the half-life of the drug depends greatly on hepatic function, the infusion rate should be lowered in patients with reduced hepatic blood flow (as in heart failure or in older individuals) or intrinsic liver disease.

The most common side effects of lidocaine are related to the CNS and include confusion, paresthesias, dizziness, and seizures.

Mexiletine, administered orally, is structurally similar to lidocaine and shares its electrophysiologic properties. Ninety percent of mexiletine is metabolized in the liver to inactive products, and the dosage of the drug should be reduced in patients with hepatic dysfunction. Dose-related side effects of mexiletine are common, especially of the CNS (dizziness, tremor, slurred speech) and the gastrointestinal tract (nausea, vomiting).

CLASS IC ANTIARRHYTHMICS

Mechanism of Action

Class IC drugs are the most potent sodium channel blockers. They markedly decrease the upstroke of the action potential and conduction velocity in atrial, ventricular, and Purkinje fibers (see Fig. 17-13). Although they have little effect on the duration of the action potential or refractory period of Purkinje fibers, they significantly prolong the refractory period within the AV node and in accessory bypass tracts. The effect of class IC drugs on decreasing the action potential upstroke tends to prolong the QRS duration on the ECG, while the QT interval is typically not prolonged since the total action potential duration is not lengthened (see Table 17-13).

Clinical Uses

Class IC agents were originally developed to treat ventricular arrhythmias. However, that use has diminished because studies have shown an *increased* mortality rate in patients taking class IC drugs for ventricular ectopy following myocardial infarction and in those who have survived cardiac arrest. In addition, in patients with underlying left ventricular dysfunction, class IC drugs can precipitate heart failure. Thus, drugs of this subclass should be avoided in patients who have other underlying heart abnormalities, such as CAD or LV dysfunction. Class IC drugs *have* been shown to be beneficial (and generally safe) in the treatment of supraventricular arrhythmias, including atrial fibrillation and AV nodal reentrant tachycardia, in patients who have otherwise structurally normal hearts (see Table 17-14).

Specific Class IC Drugs

Flecainide is well absorbed after oral administration. Approximately 40% of the drug is excreted unchanged in the urine, and the remainder is converted to inactive metabolites by the liver. Dose-dependent noncardiac side effects include confusion, dizziness, and blurred vision.

The electrophysiologic properties of **propafenone** are similar to those of flecainide, but additionally, it exhibits weak β-adrenergic blocking activity. Propafenone is metabolized by the liver, but because the level of genetic variation is high, a patient's dosage must be titrated by observing the drug's effect. Extracardiac side effects are not common and include dizziness and disturbances of taste.

CLASS II ANTIARRHYTHMICS

Mechanism of Action

Class II drugs are β-adrenergic receptor antagonists and are used in the management of both supraventricular and ventricular arrhythmias. Most of the antiarrhythmic properties of class II agents can be attributed to inhibition of cardiac sympathetic activity. Additional actions of some β-blockers, such as β_1-cardioselectivity or a membrane-stabilizing effect, seem to make no contribution to antiarrhythmic activity.

Chapter 11 describes how β-adrenergic stimulation results in a more rapid upslope of phase 4 depolarization and an increased firing rate of the SA node. β-Adrenergic antagonists inhibit these effects, thus reducing automaticity (Fig. 17-14). This action extends to the cardiac Purkinje fibers, where arrhythmias due to enhanced automaticity are suppressed. β-Blockers also

Figure 17-14. Electrophysiologic effects of the class II antiarrhythmic drugs on the pacemaker cell action potential.

decrease conduction velocity and lengthen the refractory period of the AV node, thus beneficially slowing the ventricular rate in patients with rapid atrial rhythms. In addition, because delayed afterdepolarizations may be caused by excessive catecholamines, β-blockers may prevent triggered arrhythmias induced by that mechanism.

β-Blockers may also have a beneficial antiarrhythmic effect by decreasing myocardial oxygen demand, thus reducing myocardial ischemia. Several drugs from this group have been shown to reduce mortality following myocardial infarction (see Chapter 7), which may in part relate to their antiarrhythmic effect.

Since the AV nodal conduction time is prolonged by β-blockers, the PR interval on the ECG may become prolonged (see Table 17-13). The QRS and QT intervals are usually unaffected.

Clinical Uses

β-Blockers are most useful in suppressing tachyarrhythmias induced by excessive catecholamines (eg, during exercise or emotional stimulation). They are also frequently used to slow the ventricular rate in atrial flutter and fibrillation by impairing conduction and increasing the refractoriness of the AV node. In addition, β-blockers may terminate reentrant supraventricular arrhythmias in which the AV node constitutes one limb of the reentrant pathway.

β-Blockers suppress ventricular premature beats and other ventricular arrhythmias, especially when induced by exercise. They are also effective in treating ventricular arrhythmias related to prolongation of the QT interval because, unlike group IA agents, they do not lengthen that interval.

CLASS III ANTIARRHYTHMICS

Mechanism of Action

Class III drugs are structurally dissimilar from one another but share the property of significantly prolonging the action potential of Purkinje and ventricular muscle fibers (Fig. 17-15), predominantly by blocking the outward K$^+$ current of phase 3 repolarization. Unlike class I agents, class III antiarrhythmics generally have little effect on phase 0 depolarization or conduction velocity.

Figure 17-15. Electrophysiologic effects of the class III antiarrhythmic drugs on the Purkinje cell action potential.

Specific Class III Drugs

Amiodarone

Amiodarone is a very effective antiarrhythmic that also has many potential adverse effects. Its major therapeutic action is to prolong the action potential duration and refractoriness of all cardiac regions. However, it also shares actions with each of the other antiarrhythmic classes. The slope of phase 0 depolarization may be depressed through sodium channel blockade (class I effect), it exerts a β-blocking effect (class II), and it also demonstrates weak calcium channel blockade (class IV). As a result, the electrophysiologic effects of amiodarone are to decrease the SA node firing rate, suppress automaticity, interrupt reentrant circuits, and prolong the PR, QRS, and QT intervals on the ECG (see Table 17-13).

In addition, amiodarone is a vasodilator (because of α-receptor and calcium channel–blocking effects) and a negative inotrope (β-blocker and CCB effects). The resulting vasodilation is more prominent than the negative inotropic effect, so that CO does not usually suffer.

Amiodarone is more effective than most other antiarrhythmic drugs for a wide spectrum of ventricular and supraventricular tachyarrhythmias. It is a first-line agent for the emergency treatment of ventricular arrhythmias during cardiac resuscitation (including ventricular fibrillation and ventricular tachycardia refractory to electrical shocks). It is commonly used to treat arrhythmias in patients with ventricular systolic dysfunction because it causes fewer proarrhythmic complications in that population than other agents. In addition, low-dose amiodarone is effective for long-term suppression of atrial fibrillation and flutter.

Amiodarone is absorbed slowly from the gastrointestinal tract, requiring 5-6 hours to reach peak plasma concentrations. It is highly lipophilic and extensively sequestered in tissues, and it undergoes very slow hepatic metabolism. Its elimination half-life is long and variable, averaging 25-60 *days*. The drug is excreted by the biliary tract, lacrimal glands, and skin but not by the kidney. Because the drug's action has a delayed onset and very long duration, its effects cannot be altered quickly if side effects ensue.

There are numerous potential adverse reactions of amiodarone. The most serious is pulmonary toxicity, manifest by pneumonitis leading to pulmonary fibrosis. Its origin is unclear but may represent a hypersensitivity reaction and, if recognized early, is reversible.

Other life-threatening side effects of amiodarone relate to cardiac toxicity: symptomatic bradycardia and aggravation of ventricular arrhythmias, each occurring in ~2% of patients. Because amiodarone significantly prolongs the QT interval, early afterdepolarizations and torsades de pointes can occur, though these are rare. Intravenously administered amiodarone occasionally causes hypotension.

Abnormalities of thyroid function are common during amiodarone treatment because the drug contains a significant iodine load and because it inhibits the peripheral conversion of T_4 to T_3. During the first few weeks of therapy, transient abnormalities of thyroid biochemical tests are common, without clinical findings of thyroid disease: serum TSH and T_4 rise, and serum T_3 falls. Over time, some patients develop overt hypothyroidism (owing mostly to the antithyroid effects of excessive iodine) or hyperthyroidism (because of either an iodine effect in iodine-deficient communities or a direct thyroid inflammatory process incited by amiodarone in susceptible patients).

Gastrointestinal side effects of amiodarone include anorexia, nausea, and elevation of liver function blood tests, all of which improve with lower doses of the drug. Neurologic side effects include proximal muscle weakness, peripheral neuropathy, ataxia, tremors, and sleep disturbances. Corneal microdeposits can be detected in patients receiving chronic amiodarone therapy, but these rarely affect vision.

As a result of these potential adverse effects, ECGs, thyroid and liver function blood tests, and chest radiography or pulmonary function studies are typically performed on a regular basis in patients receiving chronic therapy. Amiodarone interacts with, and increases the activity of, certain drugs including warfarin and digoxin, such that the dosages of those agents must be adjusted when used concurrently.

Other Class III Drugs

Dronedarone, a noniodinated analog of amiodarone, is used to maintain sinus rhythm in patients with a history of atrial fibrillation. Similar to amiodarone, it blocks potassium, sodium, and L-type calcium channels and inhibits β- and α-adrenergic receptors. It is administered orally and reaches a steady state in 4-8 days, much faster than oral amiodarone. It is not as potent an antiarrhythmic drug as amiodarone, but it lacks the latter's pulmonary, thyroid, and liver toxicities. The major side effects are gastrointestinal, including nausea, vomiting, and diarrhea. Dronedarone can increase the QT interval but only rarely results in torsades de pointes.

Dronedarone is *contraindicated* in patients with advanced heart failure (New York Heart Association class IV) and those with recent decompensation of heart failure, as increased mortality has been demonstrated with the drug in such patients. Furthermore, the drug increases mortality in patients with *permanent* atrial fibrillation; it should only be used over the long term to *prevent* recurrences of atrial fibrillation in patients who have converted back to sinus rhythm.

Sotalol is a nonselective β-blocker, but it is used in practice as an oral antiarrhythmic drug because of its additional class III properties. It prolongs the duration of the action potential, increases the refractory period of atrial and ventricular tissue, and inhibits conduction in accessory bypass tracts. The phase 0 upstroke velocity is not altered in the usual dosage range. It is effective in the treatment of both supraventricular and ventricular arrhythmias.

Because sotalol is excreted exclusively by the kidneys, its dosage should be adjusted in the presence of renal disease. Potential side effects include those of the β-blockers described earlier. Because the drug prolongs the QT interval, the most serious potential adverse effect is torsades de pointes. This complication occurs in ~2% of patients and is more common in patients with a history of heart failure and in women (for unknown reasons).

Dofetilide is another oral class III agent that blocks the outward potassium current, causing prolongation of the action potential duration and an increase in the effective refractory period. It is used in the management of atrial fibrillation and atrial flutter. Dofetilide is excreted by the kidney, and its dose must be adjusted in patients with renal failure. QT prolongation complicated by torsades de pointes is the major potential adverse effect.

Ibutilide is a class III drug used intravenously for the acute conversion of atrial fibrillation or atrial flutter of recent onset. This agent prolongs the action potential duration and increases atrial and ventricular refractoriness. Unlike other class III drugs, its major mechanism relates to activation of a slow inward sodium current that prolongs the plateau (phase 2) of the action potential. Because ibutilide prolongs the QT interval, torsades de pointes can be precipitated, especially in patients with underlying ventricular dysfunction.

CLASS IV ANTIARRHYTHMICS

Mechanism of Action

Class IV drugs exert their electrophysiologic effects by selective blockade of L-type cardiac calcium channels and include **verapamil** and **diltiazem**, but not nifedipine or the other dihydropyridine CCBs. They are most potent in tissues such as the SA and AV nodes in which the action potential upstroke depends on calcium currents. Within nodal tissue, calcium channel blockade decreases the rate of rise of phase 0 depolarization and conduction velocity and lengthens the refractory period of the AV node (Fig. 17-16). These agents also raise the threshold potential at the SA node. The resulting clinical effects are as follows: (1) the heart rate slows; (2) transmission of rapid atrial impulses through the AV node to the ventricles decreases, thus slowing the ventricular rate in atrial fibrillation and atrial flutter; and (3) reentrant rhythms traveling through the AV node may terminate.

↑ Threshold potential of SA node ⟶ ↓ **Heart rate**

↓ Conduction velocity of AV node ↘

↓ **Reentry**

↑ Effective refractory period of AV node ↗

Figure 17-16. Electrophysiologic effects of the class IV antiarrhythmic drugs on the pacemaker cell action potential.

In normal sinus rhythm, the PR interval on the ECG may be prolonged in a patient taking a class IV agent since AV nodal conduction time is prolonged (see Table 17-13).

Clinical Uses

One use of class IV drugs is for the treatment of reentrant SVTs (eg, AV nodal reentrant tachycardia). In the past, intravenous verapamil was the treatment of choice for acute episodes of such rhythms, but intravenous adenosine (described in the next section) has assumed that role.

The pharmacology and toxicities of CCBs were presented earlier in this chapter. The most important side effect of verapamil and diltiazem, when administered intravenously, is hypotension. In addition, these agents should be avoided, or used cautiously, in patients receiving β-blocker therapy, because the combined negative inotropic and chronotropic effects may precipitate heart failure and/or significant bradycardia.

ADENOSINE

Adenosine is an endogenous nucleoside with a very short half-life. Administered intravenously, it is the most effective drug for the rapid termination of reentrant SVT, such as AV nodal reentrant tachycardia.

Adenosine has substantial electrophysiologic effects on specialized conduction tissues, especially the SA and AV nodes. By binding to adenosine receptors on cardiac cells, it activates potassium channels that are open during diastole (Fig. 17-17). The resultant increase in the outward potassium current hyperpolarizes the membrane, which suppresses spontaneous depolarization of the SA node and slows conduction through the AV node. In addition, adenosine decreases the intracellular cAMP concentration by inhibiting adenylate cyclase. The result is a decrease in the inward pacemaker current (I_f) and the inward calcium current (Fig. 17-17). Thus, the net effect of adenosine is to slow the SA node firing rate and to decrease AV nodal conduction. By inducing transient AV nodal block, adenosine terminates reentrant pathways that include the AV node as part of the circuit. Ventricular myocytes are relatively immune to these effects, in part because the specific potassium channels responsive to adenosine are less important for conduction in those cells.

With a half-life of only 10 seconds, any side effects of adenosine (headache, chest pain, flushing, bronchoconstriction) are very transient. Because methylxanthines (caffeine, theophylline) competitively antagonize the adenosine receptor, higher doses of adenosine may be necessary for clinical effect in patients using those substances. Conversely, dipyridamole inhibits the breakdown of adenosine and amplifies its effect.

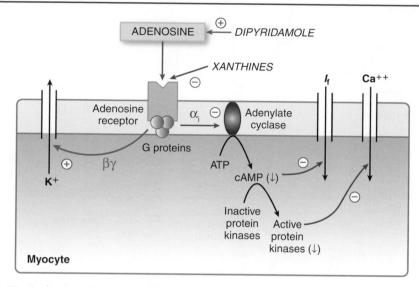

Figure 17-17. Mechanism of antiarrhythmic action of adenosine. Stimulation of the myocyte adenosine A_1 receptor activates inward rectifier potassium channels via direct binding of the G protein βγ-subunit, and the resultant outward K^+ current further hyperpolarizes the membrane during diastole, resulting in decreased automaticity. Adenosine also inhibits membrane adenylate cyclase activity, via the G protein $α_i$-subunit. The subsequent decline in cAMP has two pertinent effects: the inward pacemaker current (I_f) is diminished and the production of active protein kinases is lessened, leading to a reduction of the inward Ca^{++} current. These effects contribute to decreased automaticity and slowed conduction through the AV node. Xanthines compete for the receptor, blocking adenosine's effects. Conversely, dipyridamole interferes with cellular uptake and degradation of adenosine and therefore amplifies its effect.

DIURETICS

Diuretics are most often used to treat heart failure and hypertension. In heart failure, enhanced renal reabsorption of sodium and water, with subsequent expansion of the extracellular volume, contributes to peripheral edema and pulmonary congestion. Diuretics eliminate excess sodium and water through renal excretion and are therefore a cornerstone of therapy in heart failure patients with volume excess (see Fig. 17-1 and Chapter 9). In the treatment of hypertension, diuretics similarly reduce intravascular volume and in some cases promote vascular dilation. To better understand these intended functions of diuretics, the section begins with a brief review of normal renal transport of sodium and water.

In the kidney, the rate of glomerular filtration averages 135-180 L/d in normal adults. Most of the filtered Na^+ is reabsorbed by the renal tubules, leaving only a small quantity in the final urine (Fig. 17-18). Approximately 65%-70% of the filtered Na^+ is reabsorbed isosmotically in the proximal tubule by active transport. In the thick ascending limb of the loop of Henle, an additional 25% of the filtered sodium is reabsorbed, through a Na^+-K^+ cotransport system coupled to the uptake of two Cl^- ions. Because this region is impermeable to the reabsorption of water, it is the site of hypotonic tubular fluid formation, and the surrounding interstitium becomes hypertonic. In the distal convoluted tubule, an additional small fraction of NaCl is reabsorbed ($\sim 5\%$) via a sodium-chloride cotransporter. In the cortical collecting duct, Na^+ permeability is modulated by an aldosterone-sensitive mechanism, such that Na^+ is reabsorbed into the tubular cells in the presence of aldosterone, creating a lumen-negative potential difference that enhances K^+ and H^+ excretion. Approximately 1%-2% of sodium reabsorption takes place at this location.

Most of the distal tubule is impermeable to water. In the collecting tubule, however, water permeability and reabsorption are promoted by antidiuretic hormone and driven by the

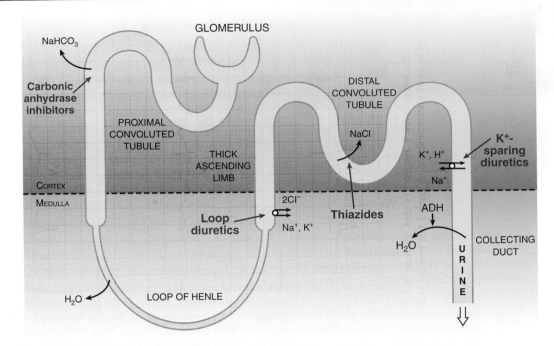

Figure 17-18. Schematic diagram of the renal tubules. Approximately 70% of filtered sodium is reabsorbed in the proximal convoluted tubule, 25% in the thick ascending limb of the loop of Henle, 5% in the distal convoluted tubule, and 1%-2% in the cortical collecting tubule (mediated by the action of aldosterone). Antidiuretic hormone (ADH) increases the permeability of the distal nephron for water. Diuretic drugs are secreted into the proximal convoluted tubule and act at the sites shown.

osmotic gradient between the tubule and the hypertonic interstitium. Therefore, substances that interfere with antidiuretic hormone, such as ethanol, have diuretic actions.

The three most commonly used groups of diuretics are loop diuretics, thiazide diuretics, and potassium-sparing diuretics (Table 17-15; Fig. 17-18). These classes are distinguished by the site of the kidney tubule where they act and by their potency. Loop diuretics impair absorption in the thick ascending limb of the loop of Henle, thiazide diuretics act on the distal tubule and collecting segment, and potassium-sparing diuretics act on the aldosterone-sensitive region of the cortical collecting tubule. Members of a fourth group, the carbonic anhydrase inhibitors, are weak diuretics that act at the proximal convoluted tubule, resulting in a loss of bicarbonate (and sodium) in the urine.

Loop Diuretics

These agents are so named because they act principally on the thick ascending limb of the loop of Henle. They are powerful diuretics that result in the excretion of 20%-25% of the filtered Na^+ load through inhibition of the Na^+-$2Cl^-$-K^+ cotransport system. Because inhibition at this site impairs the generation of a hypertonic interstitium, the gradient for passive water movement out of the collecting duct is diminished and diuresis results.

Loop diuretics are used extensively in the acute management of pulmonary edema (administered intravenously) and in the treatment of chronic heart failure or peripheral edema (taken orally). Unlike other diuretics, they tend to be effective even in the setting of impaired renal function. In addition to the diuretic effect, and even preceding it, drugs of this class may induce venous vasodilation, which is also beneficial in reducing venous return to the heart and pulmonary congestion. The mechanism of venodilation appears to involve drug-induced prostaglandin and nitric oxide generation from endothelial cells, which act to relax vascular smooth muscle.

TABLE 17-15 Commonly Used Diuretics

Diuretic	Method of Administration	Onset of Action (Hours)	Duration of Action (Hours)	Potential Adverse Effects
Thiazides and related compounds				
Chlorothiazide	po	1	6-12	Hypokalemia, hypomagnesemia, hyponatremia, hypercalcemia, hyperglycemia, hyperuricemia, hypercholesterolemia, hypertriglyceridemia, metabolic alkalosis
	IV	0.25	2	
Hydrochlorothiazide	po	2	12	
Chlorthalidone	po	2	24	
Metolazone	po	1	12-24	
Indapamide	po	1-2	16-36	
Loop diuretics				
Furosemide	po	1	6	Hypotension, hypokalemia, hypomagnesemia, hyperglycemia, hyperuricemia, metabolic alkalosis
	IV	5 min	2	
Bumetanide	po	0.5-1	4-6	
	IV	0.25	0.5-1	
Torsemide	po	<1	6-8	
	IV	10 min	6-8	
Ethacrynic acid	IV	0.25	3	
K$^+$-sparing diuretics				
Spironolactone	po	>24	2-3 d	Hyperkalemia, GI disturbances, gynecomastia (spironolactone only)
Eplerenone	po	>24	24	
Triamterene	po	2	12-16	
Amiloride	po	2	24	

GI, gastrointestinal; IV, intravenous; po, by mouth.

The most common side effects of the loop diuretics are intravascular volume depletion, hypokalemia, and metabolic alkalosis. *Hypokalemia* arises because (1) these agents impair the reabsorption of sodium in the loop of Henle, such that an increased amount of Na$^+$ is delivered to the distal tubule, where it prompts greater-than-normal exchange for potassium (and therefore more K$^+$ excretion into the urine) and (2) diuretic-induced intravascular volume depletion activates the renin-angiotensin system. The subsequent rise in aldosterone promotes additional Na$^+$-K$^+$ exchange.

Metabolic alkalosis during loop diuretic therapy results from two mechanisms: (1) increased H$^+$ secretion into the distal tubule (and therefore into the urine) due to the secondary hyperaldosteronism described earlier and (2) contraction alkalosis, in which reduced intravascular volume promotes increased sodium bicarbonate reabsorption by the proximal tubule (see Fig. 17-18).

Additional side effects may also occur during continued loop diuretic therapy. *Hypomagnesemia* may result, because magnesium reabsorption depends on NaCl transport in the thick ascending limb of the loop of Henle, which is blocked by loop diuretics. *Ototoxicity* (cranial nerve VIII toxicity, with impaired hearing and/or vestibular function) occasionally develops and is thought to arise from electrolyte disturbances of the endolymphatic system, most likely because of Na$^+$-2Cl$^-$-K$^+$ cotransport inhibition by the diuretic at that site.

The most commonly used loop diuretic is **furosemide**, the oral form of which has a short duration of action (4-6 hours) that limits its usefulness in the chronic treatment of hypertension. **Bumetanide** is similar to furosemide and shares its actions and adverse effects but has greater potency and bioavailability. It also appears to have a lower incidence of oto-toxicity than the other drugs of this class. Bumetanide is sometimes useful in heart failure patients when edema is refractory to other agents and in some patients who are allergic to furosemide. **Torsemide** is also similar to furosemide, with more complete bioavailability and a longer duration of action. **Ethacrynic acid** is the only nonsulfonamide loop diuretic, so it can be prescribed to patients with sulfonamide intolerance. It is otherwise not widely used because of its high incidence of ototoxicity.

THIAZIDE DIURETICS

Thiazides and related compounds (eg, hydrochlorothiazide, chlorthalidone, metolazone) are also commonly used diuretics. Though less potent than the loop diuretics, their sustained action makes them useful in chronic conditions such as hypertension and mild congestive heart failure (CHF).

Thiazides act at the distal tubule, where they block the reabsorption of $\sim 3\%$-5% of the filtered sodium (see Fig. 17-18). Na^+ reabsorption at this site is mediated through a Na^+-Cl^- cotransporter on the luminal membrane as described earlier. The thiazides inhibit this carrier by a mechanism that has not been elucidated but may involve competition for the Cl^- site. The antihypertensive effect is initially associated with a decrease in CO due to reduced intra-vascular volume with unchanged peripheral resistance. With long-term thiazide use, how-ever, CO often returns to normal as vasodilation leads to a reduction in vascular resistance.

Thiazides are typically administered orally. Diuresis occurs after 1-2 hours, but the full antihypertensive effect of continued therapy may not emerge for up to 12 weeks (possibly related to the vasodilator mechanism alluded to in the previous paragraph). **Chlorothiazide**, the parent compound, has low lipid solubility and hence low bioavailability; higher doses are therefore required to achieve therapeutic levels compared with the more commonly used **hydrochlorothiazide**. **Chlorthalidone** is slowly absorbed and hence has a long duration of action. **Metolazone**, unlike other drugs of this class, is sometimes effective in patients with reduced renal function.

Clinically, the thiazides differ from the loop diuretics in that they are less potent, have a longer duration of action, and (with the exception of metolazone) demonstrate poor diuretic efficacy in the setting of impaired renal function: generally, they are not effective when the GFR is <25 mL/min.

Thiazides serve as a cornerstone of antihypertensive therapy because of their low cost, effectiveness, and proven benefits in reducing the risk of stroke and cardiac events in hyper-tensive patients. They are also effective as add-on therapy for heart failure patients who have become refractory to the diuretic effect of a loop diuretic. Since they act on sequential seg-ments of the renal tubule, the combination produces a more profound natriuretic effect than either agent used alone.

Among the most important potential adverse effects of thiazides are (1) *hypokalemia* and *metabolic alkalosis*, which result from increased Na^+ delivery to the distal tubule, where exchange for K^+ and H^+ takes place, and from volume contraction and secondary hyperaldo-steronism, as previously described for the loop diuretics; (2) *hyponatremia*, during prolonged treatment because of continued Na^+ excretion in the setting of chronic free water consump-tion; (3) *hyperuricemia* (and possible precipitation of gout) owing to decreased clearance of uric acid; (4) *hyperglycemia*, because of either impaired pancreatic insulin release or decreased peripheral glucose utilization; and (5) *alterations in serum lipids* (at least transiently), charac-terized by increased low-density lipoprotein (LDL) cholesterol and triglycerides. In addition, serum calcium levels often rise slightly during thiazide therapy.

POTASSIUM-SPARING DIURETICS

These are relatively weak diuretics that antagonize physiologic Na^+ reabsorption at the distal convoluted tubule and cortical collecting tubule. Potassium-sparing agents reduce K^+ excretion; thus, unlike other diuretics, hypokalemia is not a side effect. They are used when maintenance of serum potassium levels is crucial and in states characterized by aldosterone excess (eg, primary or secondary hyperaldosteronism). Two types of drugs make up this group: (1) aldosterone antagonists (eg, spironolactone and eplerenone) and (2) direct inhibitors of Na^+ permeability in the collecting duct, which act independently of aldosterone (eg, triamterene and amiloride).

Na^+ and K^+ exchange in the collecting tubules accounts for only a small percentage of sodium reuptake, so diuretic effectiveness is modest when these agents are used alone. They are often used in combination with the loop or thiazide classes for additive diuretic effect and to prevent hypokalemia.

Spironolactone is a synthetic steroid that competes for the cytoplasmic aldosterone receptor, thereby inhibiting the aldosterone-sensitive Na^+ channel in the kidney. Because Na^+ reabsorption through the sodium channel is inhibited, no lumen-negative potential exists to drive K^+ and H^+ ion excretion at the distal nephron sites; thus, K^+ and H^+ ions are retained in the circulation. Spironolactone also displays beneficial cardiac reverse remodeling effects in patients with heart failure (see Chapter 9). In a trial of patients with severe heart failure, spironolactone (added to an ACE inhibitor and a loop diuretic) improved heart failure symptoms and reduced mortality rates.

The most serious potential complication of spironolactone is hyperkalemia, resulting from the impaired excretion of that ion. Thus, caution should be observed when administering K^+ supplements, ACE inhibitors, and ARBs concurrently with potassium-sparing diuretics because they could contribute to this complication. Spironolactone also displays antiandrogenic activity that may produce gynecomastia in men and menstrual irregularities in women.

Eplerenone is a more specific inhibitor of the aldosterone receptor that does not have the systemic antiandrogenic effects of spironolactone. Like spironolactone, it is used in the treatment of hypertension and chronic systolic heart failure. In patients with clinical evidence of heart failure and left ventricular ejection fraction <40% following myocardial infarction, eplerenone has also been shown to improve survival when added to usual care.

Triamterene and **amiloride** are structurally related potassium-sparing diuretics that act independently of aldosterone. At the distal tubules, they inhibit the reabsorption of Na^+, which subsequently diminishes the excretion of K^+ and H^+. Triamterene is metabolized by the liver, and its active product is secreted into the proximal tubule by the organic cation transport system. Amiloride is secreted directly into the proximal tubule and appears unchanged in the urine. The most important potential adverse effect of these drugs is hyperkalemia.

ANTITHROMBOTIC DRUGS

Platelets and the coagulation proteins play a key role in the pathogenesis of many cardiovascular disorders, including acute coronary syndromes, deep venous thrombosis (DVT), and thrombi that may complicate atrial fibrillation, dilated cardiomyopathy, or mechanical prosthetic heart valves. Therefore, the modulation of platelet function and of the coagulation pathway is often critically important in cardiovascular therapeutics.

The formation of a thrombus requires three events: (1) exposure of circulating blood elements to thrombogenic material (eg, unmasking of subendothelial collagen after atherosclerotic plaque rupture), (2) activation and aggregation of platelets, and (3) triggering of the coagulation cascade, ultimately resulting in a fibrin clot. Hemostasis effected by platelets and the coagulation system is closely interlinked: activated platelets accelerate the coagulation pathway, and certain coagulation proteins (eg, thrombin) contribute to platelet aggregation.

This section focuses first on drugs that interfere with platelet function and then on those that inhibit the coagulation cascade. Fibrinolytic agents, which dissolve clots that have already formed, are described in Chapter 7.

PLATELET INHIBITORS

Platelets are responsible for primary hemostasis by a three-part process: (1) adhesion to the site of injury, (2) activation via cell-surface receptors and secretion of platelet products, and (3) aggregation, in which platelets are linked together. For example, following blood vessel injury, platelets quickly adhere to exposed subendothelial collagen by means of membrane glycoprotein (GP) receptors, a process that depends on von Willebrand factor. Following adhesion to the vessel wall, platelets release the preformed contents of their granules in response to agonists (including collagen and thrombin) that bind to platelet receptors. Among these prepackaged substances are adenosine diphosphate (ADP), serotonin, fibrinogen, growth factors, and procoagulants. Concurrently within the activated platelet, there is *de novo* synthesis and secretion of thromboxane A_2 (TXA_2), a powerful vasoconstrictor (Fig. 17-19).

Certain agonists, including ADP, thrombin, and TXA_2, stimulate platelets to aggregate and form the primary hemostatic plug. During this process, platelet membrane GP IIb/IIIa receptors undergo a critical conformational change. This alteration allows the previously inactive GP IIb/IIIa receptor to bind fibrinogen molecules, an action that tightly links platelets to one another and constitutes the final common pathway of platelet aggregation. The developing clump of platelets is stabilized and tethered to the site of injury by a mesh of fibrin, which is produced by the simultaneous activation of the coagulation protein cascade.

Platelet activation is regulated to a great extent by release of stored Ca^{++} from the platelet dense tubular system. This action results in an increase in cytosolic calcium concentration, with activation of protein kinases and phosphorylation of intraplatelet regulatory proteins. The augmented cytosolic Ca^{++} also stimulates phospholipase A_2 (PLA_2), causing the release of arachidonic acid, the precursor of TXA_2 (see Fig. 17-19).

The critical release of calcium is modulated by several factors. Acting at their respective platelet membrane receptors, thrombin and other agonists generate intermediaries that *stimulate* the release of calcium from the dense tubules. TXA_2 increases the intracellular Ca^{++} by binding to its platelet receptor, which *inhibits* the activity of adenylate cyclase and thereby reduces cAMP formation, an action that augments the release of Ca^{++} from the dense tubules (see Fig. 17-19). Conversely, endothelial cell–derived prostacyclin (PGI_2) *stimulates* adenylate cyclase activity and increases platelet cAMP concentration, which *inhibits* Ca^{++} release from the dense tubular system.

Antiplatelet drugs interfere with platelet function at various points along the sequence of activation and aggregation (see Fig. 17-19). The most commonly used antiplatelet drug is aspirin, but the roles of newer antiplatelet drugs, especially $P2Y_{12}$ receptor antagonists, have rapidly expanded.

Aspirin

As described in the previous section, TXA_2 is an important mediator of platelet activation and clot formation. Aspirin (acetylsalicylic acid) acts by irreversibly acetylating (and thus blocking the action of) cyclooxygenase, an enzyme essential to TXA_2 production from arachidonic acid (see Fig. 17-19). The form of the enzyme found in platelets is cyclooxygenase-1 (COX-1), which is effectively inhibited by the nonselective action of aspirin (but it is *not* inhibited by selective COX-2 antagonists, such as celecoxib). Because platelets lack nuclei and therefore

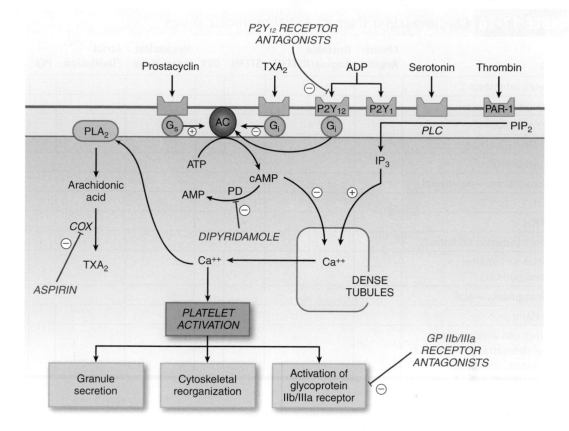

Figure 17-19. Platelet activation is mediated by cytosolic Ca^{++}. Factors that promote and inhibit calcium release from the platelet-dense tubules are shown. Thrombin and serotonin, acting at their specific receptors, stimulate the formation of inositol triphosphate (IP$_3$) from phosphatidylinositol bisphosphate (PIP$_2$) by phospholipase C (PLC). IP$_3$ subsequently enhances the intracellular release of calcium. Thromboxane A$_2$ (TXA$_2$) also facilitates calcium release. It inhibits adenylyl cyclase (AC) and reduces cyclic adenosine monophosphate (cAMP) formation. Because cAMP normally *prevents* Ca^{++} release from the dense tubules, the reduction of this effect by TXA$_2$ *increases* Ca^{++} release into the cytosol. Conversely, endothelial-derived prostacyclin has the opposite effect. It reduces intraplatelet calcium release because it *stimulates* AC activity and cAMP formation. ADP also stimulates calcium release via its two receptors (see text for details). Calcium promotes the action of phospholipase A$_2$ (PLA$_2$), which generates the precursors of TXA$_2$ from the cell membrane. Platelet activation modulated by Ca^{++} ultimately results in granule secretion, cytoskeletal reorganization, and the critical conformational change in GP IIb/IIIa receptors that is necessary for platelet aggregation. The sites of action of commonly used antiplatelet drugs are shown. COX, cyclooxygenase; PAR-1, protease-activated receptor-1.

cannot synthesize new proteins (including cyclooxygenase), aspirin *permanently* disables TXA$_2$ production in exposed cells.

The prostaglandin PGI$_2$, a major antagonist of TXA$_2$ that is produced by endothelial cells, shares a dependency on cyclooxygenase activity for its formation, and aspirin, at high doses, impairs its synthesis as well. Unlike platelets, however, endothelial cells *are* able to generate new cyclooxygenase to replace what has been deactivated by acetylation. Thus, when used at low doses, aspirin effectively inhibits platelet TXA$_2$ synthesis without significantly interfering with the presence and beneficial actions of PGI$_2$.

Because the antiplatelet effect of aspirin is limited to inhibition of TXA$_2$ formation, platelet aggregation induced by other factors (eg, ADP) is not significantly impeded.

Clinical Uses

Aspirin has many clinical benefits in patients with cardiovascular disease (Table 17-16). In individuals with unstable angina, acute myocardial infarction, or a history of myocardial

TABLE 17-16 Cardiovascular Uses of Antithrombotic Drugs

Drug	Chronic Angina	Unstable Angina/NSTEMI	STEMI	DVT	Mechanical Heart Valve	Atrial Fibrillation	PCI	HIT
Platelet inhibitors								
Aspirin	+	+	+	a			+	
P2Y$_{12}$ antagonists		+	+				b	
GP IIb/IIIa antagonists		+	+				+	
Dipyridamole					c			
Anticoagulants—parenteral								
UFH		+	+	+	d	d	+	
LMWH		+	+	+				
Direct thrombin inhibitors		e					+	+
Factor Xa inhibitor (fondaparinux)				+				
Anticoagulants—oral								
Warfarin			f	+	+	+		
Direct oral anticoagulants (eg, dabigatran, rivaroxaban, apixaban, edoxaban)	g			+		+		

aUsed in combination with warfarin.
bWhen intracoronary stent is implanted.
cSometimes used in combination with warfarin for recurrent thromboembolism.
dFor hospitalized patients unable to take warfarin.
eIf undergoing PCI.
fIf ventricular thrombus is present.
gLow-dose rivaroxaban, in combination with aspirin, has been shown to reduce rates of major cardiovascular events in individuals with chronic CAD or peripheral artery disease.
DVT, deep venous thrombosis; HIT, heparin-induced thrombocytopenia; LMWH, low-molecular-weight heparin; NSTEMI, non–ST elevation myocardial infarction (MI); PCI, percutaneous coronary intervention; STEMI, ST elevation MI; UFH, unfractionated heparin.

infarction, aspirin reduces the incidence of future fatal and nonfatal coronary events. Similarly, in patients with chronic stable angina without a history of myocardial infarction, aspirin lessens the occurrence of subsequent MI. In patients who have suffered a minor stroke or transient cerebral ischemic attack, aspirin reduces the rate of future stroke and cardiovascular events. Additionally, aspirin lowers the likelihood of graft occlusion in patients who have undergone coronary artery bypass surgery.

Less clear is the benefit of aspirin for *primary* prevention (ie, in individuals without a history of cardiovascular events or symptoms). When tested in a large cohort of healthy American middle-aged men, aspirin was associated with a reduced incidence of nonfatal myocardial infarction but an increased rate of nonfatal hemorrhagic stroke and gastrointestinal bleeding; there was no effect on total vascular mortality. More recent trials and meta-analyses have similarly concluded that aspirin is effective for primary prevention of myocardial infarction in patients with coronary risk factors, but it increases the risk of major bleeding. And in the prospective primary prevention trial known as the Women's Health Initiative, aspirin lowered the risk of ischemic stroke in women but did not reduce the incidence of MI or death from cardiovascular disease. Thus, whereas aspirin plays an extremely important role in patients with known cardiovascular disease, it is no longer advised that otherwise healthy people routinely take aspirin for "cardiovascular protection." Rather, preventive aspirin therapy should be limited to individuals at high cardiovascular risk, who do not have conditions that predispose to major bleeding complications.

Adverse Effects

The most common adverse effects of aspirin are related to the gastrointestinal system, including dyspepsia and nausea, which often can be ameliorated by prescribing low dosage (eg, 81 mg tablet) and/or using enteric-coated or buffered tablets. More serious potential side effects include gastrointestinal bleeding, hemorrhagic strokes, allergic reactions, and asthma exacerbation in aspirin-sensitive patients. Because aspirin is excreted by the kidneys and competes with uric acid for the renal proximal tubule organic anion transporter, it may also occasionally exacerbate gout.

Platelet $P2Y_{12}$ Receptor Antagonists (Table 17-17)

During platelet activation, ADP is released and extracellular ADP then contributes to further platelet activation, and promotes aggregation, by binding to two types of surface purinoceptors. The first ($P2Y_1$ receptor) acts through phospholipase C to increase intraplatelet $[Ca^{++}]$. The second purinoceptor ($P2Y_{12}$) is linked to an inhibitory G protein and reduces cAMP production, thus also raising intraplatelet $[Ca^{++}]$ and promoting continued platelet activation (see Fig. 17-19). ADP-induced platelet activation requires that ADP simultaneously activate *both* $P2Y_1$ and $P2Y_{12}$ receptors. Current antagonists of such ADP activation interfere with the $P2Y_{12}$ receptor, either irreversibly (eg, the thienopyridines) or reversibly (eg, ticagrelor). The most important side effect of all $P2Y_{12}$ receptor antagonists is bleeding.

Thienopyridines

Oral thienopyridines irreversibly block $P2Y_{12}$ by covalently binding to the receptor. Studies evaluating the combination of aspirin plus the thienopyridine **clopidogrel** in patients with unstable angina, non–ST elevation myocardial infarction (NSTEMI), ST elevation myocardial infarction (STEMI), and elective coronary stenting have demonstrated a significant benefit in cardiovascular outcomes compared with aspirin alone. However, clopidogrel is a prodrug that requires cytochrome P450–mediated biotransformation to the active metabolite, which

TABLE 17-17 Platelet $P2Y_{12}$ Receptor Antagonists

	Clopidogrel	Prasugrel	Ticagrelor	Cangrelor
Class	Thienopyridine	Thienopyridine	Nonthienopyridine	ATP analog (nonthienopyridine)
$P2Y_{12}$ receptor binding effect	Irreversible	Irreversible	Reversible	Reversible
Administration route	Oral	Oral	Oral	Intravenous
Half-life	8 h	7 h	7 h (9 h for active metabolite)	≤6 min
Benefits	Generic available	Less variable activation than clopidogrel	More rapid onset of action than clopidogrel and faster platelet recovery after discontinuation	Rapid onset of action and of platelet recovery
Limitations	Onset of action delayed; activation affected by genetic polymorphisms of cytochrome P450 2C19 alleles and some drugs	Higher bleeding risk than clopidogrel; avoid in elderly or if history of stroke or TIA	Higher bleeding risk than clopidogrel; requires twice-daily dosing; side effects include dyspnea and bradycardia; avoid concurrent aspirin dose >100 mg/d	Intravenous use only; expensive

contributes to the drug's delayed onset of action and to variability in its antiplatelet effect. For example, patients with common reduced-function polymorphisms of the cytochrome P450 2C19 (CYP2C19) gene demonstrate weakened platelet inhibition and less clinical benefit. In addition, studies have implicated proton pump inhibitors (eg, omeprazole) as drugs that can potentially interfere with hepatic CYP2C19 activation of clopidogrel.

A newer thienopyridine, **prasugrel**, addresses these shortcomings. It is metabolized to an active form more readily than clopidogrel and has a more potent antiplatelet effect. Compared to clopidogrel, it has been shown to further reduce the risk of future myocardial infarction in patients with ACS who undergo percutaneous coronary intervention. This benefit comes with an increased risk of bleeding, a complication that is more likely to occur in patients who are elderly (>age 75), those with prior cerebrovascular disease, and individuals with low body weight (<60 kg).

A limitation of thienopyridines, both clopidogrel and prasugrel, is that they are *irreversible* platelet inhibitors. If a thienopyridine-treated patient with an ACS requires coronary artery bypass surgery, a waiting period of several days is necessary to allow adequate return of platelet function to prevent perioperative bleeding complications.

Ticagrelor

Unlike the thienopyridines, **ticagrelor** is an oral *reversible* $P2Y_{12}$ receptor blocker that provides faster onset of action and greater inhibition of platelet aggregation than clopidogrel. Rather than covalently binding the $P2Y_{12}$ receptor, ticagrelor causes a conformational change of the receptor, resulting in reversible and concentration-dependent inhibition. In addition, the antiplatelet effect resolves more quickly when the drug is discontinued compared to the irreversible thienopyridines. In a large clinical trial, ticagrelor reduced the rate of MI and cardiovascular death compared with clopidogrel in patients with acute coronary syndromes, without a difference in major bleeding episodes. Of note, the dose of aspirin combined with ticagrelor should not exceed 100 mg/day, as higher dosage blunted the superiority of ticagrelor over clopidogrel in this trial.

Other occasional side effects that have been associated with ticagrelor include dyspnea and bradyarrhythmias, possibly due to ticagrelor-related stimulation of adenosine receptors.

Cangrelor

In distinction to the thienopyridines and ticagrelor, **cangrelor** is an *intravenous*, rapidly acting, and reversible $P2Y_{12}$ receptor antagonist that is sometimes utilized during percutaneous coronary intervention procedures. Like ticagrelor, cangrelor achieves greater inhibition of platelet activation than clopidogrel. Administered as an IV bolus followed by continuous infusion, cangrelor's advantages include platelet inhibition within minutes, with antiplatelet effects that resolve quickly after drug discontinuation. In a large randomized trial, cangrelor significantly reduced ischemic events in patients undergoing percutaneous coronary intervention in comparison to clopidogrel.

Glycoprotein IIb/IIIa Receptor Antagonists

The GP IIb/IIIa receptor antagonists constitute one of the most potent classes of antiplatelet agents. This group reversibly inhibits the critical and final common pathway of platelet aggregation—the binding of activated platelet GP IIb/IIIa receptors to fibrinogen and von Willebrand factor. As a result, platelets are inhibited from "sticking" to one another, impairing the formation of a hemostatic plug. Three types of GP IIb/IIIa receptor antagonists have been developed: (1) monoclonal antibodies (eg, **abciximab**, the Fab fragment of a chimeric human-mouse monoclonal antibody), (2) synthetic peptide antagonists (eg, **eptifibatide**), and (3) synthetic nonpeptide antagonists (eg, **tirofiban**).

All GP IIb/IIIa receptor inhibitors in use are administered intravenously. They were originally developed as antiplatelet agents for patients undergoing percutaneous coronary intervention and in the setting of acute coronary syndromes. However, the subsequent availability of dual antiplatelet therapy (DAPT) with aspirin plus a P2Y$_{12}$ inhibitor has rendered the use of GP IIb/IIIa receptor antagonists unnecessary in most situations. They are now prescribed occasionally for high-risk patients who manifest ongoing coronary ischemia despite DAPT, in individuals with thrombotic complications during PCI, and for those likely to require urgent cardiac surgery after cardiac catheterization, as a substitute for a P2Y$_{12}$ inhibitor.

The major side effects of the GP IIb/IIIa receptor inhibitors are bleeding and thrombocytopenia. Abciximab has a short plasma half-life (30 minutes); thus, its effects can be reversed by discontinuing the drug or by administering a platelet transfusion. Because the other GP IIb/IIIa receptor antagonists have longer half-lives, they may continue to inactivate transfused platelets. Nonetheless, bleeding complications are infrequent using current protocols.

Dipyridamole

The antiplatelet drug **dipyridamole** is uncommonly prescribed by itself. Rather, a capsule formulation that combines dipyridamole with low-dose aspirin is used for the prevention of stroke in patients with prior cerebrovascular symptomatology. Dipyridamole's mechanism of antiplatelet action involves an increase in platelet cAMP levels by (1) inhibiting the destruction of cAMP by phosphodiesterase (see Fig. 17-19) and (2) impeding cellular uptake and destruction of adenosine, thereby augmenting adenosine's availability to stimulate the platelet A$_2$ receptor, which enhances the production of cAMP via adenylate cyclase. cAMP in turn reduces intracellular Ca^{++} concentration, thus inhibiting platelet activation (see Fig. 17-19).

ANTICOAGULANT DRUGS: PARENTERAL AGENTS

Anticoagulant drugs (see Table 17-16) interfere with the coagulation cascade and impair secondary hemostasis. Because the final step in both the intrinsic and extrinsic coagulation pathways is the formation of a fibrin clot by the action of thrombin, major approaches to anticoagulation therapy are to inhibit the activation of thrombin by factor Xa (eg, using unfractionated heparin [UFH], low molecular weight heparin [LMWH], or factor Xa inhibitors), to inhibit thrombin itself (eg, UFH or direct thrombin inhibitors), or to decrease the production of functional prothrombin (eg, warfarin). This section describes anticoagulants that are administered by intravenous or subcutaneous administration, while the next section considers oral anticoagulants.

Unfractionated Heparin

UFH is a heterogeneous mixture of glycosaminoglycans. Although it has little anticoagulant action by itself, UFH associates with antithrombin (AT) in the circulation, greatly increasing its effect. AT is a natural protein that inhibits the action of thrombin and other clotting factors. When UFH complexes with AT, the affinity of AT for thrombin increases 1000-fold, markedly reducing thrombin's ability to generate fibrin from fibrinogen. The UFH-AT complex also inhibits activated factor X, additionally contributing to the anticoagulant action. Furthermore, UFH has antiplatelet properties by binding to, and blocking the action of, von Willebrand factor.

UFH is administered parenterally because it is not absorbed from the gastrointestinal tract. For most acute indications, an intravenous bolus is followed by a continuous infusion of the drug. The bioavailability of UFH varies because it is a heterogeneous collection of molecules that bind to plasma proteins, macrophages, and endothelial cells. The dosage-effect relationship is often not predictable; thus, frequent blood samples are required to monitor the degree of anticoagulation (most commonly, measurement of the activated partial thromboplastin time), so that the infusion rate can be adjusted accordingly.

The usual cardiovascular settings in which intravenous UFH is indicated include (1) acute coronary syndromes, (2) hospitalized patients with atrial fibrillation, and (3) pulmonary embolism or DVT. Among hospitalized or bedridden patients not receiving intravenous heparin, fixed low dosages of *subcutaneous* UFH are often administered to prevent DVT.

The most important side effect of heparin is *bleeding*. An overdose of UFH can be treated with intravenous **protamine sulfate**, which forms a stable complex with UFH and immediately reverses the anticoagulation effect.

Heparin-induced thrombocytopenia (*HIT*) is another potential major adverse effect and can occur in two forms. The more common type, thought to result from direct heparin-induced platelet aggregation, occurs in up to 15% of patients and is usually asymptomatic, dose dependent, and self-limited. This mild HIT rarely causes severe reductions in platelet counts and usually does not require cessation of heparin.

The less common, much more dangerous form of HIT is immune-mediated, a condition that affects 3% of UFH-treated patients. It can lead to life-threatening bleeding and, paradoxically, to thrombosis. Thrombosis is caused by the formation of antibodies directed against heparin-platelet complexes, resulting in platelet activation, aggregation, and clot production. In the immune-mediated form of HIT, the platelet count can fall markedly and is not dependent on the dose of heparin. Therapy requires immediate cessation of heparin and substitution by alternate antithrombotic therapy to prevent further clotting (eg, a direct thrombin inhibitor, described later).

Low Molecular Weight Heparins

Some of the shortcomings of UFH (eg, short half-life and unpredictable bioavailability) have been addressed by the development of LMWHs, examples of which are **enoxaparin**, **dalteparin**, and **tinzaparin**. As the name implies, LMWH molecules are smaller than UFH (approximately one-third the size). These agents interact with AT, but unlike UFH, the LMWH-AT complex preferentially inhibits factor Xa more than thrombin (thrombin inhibition requires heparin molecules larger than those in LMWHs). Selectively inhibiting factor Xa upstream in the coagulation cascade has a multiplier effect in preventing downstream formation of thrombin.

Advantages of LMWHs over UFH include (1) inhibition of platelet-bound factor Xa, contributing to a more prominent anticoagulant effect; (2) less binding to plasma proteins and endothelial cells, resulting in more predictable bioavailability and a longer half-life; (3) fewer bleeding complications; and (4) a lower incidence of immune-mediated HIT.

From a practical standpoint, the major advantages of LMWH formulations are the ease of use and more consistent level of anticoagulation. They can be administered as subcutaneous injections once or twice a day in fixed doses, without the repetitive blood monitoring required for UFH. In rare cases in which monitoring the anticoagulant effect *is* necessary (eg, in patients with renal dysfunction, because LMWHs are cleared via the kidneys), a factor Xa inhibition assay is used.

In clinical trials, LMWH therapy is at least as effective as UFH in preventing DVT and treating unstable angina. It also has a better safety profile than UFH, with lower rates of bleeding and thrombocytopenia. LMWHs should not, however, be used in patients with a history of HIT, and unlike UFH, the effects of LMWHs cannot be completely reversed by protamine. The major clinical indications for LMWH therapy are (1) prophylaxis against DVT following hip, knee, or abdominal surgery, (2) treatment of DVT (with or without pulmonary embolism), and (3) anticoagulation in acute coronary syndromes.

Direct Thrombin Inhibitors

The anticoagulation effects of UFH and LMWH are limited because their activity depends, at least in part, on AT and they inhibit only *circulating* thrombin. The large heparin-AT complex cannot inactivate thrombin that is already bound to fibrin within a clot. In contrast, intravenous direct thrombin inhibitors (eg, **bivalirudin**, **argatroban**) inhibit thrombin activity independently of AT and are effective against both circulating *and* clot-bound thrombins. They do not cause thrombocytopenia and are used to maintain anticoagulation and prevent thrombosis in patients with HIT. Bivalirudin is also approved for use as an anticoagulant in patients with unstable angina undergoing percutaneous coronary intervention. All direct thrombin inhibitors are potent anticoagulants and the major adverse effect is bleeding.

Factor Xa Inhibitor

The anticoagulant **fondaparinux** is a synthetic pentasaccharide that specifically inhibits factor Xa, thereby reducing thrombin activation. Like heparin, fondaparinux binds to AT with high affinity, greatly increasing AT's ability to inactivate factor Xa. Unlike UFH, fondaparinux does not inactivate formed thrombin, nor does it interfere with platelet actions or cause HIT. It is administered by subcutaneous injection, and its half-life is sufficiently long (17-21 hours) that it can be administered just once a day. Fondaparinux is approved for prevention of DVT after certain surgical procedures and as treatment for DVT and pulmonary embolism.

ANTICOAGULANT DRUGS: ORAL AGENTS

Warfarin

Warfarin is prescribed for long-term anticoagulation. It acts by antagonizing the enzyme vitamin K epoxide reductase that is required in usual vitamin K metabolism. Normally, the reduced form of vitamin K promotes the carboxylation of a glutamic acid residue within specific coagulation factors (factors II, VII, IX, and X), an action that is necessary for the factors to subsequently bind calcium, become functional, and participate in coagulation (Fig. 17-20). By interfering with the formation of reduced vitamin K, warfarin indirectly inhibits carboxylation of the coagulation factors, rendering them inactive. Because certain natural coagulation *inhibitors* (protein C and protein S) are also vitamin K dependent, warfarin impairs their functions as well, which in some cases may counteract the drug's anticoagulant effect.

Warfarin's action has a delayed onset of 2-7 days; thus, if immediate anticoagulation is needed, UFH or LMWH must be prescribed concurrently at first (known as anticoagulant "bridging"). The half-life of warfarin is long (37 hours), and the drug's dosage must be individualized to achieve a therapeutic effect while minimizing the risk of bleeding complications. The extent of anticoagulation is monitored by measuring the prothrombin time in blood samples, reported as an international normalized ratio (INR). There are two target ranges of anticoagulant intensity. For patients at greatest risk of pathologic thrombosis (eg, those with certain types of mechanical heart valves), the desired INR is 2.5-3.5. For others (eg, those with uncomplicated atrial fibrillation), the target INR is usually 2.0-3.0.

Many factors influence the anticoagulation effect of warfarin and require alterations in its dosage. For example, liver disease and heart failure each reduce the warfarin requirement, whereas a high dietary ingestion of foods containing vitamin K (eg, green leafy vegetables) increases the required dose. Similarly, many pharmaceuticals alter

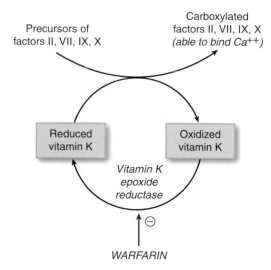

Figure 17-20. Mechanism of action of warfarin.
Normally, coagulation factors II, VII, IX, and X are converted to functional forms by carboxylation in the liver, in the presence of reduced vitamin K. During this reaction, vitamin K undergoes oxidation and must be regenerated back to the reduced state for the sustained synthesis of functional clotting factors. Warfarin inhibits the formation of reduced vitamin K by antagonizing the enzyme epoxide reductase, such that the conversion of the coagulation factors does not occur and they remain nonfunctional.

TABLE 17-18	**Examples of Drugs that Alter the Anticoagulation Effect of Warfarin**
Reduced Anticoagulation Effect	**Increased Anticoagulation Effect**
Hepatic enzyme induction	**Hepatic enzyme inhibition**
Barbiturates	Amiodarone
Rifampin	Cephalosporins
Carbamazepine	Cimetidine
Nafcillin	Erythromycin
Warfarin malabsorption	Fluconazole
Cholestyramine	Isoniazid
Sucralfate	Ketoconazole
	Metronidazole
	Propafenone
	Trimethoprim-sulfamethoxazole
	Displacement from protein-binding sites
	Allopurinol
	Gemfibrozil
	Phenytoin
	Altered vitamin K production by gut flora
	Ciprofloxacin
	Piperacillin

warfarin's anticoagulation effect (Table 17-18). Finally, the combined use of warfarin with aspirin or other antiplatelet agents increases the risk of a bleeding complication.

If serious bleeding arises during warfarin therapy, the drug's effect can be reversed within hours by the administration of vitamin K (or even more quickly by transfusing prothrombin complex concentrate or fresh frozen plasma, which directly replenish functional circulating clotting factors). In patients with mechanical heart valves, vitamin K reversal therapy should be avoided unless life-threatening bleeding occurs, because of the possibility of rebound valve thrombosis. Warfarin is teratogenic and should not be taken during pregnancy, especially during the first trimester.

Given the many limitations and inconvenience of warfarin therapy, newer oral anticoagulants have been developed with more predictable pharmacologic properties and ease of use, as described in the next section.

Direct Oral Anticoagulants

Direct oral anticoagulants (DOACs) are alternatives to warfarin that are more convenient to administer. Compared to warfarin, they offer equivalent or superior efficacy and greater safety. Specific advantages include a fixed dosing regimen (no need to monitor laboratory tests to assess the degree of anticoagulation) and very few interactions with other medications, and their effectiveness is not altered by foods that contain vitamin K. In clinical trials, several DOACs have been shown to be at least as effective as warfarin for treatment of venous thromboembolism and for prophylaxis against stroke in patients with atrial fibrillation. Yet major bleeding (eg, intracranial bleeding) complications are lower than with warfarin.

There are two pharmacologic classes of DOACs (Table 17-19): direct thrombin inhibitors (eg, **dabigatran**) and factor Xa inhibitors (**apixaban, rivaroxaban, edoxaban, betrixaban**). The mechanism of action of dabigatran is the same as the parenteral direct thrombin inhibitors described earlier in the chapter. Apixaban, rivaroxaban, edoxaban, and betrixaban differ

TABLE 17-19 Direct Oral Anticoagulant Drugs

	Dabigatran	Apixaban	Rivaroxaban	Edoxaban	Betrixaban
Mechanism	Direct thrombin inhibitor	Direct factor Xa inhibitor[a]	Direct factor Xa inhibitor[a]	Direct factor Xa inhibitor[a,d]	Direct factor Xa inhibitor
Indications	• Atrial fibrillation[a] • VTE[b,c] • VTE prevention after hip replacement surgery	• Atrial fibrillation[a] • VTE[c] • VTE prevention after hip or knee replacement surgery	• Atrial fibrillation[a] • VTE[c] • VTE prevention after hip or knee replacement surgery • Chronic CAD or PAD, in combination with aspirin (see Chapters 6 and 15)	• Atrial fibrillation[a,d] • VTE[b]	• VTE prevention for at-risk hospitalized patients with acute medical illness
Dose reduction required in renal impairment	Yes	Yes[e]	Yes	Yes	Yes
Drug interactions	• P-gp inducers[f] reduce potency • P-gp inhibitors[g] increase potency	• Combined P-gp and strong CYP3A4 inducers[h] reduce potency • Combined P-gp and strong CYP3A4 inhibitors[i] increase potency	• Combined P-gp and strong CYP3A4 inducers[h] reduce potency • Combined P-gp and strong CYP3A4 inhibitors[i] increase potency	• P-gp inducers may reduce potency—specifically, avoid concurrent use of antibiotic rifampin	• P-gp inducers[f] reduce potency • P-gp inhibitors[g] increase potency
Anticoagulation reversal methods	• Idarucizumab • PCC • Dialysis	• Andexanet alpha • PCC	• Andexanet alpha • PCC	• PCC	• PCC

[a]Not for use in patients with a mechanical heart valve or moderate-to-severe mitral stenosis.

[b]After 5-10 days of parenteral unfractionated heparin or low-molecular-weight heparin.

[c]Also indicated for extended therapy for VTE prevention in patients previously treated for acute VTE.

[d]Avoid in patients with very *high* creatinine clearance (>95 mL/min) as rapid drug clearance may reduce anticoagulation effect.

[e]If serum creatinine ≥1.5 mg/dL and either age ≥80 or weight ≤60 kg.

[f]Examples include rifampin (antibiotic) and certain anticonvulsant drugs (phenytoin, carbamazepine, barbiturates).

[g]Examples include verapamil (calcium channel blocker), dronedarone (antiarrhythmic), ketoconazole (antifungal agent), and clarithromycin (antibiotic).

[h]Examples include ketoconazole (antifungal agent) and ritonavir (protease inhibitor).

[i]Examples include rifampin (antibiotic) and certain anticonvulsant drugs (phenytoin, carbamazepine).

CAD, coronary artery disease; CYP3A4, cytochrome P450 3A4 enzyme; PCC, prothrombin complex concentrate; P-gp, p-glycoprotein; PAD, peripheral arterial disease; VTE, venous thromboembolism.

from the parenteral anti–factor Xa agent fondaparinux described earlier in that they *directly* inhibit factor Xa, without requiring AT as an intermediary.

All currently available DOACs are partially excreted via the kidneys, and dosage adjustments may be required in patients with renal insufficiency or warfarin used instead. And despite the great appeal of DOACs, there are circumstances in which they should not be used. For example, they are contraindicated in individuals with mechanical heart valves (because of a greater risk of valve thrombosis) and are not prescribed to patients with moderate-to-severe mitral stenosis, in pregnancy, or in morbidly obese individuals, as such patients were excluded from DOAC clinical trials. In addition, the shorter half-lives of DOACs compared to warfarin can result in inadequate anticoagulation (and potential thrombosis) if doses of DOACs are missed.

Antidotes for DOACs have been developed for rapid reversal of the anticoagulant effect in cases of life-threatening bleeding. **Idarucizumab** is a monoclonal antibody fragment that binds to, and neutralizes, the action of dabigatran. **Andexanet alfa** is a recombinant factor Xa decoy protein that binds to, and inactivates, factor Xa inhibitors. It has been shown to reverse the anticoagulant effects of apixaban and rivaroxaban (data are not available to assess its effectiveness in neutralizing edoxaban and betrixaban). Another means to counteract the anticoagulant effect of DOACs is by an infusion of **prothrombin complex concentrate**. Dabigatran is the only available DOAC that can be removed by dialysis.

LIPID-REGULATING DRUGS

As described in Chapter 5, abnormal serum lipid levels play a critical role in the pathogenesis of atherosclerosis. Specific groups of drugs that improve lipid abnormalities are cardioprotective; they inhibit the progression of atherosclerosis, improve cardiovascular outcomes, and, especially in high-risk patients, reduce mortality rates.

HMG-CoA REDUCTASE INHIBITORS

The HMG-CoA reductase inhibitors, commonly known as "statins," are the most commonly prescribed lipid-altering therapy by virtue of their potency, tolerability, and impact on reduction of cardiovascular events. The most frequently used agents of this group, in increasing order of potency, are **lovastatin**, **pravastatin**, **simvastatin**, **atorvastatin**, and **rosuvastatin** (Table 17-20).

Statins are competitive inhibitors of the enzyme HMG-CoA reductase, a rate-controlling factor in cholesterol biosynthesis (Fig. 17-21). By inhibiting cholesterol production in the liver, statins lower serum LDL cholesterol through three mechanisms: (1) the reduced intrahepatic cholesterol content induces increased expression of the LDL receptor gene, causing a greater number of LDL receptors to appear on the surface of the hepatocyte, which facilitates the binding and clearance of LDL from the circulation; (2) circulating LDL precursors (known as very low-density lipoprotein [VLDL] remnants and intermediate-density lipoprotein particles) are cleared more rapidly from the circulation because of their cross-recognition with the hepatic LDL receptor; and (3) hepatic VLDL production falls due to the reduced availability of intracellular cholesterol for lipoprotein assembly. Because the catabolism of VLDL in the circulation ultimately forms LDL, lowering VLDL production also decreases circulating LDL levels. The reduced production of VLDL is also likely responsible for the triglyceride-lowering effect of statins, because this lipoprotein is the major carrier of triglycerides in the circulation.

The overall effect is that statins reduce serum LDL levels by 20%-60%, depending on the specific drug and dose. Statins also decrease plasma triglyceride levels by 7%-30%, and by an unclear mechanism, HDL levels increase by 5%-15%.

TABLE 17-20	Lipid-Regulating Drugs			
Class	**LDL Effect (%)**	**HDL Effect (%)**	**Triglyceride Effect (%)**	**Adverse Effects**
HMG-CoA reductase inhibitors Atorvastatin Fluvastatin Lovastatin Pitavastatin Pravastatin Rosuvastatin Simvastatin	↓ 20-60	↑ 5-15	↓ 7-30	Transaminitis, myopathy
Cholesterol absorption inhibitor Ezetimibe	↓15-20	↑ 1-2	↓0-5	Rare upper respiratory symptoms, arthralgia
PCSK9 inhibitors Evolocumab Alirocumab	↓ 60	↑ 5-10	↓ 15	Mild injection site reactions
Bile acid–binding agents Cholestyramine Colestipol Colesevelam	↓ 15-30	↑ 3-5	May ↑	Constipation, bloating
Niacin	↓ 5-25	↑ 15-35	↓ 20-50	Flushing, hepatotoxicity, hyperglycemia,
Fibric acid derivatives Fenofibrate Gemfibrozil	↓ 0-20 *or* ↑ 0-10	↑ 10-20	↓ 20-50	Nausea, gallstones

The lowering of LDL reduces the lipid content of atherosclerotic lesions and promotes plaque stability. This lessens the vulnerability of plaque to rupture, thus decreasing the likelihood of thrombus formation and vascular occlusion. In addition to their lipid-modulating properties, statins have other potentially cardioprotective effects. They improve endothelial function as evidenced by enhanced synthesis of nitric oxide. They further promote plaque stability by inhibiting monocyte penetration into the arterial wall and reducing macrophage secretion of metalloproteinases, enzymes that degrade and weaken the fibrous caps of plaques. Statins also diminish the vulnerability of lipoproteins to oxidation, thus inhibiting the unregulated uptake of modified LDL cholesterol by macrophages (see Chapter 5). Finally, they appear to suppress inflammation, a key component of atherogenesis.

Statins are widely prescribed for secondary prevention in patients with known atherosclerotic cardiovascular disease because major trials have shown that they substantially reduce mortality, cardiac events, and strokes in this population, whether LDL cholesterol is elevated or even in the "normal" range. In studies of patients not known to have atherosclerotic cardiovascular disease statin therapy for primary prevention is recommended in individuals with LDL ≥ 190, individuals with diabetes, and individuals with an elevated 10-year risk of cardiovascular events (see Table 5-2).

Statins are well-tolerated drugs. The most significant potential adverse effects are hepatotoxicity and myopathy (skeletal muscle toxicity). *Hepatotoxicity* is dose related and occurs in fewer than 1% of patients. Those affected may experience fatigue, anorexia, and weight

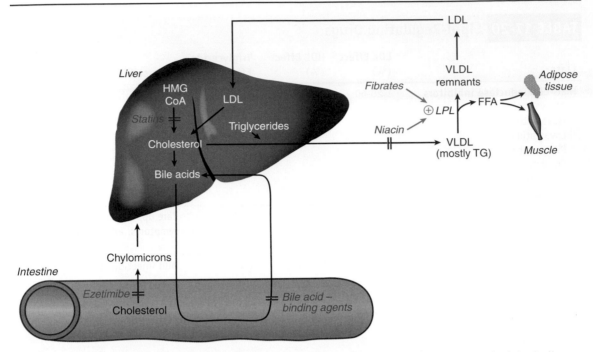

Figure 17-21. Major sites of action of lipid-regulating drugs. The *statins* inhibit cholesterol biosynthesis in the liver by competing with the enzyme HMG-CoA reductase. This action depletes intrahepatic cholesterol stores, which results in increased expression of surface low-density lipoprotein (LDL) receptors. The latter enhance clearance of LDL and very low-density lipoprotein (VLDL) remnants from the circulation. The lower intrahepatic cholesterol content leads to reduction in VLDL synthesis. *Ezetimibe* selectively inhibits cholesterol uptake in the small intestine, thereby reducing chylomicron production and cholesterol delivery to the liver. *Bile acid–binding agents* interrupt the enterohepatic circulation of bile acids in the intestine, causing more hepatic cholesterol to be diverted to new bile acid production; the reduced availability of intrahepatic cholesterol augments LDL receptor expression and LDL clearance increases. Among its effects, *niacin* inhibits VLDL production. It also increases lipoprotein lipase (LPL) activity, thus promoting triglyceride (TG) clearance from circulating VLDL particles. Niacin raises circulating high-density lipoprotein (HDL) by impairing hepatic uptake of apo AI, the HDL apoprotein (not shown). *Fibrates* enhance VLDL catabolism by increasing the synthesis of lipoprotein lipase via peroxisome proliferator–activated receptor-α (PPAR-α), a nuclear transcription factor. They also raise HDL by stimulating the production of HDL-associated apoproteins (not shown). FFA, free fatty acids.

loss. More commonly, the patient is asymptomatic, but laboratory studies show an increase in transaminase levels (ALT, AST). Symptoms resolve almost immediately after the drug is discontinued. Serious hepatic injury is very rare, occurring in ~0.001% of patients. The risk of statin-associated hepatic toxicity is higher in patients who drink excessive amounts of alcohol.

Myopathy, typically involving the proximal leg or arm muscles symmetrically, can range from vague aches to intense myalgias and muscle weakness and rarely may lead to rhabdomyolysis (destruction of muscle) with myoglobinuria and renal failure. While benign muscle aches are reported in 2%-10% of patients on statins, the risk of serious muscle injury (including rhabdomyolysis) is <0.1%. However, the incidence of muscle injury is increased by concomitant therapy with certain drugs, including other lipid-lowering agents (ie, niacin and the fibric acid derivatives) and drugs that inhibit the 3A4 isoform of cytochrome P450, which is responsible for the hepatic metabolism of many statins. Such agents include macrolide antibiotics (eg, erythromycin, clarithromycin), azole antifungal drugs (eg, ketoconazole, itraconazole), and many HIV protease inhibitors. Notably, pravastatin, rosuvastatin, and fluvastatin are not substantially dependent on the cytochrome P450 3A4 isoform for their metabolism and may be less likely to cause myopathy in combination with these other drugs.

Statins have also been associated with a slightly enhanced risk of *diabetes* (0.2%/year). However, the great benefits of statin therapy outweigh this potential risk.

As described in Chapter 5, statins form the foundation of lipid-lowering drug therapy. The following sections describe additional lipid-lowering agents that are prescribed to patients who cannot achieve target LDL reduction on statin therapy alone, to patients who are intolerant of statins, or in other special circumstances.

CHOLESTEROL ABSORPTION INHIBITOR

Ezetimibe, the first member of this class, is a selective inhibitor of cholesterol uptake at the brush border of epithelial cells in the small intestine. It acts by competitively inhibiting a transporter known as the Niemann-Pick C1–like 1 protein. Normally, a portion of dietary and biliary cholesterol taken up in this manner is esterified and incorporated into chylomicrons, which then enter the circulation and are transported to the liver (see Box 5-1). By inhibiting cholesterol uptake (see Fig. 17-21), ezetimibe results in reduced chylomicron production and therefore less cholesterol delivery to the liver. The reduced cholesterol content stimulates compensatory hepatic production of LDL receptors, which augment clearance of circulating LDL particles. The net result is lowering of circulating LDL.

Used alone, ezetimibe reduces LDL cholesterol by about 18%. When combined with a statin, more potent LDL lowering results. A prospective clinical trial of patients soon after experiencing an acute coronary syndrome showed that the combination of ezetimibe plus a statin was modestly superior to statin therapy alone at preventing subsequent cardiovascular events.

The main uses of ezetimibe are to promote LDL lowering in statin-intolerant patients or for patients who require additional LDL lowering on maximum dose statin therapy. Side effects are rare. The addition of ezetimibe to a statin regimen does not appear to significantly increase the risk of statin-associated myopathy.

PROPROTEIN CONVERTASE SUBTILISIN/KEXIN TYPE 9 (PCSK9) INHIBITORS

PCSK9 is an enzyme secreted into the circulation by hepatocytes that plays a crucial role in the life cycle of LDL receptors (Fig. 17-22). When circulating LDL binds to an LDL receptor, that complex is internalized via endocytosis, after which the LDL is released into the cell and the receptor is recycled back to the cell surface (Fig. 17-22). Individual LDL receptors may be recycled in this fashion many dozens of times during its lifespan. However, when PCSK9 binds to an LDL receptor, it targets the receptor for lysosomal destruction following endocytosis, rather than recycling back to the surface (see Fig. 17-22). Such reduction in surface LDL receptors impairs the capacity to remove LDL from the circulation.

As a result of this mechanism, patients who have gain-of-function mutations in the gene that codes for PCKS9 display decreased clearance of LDL from the circulation and high circulating LDL. Conversely, patients with loss-of-function mutations in the PCSK9 gene manifest low serum LDL, as well as a low burden of atherosclerotic disease. Therapeutic PCSK9 inhibitors have been developed to mimic the latter effect.

The two currently available PCSK9 inhibitors (**alirocumab** and **evolocumab**) consist of monoclonal antibodies directed against PCSK9. They are injected subcutaneously, once every 2 or 4 weeks, and when added to statin therapy, each of these PCSK9 inhibitors greatly reduces LDL, by 50%-60%. A large, randomized prospective study showed that alirocumab, added to statin therapy in patients with a recent acute coronary syndrome, significantly reduced subsequent cardiac events compared to placebo, especially in patients with an entry LDL cholesterol $\geq$100 mg/dL. An even larger randomized trial of patients with atherosclerotic coronary disease and baseline LDL $\geq$ 70 mg/dL on statin therapy were randomized to evolocumab vs

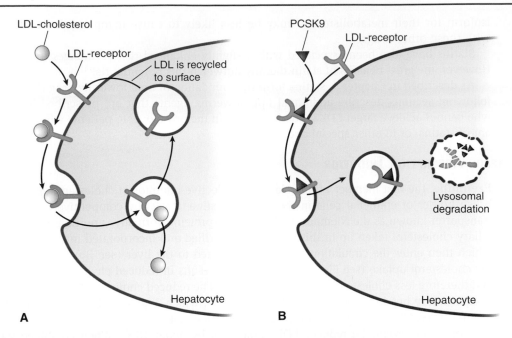

Figure 17-22. Role of PCSK9 in regulation of LDL receptors. A. Circulating LDL normally binds to surface LDL receptors, the complex is internalized into the cell, LDL is released, and the receptor is then recycled back to the cell surface. **B.** When PCSK9 binds to an LDL receptor, it targets that receptor for lysosomal destruction following internalization, rather than recycling. A reduced number of LDL receptors result, impairing the capacity to remove LDL from the circulation. Current PCSK9 inhibitors are monoclonal antibodies that bind to circulating PCSK9 and prevent its interaction and subsequent destruction of LDL receptors.

placebo. On the PCSK9 inhibitor, the average LDL fell to 30 mg/dL accompanied by a significant reduction in the combined primary endpoint of cardiovascular death, MI, stroke, hospitalization for unstable angina, or coronary revascularization.

PCSK9 inhibitors have an excellent safety profile, the most common side effect being mild injection site reactions. PSCK9 inhibitors are currently indicated primarily for patients with clinical atherosclerotic disease, or familial hypercholesterolemia, if LDL remains above target goals (see Table 5-2) on maximally tolerated statin plus ezetimibe therapies.

n-3 FATTY ACIDS

Long chain n-3 polyunsaturated fatty acids, present in fish oils, lower serum triglyceride levels by 20%-50% by inhibiting the synthesis of VLDL (see Box 5-1) in the liver and by enhancing VLDL clearance from the circulation. Meta-analyses of over-the-counter fish oil supplements have not demonstrated a cardiovascular benefit of such agents. However, a recent prospective clinical trial of adults at high cardiovascular risk (with CAD or with diabetes plus at least one other atherosclerotic risk factor) who had elevated triglyceride levels despite statin therapy showed that **icosapent ethyl**, a prescription-strength purified derivative of the n-3 fatty acid eicosapentaenoic acid, reduced the risk of subsequent ischemic events (including cardiovascular mortality) compared with placebo.

The main side effects of n-3 fatty acids are gastric upset and burping.

BILE ACID–BINDING AGENTS

This group includes the resins **cholestyramine** and **colestipol** and the hydrophilic polymer **colesevelam**. These drugs are large, highly positively charged molecules that bind bile acids (which are negatively charged) in the intestine and prevent their normal reabsorption to the liver through the enterohepatic circulation (see Fig. 17-21). As a consequence, more hepatic cholesterol is converted into newly produced bile acids. This action depletes intrahepatic cholesterol stores, thus stimulating the production of LDL receptors. Similar to the effect of the statins, an increased number of hepatic LDL receptors bind a greater amount of circulating LDL, reducing the circulating concentration of that lipoprotein. However, unlike statins, *new* hepatic cholesterol production is also stimulated by the reduced intrahepatic cholesterol content. The boost in cholesterol synthesis augments VLDL production, which likely explains the commonly observed rise in serum triglyceride levels during therapy with a bile acid–binding agent.

Drugs of this class are difficult for patients to take (eg, cholestyramine and colestipol are unappealing gritty powders that must be mixed with liquids), and their potency is much less than that of statins. Thus, bile acid–binding agents are only rarely used, in some patients who cannot tolerate statins. Because they can elevate the serum triglyceride level, they should be avoided in patients with hypertriglyceridemia.

The bile acid–binding agents interfere with the absorption of fat-soluble vitamins and certain drugs (eg, warfarin, digoxin, propranolol, and thyroid hormones). Thus, other medications should be consumed 1 hour before or 3-4 hours after these agents. The main side effects are gastrointestinal: bloating, constipation, and nausea. Because bile acid–binding agents are not absorbed into the circulation, they do not cause systemic side effects.

NIACIN

Niacin is one of the oldest lipid-regulating agents. It raises HDL cholesterol (by 15%-35%), and it reduces LDL cholesterol (by 5%-25%) and triglyceride levels (by 20%-50%).

Niacin modifies lipid levels through multiple mechanisms. It inhibits the release of fatty acids from adipose tissue. As a result, fewer fatty acids are transported to the liver and hepatic triglyceride synthesis declines. Impaired triglyceride production by the liver reduces VLDL secretion into the circulation; consequently, less LDL is formed (see Fig. 17-21). Niacin also enhances the clearance of triglycerides from circulating VLDL by promoting the activity of lipoprotein lipase at adipose and muscle cells. The net effect of these actions is a reduction in serum triglyceride and LDL levels. Niacin is thought to raise circulating HDL cholesterol levels by decreasing the hepatic uptake of its apoprotein, apo AI, thus reducing clearance of HDL particles from the circulation. This mechanism does not disturb hepatic retrieval (and disposal) of cholesterol from the HDL particles.

Prior to the era of statin therapy, a study of men with a history of myocardial infarction showed that niacin reduced the risk of future cardiac events. However, more recent large clinical trials have demonstrated no significant benefit of niacin on cardiovascular outcomes when the drug is added to patients whose LDL levels are already well controlled on statin therapy. Therefore, the use of niacin has greatly declined.

Niacin has several common side effects. Transient cutaneous flushing episodes occur in most patients. These episodes are prostaglandin mediated and can be minimized by taking aspirin prior to the daily niacin dose. Gastrointestinal side effects include exacerbation of peptic ulcer disease and hepatotoxicity. Niacin can contribute to insulin resistance and hyperglycemia. It also raises serum uric acid levels and can precipitate gout in susceptible patients.

FIBRATES

The fibric acid derivatives ("fibrates") **gemfibrozil** and **fenofibrate** are used primarily to treat marked hypertriglyceridemia. They reduce serum triglyceride levels by up to 50%, and they raise HDL cholesterol levels as much as 20%. Their effect on LDL cholesterol is more variable and less beneficial than other lipid-altering drugs (see Table 17-20). Unlike icosapent ethyl, they have not been shown to reduce cardiovascular mortality rates.

Fibrates are thought to exert their antilipid effects through interactions with peroxisome proliferator–activated receptor-α (PPAR-α), a nuclear transcription factor. Activation of PPAR-α leads to a decrease in triglycerides at least in part by augmenting fatty acid oxidation and increasing the synthesis of lipoprotein lipase (see Fig. 17-21). The latter results in increased VLDL catabolism, which may actually *raise* the circulating LDL level, especially in patients with baseline hypertriglyceridemia. Fibrates are believed to augment HDL cholesterol levels via PPAR-α activation of the gene for apoprotein AI, a key constituent of HDL particles.

Fibrates are metabolized by hepatic glucuronidation with subsequent renal excretion. Thus, they should be avoided or prescribed at lower dosages for patients with impaired liver or kidney function. Potential side effects include dyspepsia, gallstones, and myalgias. When used in combination with a statin, the risk of rhabdomyolysis is increased.

Summary

- **Inotropic drugs** are used to increase the force of ventricular contraction in some patients with systolic dysfunction and include the cardiac glycosides (digitalis), sympathomimetic amines, and phosphodiesterase-3 inhibitors.

- **Vasodilator therapy** (eg, ACE inhibitors, angiotensin receptor blockers, angiotensin receptor–neprilysin inhibitors, nitrates, hydralazine) for heart failure is directed at modulating the excessive constriction of veins and arterioles that occurs during physiologic compensation for the fall in CO, thus reducing pulmonary congestion and augmenting forward CO; in hypertension, vasodilator therapy decreases arteriolar resistance and lowers blood pressure.

- **Antiadrenergic drugs** interfere with the sympathetic nervous system.

- **Centrally acting antiadrenergic agents** (eg, methyldopa) *stimulate* CNS α_2-adrenergic receptors and thereby reduce systemic sympathetic outflow, peripheral vascular resistance, and cardiac stimulation, resulting in a fall in blood pressure and heart rate.

- **Peripheral α-antagonists** are divided into those that act on both α_1- and α_2-receptors (eg, phentolamine and phenoxybenzamine) and those that inhibit α_1 alone (eg, prazosin, terazosin, doxazosin), the latter resulting in reduced norepinephrine release and blunted reflex sympathetic side effects.

- **β-Blockers** are distinguished by their specific properties: (1) the relative affinity of the drug for β_1- and β_2-receptors, (2) whether partial β-*agonist* activity is present, (3) whether the drug also has vasodilator properties, and (4) differences in pharmacokinetic properties.

- **Antiarrhythmic drugs** can be grouped according to their primary electrophysiologic mechanisms of action: (1) class I drugs primarily block the fast sodium channel responsible for phase 0 depolarization of the action potential in cardiac muscle cells and Purkinje fibers (and are further subdivided into classes IA, eg, quinidine; IB, eg, lidocaine; and IC, eg, flecainide); (2) class II drugs are β-adrenergic receptor antagonists (β-blockers); (3) class III drugs (eg, amiodarone) predominantly block potassium channels responsible for repolarization, thereby prolonging the action potential with little effect on the rise of phase 0 depolarization; and (4) class IV drugs (eg, verapamil and diltiazem) block the L-type calcium channel.

- **Diuretics** (eg, loop, thiazide, and potassium-sparing diuretics), which eliminate excess sodium and water through renal excretion, are a cornerstone of therapy for hypertension and heart failure.

- **Antithrombotic drugs** inhibit platelet function (eg, aspirin, thienopyridines, ticagrelor, cangrelor, GP IIb/IIIa receptor inhibitors, dipyridamole) or inhibit the coagulation cascade (eg, UFH, low molecular weight heparin, direct thrombin inhibitors, factor Xa inhibitors, warfarin), thereby modulating key pathways in the pathogenesis of acute coronary syndromes, DVT, and thrombi that may complicate atrial fibrillation, dilated cardiomyopathy, or mechanical prosthetic heart valves.

- **Lipid-regulating drugs** include HMG-CoA reductase inhibitors ("statins"), a cholesterol absorption inhibitor (ezetimibe), PCSK9 inhibitors (eg, alirocumab, evolocumab), n-3 fatty acids, bile acid–binding agents (eg, cholestyramine and colestipol), niacin, and fibric acid derivatives (eg, gemfibrozil and fenofibrate).

- Of the lipid-altering agents, **statins** and **PCSK9 inhibitors** are the most potent to lower LDL cholesterol and reduce coronary event rates.

Review Questions

1. A 65-year-old man with a history of hypertension, hyperlipidemia, and type II diabetes is admitted to the hospital with worsening shortness of breath, especially with exertion or lying flat. He has also noticed edema in both lower extremities in recent months. The ECG shows normal sinus rhythm and no change compared with 6 months earlier. Transthoracic echocardiography shows a left ventricular ejection fraction of 30%. Which of the following medications has NOT been shown to improve survival in such a patient?

   a. Metoprolol succinate
   b. Captopril
   c. Spironolactone
   d. Furosemide

2. A 55-year-old woman has a history of myocardial infarction and heart failure with reduced ejection fraction (HFrEF). She presents to the hospital with increasing exertional dyspnea after eating fried chicken, seasoned turkey, and canned soup over the Thanksgiving holiday. Her physical exam is notable for prominent jugular venous distention and crackles on pulmonary exam halfway up both posterior lung fields. Labs are notable for elevated serum potassium level of 5.8 mEq/L (normal range = 3.5-5.0 mEq/L). She is treated with intravenous furosemide but demonstrates poor diuresis. Which of the following diuretics acts at the distal convoluted tubule and would be appropriate therapy to further facilitate diuresis in this patient?

   a. Lisinopril
   b. Metolazone
   c. Spironolactone
   d. Bumetanide

3. A 67-year-old woman with a history of hypertension, diabetes mellitus, hypothyroidism, and coronary artery disease comes to emergency department with a 3-day history of palpitations. The ECG in the emergency department shows an irregular rhythm without discernable P waves, with a ventricular rate of 94 beats/min. She has no history of mitral stenosis. The serum creatinine is normal. She is initially prescribed metoprolol (β-blocker) and enoxaparin (a low molecular weight heparin). At the time of discharge, she is converted from enoxaparin to oral apixaban therapy. By what mechanism does apixaban exert its anticoagulant effect?

   a. Inhibition of platelet cyclooxygenase-1
   b. Reversible inhibition of the platelet $P2Y_{12}$ receptor
   c. Direct inhibition of activated factor II (thrombin)
   d. Inhibition of activated factor X

4. Match each of the following vasoactive drugs to the receptors with which they interact. Note that each drug acts at more than one receptor.

I.	Epinephrine	A.	α-Receptor
II.	Norepinephrine	B.	$β_1$-Receptor
III.	Dobutamine	C.	$β_2$-Receptor
IV.	Isoproterenol	D.	V_1 receptor

5. A 78-year-old woman with ischemic cardiomyopathy and left ventricular ejection fraction of 40% has recurrent episodes of symptomatic atrial fibrillation. Which of the following antiarrhythmic drugs is least likely to cause proarrhythmic effects (including sudden cardiac death) in her case?

   a. Sotalol
   b. Flecainide
   c. Propafenone
   d. Amiodarone

6. A 45-year-old man with a history of diabetes mellitus and hyperlipidemia has been hospitalized for an acute coronary syndrome. His serum LDL cholesterol prior to admission on high-dose atorvastatin (80 mg daily) was 82 mg/dL. Which of the following lipid-lowering regimens would be most appropriate following discharge?

   a. Continue high-dose statin only.
   b. Continue high-dose statin and add ezetimibe.
   c. Continue high-dose statin and add a PCSK9 inhibitor.
   d. Continue high-dose statin and add niacin.

Answers to Review Questions

1. **Choice d is correct.** This patient has symptomatic heart failure with reduced ejection fraction (HFrEF). While diuretics are beneficial for relief of congestive symptoms, they have not been shown to improve long-term survival in this condition. Conversely, ACE inhibitors (eg, captopril), certain β-blockers (eg, metoprolol succinate), and aldosterone antagonists are among the pharmacologic agents that have been shown to improve symptoms and reduce mortality in HFrEF.

2. **Choice b is correct.** Metolazone is an oral thiazide-like diuretic that acts by blocking sodium reabsorption at the renal distal convoluted tubule. Since thiazides act on a more distal segment of the tubule than loop diuretics, the combination often leads to augmented diuresis. Bumetanide is a loop diuretic whose site of action is the same as furosemide, lisinopril is an ACE inhibitor, and spironolactone is a weak diuretic that antagonizes the action of aldosterone in the distal nephron. Spironolactone can raise the serum potassium level through this mechanism and should not be taken by patients who are already hyperkalemic.

3. **Choice d is correct.** The irregular rhythm without P waves is indicative of atrial fibrillation. Anticoagulation to prevent thromboembolism in atrial fibrillation is indicated for men with a CHA_2DS_2-VASc score ≥ 2 and females with a CHA_2DS_2-$VAS_c \geq 3$. Direct-acting oral anticoagulants (eg, factor Xa inhibitors apixaban, rivaroxaban, and edoxaban and the direct thrombin inhibitor dabigatran) are the preferred anticoagulants, unless the patient has moderate-to-severe mitral stenosis or a mechanical heart valve, in which case warfarin should be prescribed instead.

4. **I. A,B,C; II. A,B; III. A,B,C; IV. B,C**

5. **Choice d is correct.** Amiodarone is the most effective drug to prevent recurrences of atrial fibrillation in individuals with heart failure and, in distinction to many other antiarrhythmics, is less likely to be proarrhythmic or lead to sudden cardiac death. It can, however, cause many other side effects including pneumonitis, thyroid abnormalities, and hepatic function abnormalities.

6. **Choice b is correct.** For high-risk patients (eg, following an acute coronary syndrome), the currently recommended goal LDL cholesterol is <70 mg/dL. The addition of ezetimibe is recommended as the next step to achieve that goal, followed if necessary by the addition of a PCSK9 inhibitor. A large prospective placebo-controlled clinical trial showed that the addition of ezetimibe to statin therapy for individuals following an acute coronary syndrome leads to further reduction in LDL levels and major adverse cardiovascular events.

Acknowledgments

Contributors to previous editions of this chapter were Andrey V. Dolinko, MD; Michael T Kuntz, MD; Christopher A. Miller, MD; Cyrus K. Yamin, MD; Martin W. Schoen, MD; Mark Friedberg, MD; Chiadi E. Ndumele, MD; Steven N. Kalkanis, MD; David Sloane, MD; Andrew C. Hecht, MD; Steven P. Leon, MD; Ralph A. Kelly, MD; Elliott M. Antman, MD; and Gary R. Strichartz, PhD.

Additional Reading

Anderson I, Cifu AS. Management of bleeding in patients taking oral anticoagulants. *JAMA*. 2018;319:2032-2033.

Bhatt DL, Steg PG, Miller M, et al. Cardiovascular risk reduction with icosapent ethyl for hypertriglyceridemia. *N Engl J Med*. 2019;380:11-22.

Capodanno D, Huber K, Mehran R, et al. Management of antithrombotic therapy in atrial fibrillation patients undergoing PCI. *J Am Coll Cardiol*. 2019;74:83-99.

Gaziano JM. Aspirin for primary prevention: clinical considerations in 2019. *JAMA*. 2019;321:253.

Grundy SM, Stone NJ, Bailey AL, et al. 2018 AHA/ACC/AACVPR/AAPA/ABC/ACPM/ADA/AGS/APhA/ASPC/NLA/PCNA guideline on the management of blood cholesterol: executive summary: a report of the American College of Cardiology/ American Heart Association Task Force on Clinical Practice Guidelines. *J Am Coll Cardiol*. 2019;73:3168-3209.

Joseph P, Swedberg K, Leong DP, et al. The evolution of β-blockers in coronary artery disease and heart failure. *J Am Coll Cardiol*. 2019;74:672-682.

Layland J, Carrick D, Lee M, et al. Adenosine: physiology, pharmacology, and clinical applications. *JACC Cardiovasc Interv*. 2014;7:581-591.

Lei M, Wu L, Terrar DA, et al. Modernized classification of cardiac antiarrhythmic drugs. *Circulation*. 2018;138:1879-1896.

Leong DP, McMurray JJV, Joseph PG, et al. From ACE inhibitors/ARBs to ARNIs in coronary artery disease and heart failure. *J Am Coll Cardiol*. 2019;74:683-698.

Michos ED, McEvoy JW, Blumenthal RS. Lipid management for the prevention of atherosclerotic cardiovascular disease. *N Engl J Med*. 2019;381:1557-1567.

Sabatine MS. PCSK9 inhibitors: clinical evidence and implementation. *Nat Rev Cardiol*. 2019;16:155-165.

Verheugt FWA, ten Berg JM, Storey RF, et al. Antithrombotics: aspirin to DOACs in coronary artery disease and atrial fibrillation. *J Am Coll Cardiol*. 2019;74:699-711.

Zheng SL, Roddick AJ. Association of aspirin use for primary prevention with cardiovascular events and bleeding events: a systematic review and meta-analysis. *JAMA*. 2019;321:277.

Index

Note: Page numbers followed by *f* indicate figures; Page numbers followed by *t* indicate tables; those followed by *b* indicate boxes.

A

ABCA1 gene, 124*b*
ABCG1 gene, 124*b*
Abciximab, 190, 470
Abdominal aorta, 373, 375
Abdominal aortic aneurysm, 345
Aberrant conduction, 310–311
Accelerated-malignant hypertension, 347
Accessory pathway, 296–297, 297*f*. *See also* Bypass tract
  concealed, 318, 320
  impulse conduction and, 315
ACE inhibitors. *See* Angiotensin-converting enzyme (ACE) inhibitors
Acetylcholine (ACh), 145–146
Acoustic shadowing, 53–54
Actin, 21
Action potential
  cardiac conduction system, 16–18
  cardiac muscle cell, 16–18
  digitalis effect, 431
  early afterdepolarizations-triggered, 292–293
  electrical stimulation, 12
  pacemaker cells, 18–19, 18*f*
  of pacemaker cells, 287, 287*f*
  plateau phase of, 17–18
  refractory periods, 19, 20*f*
  specialized conduction system, 18
  spontaneous, 292
  transmembrane cardiac ionic currents, 16*t*
  triggered activity, 292–293, 292*f*–293*f*
Acute arterial occlusion, 384–385, 384*t*
Acute cholecystitis, 185*t*
Acute coronary syndromes (ACS)
  acute myocardial infarction (*see* Acute myocardial infarction (AMI))
  angina pectoris (*see* Angina pectoris)
  clinical features of, 183–187
  clotting factors inactivation, 173–174, 174*f*
  cocaine abuse and, 178
  complications of
    arrhythmias, 194–195, 194*t*
    conduction blocks, 195
    recurrent ischemia, 194
    supraventricular arrhythmias, 195
    ventricular fibrillation, 195
  diagnosis of

creatine kinase levels, 187
  echocardiography, 187
  electrocardiogram, 185–186, 186*f*
  troponins levels, 186–187
fibrin clots lysis, 174
hemostasis, 173
myocardial dysfunction, 195–196
pathogenesis of, 172–178
pathology and pathophysiology
  description of, 178
  early changes, 179–180, 179*t*, 180*f*, 181*f*
  functional alterations, 182–183
  impaired contractility and compliance, 182
  ischemic preconditioning, 182
  late changes, 180, 181*f*
  stunned myocardium, 182
  ventricular remodeling, 182–183
right ventricular infarction, 196
spectrum of, 173*t*
treatment of
  adjunctive therapy, 192–193
  anticoagulant drugs, 190
  anti-ischemic therapy, 188–189
  antiplatelet drugs, 189–190
  antithrombotic therapy, 189–190
  continuous ECG monitoring, 187
  descriptions of, 187
  fibrinolytic therapy, 192
  initial management strategies in, 188*f*
  non ST-segment elevation myocardial infarction, 102, 103, 103*f*, 104*f*
  oxygen supplemental, 187
  primary percutaneous coronary intervention, 191–192
  ST-segment elevation myocardial infarction, 191–192
Acute intramural hematoma, 377
Acute myocardial infarction (AMI)
  arrhythmias in, 194*t*
  causes of, 178*t*
  clinical presentation of, 183–184, 184*t*
  non-atherosclerotic causes of, 177–178, 178*t*
  with pericarditis, 356–357
Acute pericarditis
  with acute myocardial infarction, 356–357
  clinical history, 358–359, 359*t*

with connective tissue diseases, 357
diagnostic studies, 359–360, 360*f*
drug-induced, 357, 358*t*
etiology, 356–358
idiopathic, 356
infectious, 356
neoplastic, 357
noninfectious, 356–358
nontuberculous bacterial pericarditis, 356
pathogenesis, 357–358
pathology, 358
physical examination, 359
radiation-induced, 357
treatment, 360
tuberculous, 356
uremic, 357
viral, 356
Acute pulmonary edema, 260
Acute rheumatic fever (ARF), 203*b*
Adenosine, 460, 461*f*
Adenosine diphosphate, 144–145, 176
Adenosine triphosphate, 144–145, 179
Adrenergic nervous system, 245
Adrenocortical hormone excess, 341–342
Adventitia, 118
Afterdepolarization, 292–293, 292*f*–293*f*
Afterload, 236
  alterations in, 238–239, 239*f*
  definition, 234, 235*t*, 236
  effect of, 239*f*
Agatston score, 69
Akinetic, of wall motion abnormalities, 182
Alcohol intake, hypertension management, 348
Alcoholic cardiomyopathy, 267–268
Aldosterone antagonist
  therapy for acute MI, 193
  therapy for heart failure, 256
Alirocumab, 479–480
α_1-adrenergic receptor antagonists, for hypertension, 350–351
α_2-adrenergic agonists, for hypertension, 350–351
Ambrisentan, 445
Amiloride, 463*t*, 465
Amiodarone, 271, 451*t*, 458
Amyloidosis, as cause for restrictive cardiomyopathy, 278–279

487